DISORDERS OF THE PITUITARY

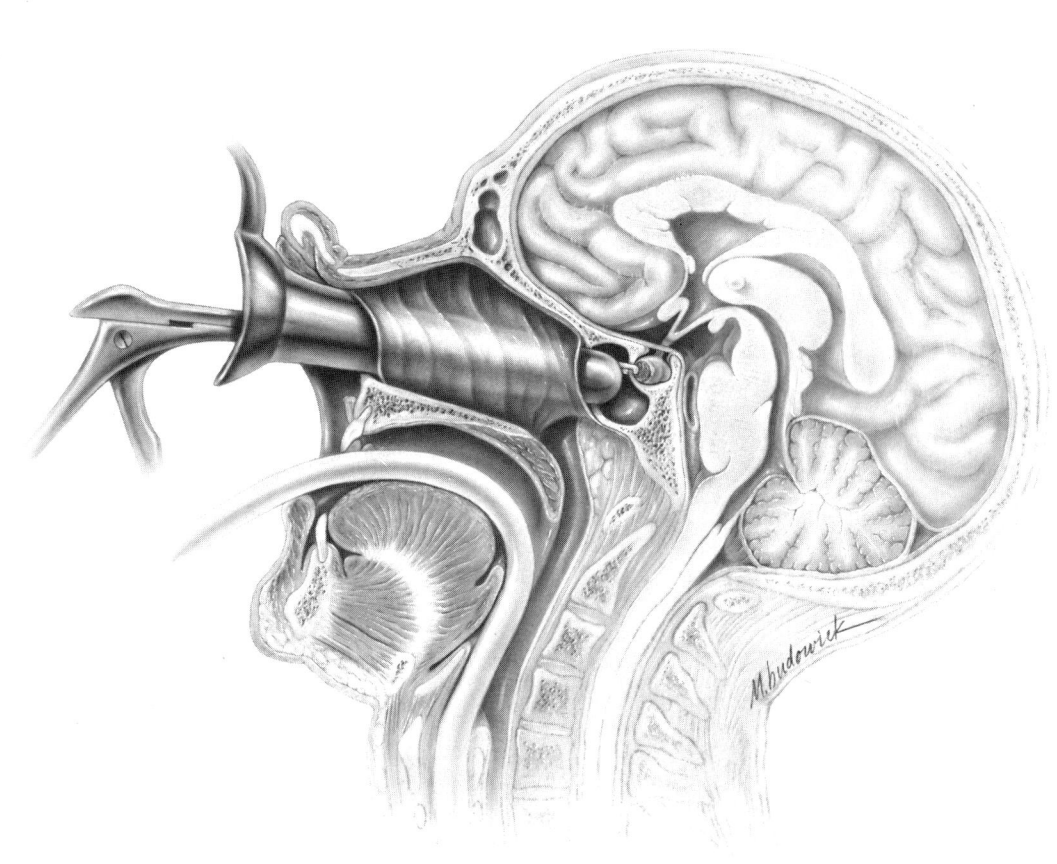

ns of
DISORDERS OF
THE PITUITARY

GEORGE T. TINDALL, M.D.

Professor of Surgery (Neurosurgery)
Department of Surgery
Emory University School of Medicine
Atlanta, Georgia

DANIEL L. BARROW, M.D.

Assistant Professor of Surgery (Neurosurgery)
Department of Surgery
Emory University School of Medicine
Atlanta, Georgia

With Chapter 2 contributed by
JOSEPH B. MARTIN, M.D., Ph.D.

Julianne Dorn Professor of Neurology, Harvard Medical School;
Chief, Neurology Service Massachusetts General Hospital
Boston, Massachusetts

With 274 illustrations and 4 4-color plates
Electron micrographs supplied by Kalmon Kovacs, M.D.

THE C. V. MOSBY COMPANY
ST. LOUIS • TORONTO • PRINCETON   1986

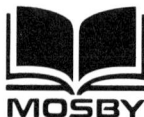

A TRADITION OF PUBLISHING EXCELLENCE

Editor-in-chief: Karen Berger
Assistant editor: Sandra L. Gilfillan
Editing supervisors: Judi Wolken, Peggy Fagen
Manuscript editor: Melissa Neves
Book design: Kay Kramer
Cover design: John Rokusek
Production: Teresa Breckwoldt

Copyright © 1986 by The C.V. Mosby Company

All rights reserved. No part of this publication may be reproduced, stored in a retrieval system, or transmitted, in any form or by any means, electronic, mechanical, photocopying, recording, or otherwise, without prior written permission from the publisher.

Printed in the United States of America

THE C.V. MOSBY COMPANY
11830 Westline Industrial Drive, St. Louis, Missouri 63146

Library of Congress Cataloging-in-Publication Data

Tindall, George T.,
    Disorders of the pituitary.

    Includes bibliographies and index.
    1. Pituitary body—Diseases.   I. Barrow, Daniel L.
II. Martin, Joseph B., 1938-   .   III. Title.
[DNLM: 1. Pituitary Diseases.   WK   550 T588d]
RC658.T56   1986   616.4′7   85-18918
ISBN 0-8016-4985-4

GW/MV/MV   9 8 7 6 5 4 3 2 1   04/B/577

To the memory of

HARVEY CUSHING

who contributed significantly to our understanding

of pituitary disorders

Preface

The pace of progress is as variable as the seasons—sometimes halting, often brisk, but seemingly inevitable. Agonizingly slow in the distant past, the tempo has accelerated in recent times, particularly during the last 50 years. Contrast, for example, the long time span between the wheel's discovery and the invention of the automobile with the short lapse from a brief flight in a flimsy aircraft on a windy Carolina beach to a spaceship voyage to the surface of the moon. Medicine has followed similar trends in its development; in some areas, advances have been scant and laborious, whereas in others, our understanding has grown at an exponential rate.

The study of pituitary disorders has witnessed some of the most startling and exciting developments in medicine. Discoveries in neuroendocrinology, ranging from the early observations of Harris and Green on blood flow direction in the pituitary stalk to current isolation and identification of hypothalamic hormones, seem to occur with astounding regularity. The many Nobel laureates in the field of neuroendocrinology over the past several years are further testimony to the numerous advances in this field, many of which have led to more effective treatment options. Breakthroughs in neuroradiology have also occurred. High-resolution CT and MRI are two recent developments in this field, and the variety of images they present, especially MRI, sometimes astound even experienced neuroradiologists.

It is difficult to keep pace with and record the many advances in this field. Scientific presentations provide one opportunity; medical journals, another. To accomplish this task in a book presents an even more formidable challenge because of the unavoidable delays inherent in the writing and publication process. Nevertheless, we believe that a book is the appropriate forum for our effort to provide an up-to-date, yet comprehensive review of pituitary disorders.

Our book presents the reader with the necessary scientific and clinical background to understand the etiology, pathogenesis, and clinical manifestations of specific pituitary disorders. Building on this foundation, we provide an in-depth analysis of treatment options, all within the perspective of clinical problem solving.

A judicious balance between basic science and clinical application runs throughout the book. Separate chapters are devoted to the topics of pathology, neuroendocrinology, neuroradiology, and radiation therapy. These subjects are also interwoven with related clinical material within other chapters to provide a meaningful correlation between clinical, radiologic, and pathologic features. We have focused all the pertinent information on acromegaly into one chapter rather than scatter it throughout the book. The same approach has been used for Cushing's disease, prolactinomas, and other disorders. True, more details on certain aspects of these subjects can be found in other sections of the book, but all important issues, especially current therapy, are found in the chapters devoted to each specific problem. We have made a special effort to minimize overlap throughout the book, although at times, to make an important point, this has been allowed.

With the exception of Chapter 2, we have chosen to write the total book ourselves. It is our belief that our goal can only be accomplished through a limited authorship. Such a work avoids the repetition, contradictions, and lack of cohesiveness that surface in a multiauthored textbook. We hope it will also provide a broader and more comprehensive perspective of the subject.

The chapter on neuroendocrinology, by Dr. Joseph B. Martin of the Massachusetts General Hospital, is the only chapter we did not write. Changes in the area of neuroendocrinology are occurring so rapidly that we felt that only an expert dedicated to that specific area could present it in an authoritative manner. Dr. Martin is such an expert, and his chapter summarizes current knowledge of this discipline and applies it to the pathogenesis, diagnosis, and management of diseases of pituitary regulation, of the hypothalamus, of brain function, and of behavior resulting from hormone disturbances.

The book is written for a relatively wide audience, including neurosurgeons and endocrinologists in academic and clinical practice. Neurologists, neuroradiologists, and neuropathologists should also find it useful, as will medical students and residents in training.

Numerous individuals contributed to the publication of this book. Dr. Joseph B. Martin deserves a special thanks for writing Chapter 2 on neuroendocrinology. Drs. Kalmon Kovacs and Eva Horvath, of the University of Toronto, kindly critiqued the chapter on pathology and provided many of the outstanding illustrations that we have used in that chapter. Dr. Gary Pearl of the Department of Pathology, Emory University School of Medicine, also contributed illustrations for the pathology chapter. We are indebted to Drs. Nelson Watts and Richard Clark of the Division of Endocrinology at Emory for reviewing Chapter 4 and to Dr. Warner Ray, a radiation therapist in Atlanta, for reviewing Chapter 13; all offered sound and practical advice.

Karen Berger, our editor at Mosby, deserves a special commendation. Not only has she been a steady source of encouragement, but she has also given inestimable editorial assistance and advice. Sandy Gilfillan, assistant editor at Mosby, and Shirley Korn, administrative assistant, also provided valued help during the final phases of writing. Melissa Neves has been a delightful copy editor to work with.

Grace Groover, Susan Scott, Doris Hammond, Daphne Eitel, and David Adams graciously devoted much of their time to library research, collection of patient data, and manuscript typing; we are truly indebted to them.

Our gratitude extends to Joe Jackson for his excellent photography and to Mike Budowick for his fine illustrations. Mike brought talent and commitment to this project, and we appreciate his splendid efforts.

The authors would like to thank the neurosurgical staff at Emory for their patience and understanding during the period that this book was being written.

Finally, the senior author would like to express his sincere appreciation to his wife, Dr. Suzie C. Tindall, for her strong support, steady encouragement, and benevolent tolerance during the entire project.

GEORGE T. TINDALL
DANIEL L. BARROW

Contents

1 Anatomy, 1
2 Neuroendocrinology, 23
   JOSEPH B. MARTIN
3 Pathology of the pituitary gland and sellar region, 64
4 Clinical and endocrinologic evaluation of patients with pituitary tumors, 123
5 Neuroradiology, 145
6 Acromegaly, 203
7 Cushing's syndrome and Nelson's syndrome, 231
8 Prolactinoma, 253
9 Nonfunctional pituitary adenomas, 281
10 Uncommon pituitary and parasellar lesions, 301
11 Craniopharyngioma, 321
12 Pituitary surgery, 349
13 Radiation therapy, 401
14 Hypophysectomy, 439
15 Pituitary deficiency states, 451
16 The "empty sella" syndrome, 473

COLOR PLATES

Plate 1. Adult patient with acromegaly, *follows page 210*

Plate 2. Adult patient with Cushing's syndrome, *follows page 218*

Plate 3. Operative appearance of microadenoma, *follows page 380*

Plate 4. Transsphenoidal operative appearance of "empty sella" syndrome, *follows page 480*

DISORDERS OF THE PITUITARY

CHAPTER 1

Anatomy

Sphenoid bone and associated bony structures
Nasal cavity and septum
Pituitary gland and stalk
Hypothalamus
Parasellar anatomic structures
    Optic chiasm
    Cavernous sinus

A thorough knowledge of anatomy of the hypothalamus, pituitary, and related structures is essential for the surgeon performing surgery in this area. This chapter considers the anatomic aspects of the sellar and parasellar regions under five major categories: (1) sphenoid bone and associated bony structures, (2) nasal cavity and septum, (3) pituitary gland and stalk, (4) hypothalamus, and (5) parasellar anatomic structures (e.g., the cavernous sinus and carotid artery).

SPHENOID BONE AND ASSOCIATED BONY STRUCTURES

The sphenoid bone is situated at the base of the skull anterior to the temporalis and basilar part of the occipital bones.[5] Figs. 1-1 and 1-2 show this structure as viewed from the superior and anteroinferior aspects, respectively. In addition, a midsagittal view is shown in Fig. 1-3. The sphenoid bone is divided into a medial portion or body, two great and two small wings extending outward from the sides of the body, and two pterygoid processes that project from the inferior surface.

The body contains the sphenoid air sinuses (Fig. 1-3), which are two large cavities separated from each other by one or more thin septae. The superior surface of the body presents the ethmoid spine rostrally, which articulates with the cribriform plate of the ethmoid. Behind this is a smooth surface, slightly raised in the midline, and grooved on either side for the olfactory lobes of the brain. Continuing posteriorly, one next encounters the chiasmatic groove, which ends on either side in the optic canal. The latter canal, or foramen, transmits the optic nerve and ophthalmic artery into the orbit. The tuberculum sella is posterior to the chiasmatic groove and immediately rostral to the sella turcica, which contains the pituitary gland and is covered by the diaphragm sella. The middle clinoid processes are two small eminences, one on either side, that complete the

2 *Disorders of the pituitary*

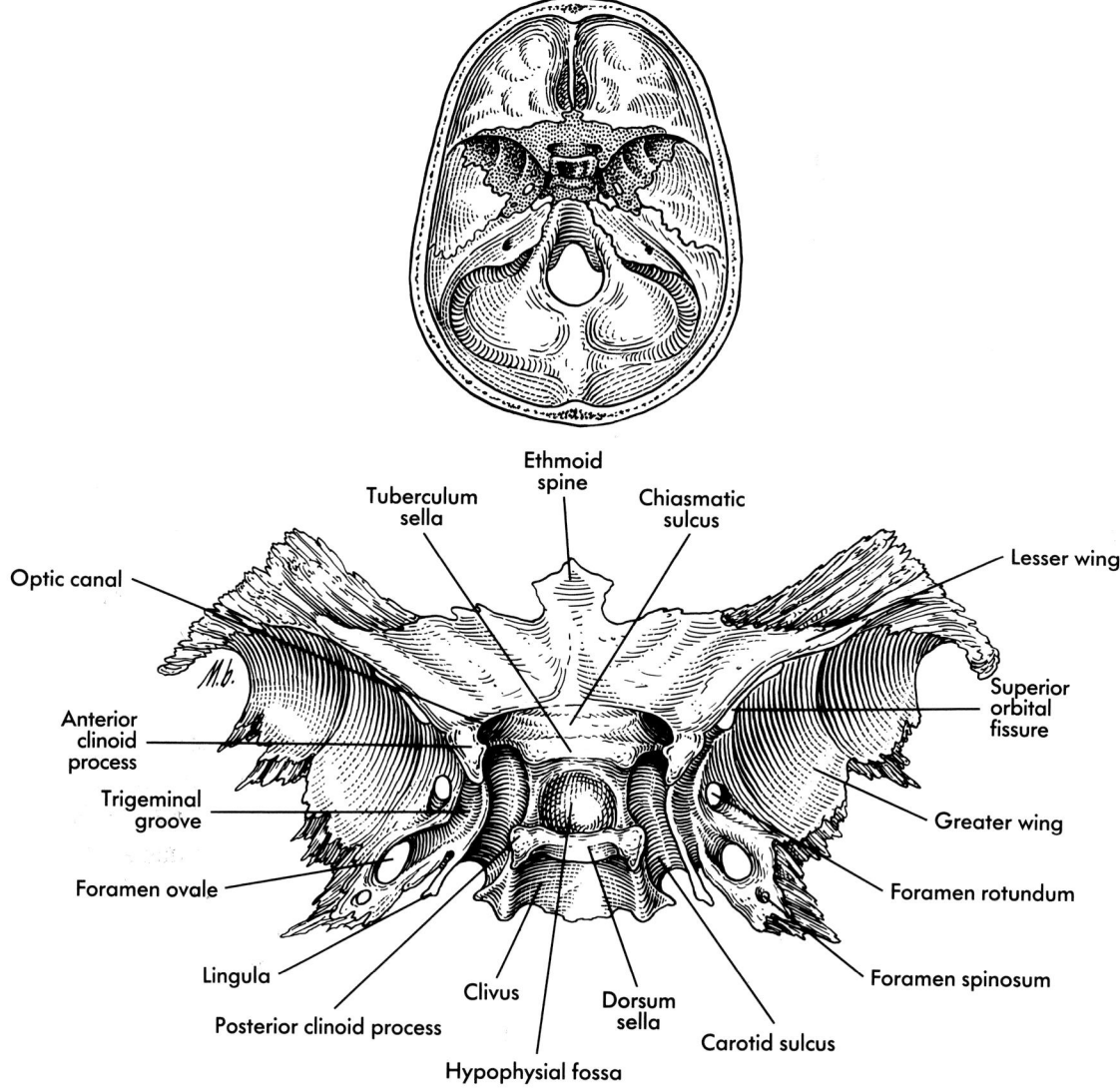

Fig. 1-1. Sphenoid bone, superior aspect.

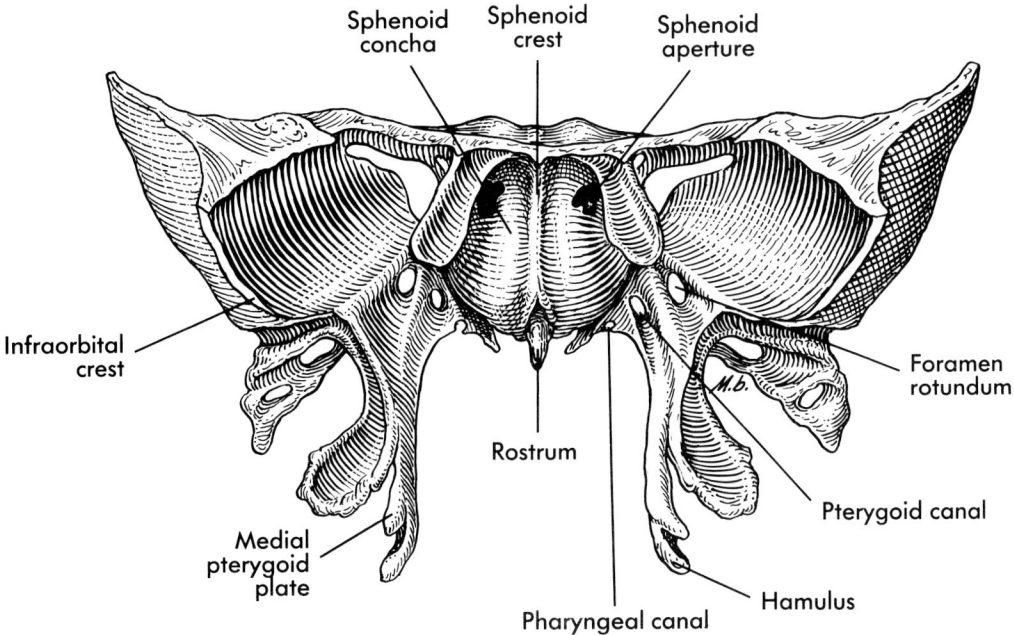

Fig. 1-2. Sphenoid bone, anteroinferior aspect.

anterior boundary of the sella turcica. The posterior boundary is formed by the dorsum sella, which extends upward and ends in two tubercles of varying size and shape—the posterior clinoid processes. These structures provide attachment for the tentorium cerebelli. The clivus is located immediately behind the dorsum sella, slopes posteriorly, and is continuous with the groove on the basilar portion of the occipital bone.

The lateral surfaces of the body are united with the great wings and the medial pterygoid plates. Above the attachment of each great wing is a groove, the carotid sulcus. Lateral and posterior to this groove is a ridge of bone called the lingula.

The anteroinferior surface of the body of the sphenoid forms the posterior wall of the nasal cavity. In the midline the sphenoid crest can be seen; it forms the posterior part of the nasal septum (see p. 6) and articulates with the perpendicular plate of the ethmoid and the vomer. Lateral and attached to the sphenoid crest are the sphenoid conchae, two thin curved plates situated at the anterior part of the body of the sphenoid. These plates are removed during the course of a transsphenoidal operation and provide access to the sphenoid sinus and floor of the sella turcica. An aperture of variable size, the sphenoid ostia, exists in the anterior wall of each concha.

The sphenoid sinuses vary in size, shape, and degree of pneumatization (see Fig. 5-5).[12,13] They are present as minute cavities at the time of birth and do not attain their full size until after puberty. When unusually large, they can extend into the base of the pterygoid processes, the greater wing of the sphenoid, and

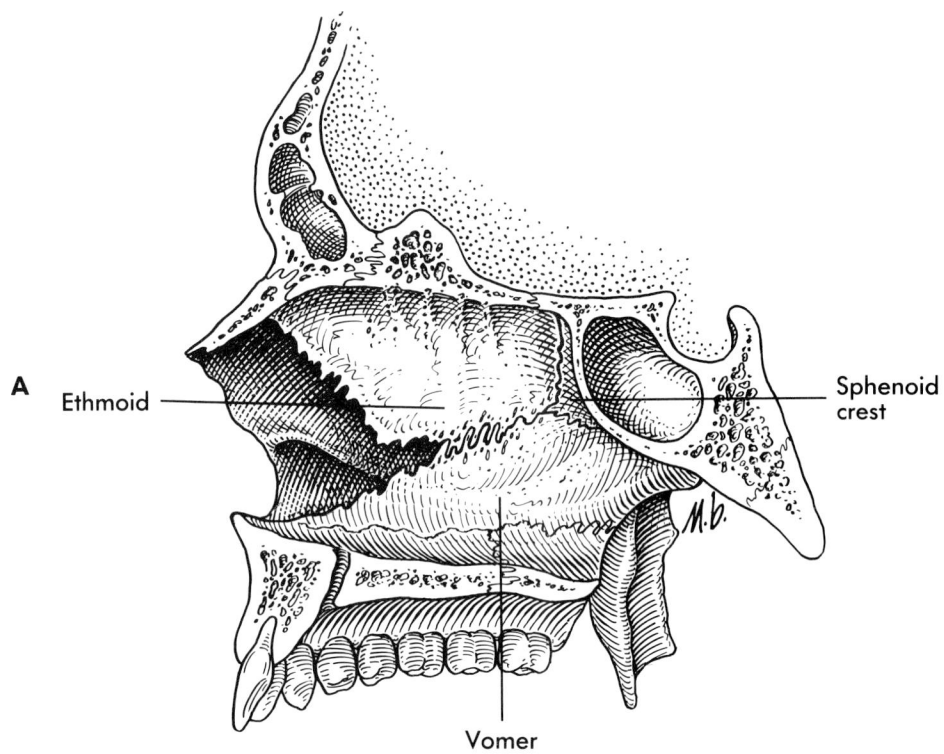
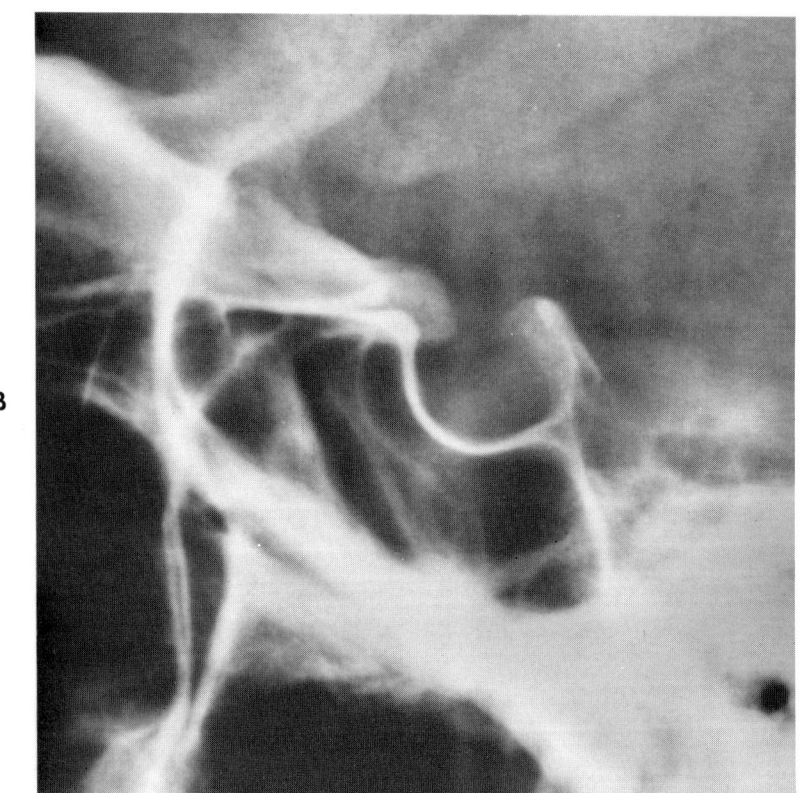

Fig. 1-3. Midline sagittal section through sphenoid bone (**A**) and lateral x-ray examination of skull centered on sella turcica (**B**) to illustrate bony structures.

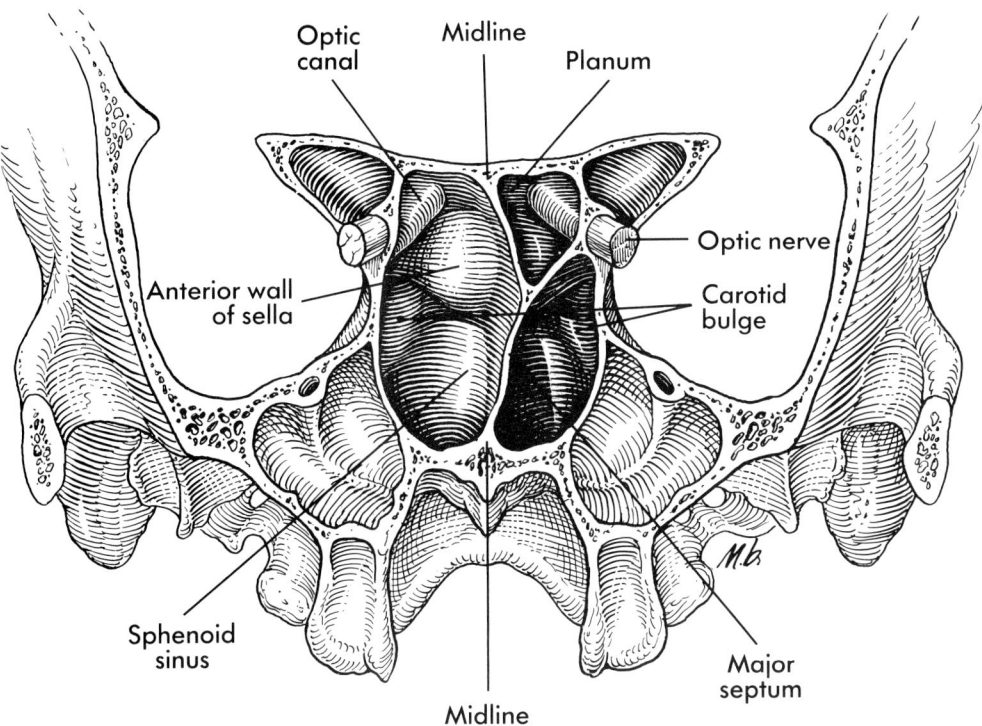

Fig. 1-4. Interior view of sphenoid sinus looking toward floor of sella. Major septum is located off midline and divides, separating sinus into asymmetric cavities. Carotid bulge can be seen bilaterally.

even the basilar part of the occipital bone. Infrequently, there are gaps in the bone with the mucous membrane lying directly against the dura. The paired sphenoid sinuses are divided from each other by the sphenoid septae. These structures are bony and vary considerably in size, shape, location, and relation to the floor of the sella. The septae are often located off the midline (Fig. 1-4) as they cross the floor of the sella, and for this reason the surgeon should never rely on the position of the septae to indicate the midline of the floor of the sella turcica. In fact, a major septum may be found as much as 8 mm off the midline.[12,13] It is common for the sphenoid sinuses to have multiple small cavities in the large paired sinuses, and these smaller cavities are separated by septae oriented in all directions.

There are several important anatomic structures located adjacent to the lateral wall of the sphenoid sinus. As shown in Fig. 1-5, the dura covering the medial wall of the cavernous sinus and optic canal lies adjacent to the thin lateral wall of the sphenoid sinus. Removal of this layer of dura mater exposes the internal carotid artery as it curves forward and then upward, the optic nerve superiorly, and the second (maxillary) division of the trigeminal nerve inferiorly. Further dissection in a lateral direction would expose the remaining structures (third, fourth, and sixth cranial nerves) within the cavernous sinus (see Fig. 1-17).

The sphenoid sinuses are the portal of entry into the sella turcica and as

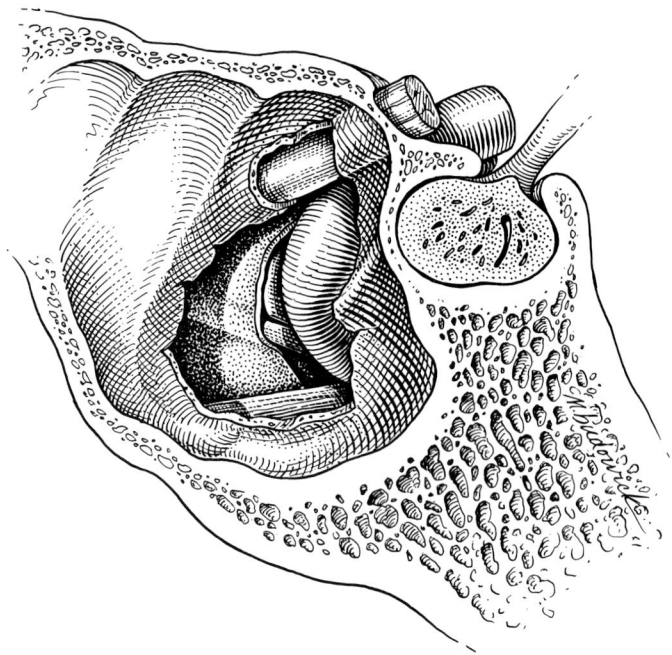

Fig. 1-5. Anatomic structures adjacent to lateral wall of sphenoid sinus. Removal of thin lateral bony wall of sinus and adjacent dura exposes internal carotid artery as it curves forward and then upward, optic nerve superiorly, and second division of trigeminal nerve inferiorly.

such are important to the surgeon using the transsphenoidal approach to the pituitary (see Fig. 5-5).

The inferior surface of the sphenoid bone also forms part of the posterior wall of the nasal cavity and appears as a triangular spine, the sphenoid rostrum, in the midline. This structure is continuous with the inferior portion of the sphenoid crest. When the sphenoid rostrum is exposed, it indicates to the surgeon that the surgical approach to the sella is directed too much in an inferoposterior direction and the operation needs to be redirected in a more anterosuperior plane.

The great wings arise from the sides of the body and the superior surface of each forms part of the middle cranial fossa. The foramen rotundum is located anteriorly and medially. The maxillary division of the trigeminal nerve (V_2) passes through this structure. Posterior and lateral to the foramen rotundum is the foramen ovale, which transmits the mandibular division of the trigeminal nerve (V_3), accessory meningeal artery, and sometimes the lesser petrosal nerve. Just behind and slightly lateral to the foramen ovale is the foramen spinosum through which pass the middle meningeal vessels and the recurrent branch from the mandibular nerve.

The orbital surface of the great wing forms the posterior part of the lateral wall of the orbit. Its inferior rounded border forms the posterior lateral boundary of the inferior orbital fissure, and its medial margin forms the inferior boundary of the superior orbital fissure. Superiorly, the orbital surface of the great wing articulates with the orbital plate of the frontal bone.

Laterally at the tip of the great wing is a triangular portion for articulation with both the parietal and frontal bones. This region, the pterion, is the pivotal point for many frontotemporal craniotomy approaches to aneurysms and other lesions such as craniopharyngiomas and occasionally pituitary adenomas.

The small wings are two thin triangular plates that arise from the superior and anterior parts of the body of the sphenoid. The superior surface of each small wing is flat and supports part of the frontal lobes. The inferior surface forms the posterior part of the roof of the orbit and the superior boundary of the superior orbital fissure. The posterior border, known also as the sphenoid ridge, fits into the lateral fissure of the brain. The medial end of this border forms the anterior clinoid processes. The small wing is connected to the body by two struts of bone, superior and inferior, between which is the optic foramen.

The pterygoid process on either side projects perpendicularly from the inferior portion where the body and great wing unite. The pterygoid process consists of a medial and a lateral plate. The lateral pterygoid plate, which is broad and thin, forms part of the medial wall of the infratemporal fossa. The medial pterygoid plate is narrower and longer than the lateral. The lateral surface of this plate forms part of the pterygoid fossa, and the medial surface constitutes the lateral boundary of the posterior aperture of the corresponding nasal cavity. The pterygoid canal, which transmits the pharyngeal branch of the maxillary artery and the pharyngeal nerve (vidian nerve) from the pterygopalatine nerves, can be seen on the anteroinferior surface of the sphenoid bone.

The sphenoid bone is joined to 12 other bones: four single—the vomer, ethmoid, frontal, and occipital; and four paired—the parietal, temporal, zygomatic, and palatine. It also sometimes articulates with the tuberosity of the maxilla. From its position and relationship to so many important structures, it is the centerpiece of the base of the skull.

NASAL CAVITY AND SEPTUM

The nasal cavities open on the face through the anterior nasal aperture and posteriorly into the nasal part of the pharynx through the posterior openings, the choanae. Each nasal cavity is bounded by a roof, a floor, and a lateral wall (Fig. 1-6). The roof is formed anteriorly by the nasal bone and the spine of the frontal; in the middle by the cribriform plate of the ethmoid; and posteriorly by the body of the sphenoid, the sphenoid concha, the ala of the vomer, and the sphenoid process of the palatine bone. The floor is formed by the palatine process of the maxilla and the horizontal part of the palatine bone. Anteriorly, there is the opening of the incisive canal. The lateral wall is formed anteriorly by the frontal process of the maxilla and by the lacrimal bone; in the middle, by the ethmoid, maxilla, and inferior nasal concha; posteriorly, by the vertical plate of the palatine bone and the medial pterygoid plate of the sphenoid. On the lateral wall, there are three irregular openings termed the superior, middle, and inferior meatus of the nose. These openings connect with the paranasal sinuses.

For the surgeon, the medial wall or nasal septum is the most important wall of the nasal cavity (Fig. 1-7).[1] It is often deviated to one side, usually to the left.

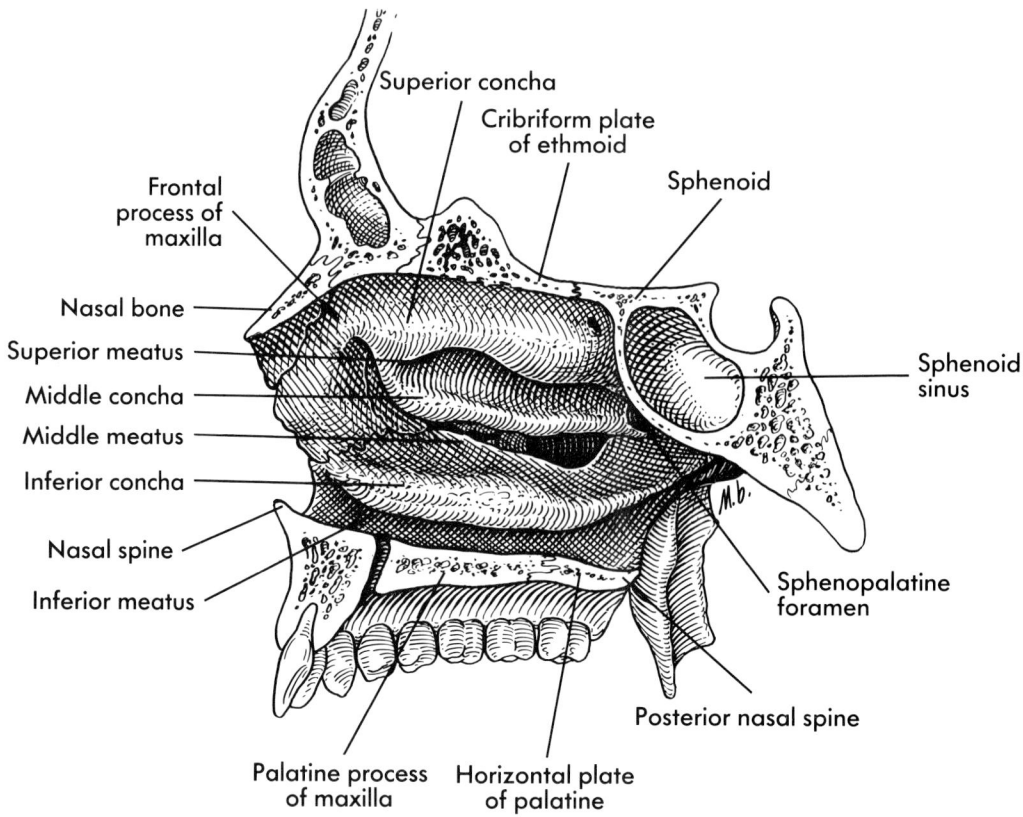

Fig. 1-6. Roof, floor, and lateral wall of nasal cavity.

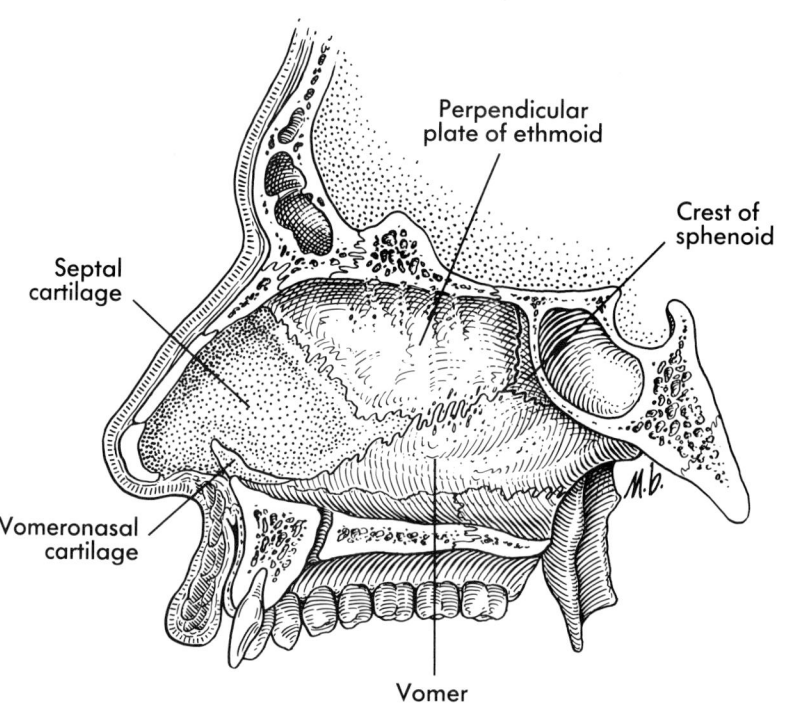

Fig. 1-7. Nasal septum, sagittal view. Primary components consist of septal cartilage, perpendicular plate of ethmoid, and vomer. Adjacent bones (frontal, maxillary, palatine, and sphenoid) make minor contributions.

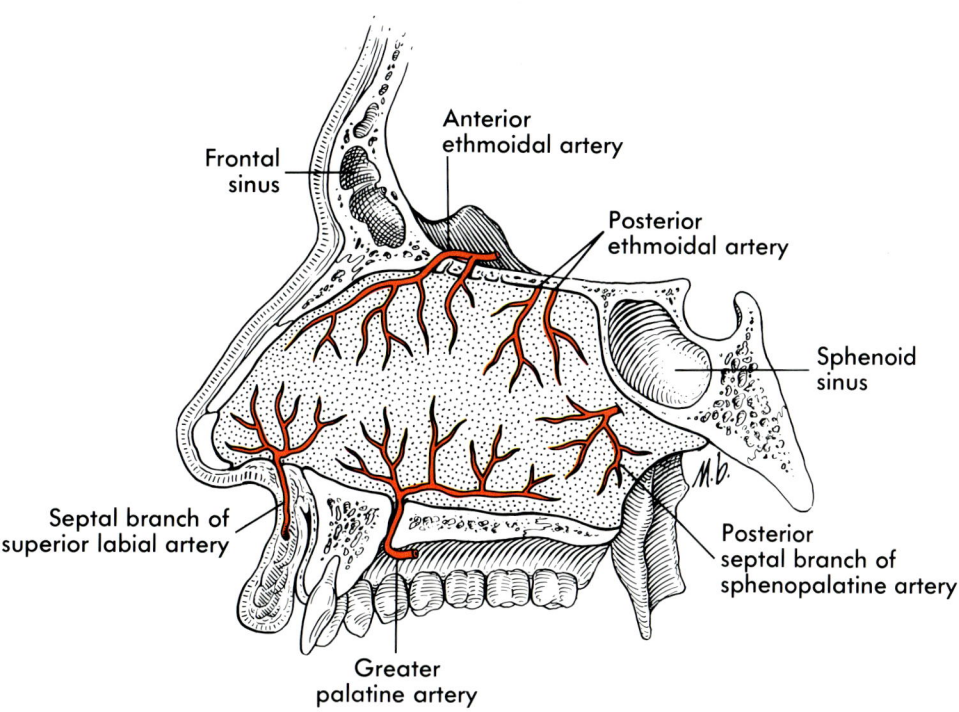

Fig. 1-8. Arterial supply of nasal septum.

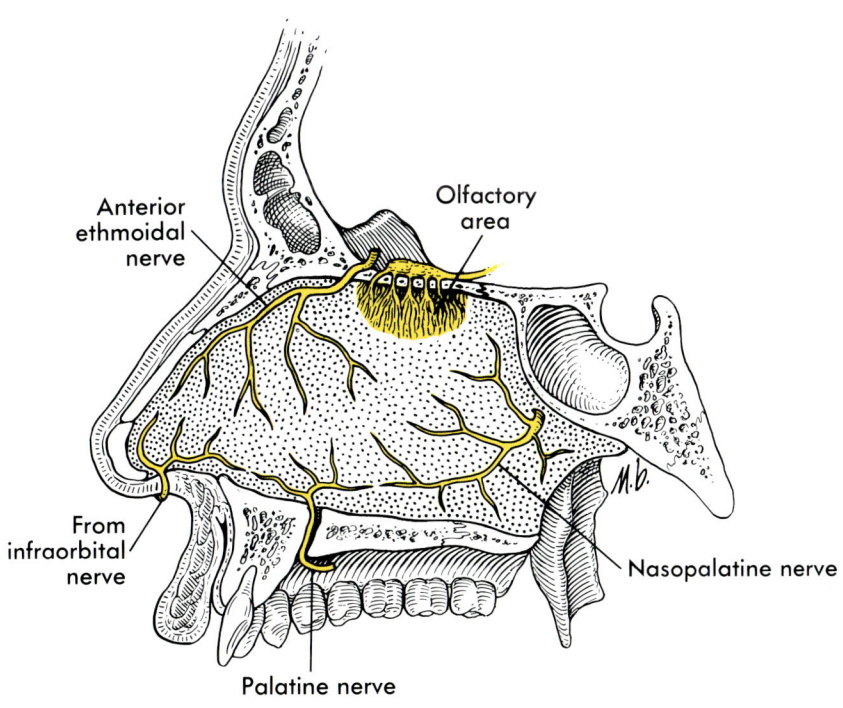

Fig. 1-9. Nerves of nasal septum.

The nasal septum consists mainly of the septal cartilage, the perpendicular plate of the ethmoid and the vomer. Adjacent bones such as the frontal, maxillary, palatine, and sphenoid make minor contributions.

The septal cartilage is thicker at its margins than at its center. Its anterior margin is connected with the nasal bones and is continuous with the anterior margins of the lateral nasal cartilages. Inferiorly, the septal cartilage is connected by fibrous tissue to the medial crura of the greater alar cartilages. Its posterior margin is connected with the perpendicular plate of the ethmoid, and its inferior margin with the vomer and the palatine processes of the maxillae. The vomer is situated in the median plane and forms the posterior and inferior part of the nasal septum. Its surfaces are marked by small furrows for blood vessels, and on each surface is the nasopalatine groove, which contains the nasopalatine nerve and vessels. The inferior border connects with the crest formed by the maxillae and palatine bones, and its superior half is fused with the perpendicular plate of the ethmoid. Its inferior half is grooved for the inferior margin of the septal cartilage of the nose. The posterior portion of the vomer joins the sphenoid crest, which in turn blends with the conchae that form the anterior bony wall of the sphenoid sinus. The perpendicular plate of the ethmoid articulates anteriorly with the spine of the frontal bone and the crest of the nasal bones. The posterior border joins the sphenoid crest and its inferior border, the vomer. The inferior border is thicker than the posterior and serves for the attachment of the septal cartilage.

The arterial supply to the septum is illustrated in Fig. 1-8. Anterior and posterior ethmoid branches of the ophthalmic artery enter through the cribriform plate. These are the only arteries supplying the septum that are derived from the internal carotid artery. The posterior septal branch of the sphenopalatine artery supplies the posterior portion; and the septal branch of the superior labial artery, the anteroinferior portion of the septum. This latter vessel, which arises from the facial artery, is usually encountered during the initial portion of a transsphenoidal operation when the nasal mucosa is being separated from the septum inferiorly. The greater palatine artery also arises from the facial artery.

The nerve supply of the nasal septum is shown in Fig. 1-9. The pterygopalatine ganglion sends the nasopalatine nerves through canals of the same name, and the pharyngeal nerve through the pharyngeal (palatovaginal) canal.

PITUITARY GLAND AND STALK

The adenohypophysis (pars anterior, anterior pituitary, pars distalis) and neurohypophysis (pars nervosa, posterior pituitary) each have a distinct embryologic origin (Fig. 1-10).[4] During the third or fourth week of gestation, a midline diverticulum, Rathke's pouch, forms as an outgrowth of the primitive stomodeum. The cells of Rathke's pouch grow cranially toward the neural tube to form the craniopharyngeal duct. The proximal portion of this duct is obliterated by the twelfth week of gestation and loses its connection with the buccal cavity. Small remnants of tissue derived from Rathke's pouch may persist into adult life, the so-called pharyngeal pituitary. Subsequent proliferation of the distal anterior wall of Rathke's pouch forms the pars distalis, which comprises the majority (90%

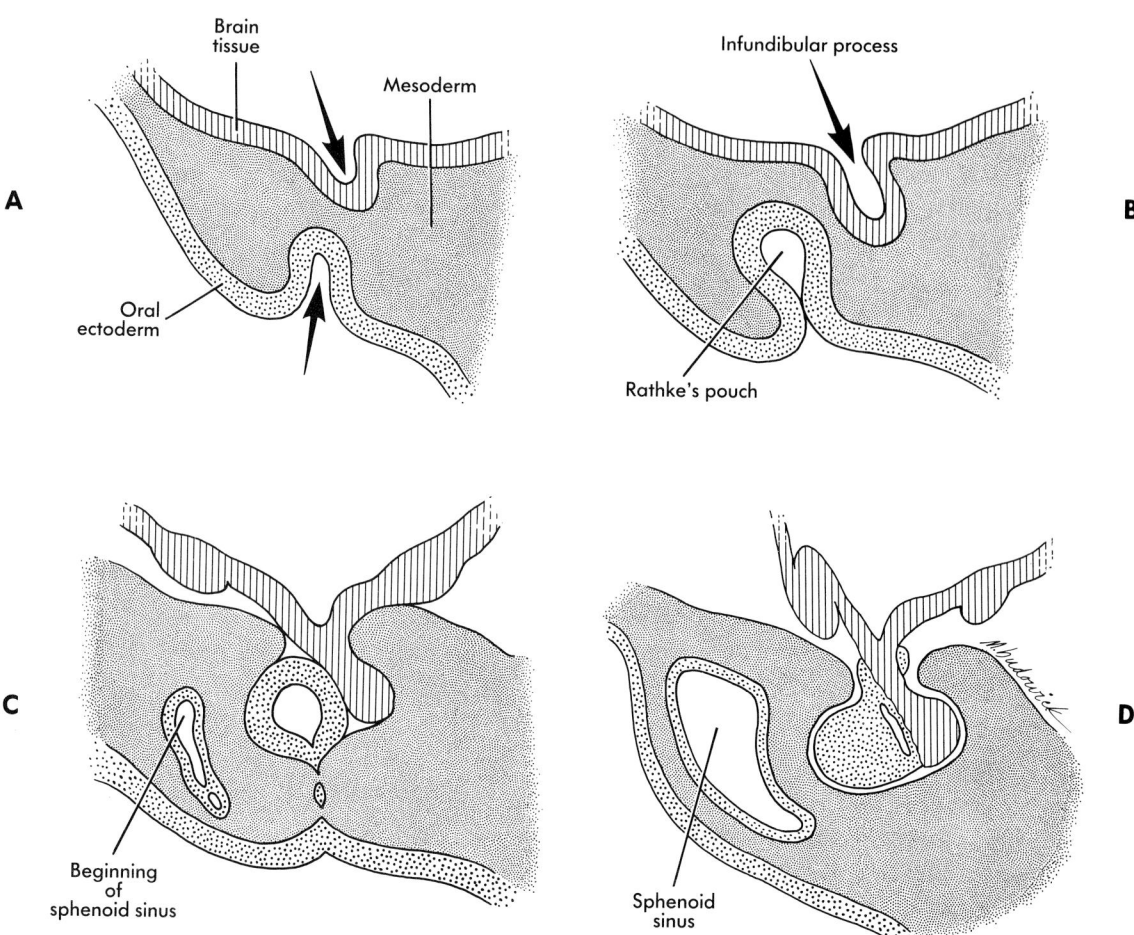

Fig. 1-10. Embryogenesis of pituitary gland. **A,** Early invagination of primitive stomodeum and infundibular process. **B,** Growth of mesoderm constricts Rathke's pouch. **C,** Further development allows Rathke's pouch to be "pinched off" from oral cavity. **D,** Rathke's cleft components develop into pars distalis, pars tuberalis, and (?) pars intermedia. Infundibular process develops into infundibular stalk and pars nervosa.

to 95%) of the adult anterior pituitary. The posterior wall of Rathke's pouch becomes the pars intermedia, which is in immediate contact with the posterior pituitary. The lumen between the anterior and intermediate parts is obliterated by epithelial infoldings in the majority of pituitary glands, although a few colloid-filled cysts may persist. There is also a thin layer of cells from the anterior pituitary anlage that surrounds the lower end of the stalk. This collection of anterior pituitary cells, the pars tuberalis, forms a thin layer of cells on the anterior surface of the stalk and extends a short distance above the diaphragm sella.

The posterior pituitary is formed early in embryonic life from a hollow ectodermal process of a separate primordium. A downpouching of the diencephalon in the floor of the third ventricle forms the infundibulum. The hollow upper portion of the infundibulum fuses to become the pituitary stalk, and the distal end enlarges to form the posterior pituitary.

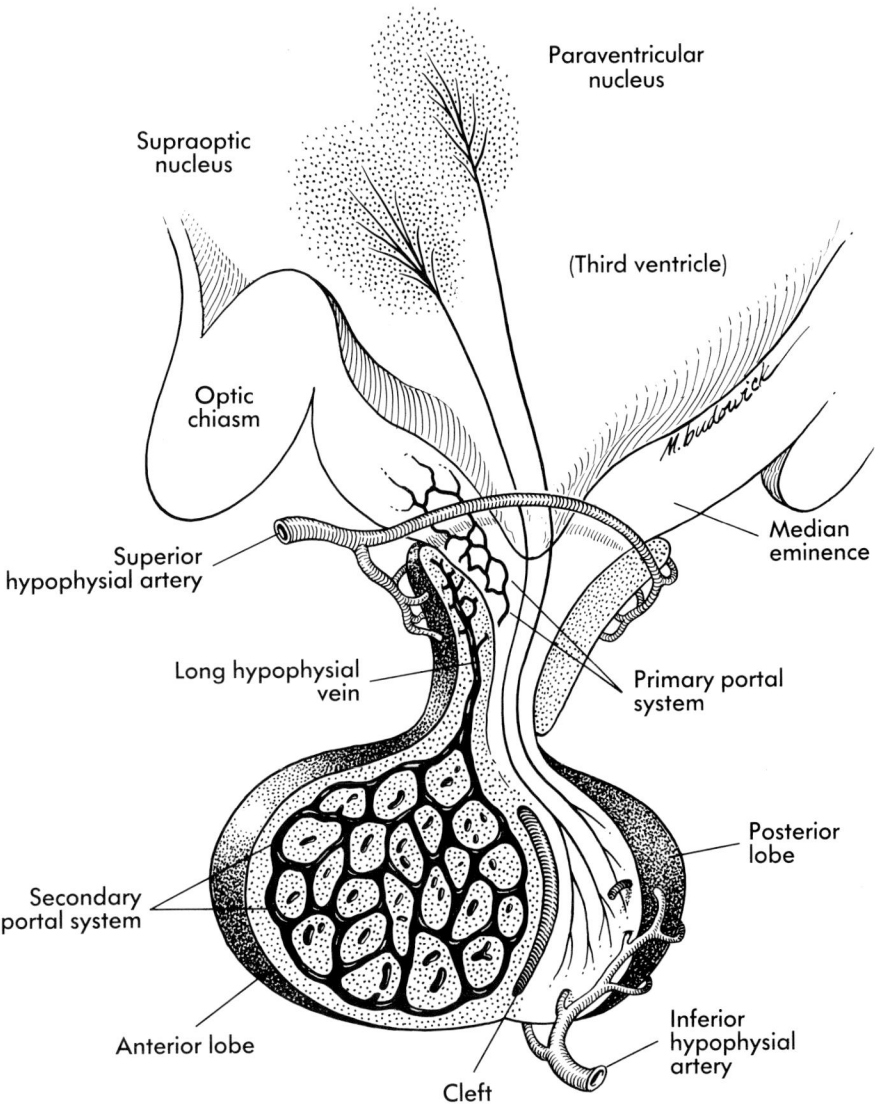

Fig. 1-11. Sagittal diagram of pituitary and some of its important anatomic features.

The pituitary gland (Fig. 1-11) is a relatively small gland measuring 1.2 to 1.5 cm in its greatest or transverse diameter (side to side), about 1 cm in its rostrocaudal, and approximately 0.5 cm in thickness. It weighs from 0.5 to 0.6 g in adult men and is somewhat larger in women. The gland resides in the sella turcica and is attached to the hypothalamus by the stalk, or infundibulum. The stalk reaches the gland through an opening in the diaphragm sella, which consists of a shelf of dura stretched between the clinoid processes. In effect, this structure covers the pituitary gland and usually isolates the gland from the brain and cerebrospinal fluid (CSF) pathways. However, the opening in the diaphragm varies in size (see Fig. 16-1) and in some cases may be unusually large, which in turn allows the suprasellar arachnoid lined cistern (which contains CSF) to bulge into the sella turcica. The "incompetent" diaphragm and the presence of the CSF-filled cistern in the sella turcica are considered to be the anatomic bases setting the stage for the "empty sella" syndrome (see Chapter 16).

The anterior lobe is larger than the posterior, occupying about 75% of the gland, and appears darker than the posterior lobe on cut section. The anterior lobe is divided into the pars tuberalis, pars distalis, and pars intermedia, although some authorities classify the latter entity with the neurohypophysis. The pars tuberalis consists of a small amount of glandular adenohypophysial tissue that is situated around the stalk, particularly its lower portion. Interestingly, the pars tuberalis is capable of hormone production. The intermediate lobe is rudimentary in man and makes up less than 1% of the total weight of the entire gland. However, this figure of less than 1% underestimates the mass of intermediate lobe cells because of the significant number of these cells that are diffusely distributed in the anterior and posterior lobes of humans.[10,14] The microscopic anatomy of the anterior lobe is discussed in Chapter 3 in connection with pathologic lesions in and about the pituitary gland.

The neurohypophysis consists of the median eminence of the hypothalamus, the infundibulum (stalk), and the posterior lobe. As indicated above, some authorities classify the intermediate lobe with the neurohypophysis. From a practical standpoint, whether to classify this structure with the neurohypophysis as opposed to the adenohypophysis is an academic issue, since the intermediate lobe, as pointed out previously, is largely rudimentary in humans. The only possible clinical significance of this structure is that current evidence suggests that its cells may serve to give origin to some of the adenomas that cause Cushing's disease (see Chapter 7).[7]

The neurohypophysis is supplied by nerve fibers from the supraoptic and paraventricular nuclei (see p. 13) of the hypothalamus (Fig. 1-11). These fibers arise from neurosecretory cells that produce the two hormones of the neurohypophysis—vasopressin, or antidiuretic hormone (ADH), and oxytocin. Further discussion of the actions of these hormones, and importantly, the clinical conditions resulting from abnormalities of ADH secretion can be found in Chapters 2 and 15. Other than this system, the pituitary has no specific innervation. Sympathetic fibers from the superior cervical ganglion have been traced along blood vessels but are not associated with glandular secretion.

The arteries to the hypophysis are the superior and inferior hypophysial arteries (Fig. 1-11). The superior hypophysial arises from the internal carotid or posterior communicating artery; and the inferior hypophysial, from the internal carotid within the cavernous sinus. The superior hypophysial supplies primarily the median eminence and stalk; and the inferior hypophysial, the posterior lobe. The blood from the capillaries of the median eminence and stalk collect into the veins (portal system) that pass down the stalk and break up into the numerous sinusoid capillaries of the adenohypophysis. The portal system performs a dual task—it nourishes the cells of the adenohypophysis and serves as a conduit for releasing and inhibiting factors and hormones from the hypothalamus to the target cells in the anterior lobe. The veins of the hypophysis, the lateral hypophysial veins, drain into the cavernous and intercavernous sinuses.

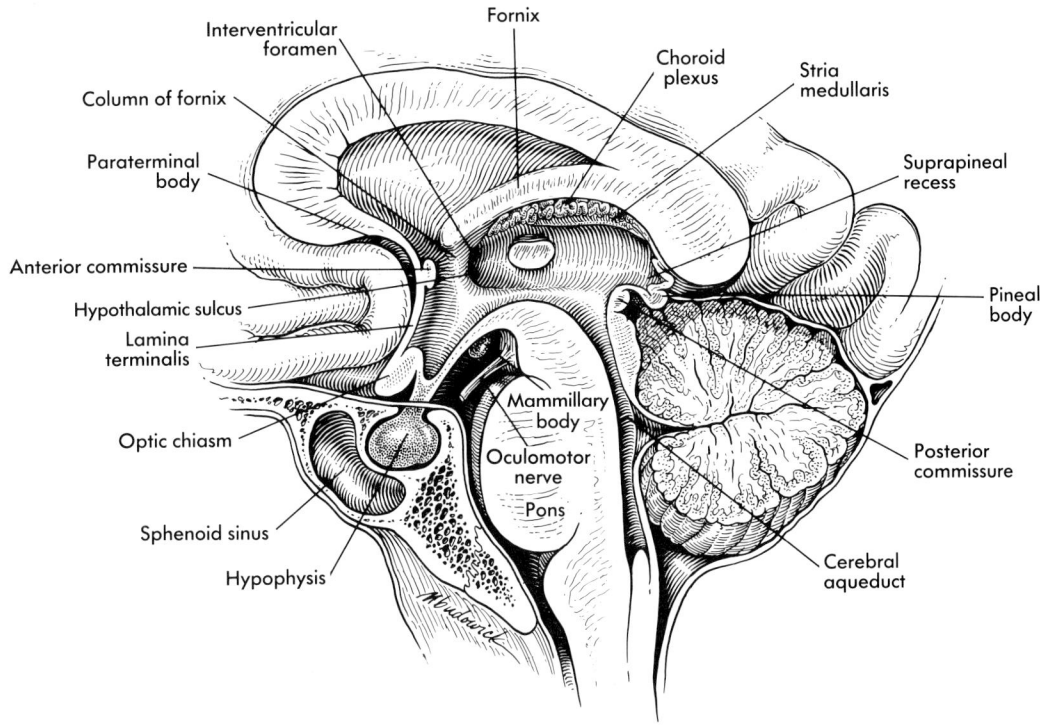

Fig. 1-12. Median sagittal section of region of hypothalamus and third ventricle.

HYPOTHALAMUS

The hypothalamus lies in the walls of the third ventricle below the hypothalamic sulcus (Fig. 1-12).[3] Its borders are relatively ill defined. Anteroinferiorly, it is limited by the optic chiasm and tracts; and posteriorly, it is bounded by the posterior perforated substance and the cerebral peduncles. On sagittal section, it can be seen to be separated from the thalamus by the hypothalamic sulcus on the wall of the third ventricle. Anteriorly, it merges with the preoptic septal region; and posteriorly, with the tegmental area of the midbrain. Its lateral relations are the subthalamus and the internal capsule.

On the ventral surface, the infundibulum, to which the hypophysis is attached, emerges posterior to the optic chiasm. A slightly bulging region posterior to the infundibulum is the tuber cinereum. The mammillary bodies are located posteriorly near the interpeduncular fossa. The area forming the floor of the third ventricle is called the median eminence of the tuber cinereum. The portion rostral to the infundibular stem is the anterior median eminence, and the portion behind the infundibular stem forms the posterior median eminence. The ventral protrusion of the hypothalamus and the third ventricle recess form the infundibulum. The median eminence represents the final point of convergence of pathways from the central nervous system on the peripheral endocrine system. It is the anatomic site of the interface between brain and the anterior pituitary. Capillaries of the hypophysial portal vessels vascularize the median eminence. The vascular system

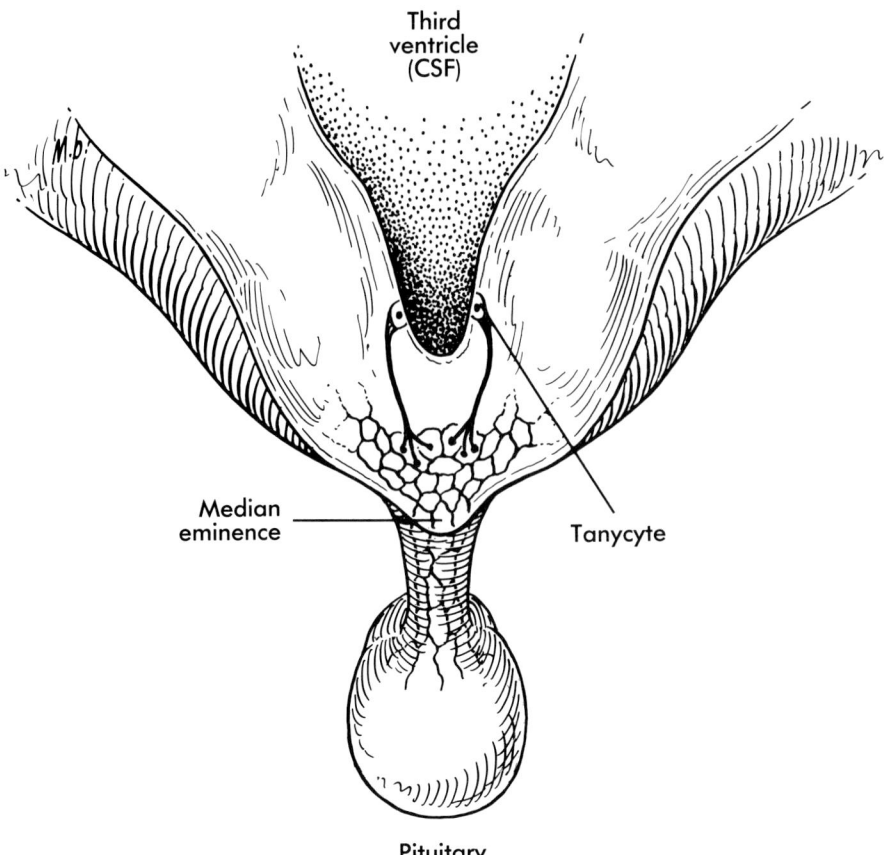

Fig. 1-13. Tanycyte, a highly specialized ependymal cell found in floor of third ventricle, is illustrated sending a process that terminates adjacent to perivascular spaces of median eminence.

of the median eminence collects the various releasing and inhibitory hormones and factors and transports them via the portal system to the target cells of the anterior pituitary. Also a connection between the median eminence and the CSF of the third ventricle is provided by ependymal cells (tanycytes). These cells line the floor of the third ventricle and send processes that traverse the width of the median eminence and terminate near the perivascular spaces of the portal vessels (Fig. 1-13).

A number of more or less distinct cellular masses known as hypothalamic nuclei are found throughout the entire area (Figs. 1-14 and 1-15). A sagittal plane passing through the anterior pillar of the fornix roughly separates the medial and the lateral hypothalamic areas. The lateral area is bounded medially by the mammillothalamic tract and the anterior column of the fornix, and the lateral boundary is the medial margin of the internal capsule and the subthalamic region. This area contains the lateral hypothalamic nucleus and two or three cell groups known as the tuberal nuclei. The preoptic area constitutes the periventricular gray and is the most rostral part of the third ventricle. Within this area are the preoptic

Anatomy 15

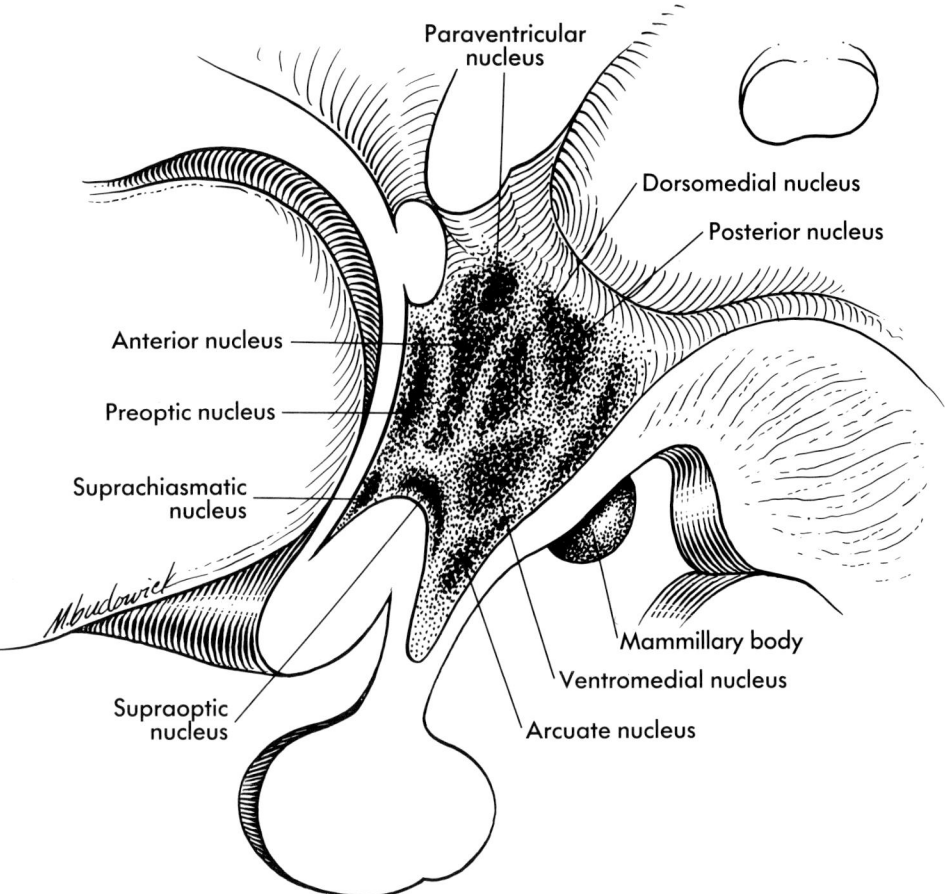

Fig. 1-14. Nuclei of hypothalamus illustrated in lateral, or sagittal, dimension.

periventricular, the medial preoptic, and the lateral preoptic nuclei. Caudal to the preoptic are three hypothalamic regions: (1) an anterior, or supraoptic, region that lies above the optic chiasm and is continuous rostrally with the preoptic area; (2) a middle, or tuberal, region; and (3) a caudal, or mammillary, region, which is continuous caudally with the central gray of the aqueduct. The supraoptic region contains the paraventricular, supraoptic, anterior hypothalamic, and suprachiasmatic nuclei. The paraventricular and supraoptic nuclei, which are two of the most striking and sharply defined hypothalamic nuclei, both send fibers to the posterior lobe of the hypophysis. In the tuberal region the hypothalamus reaches its widest extent. A number of nuclei including the ventromedial, dorsomedial, arcuate, posterior hypothalamic, and the mammilloinfundibular nuclei are found in this area. The mammillary region consists of the mammillary bodies and the dorsally located cells of the posterior hypothalamic nucleus. In man, the mammillary body consists almost entirely of the large medial mammillary nucleus.

The major influences of the hypothalamus on the pituitary are through the supraoptic hypophysial tract and the tuberohypophysial tract. The *supraoptic*

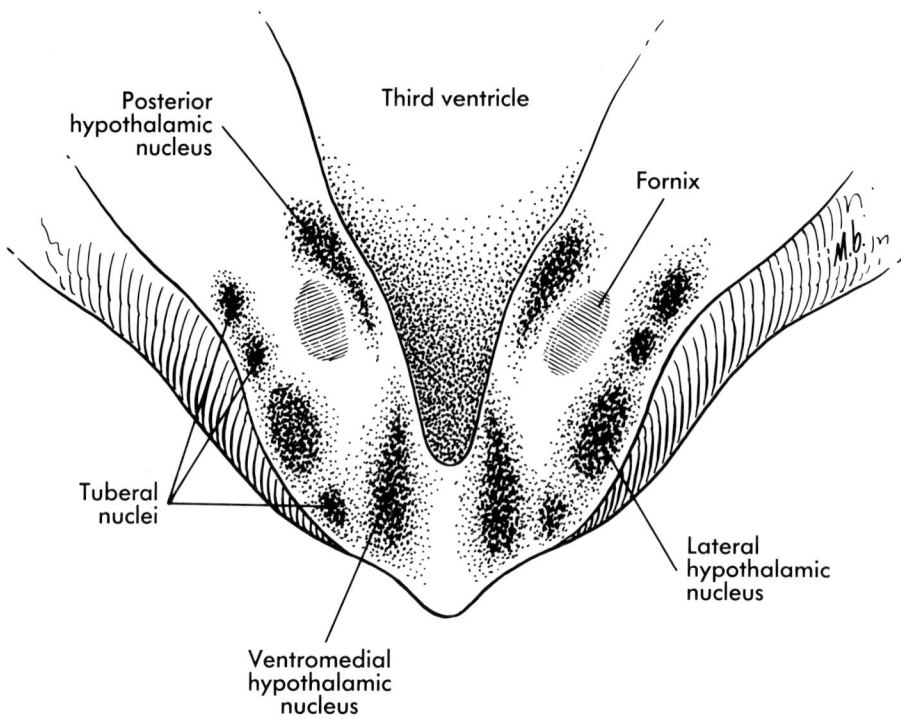

Fig. 1-15. Nuclei of hypothalamus seen in transverse, or coronal section, at level of infundibular region.

hypophysial tract is the term used to designate the fibers arising from the supraoptic and paraventricular nuclei and projecting to the posterior lobe of the pituitary. This system is specifically concerned with the maintenance of body water balance. The *tuberohypophysial tract* arises from the tuberal region, mainly from the arcuate nucleus, and can be traced only to the median eminence and the infundibular stem. Functionally, this tract and the hypophysial portal system establish the neurohumoral link between the hypothalamus and the anterior pituitary.

PARASELLAR ANATOMIC STRUCTURES

A number of important structures are situated adjacent to or in close proximity to the pituitary gland and sella turcica (Figs. 1-16 and 1-17). These structures include among others the optic nerves, chiasm, and tracts; the internal carotid artery and two of its major branches, the anterior cerebral and ophthalmic arteries; the cavernous sinus, which contains a number of important anatomic structures; and the medial portion of the temporal lobe.

The optic nerve consists mainly of the axons or central processes of the neurons in the ganglionic layer of the retina. These axons converge toward the optic disc, which is located 3 mm medial to the posterior pole of the globe, and are gathered there into small bundles that pierce the choroid and sclerotic coats of the globe to become the optic nerve. The nerve, as it courses posteriorly toward

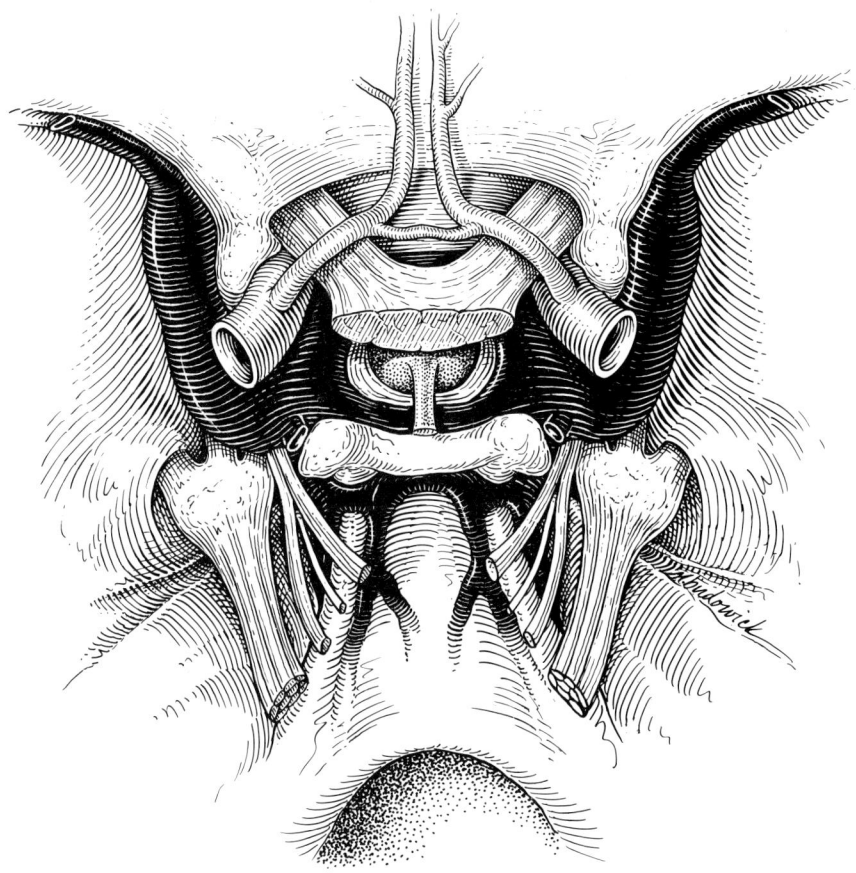

Fig. 1-16. Superior view, parasellar region, showing relationship between cavernous sinus, cranial nerves, internal carotid and anterior cerebral arteries, pituitary gland and stalk, and optic nerves and chiasm.

the brain, passes through the optic foramen and then joins the nerve of the opposite side to form the optic chiasm. The nerve in the orbit is 3 to 4 mm in diameter and 20 to 30 mm long. Except for the initial intraocular portion, which is only 1 mm in length, the optic fibers are myelinated and supported by neuroglia. The orbital portion of the nerve is invested by sheaths derived from the dura, arachnoid, and pia mater, all three of which fuse and become continuous with the sclera at the lamina cribrosa. The dura extends as far back as the intracranial cavity, the arachnoid somewhat farther, and the pia all the way to and including the chiasm. Thus the optic nerve is surrounded by a subarachnoid space continuous with the intracranial subarachnoid space. The presence of this space around the orbital portion of the optic nerve, which extends all the way to the globe, provides the anatomic basis for papilledema that usually occurs in instances of increased intracranial pressure. The optic nerves share the relatively small optic foramen with the ophthalmic artery. The latter is the first major branch of the internal

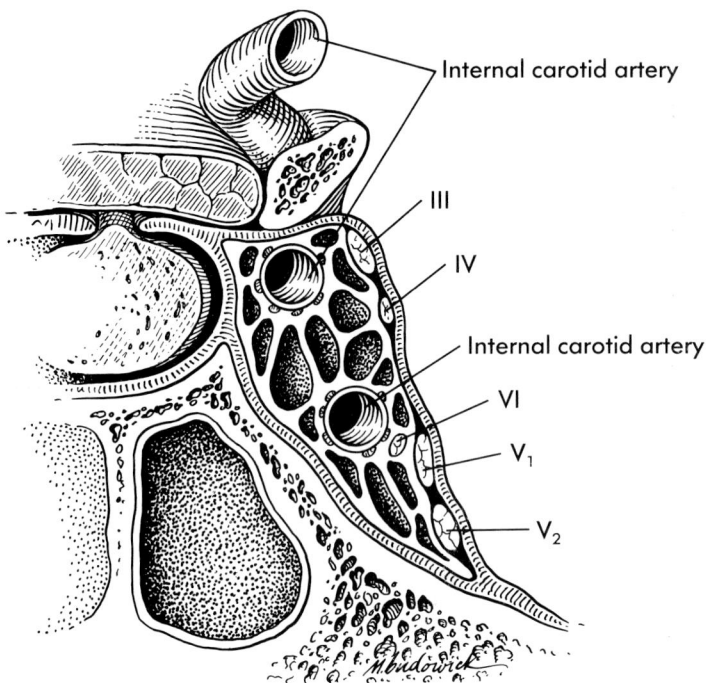

Fig. 1-17. Cavernous sinus, transverse or coronal view. Note relationship between internal carotid artery and cranial nerves III, IV, and V (V_1 and V_2), all of which are in a sheath in lateral wall of sinus. Cranial nerve VI is situated below artery and is suspended by fibrous trabeculae between lateral wall of sinus and sphenoid bone.

carotid artery and is the major arterial supply of the globe and other orbital structures.

Optic chiasm

The optic chiasm, a flattened oblong structure formed by the union of the optic nerves, usually measures 12 mm in transverse diameter, 8 mm in anteroposterior diameter, and 4 mm in thickness. The chiasm forms the anteroinferior wall of the third ventricle, and at this point it is tilted about 45° from the horizontal plane. Its anatomic relations superiorly are the lamina terminalis, anterior commissure, and the third ventricle; posteriorly, the pituitary stalk, tuber cinereum, mammillary bodies, and oculomotor nerves; and inferiorly, the diaphragm sella and pituitary gland. From a clinical viewpoint, the close anatomic relationship between the optic chiasm and the underlying pituitary gland provides an explanation for the frequency of visual impairment seen with pituitary tumors that progressively grow and produce mass effects. An appreciation of the variability in the position of the chiasm in relation to the underlying gland is also important, particularly since this variability can affect the surgical approach to the pituitary gland if transcranial operative procedures are used.[11] In the majority of cases (80%), the chiasm lies directly above the central portion of the diaphragm sella and the gland (Fig. 1-18). However, in 9% of individuals the chiasm is anteriorly

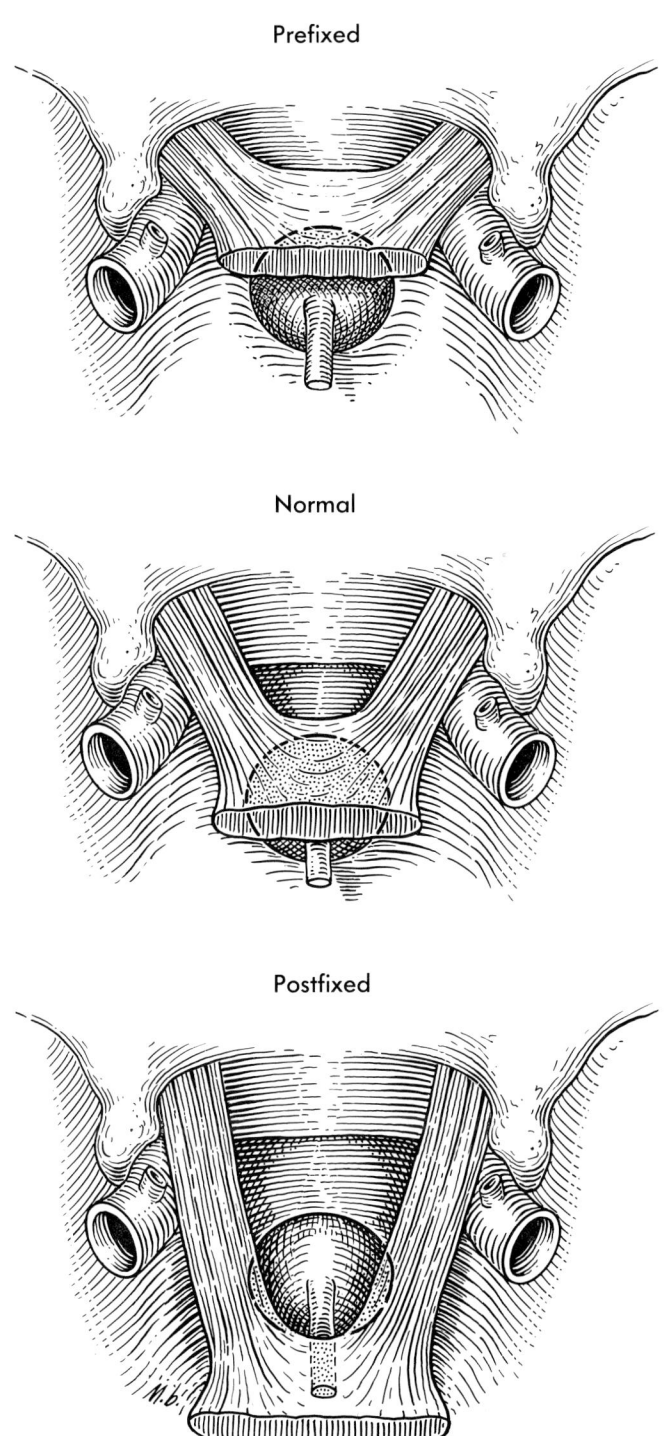

Fig. 1-18. Optic chiasm, superior view. *Top,* Prefixed chiasm that overlies tuberculum sella. *Middle,* Chiasm directly above central portion of diaphragm sella, which is usual position. *Bottom,* Postfixed chiasm is situated over posterior clinoids.

situated and overlies the tuberculum sella, in which case it is termed a prefixed chiasm. A postfixed chiasm overlies the posterior clinoids and was found in 11% of the Bergland et al series.[2] Technical difficulties in the transcranial approach to the pituitary gland may be encountered in cases in which the chiasm is prefixed in position, thus markedly obscuring the surgeon's view of the sella.

The position of the chiasm in reference to the pituitary gland and diaphragm sella may also affect the pattern of visual field changes in patients with pituitary tumors. For instance, with a prefixed chiasm, an expanding tumor may result in a bitemporal scotomatous hemianopsia rather than the classic superior bitemporal quadrantanopsia as a result of posterior infrachiasmal compression.[6] Furthermore, pituitary tumors in patients with a postfixed chiasm involve the junction of the optic nerve with the chiasm and thus may present with the anterior chiasmal syndrome, which consists of an ipsilateral visual field loss and a contralateral superior temporal quadrantanopsia (junctional scotoma) (see Fig. 4-2).[8]

The optic tract leaves the chiasm, diverges from its fellow of the opposite side, and winds obliquely across the undersurface of the cerebral peduncle. Each tract contains the temporal fibers from the ipsilateral eye and the nasal fibers from the contralateral eye.

Cavernous sinus

One of the more important structures in close proximity to the sella and pituitary gland is the cavernous sinus (Figs. 1-16 and 1-17). It is especially important to the neurosurgeon performing pituitary surgery, particularly transsphenoidal surgery, because the medial border is usually exposed at surgery. Bleeding from the cavernous sinus is not uncommon during a transsphenoidal operation and can be a significant factor in making the operation technically difficult. Another important aspect of this structure, particularly in relation to pituitary tumors, is its predisposition toward tumor invasion. When this occurs, it usually means that the lesion cannot be cured by surgery.

Anatomically, the cavernous sinus is irregular in shape and fits into the space between the body of the sphenoid bone and the dura forming the medial boundary of the middle cranial fossa. In an anteroposterior direction (Fig. 1-16), it extends from the superior orbital fissure to the apex of the temporal bone. As shown in Fig. 1-17, in the lateral wall of the cavernous sinus are several important cranial nerves. From top to bottom, one can identify the oculomotor (III), trochlear (IV), and the ophthalmic (V_1) and maxillary (V_2) divisions of the trigeminal (V). Suspended by fibrous trabeculae between the lateral wall of the sinus and the sphenoid bone are the abducens nerve (VI) and the internal carotid artery with its surrounding plexus of sympathetic fibers. The cavernous sinus receives the inferior and superior ophthalmic veins, some of the cerebral veins, and the sphenoparietal sinus. It anastomoses with other venous sinuses, and the two cavernous sinuses anastomose with each other through the intercavernous sinuses. The cavernous sinus drains into the inferior petrosal sinus, which drains into the internal jugular vein. In clinical practice, it is possible to catheterize the inferior petrosal sinus via the transfemoral route. Since the inferior petrosal contains the venous

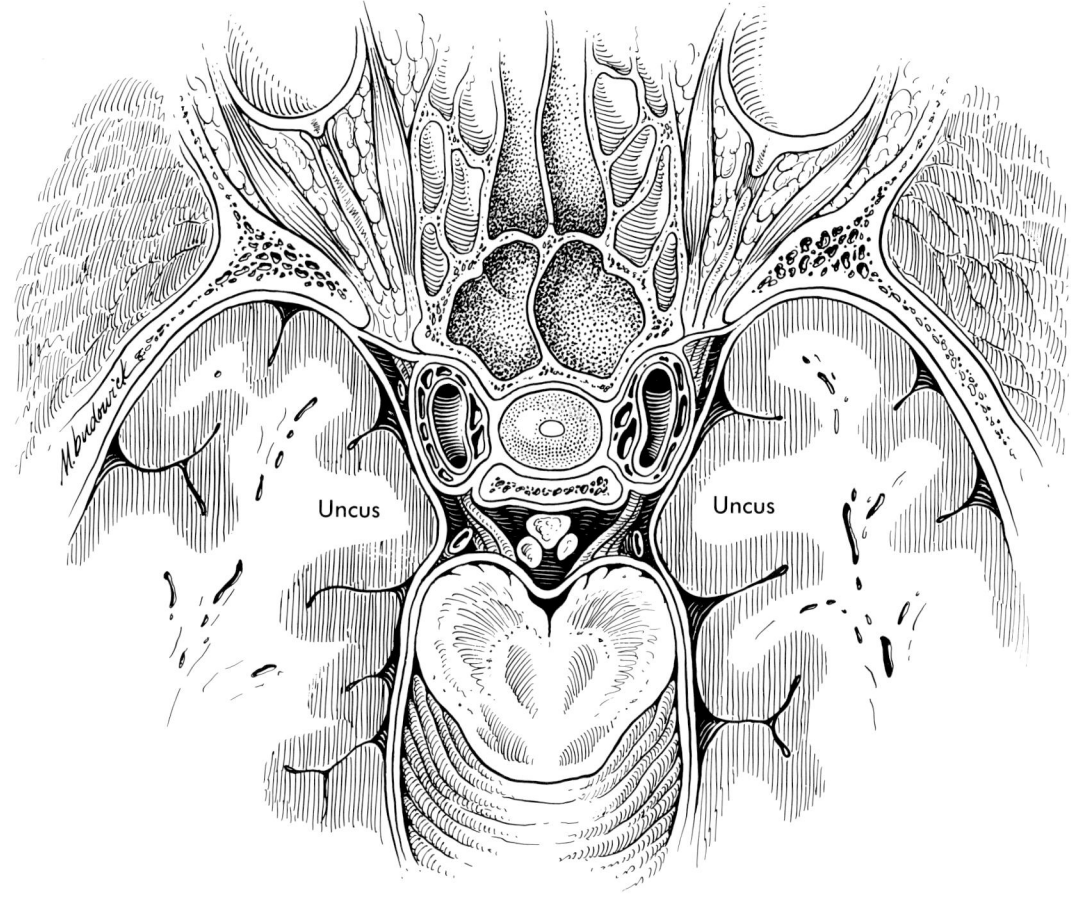

Fig. 1-19. Axial section through brain in plane of sella and pituitary gland to illustrate proximity of various anatomic structures to pituitary. Note relatively close relationship of medial portion of temporal lobe to sella and pituitary gland.

effluent from the cavernous sinus (which in turn drains the pituitary), the technique of petrosal sampling may have significant clinical value in certain instances of Cushing's syndrome in terms of identifying the pituitary as the source for the abnormal hormone (ACTH) secretion (see Chapter 7).[9]

The internal carotid artery arises at the bifurcation of the common carotid artery in the neck, traverses the upper portion of the neck, and enters the middle cranial fossa through the foramen lacerum. After passing through the latter, it curves upward and lies between the lingula and petrosal processes of the sphenoid bone. It enters the cavernous sinus, curves forward and upward (Fig. 1-17), and then perforates the part of the dura that forms the roof of the cavernous sinus on the medial side of the anterior clinoid process. The anterior cerebral artery is a major branch of the internal carotid and arises at the medial extremity of the sylvian fissure (Fig. 1-16). It passes forward and medial across the anterior perforated substance, above the optic nerve to the commencement of the longitudinal fissure, at which point it comes into close relationship with the opposite artery. The two arteries connect through a short trunk, the anterior communicating artery. The anterior cerebral artery thus lies in close proximity to the pituitary gland, optic nerves and chiasm, diaphragm sella, pituitary stalk, and hypothalamus.

Although not in direct contact, the medial portion of the temporal lobe is relatively close to the sella turcica and pituitary gland (Fig. 1-19). The clinical importance of this relationship is that on occasion a large pituitary tumor with significant suprasellar extension, particularly with a lateral component, may cause temporal lobe seizures presumably from a compressive-irritative lesion involving the hippocampal gyrus.

REFERENCES

1. Anderson JE: *Grant's Atlas of Anatomy*, ed 7. Baltimore, Williams & Wilkins, 1978.
2. Bergland RM, Ray BS, Torack RM: Anatomical variations in the pituitary gland and adjacent structures in 225 human autopsy cases. *J Neurosurg* 28:93, 1968.
3. Carpenter MB: *Core Text of Neuroanatomy*, ed 2. Baltimore, Williams & Wilkins, 1978.
4. Conklin JL: The development of the human fetal adenohypophysis. *Anat Rec* 160:79, 1968.
5. Gray H: *Anatomy of the Human Body*, ed 29, Goss CM (ed). Philadelphia, Lea & Febiger, 1973.
6. Hoyt WF: Correlative functional anatomy of the optic chiasm—1969. *Clin Neurosurg* 17:189, 1970.
7. Lamberts SWJ, de Lange SA, Stefanko SZ: Adrenocorticotropin-secreting pituitary adenomas originate from the anterior or the intermediate lobe in Cushing's disease: Differences in the regulation of hormone secretion. *J Clin Endocrinol Metab* 54:286, 1982.
8. Newman M: The chiasmal syndrome, in Gay AJ, Burde RM (eds): *Clinical Concepts in Neuro-Ophthalmology*. Boston, Little Brown & Co Inc, 1967.
9. Oldfield EH, Chrousos GP, Schulte HM, et al: Preoperative lateralization of ACTH secreting pituitary microadenomas by bilateral and simultaneous inferior petrosal venous sinus sampling. *N Engl J Med* 312:100, 1985.
10. Reichlin S: Anatomical and physiological basis of hypothalamic-pituitary regulation, in Post KD, Jackson IMD, Reichlin S (eds): *The Pituitary Adenoma*. New York, Plenum Medical Book Co, 1980.
11. Renn WH, Rhoton AL Jr: Microsurgical anatomy of the sellar region. *J Neurosurg* 43:288, 1975.
12. Rhoton AL Jr, Hardy DG, Chambers SM: Microsurgical anatomy and dissection of the sphenoid bone, cavernous sinus and sellar region. *Surg Neurol* 12:63, 1979.
13. Rhoton AL Jr, Harris FS, Renn WH: Microsurgical anatomy of the sellar region and cavernous sinus. *Clin Neurosurg* 24:54, 1977.
14. Wingstrand KG: Microscopic anatomy, nerve supply and blood supply of the pars intermedia, in Harris GW, Donovan BT (eds): *The Pituitary Gland*. Berkeley, Calif., University of California Press, 1966, vol 3.

CHAPTER 2

Neuroendocrinology

Joseph B. Martin

Neural control of glandular secretion
    Neurosecretion
Hypothalamic-pituitary unit
    Pituitary
Hypothalamus
    Gross anatomy
    Median eminence
    Tuberoinfundibular neurons
    Hypophysiotropic hormones of the hypothalamus
Extrahypothalamic regulation of the hypothalamic-adenohypophysial system
Neuropharmacology of anterior pituitary regulation
    Aminergic innervation of the hypothalamus
    Dopamine
    Norepinephrine
    Epinephrine
    Serotonin

Functions of the biogenic amines
Neurohypophysis: physiology
    Neurohypophysis
    Neurohypophysial hormones
    Regulation of ADH secretion
        Osmolarity
        Volume regulation
        Stress and nausea
    Neuropharmacology of vasopressin
Brain-gut peptides: regulatory peptides
    Concentration of peptides in brain
    Evolutionary and embryologic aspects of neuropeptides
    Validity of peptide measurements
    Postmortem studies
        Alzheimer's disease
        Huntington's disease
        Parkinson's disease
    CSF neuropeptides

Neuroendocrinology is the study of the relationship between the nervous and endocrine systems, which, operating in coordination, regulate most of the metabolic and homeostatic activities of the body.[49] In recent years, significant, almost unbelievable, advances have been made in the field of neuroendocrinology. The identification and synthesis of hypothalamic releasing hormones such as thyrotropin-releasing hormone (TRH) and gonadotropin-releasing hormone (GnRH), the identification of a myriad of important peptides, and the isolation of growth hormone–releasing factor (GHRF) from a pancreatic tumor are among the more important achievements. A sound knowledge of the many facets of neuroendocrinology such as the actions of the hypothalamus on the pituitary, neurotransmitters that ultimately effect hormone release and/or inhibition, and the chemistry and action of the many peptides that have been identified over the past several years are vital to the scientist who explores new fields in this discipline and to the clinician in treating patients with hypothalamic-pituitary disorders.

Neuroendocrine mechanisms are involved in the regulation of growth and differentiation of tissues, reproduction, and a wide variety of behaviors. The two regulatory systems interact; many hormones act on the central nervous system (CNS), and the secretion of virtually every hormone is regulated directly or indirectly by the brain. Dysfunction of these systems is involved primarily, or secondarily, in an extraordinary range of human diseases.

Although they are interactive, the endocrine and nervous systems were considered to be separate in the past. Recent studies have shown that many of the same substances found in the nervous system of higher animals are also found in endocrine glands and in the gastrointestinal tract.[23,82,84,85,156] Hormones, neuropeptides, and neurotransmitters have been identified in simple organisms, including single-celled animals.[144,145] Moreover, hormones originally isolated from the gut are now known to be present in the brain. Several glandular structures have been shown by embryologic studies to arise developmentally from primitive ectoderm as does the nervous system. These findings strongly suggest that the two principal regulatory systems of higher animals, endocrine and nervous, have evolved in parallel from primitive, single-celled organisms. The various parts of the two systems often use interchangeable components and messengers for communication.

The basic functional unit of the endocrine system is the secretory cell, which provides its regulatory influence through the circulating blood. The basic functional unit of the nervous system is the neuron, which provides an organized network of point-to-point connection. Specificity within the endocrine system is conveyed by specialized receptors on target cells; specificity within the CNS is conveyed by neurotransmitter specificity, receptor specificity, and point-to-point hardwiring.

NEURAL CONTROL OF GLANDULAR SECRETION

Secretory cells can be classified into three types: *exocrine*, which secrete into a hollow lumen that communicates with the exterior of the body; *endocrine*, which secrete into the circulation; and *neuronal*, which secrete either into the circulating blood (neurohormonal) or at synaptic contacts (neurotransmitters, neuromodulators). Exocrine glands are regulated mainly by *secretomotor* nerve fibers. The endocrine system is regulated by the pituitary, which in turn is regulated by *neurosecretory* cells of the hypothalamus (Fig. 2-1).

Neurosecretion

The term *neurosecretion* refers to the release of a hormone into the circulation from a nerve terminal. The idea that a neuron could possess secretory functions was proposed by Ernst Scharrer in 1928 based on a morphologic study

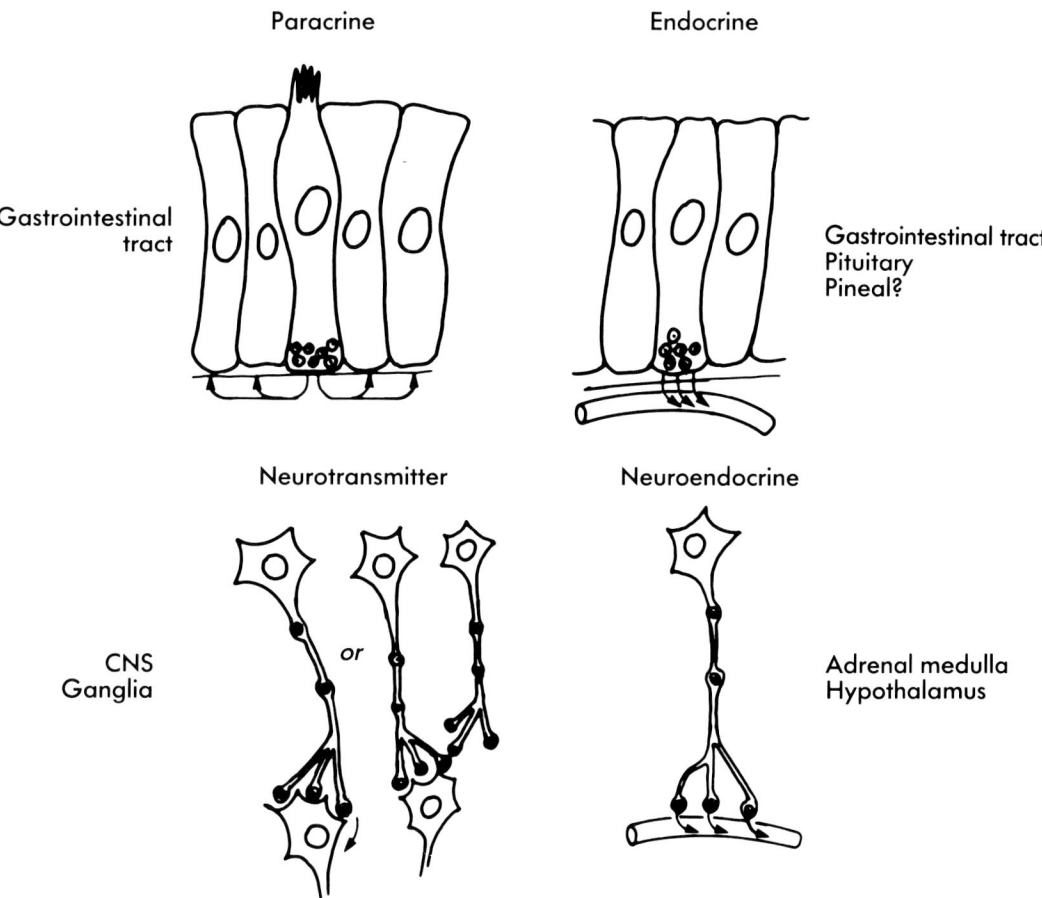

Fig. 2-1. Possible modes of peptide secretion. Peptides occur in various tissues, including gastrointestinal tract, pancreas, pituitary, and neural tissue. In gastrointestinal tract and pancreas, peptide may be secreted locally to affect a neighboring cell (paracrine secretion), or same peptide can exist in either an endocrine or gastrointestinal cell and be secreted into the bloodstream as a hormone. Same peptide may be synthesized by neuron in CNS or autonomic ganglia and be released into synaptic cleft through axodendritic synapse or may terminate presynaptically through axoaxonic synapse; in these cases it is termed a neurotransmitter or a neuromodulator. However, if neuronal product is released into bloodstream—(i.e., from the adrenal medulla or hypothalamus), it is termed a neurohormone.

From Krieger DT: Brain peptides. What, where, and why? *Science* 222:975, 1983. Copyright 1983 by the AAAS.

of certain hypothalamic cells in fish.[149,150] Later he and his colleagues observed analogous structures in the mammalian hypothalamus, recognized that the appearance of certain groups of neurons was modified by changes in the state of hydration, and showed that extracts of the hypothalamus contained bioassayable antidiuretic hormone (ADH). They proposed that the secretions of the neural lobe actually arose in the hypothalamus.

The classic example of a neurosecretory gland in the mammal is the neurohypophysis. In this structure neurosecretions (vasopressin and oxytocin) formed in cell bodies located in the supraoptic and paraventricular nuclei are transported to the neural lobe by axoplasmic flow where they are released into the blood as true hormones to regulate the function of organs at a more remote site. Similarly, other hypothalamic neurons synthesize and release peptides (releasing factors), which regulate anterior pituitary hormone secretion. Neurosecretory cells, regardless of their location, retain the functional and structural properties of neurons. They display electrophysiologic characteristics similar to other neurons, have neuron-type organelles and other cell constituents, are acted on by other neurons through synapses, and react to neurotransmitter substances such as acetylcholine. The specialized neuronal structures that secrete hormones into the blood are major links by which the brain regulates metabolic and reproductive activities. Wurtman and Anton-Tay[176] applied the term *neuroendocrine transducer* to nerve cells of this type because they are capable of translating neural activity to a hormonal output. Neurosecretory neurons provide a final common pathway for endocrine regulation, analogous to the anterior horn cell, which as formulated by Sherrington forms the final common pathway from the nervous system to the locomotor system.

HYPOTHALAMIC-PITUITARY UNIT

Early in the twentieth century, clinicians recognized that pituitary insufficiency resulted from disease in the region of the hypothalamus but were unable to resolve whether the effects resulted from direct damage to the adjacent pituitary gland.[3,4,9] On the basis of careful pathologic study, Erdheim and Stumme[48] concluded that these changes could be caused by hypothalamic damage alone; and Aschner[6] in 1912 demonstrated that gonadal deficiency (now recognized as being a result of gonadotropin failure) could be produced in dogs by hypothalamic lesions, which spared the pituitary. Over the following four decades, many workers studied the effects of "isolation" of the pituitary by surgical section of the pituitary stalk, but the results were ambiguous and controversial. In a series of important experiments, Harris and Jacobsohn[63] demonstrated the crucial role of the blood vessels of the stalk in this regulation. Pituitary stalk section in the rat caused loss of sexual function, which returned when the hypophysial-portal vessels regenerated. When a paper plate was inserted into the stalk section so as to prevent regeneration of the vessels, sexual function failed to return. They also showed that pituitaries transplanted to the pituitary fossa functioned normally, whereas pituitary transplants in other sites remained devoid of activity. These observations showed that the pituitary fossa was a privileged site for the growth and function of the pituitary and indicated that the crucial factor was the special blood supply from the hypothalamus. Nikitovitch-Winer and Everett[109] demonstrated in rats that the pituitary failure resulting from transplantation of the gland to the renal capsule was corrected by retransplantation of the same pituitary to the region beneath the basal hypothalamus, if anatomic reconnection of the blood vessels occurred. Reconstitution of pituitary function did not occur in control experiments in which the pituitary was retransplanted to the temporal lobe.

The hypophysial vessels themselves, now known to be the conduit of the hypothalamic-hypophysiotropic hormones, were first described in 1930 by Popa and Fielding.[127] The vessels were characterized by a peculiar group of coiled capillaries at the inferior extent of the hypothalamus that left the brain and joined to form long vessels that traversed the pituitary stalk. The blood in these vessels was incorrectly asserted by Popa and Fielding to flow from the pituitary upward to the base of the brain. In 1936 Wislocki and King[174] described similar vessels in the monkey and suggested on the basis of anatomic features that blood probably flowed from the hypothalamus to the pituitary. In 1947 Green and Harris[58,59,62] confirmed this suggestion by direct observation in the rat that blood in the hypothalamic portal veins did indeed flow to the anterior pituitary. Green and Harris proposed that the hypothalamus secretes into the portal capillaries of the median eminence specific pituitary-regulatory substances that are transported to the adenohypophysis by the portal vessels. This *portal vessel-chemotransmitter hypothesis* has continued to serve as the model for studies undertaken to clarify the details of this control.

The blood supply to the median eminence and anterior pituitary comes principally from the paired superior hypophysial arteries, which arise directly from the internal carotid. The portal vessels are formed by the confluence of capillary loops of the median eminence into veins (6 to 10 in number) that are visible on the anterior surface of the pituitary stalk. Portal vessels also anastomose with capillaries of the neurohypophysis, which receives a direct arterial supply from the inferior hypophysial arteries.[14,15,113] Although direct observation in anesthetized animals indicated that the predominant direction of blood flow in these vessels was downward from hypothalamus to anterior pituitary, Bergland and Page[15,113] marshaled anatomic evidence for other patterns of flow, including flow from the pituitary upward to the hypothalamus. This pattern of blood flow has not been proved by direct study, and indeed recent observations by Page[112] in the pig have confirmed the traditional view of the downward direction of blood flow.

Thus although the anterior pituitary gland lacks a direct nerve supply, the secretion of each of its hormones is under the control of the CNS. The pituitary and in turn its target glands respond to changes in the external and internal environments through neurosecretory neurons localized in the ventral hypothalamus. In addition, hypothalamic regulation of the anterior pituitary is responsive to feedback regulation by a number of hormones such as cortisol, the gonadal steroids, and thyroxine.

Pituitary

The pituitary gland, or hypophysis, lies in close proximity to the medial basal hypothalamus, to which it is connected by the highly vascular stalk (Figs. 2-2 and 2-3). It is divided into two lobes, the anterior, or *adenohypophysis,* and the posterior, or *neurohypophysis*. The adenohypophysis develops from Rathke's pouch. This pouch, which in the past has been described as an evagination of the primitive buccal ectoderm, has more recently been postulated to arise from

28 *Disorders of the pituitary*

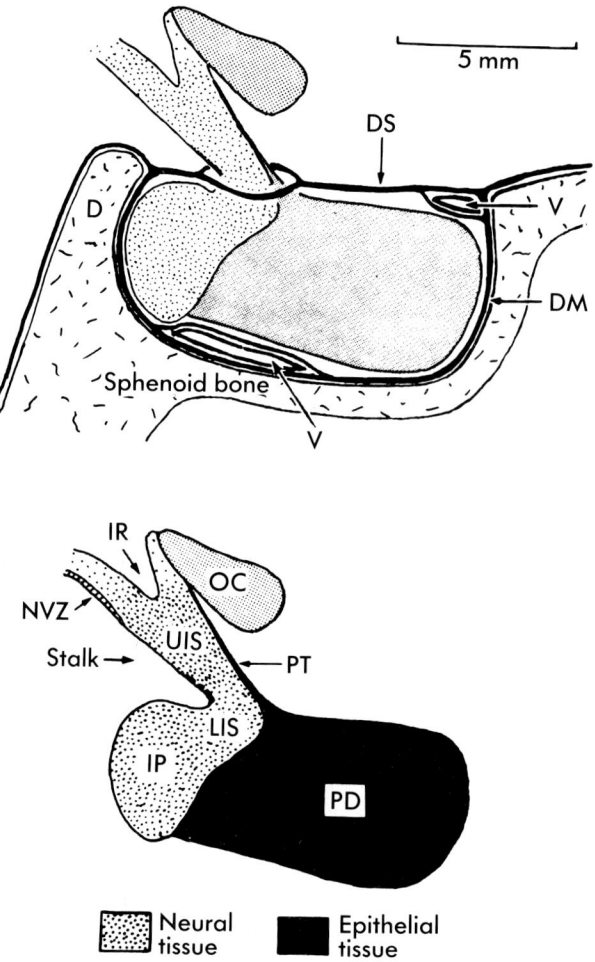

Fig. 2-2. Diagram of human pituitary within sella turcica. Upper infundibular stalk *(UIS)*, lower infundibular stalk *(LIS)*, and infundibular process *(IP)* are of neural origin. Pars distalis *(PD)* and pars tuberalis *(PT)* arise from epithelial tissue. *DS*, Diaphragm sella; *V*, veins; *DM*, dura mater lining sella turcica; *IR*, infundibular recess of third ventricle; *NVZ*, neurovascular zone of median eminence; *OC*, optic chiasm.

From Daniel PM, Prichard MML: Studies of the hypothalamus and the pituitary gland with special reference to the effects of transection of the pituitary stalk. *Acta Endocrinol.* 80(suppl):1, 1975.

ventral neural ridges in the same region from which the diencephalon and pineal gland arise. The neurohypophysis forms as a diverticulum that grows downward from the base of the hypothalamus.

The adenohypophysis is made up of three parts. The *pars distalis* is the primary source of the classic anterior pituitary hormones, thyrotropin (thyroid-stimulating hormone, TSH), adrenocorticotropin (ACTH), growth hormone (GH, somatotropin), prolactin (PRL, luteotropic hormone), luteinizing hormone (LH, interstitial cell-stimulating hormone [ISCH]), and follicle stimulating hormone (FSH); several other pituitary hormones have also been described. The *pars*

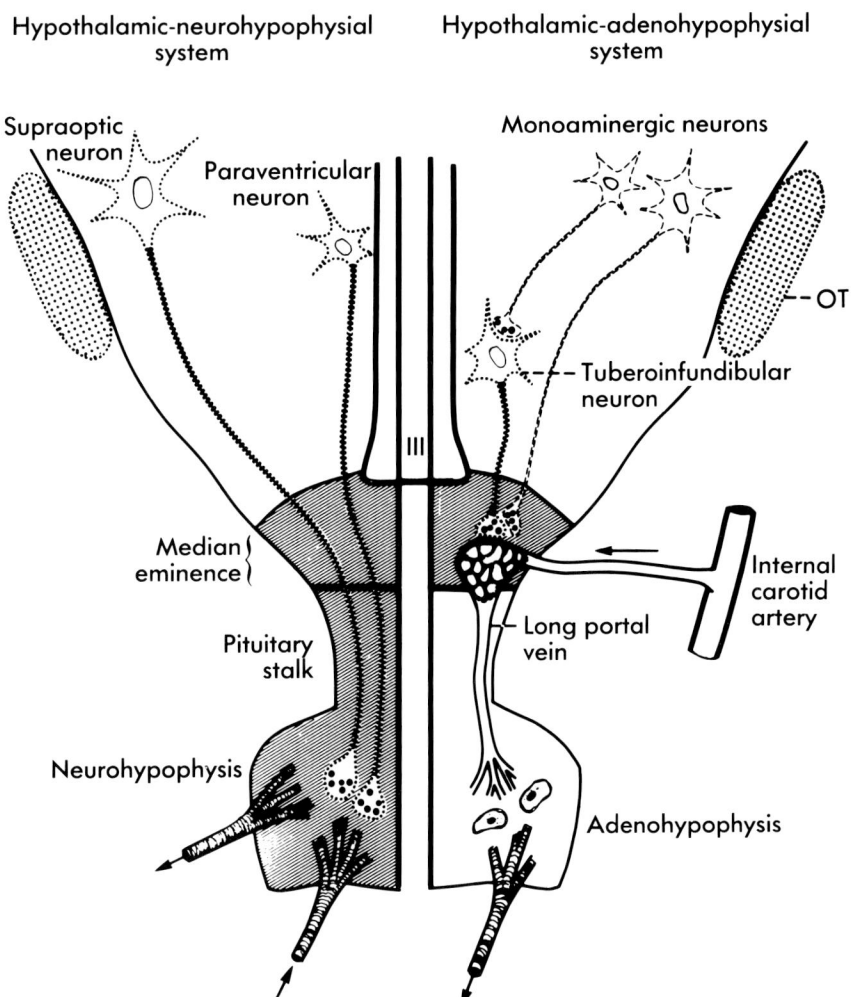

Fig. 2-3. Diagram of hypothalamic-pituitary axis in coronal section. *Left,* Hypothalamic-neurohypophysial system. Supraoptic and paraventricular axons terminate on blood vessels in posterior pituitary (neurohypophysis). *Right,* Hypothalamic-adenohypophysial system. Tuberoinfundibular neurons, believed to be source of hypothalamic regulatory hormones, terminate on capillary plexus in median eminence. Pituitary portal system is derived from branches of internal carotid, which form primary capillary bed in median eminence. Portal veins drain capillary plexus into sinusoids of anterior pituitary. Supraoptic, paraventricular, and tuberoinfundibular neurons are classed as neurosecretory cells. Activity of tuberoinfundibular neurons is influenced by monoaminergic cells.

Reprinted with permission from F.A. Davis Co.: *Clin Neuroendocrinol,* 1977.

intermedia, or intermediate lobe, is vestigial in adult man but is quite well defined in the fetus and in lower mammals, including rodents. It is the source of melanocyte-stimulating hormone (MSH) in lower mammals, whereas in adult man MSH is not secreted as such by cells of the pars distalis.[66] The *pars tuberalis* consists of secretory cells identical in appearance to those of the pars distalis, which envelop the pituitary stalk and cover the surface of the median eminence.

Microscopically, the pars distalis consists of cuboid secretory cells arranged around sinusoids lined with fenestrated endothelium. Immunocytochemical studies have demonstrated that each of the anterior pituitary hormones is produced by a separate set of cells.[69,80,81] The exceptions are some cells that contain both LH and FSH; cells that produce ACTH also produce other peptides of the opiomelanocortin family. Each cell type has a distinctive appearance by electron microscopy, distinguished primarily on the basis of the size, shape, and electron density of the secretory granules. In pituitary tumors, on the other hand, the same cell may secrete more than one hormone.

HYPOTHALAMUS
Gross anatomy

Seen from below, the ventral surface of the hypothalamus forms a convex bulge termed the tuber cinereum. Its gray color derives from the richness of cell bodies and unmyelinated fibers. Arising from it in the midline is the median eminence, readily recognized by its intense vascularity, which corresponds to the distribution of the primary hypophysial-portal plexus. The median eminence also forms the floor of the third ventricle and constitutes the infundibulum. The pituitary stalk is attached to and forms a direct extension of the infundibulum.

Hypothalamic boundaries are somewhat arbitrary, as the hypothalamus merges imperceptibly with surrounding areas (see Figs. 1-12, 1-14, and 1-15). Its anterior limits are defined as the optic chiasm and lamina terminalis, where it is continuous with the preoptic area (which is developmentally and functionally similar to the hypothalamus) and with the substantia innominata and the septal region. Posteriorly, it is bounded by an imaginary plane defined by the posterior border of the mammillary bodies ventrally and by the posterior commissure dorsally. Caudally, the hypothalamus merges with the midbrain periaqueductal gray and tegmental reticular formation. The dorsal limit of the hypothalamus is taken to be the horizontal level of the hypothalamic sulcus on the medial wall of the third ventricle, roughly at the horizontal level of the anterior commissure. Here, the hypothalamus is continuous with the subthalamus and zona incerta. Laterally, the hypothalamus is bounded by the internal capsule and the basis pedunculi, being continuous with the subthalamus caudodorsally.

The arterial blood supply of the hypothalamus varies in its detail from species to species but is similar in all mammals in being derived from small branches of the internal carotid artery.[35] In man the median eminence is also supplied by the paired superior hypophysial arteries.

Median eminence

The median eminence, or *infundibulum*, is a specialized region of the floor of the third ventricle that gives rise to the pituitary stalk. Stalk and median eminence together comprise the *contact zone* between the terminals of the tuberoinfundibular (releasing factor) neurosecretory neurons and the capillaries of the hypophysial portal circulation. The median eminence contains capillaries with fenestrated capillary endothelium, has a virtually complete lack of neuronal peri-

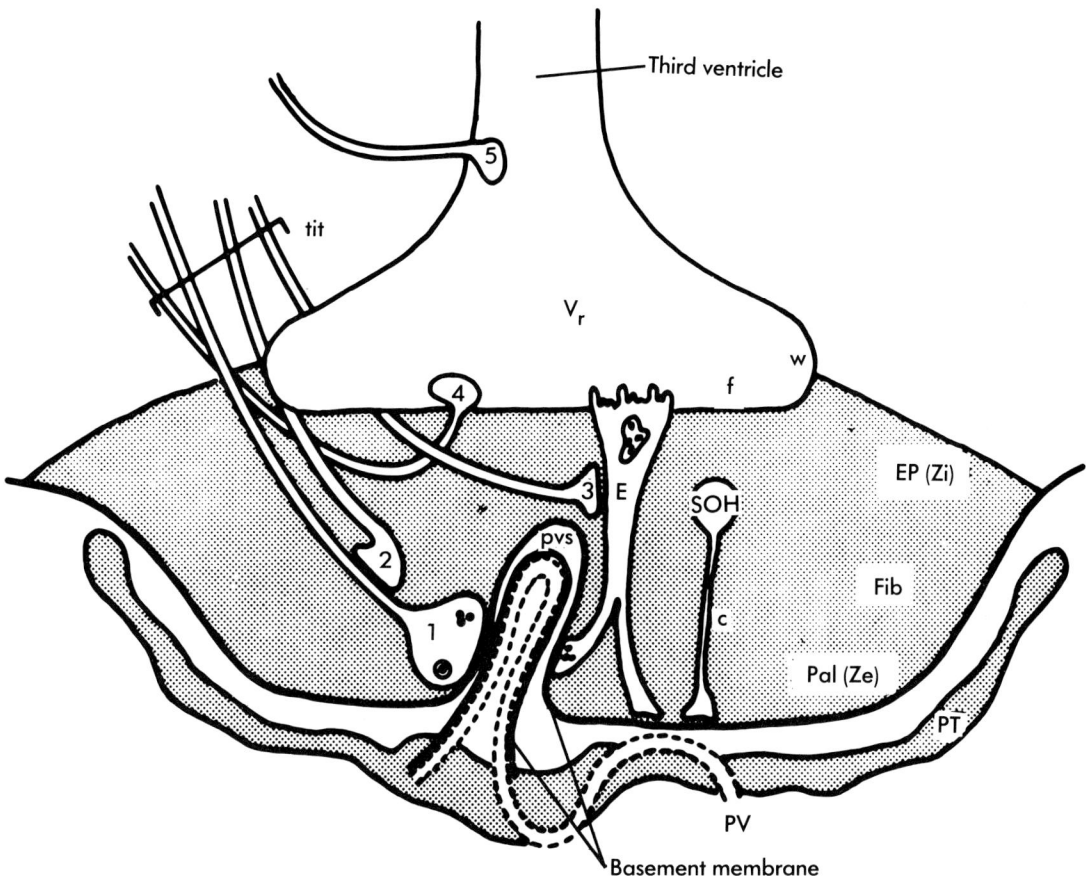

Fig. 2-4. Basic structural arrangement and cellular composition of median eminence. It is defined externally as that portion of tuber cinereum in contact with pars tuberalis *(PT)* of anterior lobe and vascularized by pituitary portal vessels *(PV);* internally it is demarcated by the wall *(w)* and floor *(f)* of ventricular recess *(V_r)*. Tissue between these two boundary planes constitutes median eminence. No barrier exists between portal blood and substance of median eminence. It is generally organized into inner ependymal *[Ep. (Zi)]*, middle fibrous *(Fib.)*, and outer palisade *[Pal. (Ze)]* layers. Tuberoinfundibular tract constitutes major afferent system; its terminals (1) abut in palisade zone on perivascular space *(pvs)*, (2) may form axoaxonic contacts, (3) make "synaptoid" contacts with ependymal cells, and (4) also have terminals that protrude into third ventricle. Ependyma *(E)* line floor of third ventricle and extend processes that traverse width of median eminence to terminate on portal perivascular space. Middle fibrous layer *(Fib.)* contains axons of supraopticohypophysial tract *(SOH)* in transit to their termination in neural lobe; some physiologic evidence, but no substantive morphologic data, suggests possibility of collaterals *(c)* terminating in palisade zone.

From Knigge KM: Anatomy of the endocrine hypothalamus, in Greep RO, Astwood EB (eds): *Handbook of physiology,* Section 7: Endocrinology, vol. 4, part 1. American Physiological Society. Bethesda, MD, 1974.

karya, and contains specialized ependymal cells known as *tanycytes* (Fig. 2-4 and see also Fig. 1-13).

The fenestrated endothelium of the capillary loops of the median eminence creates an open zone for diffusion of substances from the circulation to the intracellular spaces of the median eminence, where they potentially can modulate the release of releasing factors. However, experiments with the direct application of horseradish peroxidase (HRP) into the median eminence[88,89,173] suggest the presence of a diffusion barrier between the median eminence and the adjacent medial basal hypothalamus. This observation indicates that the releasing factors released into the extracellular space of the median eminence are not able to diffuse into the arcuate or ventromedial nuclei or into other regions of the adjacent brain.

The median eminence is composed of three zones, or layers: the *inner ependymal zone* and two palisade zones—the *inner palisade zone* and the *outer palisade zone*.[76] The outer palisade zone contains unmyelinated nerve fibers, axon terminals, glial cells, and basal processes of tanycytes (Fig. 2-4). Few or no synapses are seen between neuronal processes. The nerve terminals are separated from the capillary lumen by the fenestrated endothelium and by two basement membranes that surround the capillaries.

Axon terminals within the median eminence cocontain both dense core and small clear vesicles.[76,121] About 20% of the terminal boutons in the median eminence contain catecholamines and catecholamine-synthesizing enzymes packaged in dense core vesicles of about 60 nm diameter. These terminals are concentrated in the lateral third of the median eminence.[1] Another population of terminals contains larger dense core vesicles, up to 150 nm in diameter, shown by differential centrifugation and immunohistochemistry to contain the peptide releasing factors.[72] Other nerve terminals of the external palisade zone also contain electron dense, 170 to 260 nm diameter secretory granules typical of the vasopressin and oxytocin magnocellular systems and react immunocytochemically with antibodies to vasopressin, oxytocin, and neurophysin.[178] These findings imply that the neurohypophysial hormones themselves may also be released into the hypophysial portal circulation to act on the anterior pituitary as releasing factors. Indeed, arginine vasopressin (AVP) is an important component in regulating release of ACTH, β-endorphin, and GH. A role for oxytocin in anterior pituitary function has not been established. All the terminal boutons of the external palisade zone, plus those of the neurohypophysis, also contain small clear vesicles whose composition and functions are unknown.

The inner palisade zone of the median eminence contains the unmyelinated axons of the magnocellular neurosecretory neurons enroute from the hypothalamus to the neurohypophysis. This zone is also highly vascular, containing capillary loops that communicate with those of the external zone.

The inner ependymal zone forms the floor of the third ventricle. It contains a capillary plexus separate from that of the palisade zones and is composed primarily of the cell bodies of the tanycytes, the specialized ependymal cells lining the ventral part of the third ventricle. Unlike the ependyma of the dorsal third ventricle, the ventricular surface of the tanycytes is not ciliated but rather is covered with microvilli. Numerous blebs are apparent in scanning electron micrographs of tanycyte membranes lining the ventricle; these blebs have been taken as evidence for secretory activity. The tanycytes are connected by tight junctions and thereby form a barrier to diffusion between the ventricular cerebrospinal fluid (CSF) and the extracellular space of the median eminence. They have long basal processes that pass through both palisade zones of the median eminence to end on capillaries, where the basal surface of the processes contain numerous infoldings. The tanycyte processes contain numerous vacuoles and vesicles, but little direct evidence of pinocytotic activity is seen in electron micrographs. Terminal boutons of axons in the outer palisade zone occasionally make synapselike contacts with tanycyte processes suggesting the existence of a trophic function of this supporting cell.

The function of the tanycytes remains a matter of speculation. Because of their striking morphology, they have been invoked as potential conduits for transfer of hormones from CSF to capillaries of the median eminence[13] and vice versa. However, as Mezey and Palkovits[100] point out, the anatomy of tanycytes is more suggestive of a barrier than of a conduit.

Tuberoinfundibular neurons

The location of neurons whose terminals project to the external zone of the median eminence (thus constituting the *tuberoinfundibular neurons*) has been studied using a variety of techniques.[89,173] Most of the cell bodies are located in the medial basal hypothalamus in the arcuate nucleus (ARC), the anterior periventricular area, and the medial preoptic area (mPOA) (Fig. 2-5). Using sensitive techniques including the application of the tracer wheat germ agglutinin[88] to the median eminence, it has been possible to show that cells in the medial septum and diagonal band of Broca are also labeled, as are some cells in the magnocellular area of the paraventricular nucleus, presumably those containing vasopressin and oxytocin. Retrograde flow studies have failed to reveal projections from the amygdala, ventromedial nucleus (VMN), or aminergic nuclei of the brainstem; but studies using specific antisera directed against growth hormone–releasing hormone (GHRH) have shown both an ARC and a direct VMN projection.[19,87]

Electrophysiologic studies have demonstrated single units that can be activated antidromically by stimulation of both median eminence and other hypothalamic regions, including the paraventricular nucleus and the anterior hypothalamic nucleus.[131,132] Moreover, stimulation of the median eminence induces, in addition to antidromic invasion of the tuberoinfundibular neurons, a poststimulation inhibition of activity lasting 100 to 150 msec, consistent with recurrent inhibition by axon collaterals. The presence of recurrent collaterals from tuberoinfundibular neurons is also important in providing evidence for a CNS neurotransmitter function for hypothalamic releasing peptides. If Dale's principle holds, the same neurohumors released into portal vessels by tuberoinfundibular neurons will be released by their axon collaterals ending on CNS neurons.

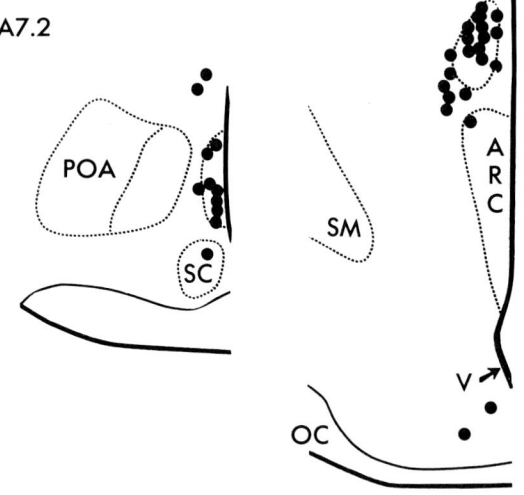
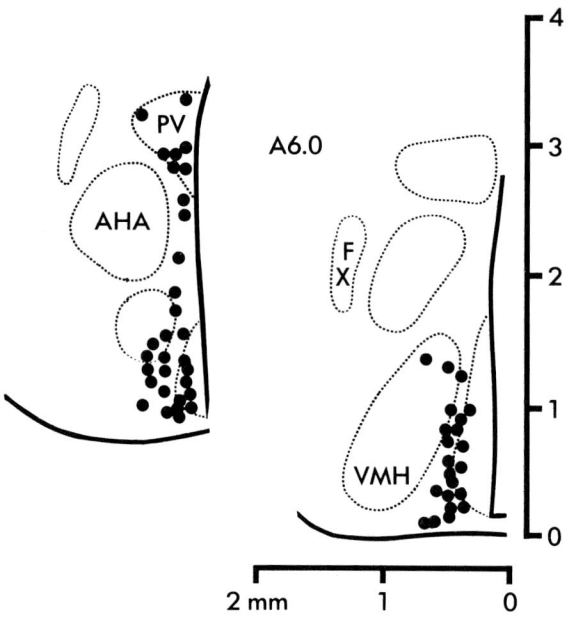

Fig. 2-5. Schematic coronal sections through rat brain between 6 and 7.2 mm anterior to interaural line. Superimposed dots depict approximate locations of neurons that display antidromic identifications from median eminence (i.e., tuberoinfundibular neurons). *AHA*, Anterior hypothalamic area; *ARC*, arcuate nucleus; *FX*, fornix; *OC*, optic chiasm; *POA*, preoptic area; *PV*, paraventricular nucleus; *SC*, suprachiasmatic nucleus; *V*, third ventricle; *VMH*, ventromedial nucleus.

Hypophysiotropic hormones of the hypothalamus

The task of identifying the chemical structures of the hypophysiotropic releasing factors was taken up by Schally and Guillemin and their collaborators beginning in the mid-1950s. The Guillemin group used sheep hypothalami[60] as their starting material, and the Schally group used hypothalami from the pig.[148] Their success depended on the organization of massive and well-focused efforts, on the development of convenient and reliable bioassays for the releasing factors, and on the application of innovative techniques of peptide chemistry. Five peptides have been isolated from hypothalamic extracts on the basis of their ability to specifically and potently stimulate or inhibit the release of anterior pituitary hormones in vitro (Table 2-1). One of the releasing factors (GHRH) was first identified as an ectopic secretion of a pancreatic adenoma that caused acromegaly,[61,133] but an identical factor was subsequently demonstrated in the human hypothalamus.[92] The first releasing factor to be identified was TRH, whose structure was reported virtually simultaneously by the two laboratories of Guillemin and Schally in 1969. In 1971 Schally and co-workers characterized luteinizing hormone–releasing hormone (LHRH, now most often termed GnRH); in 1973 Guillemin and his co-workers characterized somatostatin (somatotropin release-inhibiting factor, SRIF), which inhibits GH release.[20] The structures of all three of these small peptides

Table 2-1
Anterior pituitary and hypophysiotropic hormones

Pituitary hormone	Hypophysiotropic hormones	
	Name	Structure
Thyrotropin (TSH)	Thyrotropin-releasing hormone (TRH)	Tripeptide
Adrenocorticotropin (ACTH)	Corticotropin-releasing factor (CRF)	41-amino acids
Luteinizing hormone (LH)	Luteinizing hormone-releasing hormone (LHRH) OR	Decapeptide
Follicle-stimulating hormone (FSH)	Gonadotropin-releasing hormone (GNRH)	
Growth hormone (GH)	Growth hormone-releasing factor (GRF)	44-Amino acids
	Growth hormone release-inhibiting hormone* (somatostatin, GIH)	14-amino acids
Prolactin (PRL)	Prolactin release-inhibiting factor (PIF)	Dopamine (DA)
	Prolactin-releasing factor (PRF)†	? Vasoactive intestinal polypeptide (VIP)

*Somatostatin also inhibits TRH-stimulated TSH release.
†TRH stimulates prolactin release.

proved identical in sheep and pigs. In 1981 Vale and co-workers reported the sequence of corticotropin-releasing hormone (CRH, CRF), a 41-amino acid peptide from sheep hypothalami that stimulates corticotropin (ACTH) and beta endorphin release in vitro.[166] More recently, rat CRH has been characterized and is known to be identical[50] in structure to human CRH. In the case of pituitary prolactin (PRL), which is under a tonic inhibitory influence by the hypothalamus, current evidence indicates that dopamine (DA) serves as the principal PRL inhibiting factor(s) (PIF),[93,107,167] while the principal candidates for the PRL-releasing factor(s) are vasoactive intestinal polypeptide (VIP), peptide histidine isoleucine (PHI),[73,171] and TRH (Table 2-1).

The availability of pure hypothalamic hormones has permitted the development of immunoassays and immunohistochemical studies, the demonstration of substantial amounts of releasing hormone in extrahypothalamic tissues, and extensive clinical trials in diagnoses and therapy.

Although it was initially thought that the releasing factors were entirely specific, it is now clear that there are several crossover effects with individual hypothalamic hormones. TRH is a potent stimulus for PRL release and may also function physiologically as a PRL-releasing factor, but it does not cause release of GH, ACTH, FSH, or LH in normal individuals. TRH releases GH in acromegaly and in certain other clinical conditions such as malnutrition and depression. Somatostatin, which inhibits GH release, also inhibits TSH secretion and prevents TRH-stimulated TSH release without affecting TRH-induced PRL release. Somatostatin also has effects on other hormone-secreting tissues such as the gut and pancreas, where it inhibits insulin, glucagon, and gastrin secretion. These observations, which indicate more widespread effects of the hypothalamic hormones, have increased the complexity of our understanding of hypothalamic-pituitary control functions.

Thus the effects of the hypothalamus on the anterior pituitary are mediated by the interaction of several factors. GH secretion is stimulated by GHRH and inhibited by somatostatin; PRL release is stimulated by several prolactin-releasing factor(s) (PRFs) and inhibited by DA; and the secretion of ACTH is mediated by CRF, interacting in a synergistic way with vasopressin, and epinephrine. As far as is now known, there is only a stimulatory hypothalamic control of gonadotropin secretion. The effects of the hypothalamic factors interact at the level of the pituitary with the feedback effects of circulating target gland hormones. For example, TSH secretion is inhibited by thyroxine; ACTH secretion is inhibited by cortisol; GH secretion is sensitized by estrogens and thyroxine; and the secretion of the gonadotropins is regulated by a complex interaction with estrogens, progesterone, and androgens. In addition, the secretion of each of the hypothalamic releasing hormones is subject to feedback control by peripheral hormones interacting with central neurotransmitters and other neuroregulators.

EXTRAHYPOTHALAMIC REGULATION OF THE HYPOTHALAMIC-ADENOHYPOPHYSIAL SYSTEM

Neurosecretory neurons of the medial basal hypothalamus form the final common pathway for neuroendocrine regulation. Inputs from other regions of the hypothalamus and ascending and descending pathways from other brain regions converge on these neurons to subserve neuroendocrine responses. Certain neuroendocrine reflexes are mediated over quite specific and well-defined anatomic pathways. For example, suckling stimulates breast receptors that signal via segmental nerves to the spinal cord, where impulses ascend to the midbrain and reach the hypothalamus via the medial forebrain bundle or the dorsal longitudinal bundle of Schutz. Input to the paraventricular nuclei stimulates oxytocin release, and other connections to ARC and/or anterior periventricular neurons elicit PRL release.

With the exception of the olfactory radiation to the hypothalamus and the fibers comprising the retinohypothalamic tract, the hypothalamus receives few if any direct connections from generally recognized sensory pathways. Its most massive associations are the limbic forebrain structures and the paramedial region of the mesencephalon. In addition to the pituitary control system, the hypothalamus affects visceral motor function (i.e., parasympathetic and sympathetic outflow) by pathways through the reticular formation of the mesencephalon and lower brainstem. Of the inputs to the hypothalamus demonstrated to have an effect on anterior pituitary control, as will be discussed in the following section, those containing the biogenic amines are of particular importance.

In terms of neuroendocrine regulation, the various hypothalamic and extrahypothalamic pathways are assumed to mediate (1) circadian rhythms in hormonal secretion; (2) stress-induced alterations in hormone secretion; (3) integration of neuroendocrine activity with autonomic nervous system responses; (4) neuroendocrine effects triggered by olfactory and peripheral sensory responses; and (5) elaboration of neurosecretomotor activation for regulation of organs such as the gut, pancreas, adrenal medulla, pineal gland, and the renal juxtaglomerular apparatus.

NEUROPHARMACOLOGY OF ANTERIOR PITUITARY REGULATION

The hypothalamic releasing factor neurons are regulated by numerous convergent inputs from other brain regions. Of particular importance in this regard are the biogenic amine systems. The majority of monoaminergic neuronal cell bodies that synthesize the biogenic amines are located in the mesencephalon and lower brainstem[27] (Fig. 2-6). Their axons ascend in the medial forebrain bundle to terminate in various forebrain structures including the hypothalamus, striatum, hippocampus, amygdala, and cortex. Terminals of these systems end directly on hypophysiotropic neurons, thereby providing an anatomic pathway by which noradrenergic impulses can act directly to modulate releasing factor secretion.

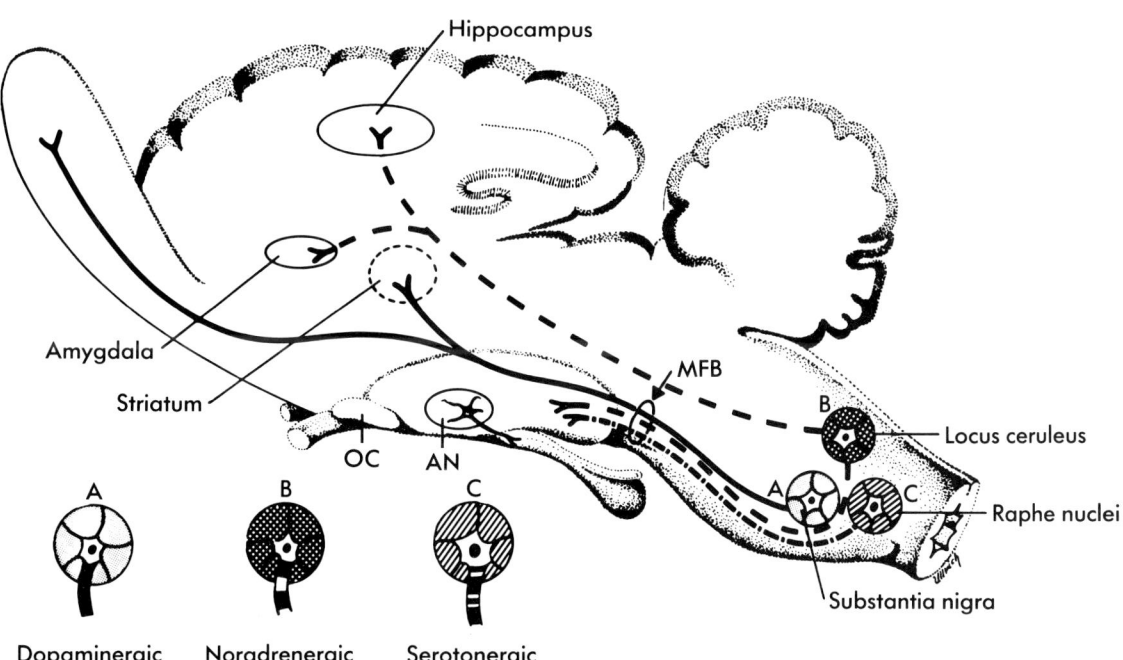

Fig. 2-6. Monoaminergic pathways in mammalian brain. Principal localization of neurons containing NE, DA, and serotonin is in mesencephalon and pons. Axons of these cells are distributed to widespread areas of cortex, limbic system, and striatum. Dopaminergic system of arcuate nucleus is exception to this general scheme of distribution. *MFB,* Medial forebrain bundle; *AN,* arcuate nucleus; *OC,* optic chiasm.

Reprinted with permission from F.A. Davis Co.: *Clin Neuroendocrinol,* 1977.

Aminergic innervation of the hypothalamus

Dopamine. DA in the hypothalamus is found in highest concentrations in the median eminence and ARC, with smaller amounts in other regions.[114,115] Median eminence DA is present in a dense plexus of DA-containing terminals, which is densest in the lateral third of the external lamina, where they account for one third of the axon terminals present.[1] A less dense band of DA-containing terminals is located in the medial part of the external lamina. DA-containing terminals, like the peptidergic terminals of the median eminence, do not make classic synapses with other terminals but instead appear to release DA into the extracellular space in the neurovascular contact zone of the stalk and median eminence. DA can thus act on receptors located on nearby peptidergic terminals or diffuse into the adjacent capillaries of the portal circulation to act on the anterior pituitary.

The majority, and perhaps all, of the DA-containing terminals of the median eminence arise from cell bodies in the ARC nucleus to form the tuberoinfundibular dopamine (TIDA) system. Only 3% to 5% of the neurons of the ARC nucleus contain DA (A_{12} cell group of Dahlstrom and Fuxe).[34] Axon collaterals of TIDA neurons synapse in the ARC itself, as well as in the VMN and the premammillary nuclei.

There is convincing evidence that DA secretion by the TIDA neurons is the principal PRL-inhibiting factor. Activity of the TIDA cells is regulated physiologically by PRL. This action of PRL, which has little or no effect on other brain DA systems, is an important mechanism in the feedback control of PRL secretion, whereby increased circulating levels of PRL stimulate increased DA secretion, which then acts to suppress PRL secretion. Decreased levels of PRL diminish DA output, tending to raise PRL levels. This is an example of a *positive feedback system* responsible for maintenance of inhibitory control of pituitary secretion. This system is also affected by drugs that alter synthesis and release of DA (such as alpha methyl paratyrosine and reserpine) and by morphine (which inhibits the secretion of DA thus accounting at least in part for the morphine-induced stimulation of PRL secretion).

DA-containing cell bodies are also located in the anterior periventricular region of the hypothalamus, (the A_{14} cell group). These cells may project to the preoptic area and the median eminence.[39] Together with the DA-containing cells of the more rostral ARC, A_{14} cells project axons to neural and intermediate lobes of the pituitary in those species with well-defined intermediate lobes. The DA nuclear groups A_{12} and A_{14} can be viewed as a single nucleus organized so that the most rostral cells project to the intermediate lobe, the next caudal group project to the neural lobe, and the most posterior project to the median eminence. DA terminals of the median eminence lack a high affinity uptake system of DA.[40] This attribute, which is in contrast to other central dopaminergic systems (mesolimbic, mesocortical), means that the DA terminals are not subject to presynaptic feedback inhibition by DA.

Norepinephrine. Norepinephrine (NE) is present in all hypothalamic nuclei but in a nonuniform distribution with highest concentrations in the paraventricular nuclei, the retrochiasmatic area, and in the ventromedial and dorsomedial nuclei.[144] Concentrations of NE in the median eminence are moderate, about one fifth that of DA. Deafferentation of the medial basal hypothalamus produces an 80% fall in NE concentration in the median eminence, implying an origin for a majority of the NE in the median eminence from outside the medial basal hypothalamus.[21] More specific lesion studies indicate that the origin of the NE is from brainstem noradrenergic cell groups, the region of the lateral reticular nucleus of the medulla and the locus ceruleus making the largest contributions.[118] Most of the noradrenergic innervation of the hypothalamus is carried by the ventral bundle.[79]

Terminals and fibers positive for immunoreactive dopamine-β-hydroxylase (the enzyme responsible for NE synthesis) are present in the median eminence primarily in the internal palisade zone, with only rare terminals found in the external lamina.[66] However, all hypothalamic nuclei contain noradrenergic fibers and terminals. This distribution allows the interpretation that noradrenergic effects on anterior pituitary function are mediated by synapses on neurons within the hypothalamus, whereas DA exerts its effect primarily at the pituitary by being released into the portal circulation.

Epinephrine. Epinephrine and its synthetic enzyme, phenylethylamine N-methyl transferase (PNMT), are found in the hypothalamus, but the overall content of epinephrine is only about 10% that of NE.[114]

The highest concentration is in the dorsomedial nucleus (DMN), paraventricular nucleus, periventricular region, ARC, and supraoptic nucleus (SON). By immunocytochemistry directed at PNMT, terminals are stained throughout the hypothalamus, but primarily in DMN, ARC, the medial parvicellular division of the paraventricular nucleus, the perifornical region, and the periventricular region.[67] There are few PNMT-containing terminals in the median eminence, and none have been seen in the external lamina.

All epinephrine-containing cell bodies of the brain are thought to be located in the medulla; however, deafferentation of the medial basal hypothalamus produces only about a 60% fall in epinephrine content, suggesting an intrinsic origin for many fibers.[114]

Serotonin. Serotonin (5-hydroxytryptamine, 5-HT) is found in many tissues throughout the body. About 90% is in enterochromaffin cells of the intestinal tract, and only 1% to 2% is present in the CNS and pineal gland. This indolalkylamine is formed from the precursor tryptophan, an essential amino acid. The concentration of plasma tryptophan, as shown by Wurtman and Fernstrom[177] determines the rate of synthesis of serotonin, and this plasma level varies markedly with diet. In the neuron, tryptophan is converted by the enzyme tryptophan hydroxylase to 5-hydroxytryptophan and thence to serotonin by the enzyme, amino acid decarboxylase.

The serotonergic neural pathways in the CNS arise in the raphe nuclei of the lower pons and upper brainstem and are distributed to the forebrain and to the hypothalamus.[146] A rich innervation of serotonergic fibers reaches the median eminence and the suprachiasmatic nucleus; the highest concentration of 5-HT within the hypothalamus is in the suprachiasmatic nuclei, suggesting a role for 5-HT in circadian rhythmicity. The arcuate and the basal and posterior regions of the hypothalamus are also rich in 5-HT; but only moderate levels are found in the median eminence.

Hypothalamic deafferentation produces only a 60% fall in 5-HT within the medial basal hypothalamus, suggesting a combination of intrinsic and extrinsic sources.[117] The intrinsic source is not known with certainty, but small clusters of neuronal perikarya fluorescent for serotonin are located within the hypothalamus.

Functions of the biogenic amines

DA acts at the level of the pituitary to inhibit PRL secretion, and to a lesser extent that of TSH and the gonadotropins. Norepinephrine acts synergistically with CRH to facilitate ACTH secretion. More importantly, NE acts in the hypothalamus to synchronize pulsatile secretion of GH, the gonadotropins, and possibly PRL and TSH. Serotonin stimulates release of ACTH and of GH by effects mediated through the hypothalamus.

Although various manipulations of the biogenic amines were widely used in the past to study hypothalamic-pituitary control in man, they have now been largely replaced by the direct use of synthetic hypothalamic releasing factors.

NEUROHYPOPHYSIS: PHYSIOLOGY
Neurohypophysis

The neural lobe develops embryologically as a downgrowth from the ventral diencephalon and retains its neural connections and neural character in adult life. The dominant features of the neurohypophysis are the supraoptic-hypophysial and paraventricular-hypophysial nerve tracts.[84,85,156] These unmyelinated nerve tracts arise from the supraoptic and paraventricular nuclei within the hypothalamus and descend through the infundibulum and neural stalk to terminate in the posterior pituitary (neurohypophysis). The hormones, vasopressin and oxytocin, are released from the nerve terminals into fenestrated capillaries of the neurohypophysis (Figs. 2-3 and 2-4).

Cells of origin of these tracts are relatively large (hence the term, *magnocellular*) and are consolidated into well-characterized groups situated in paired nuclei above the optic tract (supraoptic) and on each side of the ventricle (paraventricular). A few cells of this system are also distributed between the two nuclei and are also found in the paired suprachiasmatic nuclei.[41] Most of the cell bodies in the supraoptic nucleus contain vasopressin, but some contain oxytocin. A somewhat smaller percentage (but still the majority of stainable cells) in the paraventricular nucleus contain vasopressin. Cells contain either one peptide or the other. This is also true for the respective prohormones.

Although the principal projections of the magnocellular nuclei are to the neural lobe, vasopressin-containing nerve endings also terminate on the primary plexus of the hypophysial-portal circulation.[179] From these anatomic observations and from direct measurements of vasopressin in portal blood, it has been inferred that neurohypophysial neurons may have a role in anterior pituitary regulation

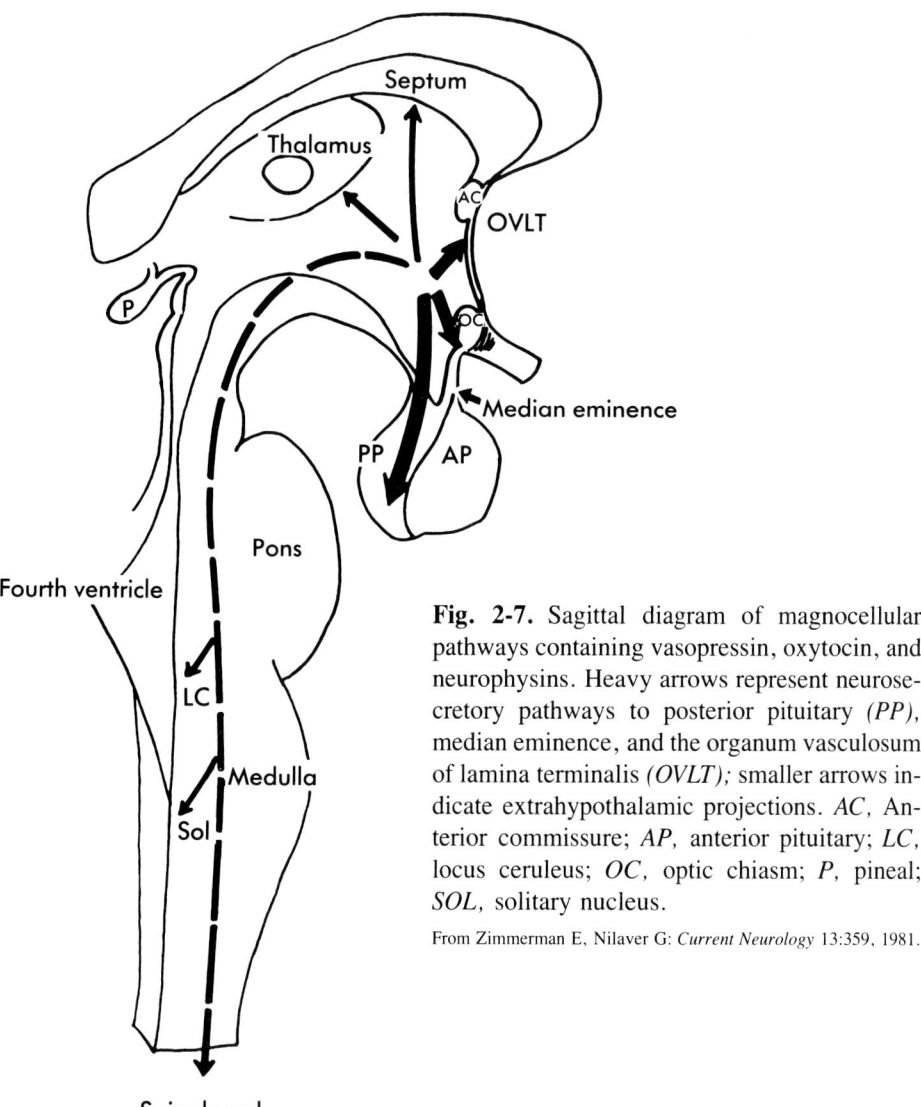

Fig. 2-7. Sagittal diagram of magnocellular pathways containing vasopressin, oxytocin, and neurophysins. Heavy arrows represent neurosecretory pathways to posterior pituitary *(PP)*, median eminence, and the organum vasculosum of lamina terminalis *(OVLT)*; smaller arrows indicate extrahypothalamic projections. *AC*, Anterior commissure; *AP*, anterior pituitary; *LC*, locus ceruleus; *OC*, optic chiasm; *P*, pineal; *SOL*, solitary nucleus.

From Zimmerman E, Nilaver G: *Current Neurology* 13:359, 1981.

and in neural lobe secretion. Indeed, recent work has shown that vasopressin synergizes with CRH to bring about stress-related ACTH release. Vasopressin also stimulates GH secretion.

Vasopressin- and oxytocin-containing fibers arising in the paraventricular nucleus are also distributed to many other regions of the CNS including the brainstem, spinal cord, hippocampus, and amygdala (Fig. 2-7). Within the spinal cord these fibers terminate on the cells of origin of the autonomic nervous system and hence can influence blood pressure. Within the brainstem, they end in the sensory nuclei of the vagus and glossopharyngeal nerve, which convey information concerning blood pressure and blood volume. The central fibers of these "vasopressinergic" and "oxytocinergic" pathways function independently of those that innervate the neurohypophysis. This has been shown by comparing

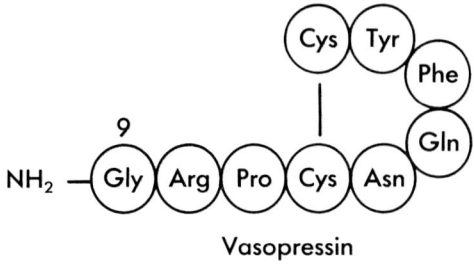

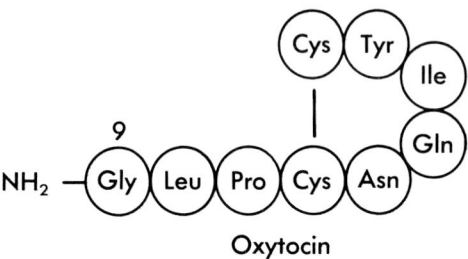

Fig. 2-8. Chemical structure of vasopressin and oxytocin.

changes in CSF vasopressin with those of blood vasopressin. Central vasopressin levels show a circadian rhythm independent of the state of hydration.[122] In contrast, peripheral vasopressin levels, which reflect the secretion of the neurohypophysis, do not follow a circadian pattern and are related to blood volume and plasma osmolarity (see p. 32). Oxytocin levels in CSF also follow a time-dependent pattern independent of blood levels.[2]

Neurohypophysial hormones

The chemical nature of vasopressin and oxytocin was identified by Nobel laureate, Du Vigneaud et al.[43] This landmark work, which established that the neurohypophysial hormones were small polypeptides composed of nine amino acids, paved the way for the structural elucidation of larger, more complex polypeptide hormones of the pituitary and of other glands. Du Vigneaud's studies were the model for the study of the structure of the hypophysiotropic hormones of the hypothalamus.

The structures of vasopressin and oxytocin are remarkably similar, differing by only two amino acids. Both have a Cys-Cys bridge in the 1-6 position (Fig. 2-8). Vasopressin and oxytocin are each associated with a distinct neurophysin, now recognized to be part of their prohormones, termed propressophysin and prooxyphysin, respectively.[22,51,86] The neurophysins are released simultaneously with their respective neurohypophysial peptide.[135,136]

Vasopressin and its related neurophysin (designated neurophysin II) and oxytocin and its related neurophysin (neurophysin I) are synthesized as prohormones in the cell bodies of the supraoptic and paraventricular neurons (Fig. 2-3). The prohormones are transported in membrane-bound vesicles through the axons to the neural lobe, where they are stored until released. Processing of the prohormone to the secreted products—vasopressin, oxytocin, and the two neurophysins—takes place in the granules during the course of transport.

Nerve action potentials arising in the cell body are propagated along the axon and trigger hormone discharge. The neurohypophysial hormones leave the cell together with neurophysin in a fixed ratio.

Regulation of ADH secretion

The association of pathologic conditions of the neural stalk and pituitary with the syndrome of diabetes insipidus (DI) prompted physicians to postulate that DI was a deficiency disease. In 1924 Starling and Verney[168] identified the site of action of posterior pituitary extracts on water excretion by perfusing the isolated kidney and demonstrating an antidiuretic effect. In the early 1930s Verney demonstrated the influence of hyperosmolar stimuli on antidiuresis by perfusing the carotid artery with hypertonic saline. From these observations, he concluded that the brain was sensitive to alterations in osmolarity. Verney[168] localized the region of the brain critical for this antidiuretic effect to the anterior hypothalamus in the region of the supraoptic and paraventricular nuclei. As a consequence of Verney's work, the term *osmoreceptor* was applied to cells within the brain that monitor extracellular osmolality. Characteristically, such cells show alterations in electrical firing rates in association with osmotic stimuli. Verney pioneered in his delineation of neural control of osmotic balance, but his work was also important in the development of a strategy in neuroendocrine investigations. He showed that emotional factors were important in ADH regulation, thus pointing out, for the first time, the role of stress in neuroendocrine regulation. He also adapted the classic Sherringtonian approach of the neurologist to identify a neuroendocrine reflex analogous to a spinal reflex. This involves the identification of a receptor for afferent stimuli and a motor component effecting hormone secretion. Like Sherrington, Verney emphasized the use of selective neurologic ablations to identify neural pathways of neuroendocrine control. This approach, now taken for granted, has been widely used for studies of anterior and posterior pituitary secretion.

The most important factors regulating vasopressin secretion are plasma osmolarity and "effective" circulating blood volume. Blood pressure, nausea, and various forms of stress also influence vasopressin release.[64,101,102,130,134]

Osmolarity. Maintenance of normal blood water concentration is the major homeostatic function of the neurohypophysis. Blood osmolality is zealously guarded over a relatively narrow range ($\pm 1.8\%$). Detailed studies of osmotic control of vasopressin release show that the set point of plasma osmolality for normal individuals is 280 mOsm/kg and that vasopressin release is initiated after infusion of hypertonic saline has led to an increase to 287.3 mOsm/kg, a value termed the osmotic threshold.[101-103,134] Plasma ADH levels are 2 pg/ml at this plasma osmolality. Above this value, vasopressin secretion increases rapidly and progressively with increasing plasma osmolarity. On the other hand, water loading inhibits vasopressin release. The exquisite sensitivity of the osmoreceptor-ADH-renal reflex can be demonstrated by combining radioimmunoassay (RIA) measurements of ADH in blood with plasma osmolality. An increase of 1% in total body water causes a fall of 2.8 mOsm/kg water, a decrease in ADH levels to 1 pg/ml, and a fall in urine osmolality from 500 to 250 mOsm/kg water. An increase in total body water by 2% suppresses ADH maximally (<0.25 pg/ml). In the opposite direction, a 2% decrease in total body water will increase plasma osmolality by 2% (5.6 mOsm/kg). Plasma ADH will rise from 2 to 4 pg/ml and urine will be maximally concentrated (>1000 mOsm/kg).[4] These observations on the extraordinary sensitivity of this regulatory system help to explain the common occurrence of the syndrome of inappropriate ADH secretion (see Chapter 15); minor deviations in regulation may have profound effects with water retention leading to hyponatremia.

This precise osmotic regulatory system operates through a hypothalamic osmoreceptor neuron system. Although a number of neurons in both supraoptic and paraventricular nuclei (including some that project directly to the neural lobe) show increased frequency of electrical discharge immediately following intracarotid injections of hypertonic saline, the possibility also exists that another population of osmoreceptor cells may activate the vasopressin secreting cells transsynaptically. This idea is supported by observations that, under some clinical conditions, osmoreceptor control of vasopressin secretion can be lost while other forms of control remain. The neuronal basis of osmoreception remains obscure. Any particle that exerts osmotic effects and does not enter nerve cell bodies can stimulate vasopressin release.

Volume regulation. Hemorrhage or decreased blood volume resulting from any cause, if sufficient in degree, is followed by release of vasopressin. The change in volume (as contrasted with the change in osmolarity) must be relatively large. For example, phlebotomy, which reduces blood volume by 6% to 9%, or assumption of the upright posture, which reduces central blood volume by 10% to 15%, has no effect on vasopressin release.[103] On the other hand, a change of blood volume of more than 10%, which can be produced by the combination of phlebotomy and assumption of the erect position, will elicit vasopressin release. Although plasma osmolality is the prime determinant of vasopressin secretion under usual conditions, severe volume depletion can override the osmoreceptor control. With less severe degrees of volume change, osmotic control is precisely exerted, but there is a shift of the "osmotic set point" so that a lower osmotic threshold is required to trigger vasopressin secretion in the volume-depleted animal.

Glucocorticoids also modulate the "set point" of neurohypophysial control.

Adrenal deficiency raises it and thereby induces a relative increase in vasopressin secretion that may contribute to the lower serum sodium in patients with this disorder.[7]

Receptors for volume control are located in the left atrium and in the baroreceptors of the carotid sinus and perhaps elsewhere. Modest degrees of volume depletion, insufficient to lower blood pressure, activate the atrial receptors, whereas depletion sufficient to cause hypotension mobilizes baroreceptor reflexes. Because even high amounts of vasopressin are not associated with hypertension in man, it appears likely that the neurohypophysis has only a modest role in blood pressure regulation but that vasopressin plays a complex role in cardiovascular regulation under special conditions such as shock and volume depletion.[155]

Neural reflexes involved in volume and pressure control reach the brainstem by way of cranial nerve afferents terminating in the midbrain, ascend through multisynaptic pathways, and ultimately impinge on the nuclei of the neurohypophysial system. Presumably, the principal activating pathways are mediated by cholinergic neurotransmitters, but other pathways could be involved in view of the wealth of potential neurotransmitters in the supraoptic nucleus.[155]

A novel additional endocrine function of the left atrium in blood volume control (separate from the reflex activation of the neurohypophysis) has recently been proposed. Several peptides with potent natriuretic activity (designated *cardionatrins* or *atriopeptins*) have been isolated from atrial muscle.[32,33,153] They have been postulated to be part of a homeostatic feedback loop for the regulation of intravascular volume.

Stress and nausea. The secretion of vasopressin is affected by inputs from various parts of the "visceral brain" and the reticular activating system, which are regions involved in the maintenance of consciousness and in emotional expression. Nausea is accompanied by intense vasopressin release, presumably by reflex stimulation from the medullary vomiting center.

When Verney began his studies of water regulation in the dog, he was struck by the marked effect of emotional stress on antidiuretic activity. It has been generally believed that humans and rats also release vasopressin in response to emotional stress; but Robertson has shown by immunoassay methods that pain or other stresses incidental to physiologic experiments in man rarely influence plasma vasopressin levels, nor does deliberately applied severe stress in rats.[134] Nevertheless, the influence of "higher" neural centers on vasopressin secretion can be demonstrated by the experimental induction of diuresis or antidiuresis by hypnotic suggestion in man or by psychologic conditioning of dogs. Other examples of neurogenic disturbance in regulation of vasopressin secretion are the disturbed osmolar control of water excretion in patients with anorexia nervosa and in some schizophrenic persons[56] who have succeeded in overhydrating themselves to the point of water intoxication.[70]

Other stimuli can elicit vasopressin release in experimental animals. Endotoxin, a substance that elicits fever and blood pressure changes by acting directly on hypothalamic thermoregulatory centers, causes release of vasopressin in rats.[77,78] This response, which may be triggered in part by changes in blood volume and blood pressure, may serve as a homeostatic mechanism to regulate these important physiologic functions.

Neuropharmacology of vasopressin

In addition to the direct osmotic control of ADH by osmoreceptors, there is evidence that cholinergic and adrenergic inputs to the magnocellular neurons influence cellular activity and mediate reflex control of secretion.[9,42,104] An excitatory role for acetylcholine in ADH release was proposed as early as 1939 when Pickford[126] reported that intravenous administration of acetylcholine caused inhibition of water diuresis in dogs, a response dependent on an intact neurohypophysis. She later reported that injection of acetylcholine into the supraoptic region of anesthetized dogs also caused antidiuresis. Intracarotid or intraventricular injection of acetylcholine or its analogs, carbachol and methylcholine, caused an increased firing rate of the supraoptic neurons that was accompanied by release of ADH.

In contrast to the excitatory effects of cholinergic agents, adrenergic drugs such as norepinephrine inhibit the release of ADH.[9,104] Systemic administration of epinephrine or NE causes inhibition of ADH release, predominantly by effects mediated through peripheral baroreceptor mechanisms; however, central adrenergic mechanisms are also important, since NE administered into the third ventricle also will inhibit ADH release.

Anatomic studies using the Falck fluorescence method show that noradrenergic fibers terminate directly on neurons of the supraoptic and paraventricular nuclei. Since similar terminals are not found in the neurohypophysis, it is likely that the effects of noradrenergic agents are mediated by direct effects on the perikarya of neurosecretory cells.

Studies using direct iontophoresis of these putative neurotransmitters on cells of the supraoptic nuclei have provided additional evidence for their role in synaptic regulation of ADH secretion. Barker and co-workers using antidromically identified neurosecretory cells in the cat, found that the monoamines—DA, NE, and serotonin—uniformly reduced the activity of these cells.[8] The inhibition of activity was blocked by adrenergic blocking agents. Acetylcholine, on the other hand, produced a dual effect. These workers postulated that supraoptic neurons may have both excitatory (nicotinic) and inhibitory (muscarinic) cholinergic receptors. Recent studies by Arnaud and co-workers in the rat support these observations.[4] They found that nicotine and acetylcholine stimulated phasically-active cells (believed to be vasopressin secreting), whereas NE inhibited cellular firing. These experimental observations appear to also hold true in man. Hence tobacco smoking releases vasopressin in response to nicotinic receptor stimulation.

Acetylcholine also stimulates oxytocin secretion. It is likely that the stress-induced inhibition of the "milk let-down" reflex, well known from both animal husbandry and human nursing experience, results from adrenergic inhibition of oxytocin release. The same kind of reaction may be responsible for stress-induced diuresis (i.e., adrenergic substances acting to inhibit ADH secretion).

Secretion of vasopressin and electrophysiologic activation of supraoptic neurons are also modified by certain neuropeptides. Direct intrahypothalamic application of angiotensin-II releases vasopressin and influences drinking behavior.[53] Neurohypophysial neurons are also stimulated by endogenous opioids (endorphins). The well-known antidiuretic action of morphine is caused by the release of vasopressin, an effect that can be duplicated by the intracerebroventricular administration of β-endorphin. That the endorphins may be involved in vasopressin secretion regulation is further supported by the observation that naloxone, an opiate antagonist, reverses neurogenically inappropriate ADH secretion in some cases.

Other drugs exert important effects on ADH secretion. Alcohol strongly inhibits ADH release, both decreasing basal levels and preventing normal ADH responses to stimuli such as reduced blood volume. Phenytoin also inhibits ADH release transiently. On the other hand, ADH release is stimulated by morphine, barbiturates, and other hypnotics; these agents can cause significant antidiuresis. From a practical point of view, drug-induced ADH release leads to impaired water excretion and may be responsible in part for water intoxication in hospitalized patients given intravenous fluids. Pain and stress, which also stimulate ADH secretion, can intensify the defect in water clearance.

The clinical disorders, DI, and the syndrome of inappropriate ADH secretion (SIADH), are discussed in Chapter 15.

BRAIN-GUT PEPTIDES: REGULATORY PEPTIDES

The discovery that identical peptides are present as secretory products in defined populations of neurons in the CNS and peripheral nervous system and in certain glandular cells of the pancreas and gut has been one of the most important advances in regulatory biology in the last decade. This finding, together with new insights into the molecular evolution of neuropeptides, has broken down previous rigid classifications of the ways in which cellular function is integrated and has made it possible for scientists to apply the powerful tools of molecular biology to the understanding of brain function.[22,83,106,151]

Substance P was the first of the peptides to be found in both gut and brain. It was first isolated in crude form from intestinal extracts by Von Euler and Gaddum in 1931 on the basis of its biologic effects on smooth muscle function, but its structure was not elucidated.[169] More than 35 years later, while searching for CRF in hypothalamic extracts, Leeman et al.[26,91] noted that a particular fraction induced intense salivation in assay animals. Using the sialogogic effect as a bioassay, these workers were able to isolate the active principle, determine its structure, and synthesize a peptide that had identical chemical and biologic properties. Further study of the pharmacologic effects of this compound led to the recognition that it was similar to the previously described substance P of Von Euler, which was then shown to be an active sialogogue. By this time, specific immunologic techniques were available to show that intestinal substance P was immunologically identical to Leeman's "sialogen." The chemical structure of the gut substance is now known to be identical to hypothalamic substance P.

Immunohistochemical techniques demonstrated the presence of substance P in many different kinds of neurons and in certain glandular cells of the gut, thus establishing what appeared to be a new class of *brain-gut peptides*.

The next advance in broadening our concepts of the significance of neuropeptides was the discovery in 1973 that TRH, functioning in the hypothalamus as the thyrotropin-releasing hormone, had a wide distribution in the extrahypothalamic brain of all mammalian species and in the brains of representatives of all animal classes down to the snail.[74,75] TRH has more recently been demonstrated to be present in the pancreas and gut and thus can be included in the list of classic brain-gut peptides.[75]

The concept of the brain-gut peptides was broadened by discovery of somatostatin, reported in 1973 by Brazeau et al.[20] Initially isolated from the hypothalamus, where it functions as a hypophysiotropic hormone to inhibit GH and TSH release, somatostatin was found to inhibit pancreatic cells.[129,137]

Perhaps the most electrifying advance in regulatory peptide physiology was the discovery of the endogenous opioids, including the enkephalins by Hughes et al.[71] and the subsequent identification of β-endorphin and of the family of molecules contained in the opiomelanocortin precursor.[94] Recognition of the widespread occurrence of peptides in brain and gut has led workers throughout the world to an enthusiastic effort to isolate traditional gut peptides from brain and brain peptides from gut. In fact, it has now become a matter of routine as new peptides are discovered for workers in this field to test for their presence in all tissues.[65,105]

Additional new peptides continue to be described because of advances in peptide purification, sequencing, and synthesis procedures and of development of new antibodies for RIA and immunocytochemistry. The development of molecular biology has revealed a new universe of potential neuropeptides, present in the sequences of prohormones, some of which have already been shown to have biologic activity.

There are few if any examples of regulatory peptides distributed in only one type of cell. Since it is estimated that conventional nonpeptide neurotransmitters may account for only 40% of the synapses in the CNS, it is apparent that elucidation of the role of peptides, both discovered and unknown, will provide major new insights into CNS function.

The peptides that can be found in both gut and brain are listed as follows:

Hypothalamic releasing hormones
    Thyrotropin-releasing hormone (TRH)
    Gonadotropin-releasing hormone (GNRH)
    Somatostatin
    Corticotropin-releasing factor (CRF)
    Growth hormone releasing factor (GRF)
Neurohypophysial hormone
    Vasopressin
    Oxytocin
    Neurophysin(s)
Gastrointestinal peptides
    Vasoactive intestinal polypeptide (VIP)
    Cholecystokinin (CCK-8)
    Gastrin
    Substance P
    Neurotensin
    Methionine enkephalin
    Leucine enkephalin
    Insulin
    Glucagon
    Bombesin

Gastrointestinal peptides *(cont'd)*
    TRH
    Secretin
    Somatostatin
    Pancreatic polypeptide—Neuropeptide Y
    Motilin
Pituitary peptides
    Adrenocorticotropic hormone (ACTH)
    β-endorphin
    Melanocyte-stimulating hormone (MSH)
    Prolactin (PRL)
    Growth hormone (GH)
    Luteinizing hormone (LH)
    Thyrotropin
Others
    Angiotensin
    Bradykinin
    Calcitonin
    Carnosine
    Neuropeptide Y
    Sleep peptide(s)

Concentration of peptides in brain

All the peptides are found in brain in significantly lower concentrations (10^{-12} to 10^{-15} M/mg protein) than is the case with the classic biogenic amine neurotransmitters such as acetylcholine, NE, and DA, which are found in concentrations of 10^{-9} to 10^{-10} M/mg protein. The amino acid neurotransmitters—gamma amino butyric acid (GABA), glycine, and glutamate—are found in even higher concentrations (10^{-6} to 10^{-8} M/mg protein). Hypothalamic and pancreatic concentrations of somatostatin are approximately equivalent; whereas the concentrations of brain ACTH is about 1/1000 that found in the anterior pituitary, and that of brain insulin is approximately 1/1000 that present in the pancreas. Cholecystokinin (CCK) seems thus far to be the only peptide whose CNS concentration is greater than that described in the gastrointestinal tract. Recently discovered neuropeptide Y (NPY), which appears to be found exclusively in neural tissues, is present in unusually high concentrations in the CNS, about 10 times that of CCK. In general, however, CNS concentrations of peptides derived from homogenized tissue do not reliably indicate their functional importance. Concentration does not indicate turnover; additionally, regional, cellular, and subcellular distribution of peptides are likely of greater biologic importance than overall determinations of concentrations in whole regions of the brain or spinal cord.

Evolutionary and embryologic aspects of neuropeptides

Neuropeptides have undergone a fascinating evolutionary development. The families of neurohypophysial hormones illustrate this principle, in which evolution apparently gives rise to modifications of a common ancestral peptide. Vasotocin, the ancient form of vasopressin, has only a single amino acid substitution when compared with vasopressin. Lysine vasopressin, which also arose early in evolution, persists in the pig, where it exists as the major form. It is now known that marsupials, whether found in Australia, in Africa, or in North or South America are unique in containing both arginine and lysine vasopressin in the neural lobe of the pituitary, indicating their common ancestry.

The family of tachykinins (which includes substance P, physalemin, phyllomedusin, and kassinin) also occurs as a heterogenous group of peptides, many of which are found in high concentrations in amphibian skin. These patterns of peptide changes give valuable clues to the very nature and process of evolution.

Molecular biologic analysis has also traced divergent evolution of the neuropeptides. One example is that of somatostatin, represented by seven different genes in some species. It has been calculated that there is about 70% homology of somatostatin prohormones between fish and rat—species that may have diverged from a common ancestor 400 million years ago.

The presence of similar peptides in different tissues and in different species also indicates common evolutionary mechanisms, providing insight into gene structure and function and gene mutation and duplication. Neurotransmission and neurosecretion of peptides occurs in Coelenterates and annelids that have no recognizable endocrine tissue. The presence of CCK and somatostatin in the gastrointestinal tract and brain has been noted as early in invertebrate evolution as the lamprey.[129] Even more striking is the demonstration of substances similar to mammalian insulin, ACTH, and β-endorphin in unicellular eukaryotes (*Tetrahymena pyriformis, Neurospora crassa, Aspergillus fumigatus, Escherichia coli*). These observations raise the possibility that most cells have a capacity for a low level of expression of many peptides. In simpler organisms, peptides may have functions other than those that have evolved in higher organisms; with increasing evolutionary complexity, there may be selective enhanced expression of peptide biosynthesis in specific tissue.

Reports of similar peptides in different tissues also raise questions concerning the embryologic origins of peptides. Observations that peptide expression may be a common feature of many cells no longer make it necessary to attempt, as has been done previously, to establish a common embryologic origin for tissues that express the same peptides. For example, Pearse[120] postulated that all tissue containing similar peptides were of neural crest origin. It is now realized that many cells, regardless of embryologic origin can express peptide-producing mechanisms.

Validity of peptide measurements

The primary tools of peptide research, RIA and immunocytochemistry, have been applied to human brain tissue obtained at surgery and at autopsy. In addition, there are numerous studies of neuropeptide concentrations in human CSF determined by RIA or, in the case of endorphins, by receptor binding assay.

Measurements of neuropeptides in postmortem tissue show considerable biologic variations in concentration; consequently, studies must include sufficient numbers of cases to be able to detect significant differences. Antemortem factors such as age, sex, time of death, drug treatment, other coincident illnesses, and cause of death must be considered as sources of peptide alterations. For instance, virtually all patients dying with Huntington's disease or schizophrenia have been treated with long-term neuroleptic therapy. It is necessary therefore to either control such therapy or demonstrate that it is not the cause of any abnormalities recognized.

Peptides in postmortem tissue have been demonstrated to be quite stable. This stability is probably related to vesicular storage and protection from lysosomal peptidases. Many studies show no correlation of peptide concentration with delay to autopsy. Substance P,[24,28,31,52] somatostatin,[24,28,37,55] cholecystokinin octapeptide (CCK-8),[47,124,143] met-enkephalin,[57] TRH,[16,111] GnRH,[18,111] neurotensin,[16,24,28,95] and VIP[124] have been shown to be stable in the human brain by this criterion.

Investigators have used chromatographic techniques to look for peptide degradation products in postmortem tissue and have generally failed to find them. Immunoreactive substance P,[5,44,98] CCK,[124,165] VIP,[45] met-enkephalin,[44] and neurotensin[95] in extracts of human brain have all been shown to migrate as single chromatographic peaks. In the case of somatostatin, where higher molecular weight forms of immunoreactive material can generally be found in extracts of animal tissue, it is encouraging that such presumed precursor forms are also present in extracts of human postmortem brain,[5,37,55] although conversion of high molecular precursors to somatostatin-14 may continue slowly after death.[55]

The most convincing evidence of postmortem stability of neuropeptides has come from animal experiments. Substance P,[44] somatostatin,[36,38,55,90] CCK-8,[142] VIP,[45] and met-enkephalin,[44] have all been shown to be stable in animal brains for at least 24 hours and in some studies for as long as 72 hours postmortem.

CSF levels of neuropeptides have also been shown to be stable after withdrawal. Immunoreactive substance P,[110] somatostatin,[119] CCK,[128] TRH,[154] and β-endorphin[25] are stable under conditions of storage expected for clinical CSF samples, with no more precaution required than refrigerating the samples. In addition, immunoreactive somatostatin[11] and substance P[110] in human CSF behave chromatographically as expected for the authentic peptides.

Postmortem studies

Alzheimer's disease. In Alzheimer's dementia and Alzheimer's-type senile dementia (AD), there is a loss of acetylcholine and the enzyme choline acetyltransferase (CAT) in the cerebral cortex to 60% to 90% of levels found in control brains.[139] This neurochemical abnormality reflects a loss of cholinergic terminals in the cortex and hippocampus. The cell bodies of origin of these terminals are found in the basal nucleus of Meynert[143,172] where loss of neuronal perikarya has been documented in AD. Senile plaques, one of the cardinal neuropathologic signs of AD, contain degenerating cholinergic nerve terminals.[164] The degree of loss of CAT activity in the cerebral cortex correlates with the density of senile plaques, and both correlate with the degree of dementia.[29]

Measurements of neuropeptide concentrations in human brain regions dissected at autopsy have shown a selective loss of somatostatin-like immunoreactivity (SLI) in the neocortex and hippocampus of patients with AD when compared to controls.[36,138] No consistent abnormalities of SLI concentration have been found in basal ganglia or hypothalamus in AD. In normal aging, there seems to be no loss of SLI from human cortex.[24,123] Arginine vasopressin, substance P, VIP, and CCK concentrations, as determined by RIA, have not been found altered in AD.[29,123,124,141,142] The lack of alteration of VIP and CCK is of particular interest. These peptides are found in highest concentration in the cerebral cortex and in rats are present in intrinsic neurons of the cortex, as demonstrated by immunocytochemistry.[45-47,54,125,141]

The degree of loss of SLI in cerebral cortex in AD correlates with the diminution in CAT activity.[37] The fall in SLI is presumed to represent a loss of somatostatin-containing neuronal elements in the cortex, but whether it reflects a loss of intrinsic cortical neurons or of fibers and terminals projecting to the cortex from an extrinsic source is not known. In the normal human brain, immunocytochemistry demonstrates SLI-containing neuronal perikarya in the cerebral cortex.[158] In the rat hippocampus, surgical section of the fornix produces a 63% fall in CAT activity in the hippocampus, consistent with the well-known extrinsic origin of cholinergic innervation of the hippocampus but no changes in SLI concentration.[99] On the other hand, the direct injection of excitotoxin kainic acid into the rat hippocampus produces a 60% decrease in SLI concentration and a corresponding decrease in glutamate decarboxylase (GAD) activity but no fall in CAT activity. In the rat hippocampus, therefore, this evidence favors an intrinsic source of somatostatin. If the same holds true for human cerebral cortex, the selectivity of AD for somatostatin, with sparing of other intrinsic peptidergic neurons containing CCK and VIP, may be a clue to the pathogenesis of neuronal loss in AD.

Huntington's disease. Huntington's disease (HD) is an autosomal dominant disorder marked by the development, usually in adult life, of a choreic movement disorder and psychiatric and intellectual impairment. The striking neuropathologic finding is atrophy of the head of the caudate nucleus. On microscopic examination, there is cell loss and gliosis of the caudate. Although there is often atrophy of the cerebral cortex on gross examination, numbers of neurons in the frontal cortex of patients dying with HD do not differ from controls.[170] The pathologic correlate of the psychiatric and intellectual manifestations of HD is therefore unknown.

Presynaptic markers of GABAergic and cholinergic neurons are diminished in the caudate of patients dying with HD, but dopaminergic markers in the caudate are increased in concentration.[17,163] These findings support the view of a specific loss of intrinsic striatal neurons in HD, with preservation of terminals from sources extrinsic to the caudate. The chorea of HD can often be suppressed by the administration of DA receptor blockers such as haloperidol, consistent with the concept of a relative excess of striatal dopaminergic function.

Peptide markers for intrinsic striatal neurons are also altered in the caudate of patients dying of HD. Three studies agree that in HD brains the concentration of immunoreactive substance P is decreased in the globus pallidus and substantia nigra, the sites of projection of striatal substance P–containing fibers.[4,44,52] Only one of these studies, however, found substance P to be significantly diminished in the striatum in HD; this discrepancy may represent variations in the stages of the disease in which the brains were obtained. Met-enkephalin immunoreactivity is diminished in the globus pallidus and substantia nigra.[44] Immunocytochemistry documents for both substance P and metenkephalin a decrease in the density of immunostained cell bodies in the striatum and a decrease in stained fibers in the globus pallidus and substantia nigra.[96] CCK-like immunoreactivity is reduced about 50% in the globus pallidus and substantia nigra but has been found to be normal in the cerebral cortex, caudate, and putamen.[47]

In contrast to substance P and met-enkephalin, both somatostatin and TRH immunoreactivities, when expressed per mg protein or per mg net weight, are increased in the basal ganglia in HD.[5,162] It is not clear if these increases in concentration represent true increases in regional peptide content or a relative preservation of peptide content in face of atrophy of total tissue mass. It is of note that, whereas DA is increased by 30% to 60% in the caudate of HD brains compared to controls, the concentrations of somatostatin and TRH are increased over twofold. Assuming no loss of nigra-striatal dopaminergic terminals in HD, this implies a true increase in both somatostatin and TRH content. Furthermore, there is an approximately 2½-fold increase in concentration of SLI in the nucleus accumbens, a region that does not atrophy in HD.[10,97]

Immunocytochemistry has demonstrated no obvious difference in the proportion of striatal cells staining for somatostatin in HD compared to control brains.[97] However, the density of stained varicose fibers in the caudate is increased in HD relative to normals. The origin of these fibers is uncertain at the present. Lesion studies in the rat suggest that about half the somatostatin in the caudate arises from intrinsic striatal somatostatin-containing neurons and half is from an extrinsic source.[12] In the normal human brain, immunocytochemistry is consistent with this observation in that many somatostatin-containing perikarya and fibers are seen in the nucleus accumbens and basal forebrain. A dense collection of somatostatin-containing fibers can be observed in the head of the caudate immediately adjacent to the nucleus accumbens. These fibers are continuous with and comparable in density to somatostatin fibers in regions near the accumbens, thus raising the possibility that some of the fibers observed in the caudate may be extrinsic in origin.[97]

There are two regions in both rat and human basal forebrain rich in somatostatin: the amygdala and the substantia innominata. In rats, excision of the amygdala leads to no change in striatal concentration of immunoreactive somatostatin. Knife cuts made in the coronal plane at the level of the anterior tip of the rat caudate, thereby disconnecting the caudate from inputs from the medial basal forebrain, produce a 70% fall in SLI in the caudate.[116] Therefore the most likely source for the increased somatostatin is the substantia innominata. Assuming that the increased concentration of somatostatin reflects a true increase in regional peptide content, it is still not clear if this represents a proliferation of fibers and terminals or an increase in the somatostatin content of individual processes.

Two negative results are of note in HD. The concentration of VIP is unchanged in both frontal cortex and basal ganglia of patients dying with HD.[45] Secondly, no alteration in cerebral cortical concentrations of somatostatin have been demonstrated in HD, distinguishing the dementia of HD from that of AD.[5,52]

Parkinson's disease. Idiopathic Parkinson's disease (PD) is in many ways the archetypic neurodegenerative disease. In PD there is a remarkably specific loss of the pigmented DA-containing neurons from the substantia nigra pars compacta and of their terminals in the caudate and putamen. Correlated with this loss is a depletion of DA, homovanillic acid, and tyrosine hydroxylase activity in substantia nigra and striatum.[161] Treatment of patients with PD with either the DA precursor levodopa or with DA agonists improves their symptoms but does not alter the progression of their disease.

In animals, a striatonigral substance P–containing pathway has been demonstrated.[108] This pathway is thought to exert an excitatory influence of dopaminergic activity in the substantia nigra. In brains of patients dying with PD, significant decreases in concentrations of substance P–like immunoreactivity (SPLI) of the substantia nigra (both pars compacta and pars reticulata) and globus pallidus externa have been observed.[98] In this study, the SPLI concentrations in caudate and putamen were reduced 24% and 27% respectively, but these differences were not statistically significant. It is also of note that the significant depletions of SPLI observed, ranging from 32% in the pars compacta of substantia nigra to 46% in the external division of the globus pallidus, are less than the 90% depletion of dopaminergic markers observed in PD. However, it may well be that a loss of excitatory substance P input to the substantia nigra contributes to the symptoms of PD.

CCK-8 is of interest in PD in view of the evidence that a subset of DA-containing cells of the ventral midbrain tegmentum, the mesolimbic neurons projecting to the nucleus accumbens, and frontal cortex contain CCK-8.[68] In PD the pathologic observations of a virtual complete loss of pigmented neurons in the substantia nigra and ventral tegmentum and the almost complete depletion of dopaminergic markers from the midbrain suggest that all subdivisions of the midbrain dopaminergic system are involved in the disease. One would hypothesize therefore that PD would be associated with a loss of immunoreactive CCK-8 from the substantia nigra and ventral tegmentum and from the nucleus accumbens and frontal cortex, the areas of projection of the mesolimbic dopaminergic neurons thought to contain CCK-8 in rats. This hypothesis has only been partially verified. The concentration of CCK-like immunoreactivity has been shown to be reduced about 40% in the substantia nigra in PD but is normal in the nucleus accumbens, frontal cortex, and striatum.[165] Whether this loss from the substantia nigra reflects the degeneration of some groups of neurons containing both DA and CCK-8 remains to be determined.

Met-enkephalin–like immunoreactivity is also reduced in the putamen, globus pallidus externa, substantia nigra pars compacta (but not the pars reticulata), and ventral tegmental area in PD.[124] Concentrations of met-enkephalin were found to be normal in the caudate, nucleus accumbens, globus pallidus interna, and other forebrain areas examined. The clinical significance of the alteration in met-enkephalin concentration is unknown. No alteration of extrahypothalamic concentrations of immunoreactive arginine vasopressin was found in PD.[140]

In the dementia sometimes associated with PD, the pathologic findings are similar to those in AD, including the presence of senile plaques, neurofibrillary tangles, and neuronal loss from the basal nucleus of Meynert.[160] It will be of interest to determine if somatostatin in the cerebral cortex is reduced in the dementia of PD as it is in AD.

CSF neuropeptides

As was discussed previously, CSF peptide assays are valid in the sense that neuropeptides apparently are quite stable in the CSF and the immunoreactive material in CSF is chromatographically indistinguishable from the native peptide. However, there are many reservations concerning the interpretation of CSF peptide concentrations. The evidence is clear that in the circumstances studied thus far CSF peptides originate in the nervous system and do not leak in from the circulation. CSF peptide levels may vary quite independently of circulating blood levels and even large doses of peptides administered into the peripheral circulation fail to appear in the CSF. Therefore there is a blood-CSF barrier, and presumably a blood-brain barrier, for peptides.

The difficult issue is to identify which CNS regions contribute to the CSF peptide pool. It may well be that regions deep in the brain supply a smaller proportion of CSF peptides than do regions close to the subarachnoid space. In one study[160] in which lumbar punctures were performed and a total of 12 ml of CSF withdrawn, there was no difference in mean somatostatin concentration assayed in the first 2 ml and the final 2 ml, whereas albumin and gamma globulin concentrations were 20% less in the final milliliter than in the first milliliter.[160] The authors' conclusion from this data was that CSF somatostatin is supplied diffusely from the CNS, although it is also consistent with a predominant spinal cord source. A comparable study performed with substance P produced a similar result.[110] Consequently, peptides measured in lumbar CSF may well be a more sensitive indicator of spinal cord than of brain disease.

The kinetics of peptide accumulation and clearance in the CSF has not been well studied. Some neuropeptides may be specifically released into the CSF and may use the CSF as a medium for transport to target sites,[57] whereas others may overflow passively into CSF. Several investigators have suggested that the tanycytes lining the third ventricle transport peptides from the median eminence to CSF, although on anatomic grounds these cells more likely seem to be barriers than conduits, and direct evidence for such transport is lacking.[152]

Despite these uncertainties, there are several interesting observations concerning CSF peptide concentrations in neurologic disease. A group of patients with advanced AD was found to have a mean CSF somatostatin concentration 42% less than a control group, suggesting that the diminished level of cerebral cortical somatostatin is reflected in lumbar CSF.[175] CSF somatostatin has also been reported to be reduced in multiple sclerosis during relapse[159] and in HD,[30] but the pathophysiology underlying these abnormalities is unclear.

Substance P levels in lumbar CSF have been found decreased in patients with peripheral neuropathy and with Shy-Drager syndrome, which includes autonomic malfunction in its manifestations.[110] The finding of low CSF substance P in cases of peripheral neuropathy reinforces the hypothesis that lumbar CSF abnormalities predominantly reflect spinal cord and nerve root pathology.

ACKNOWLEDGMENTS

The author thanks those collaborators—Drs. Flint Beal, Steve Sagar, and Seymour Reichlin—whose contributions have made much of this work possible. Excellent secretarial assistance was given by Kathy Kreatz and Pat Clougherty.

REFERENCES

1. Ajika K, Hökfelt T: Ultrastructural identification of catecholamine neurons in the hypothalamic periventricular-arcuate nucleus median eminence complex with special reference to quantitative aspects. *Brain Res* 57:97, 1973.
2. Amico JA, Tenicela R, Johnston J, et al: A timedependent peak of oxytocin exists in the cerebrospinal fluid but not in the plasma of humans. *J Clin Endocrinol Metab* 57:947, 1982.
3. Anderson E, Haymaker W: Breakthroughs in hypothalamic and pituitary research. *Prog Brain Res* 41:1, 1974.
4. Arnauld E, Cirino M, Layton BS, et al: Contrasting actions of amino acids, acetylcholine, noradrenaline and leucine enkephalin on the excitability of supraoptic vasopressin-secreting neurons: A microiontophoretic study in the rat. *Neuroendocrinology* 36:187, 1983.
5. Aronin N, Cooper PE, Lorenz LJ, et al: Somatostatin is increased in the basal ganglia in Huntington disease. *Ann Neurol* 13:519, 1983.
6. Aschner B: Über die Funktion der Hypophyse. *Pfluegers Arch* 146:1, 1912.
7. Aubry RH, Nankin HR, Moses AM, et al: Measurement of the osmotic threshold for vasopressin release in human subjects, and its modification by cortisol. *J Clin Endocrinol Metab* 25:1481, 1965.
8. Barker JL, Crayton JW, Nicoll RA: Antidromic and orthodromic responses of paraventricular and supraoptic neurosecretory cells. *Brain Res* 33:353, 1971.
9. Barker JL, Crayton JW, Nicoll RA: Noradrenaline and acetylcholine responses of supraoptic neurosecretory cells. *J Physiol* 218:19, 1971.
10. Beal MF, Bird ED, Langlais lPJ, et al: Somatostatin is increased in the nucleus accumbens in Huntington's disease. *Neurology* 34:663, 1984.
11. Beal MF, Growdon JH, Mazurek MF, et al: CSF somatostatin-like immunoreactivity in dementia. *Neurology* (in press).
12. Beal MF, Martin JB: Effects of lesions on somatostatin-like immunoreactivity in the rat striatum. *Brain Res* 266:67, 1983.
13. Ben-Jonathan N, Mical RS, Porter JC: Transport of LRF from CSF to hypophysial portal and systemic blood and the release of LH. *Endocrinology* 95:18, 1974.
14. Bergland RM, Page RB: Can the pituitary secrete directly to the brain? (Affirmative anatomical evidence). *Endocrinology* 102:1325, 1978.
15. Bergland RM, Page RB: Pituitary-brain vascular relations: A new paradigm. *Science* 204:18, 1979.
16. Biggins JA, Perry EK, McDermott JR, et al: Postmortem levels of thyrotropin-releasing hormone and neurotensin in the amygdala in Alzheimer's disease, schizophrenia and depression. *J Neurol Sci* 58:117, 1983.
17. Bird ED: Chemical pathology of Huntington's disease. *Annu Rev Pharmacol Toxicol* 20:533, 1980.
18. Bird ED, Chiappa SA, Fink G: Brain immunoreactive gonadotropin-releasing hormone in Huntington's chorea and in nonchoreic subjects. *Nature* 260:536, 1976.
19. Bloch B, Brazeau P, Ling N, et al: Immunohistochemical detection of growth hormone–releasing factor in brain. *Nature* 301:607, 1983.
20. Brazeau P, Vale W, Burgus R, et al: Hypothalamic polypeptide that inhibits the secretion of immunoreactive pituitary growth hormone. *Science* 179:77, 1973.
21. Brownstein MJ, Palkovits M, Tappaz ML, et al: Effects of surgical isolation of the hypothalamus on its neurotransmitter content. *Brain Res* 117:287, 1976.
22. Brownstein MJ, Russell JT, Gainer H: Synthesis, transport, and release of posterior pituitary hormones. *Science* 207:373, 1980.
23. Buchanan, KD: Gut hormones and the brain, in Besser GM, Martini L (eds): *Clinical Neuroendocrinology*. New York, Academic Press Inc, 1982, vol 2.
24. Buck SH, Deshmukh PP, Burks TF, et al: A survey of substance P, somatostatin, and neurotensin levels in aging in the rat and human central nervous system. *Neurobiol Aging* 2:257, 1981.
25. Burbach JPH, Loeber JG, Verhoef J, et al: Schizophrenia and degradation of endorphins in cerebrospinal fluid. *Lancet* 2:480, 1979.
26. Chang MM, Leeman SE, Niall HD: Aminoacid sequence of substance P. *Nature* 232:86, 1971.
27. Cooper JR, Bloom FE, Roth RH: *The Biochemical Basis of Neuropharmacology*. New York, Oxford University Press Inc, 1984.
28. Cooper PE, Fernstrom MH, Rorstad OP, et al: The regional distribution of somatostatin, substance P and neurotensin in human brain. *Brain Res* 218:219, 1981.
29. Coyle JT, Price DL, DeLong MR: Alzheimer's disease: A disorder of cortical cholinergic innervation. *Science* 219:1184, 1983.

30. Cramer H, Kohler J, Oepen G, et al: Huntington's chorea—Measurements of somatostatin, substance P and cyclic nucleotides in the cerebrospinal fluid. *Brain Res* 225:183, 1981.
31. Crystal HA, Davies P: Cortical substance P–like immunoreactivity in cases of Alzheimer's disease and senile dementia of the Alzheimer type. *J Neurochem* 38:1781, 1982.
32. Currie MG, Geller DM, Cole BR, et al: Bioactive cardiac substances: Potent vasorelaxant activity in mammalian atria. *Science* 221:71, 1983.
33. Currie MG, Geller DM, Cole BR, et al: Purification and sequence analysis of bioactive atrial peptides (atriopeptins). *Science* 223:67, 1984.
34. Dahlström A, Fuxe K: Evidence for the existence of monamine-containing neurons in the central nervous system: I. Demonstration of monoamines in the cell bodies of brain stem neurons. *Acta Physiol Scand* 62 (suppl):1, 1964.
35. Daniel PM, Prichard MML: Studies of the hypothalamus and the pituitary gland with special reference to the effects of transection of the pituitary stalk. *Acta Endocrinol* 80(suppl):1, 1975.
36. Davies P, Katzman R, Terry RD: Reduced somatostatin-like immunoreactivity in cerebral cortex from cases of Alzheimer disease and Alzheimer senile dementia. *Nature* 288:279, 1980.
37. Davies P, Terry RD: Cortical somatostatin-like immunoreactivity in cases of Alzheimer's disease and senile dementia of the Alzheimer type. *Neurobiol Aging* 2:9, 1981.
38. Davies P, Thompson A: Postmortem stability of somatostatin-like immunoreactivity in mouse brain under conditions simulating handling of human autopsy material. *Neurochem Res* 6:787, 1981.
39. Day TA, Blessing W, Willoughby JO: Noradrenergic and dopaminergic projections to the medial preoptic area of the rat: A combined horseradish peroxidase/catecholamine fluorescence study. *Brain Res* 193:543, 1980.
40. Demarest KT, Moore KE: Lack of a high affinity transport system for dopamine in the median eminence and posterior pituitary. *Brain Res* 171:545, 1979.
41. Dierickx K, Vandesande F: Immunocytochemical demonstration of separate vasopressin-neurophysin and oxytocin-neurophysin neurons in the human hypothalamus. *Cell Tissue Res* 196:203, 1979.
42. Dreifuss JJ, Kelly JS: The activity of identified supraoptic neurones and their response to acetylcholine applied by iontophoresis. *J Physiol* 220:105, 1972.
43. Du Vigneaud V: Hormones of the posterior pituitary gland: Oxytocin and vasopressin. *Harvey Lect* 50:1, 1954-1955.
44. Emson PC, Arregui A, Clement-Jones V, et al: Regional distribution of methionine-enkephalin and substance P–like immunoreactivity in normal human brain and in Huntington's disease. *Brain Res* 199:147, 1980.
45. Emson PC, Fahrenkrug J, Spokes EGS: Vasoactive intestinal polypeptide (VIP): Distribution in normal human brain and in Huntington's disease. *Brain Res* 173:174, 1979.
46. Emson PC, Hunt SP: Anatomical chemistry of the cerebral cortex, in Schmitt FO, Worden FG, Adelman G, et al (eds): *The Organization of the Cerebral Cortex*. Cambridge, Mass., The MIT Press, 1981.
47. Emson PC, Rehfeld JF, Langevin H, et al: Reduction in cholecystokinin-like immunoreactivity in the basal ganglia in Huntington's disease. *Brain Res* 198:497, 1980.
48. Erdheim J, Stumme E: Über die Schwangerschaftsveränderung der Hypophyse. *Beitr Pathol Anat Allgem Pathol* 46:1, 1909.
49. Evans HM: Clinical manifestations of dysfunction of the anterior pituitary, *JAMA* 104:464, 1935.
50. Furutani Y, Morimoto Y, Shibahara S, et al: Cloning and sequence analysis of cDNA for ovine coricotropinreleasing factor precursor. *Nature* 301:537, 1983.
51. Gainer H: Biosynthesis of vasopressin and neurophysin, in Reichlin S (ed): *The Neurohypophysis: Physiological and Clinical Aspects*. New York, Plenum Medical Book Co, 1984.
52. Gale JS, Bird ED, Spokes EG, et al: Human brain substance P: Distribution in controls and Huntington's chorea. *J Neurochem* 30:633, 1978.
53. Ganten D, Fuxe K, Phillips MI, et al: The brain isorenin-angiotensin system: Biochemistry, localization, and possible role in drinking and blood pressure regulation, in Ganong WF, Martini L (eds): *Frontiers in Neuroendocrinology*. New York, Raven Press, 1978, vol 5.
54. Geola FL, Hershman JM, Warwick R, et al: Regional distribution of cholecystokinin-like immunoreactivity in the human brain. *J Clin Endocrinol Metab* 53:270, 1981.

55. Geola FL, Yamada T, Warwick RJ, et al: Regional distribution of somatostatin-like immunoreactivity in the human brain. *Brain Res* 229:35, 1981.
56. Gold PW, Kaye W, Robertson GL, et al: Abnormalities in plasma and cerebrospinal fluid arginine vasopressin in patients with anorexia nervosa. *N Engl J Med* 308:1117, 1983.
57. Gramsch C, Höllt V, Mehraein P, et al: Regional distribution of methionine-enkephalin and beta-endorphin–like immunoreactivity in human brain and pituitary. *Brain Res* 171:261, 1979.
58. Green JD: The comparative anatomy of the hypophysis, with special reference to its blood supply and innervation. *Am J Anat* 88:225, 1951.
59. Green JD, Harris GW: The neurovascular link between the neurohypophysis and adenohypophysis. *J Endocrinol* 5:136, 1947.
60. Guillemin R: Peptides in the brain: The new endocrinology of the neuron. *Science* 202:390, 1978.
61. Guillemin R, Brazeau P, Böhlen P, et al: Growth hormone–releasing factor from a human pancreatic tumor that caused acromegaly. *Science* 218:585, 1982.
62. Harris GW: Neural control of the pituitary gland. *Physiol Rev* 28:139, 1948.
63. Harris GW, Jacobsohn D: Functional grafts of the anterior pituitary gland. *Proc R Soc Lond* 139:263, 1952.
64. Hayward JN: Functional and morphological aspects of hypothalamic neurons. *Physiol Rev* 57:574, 1977.
65. Hendricks SA, Roth J, Rishi S, Becker KL: Insulin in the nervous system, in Krieger DT, Brownstein MJ, Martin JB (eds): *Brain Peptides*. New York, John Wiley & Sons Inc, 1983.
66. Herbert E, Roberts J, Phillips M, et al: Biosynthesis, processing, and release of corticotropin, β-endorphin, and melanocyte-stimulating hormone in pituitary cell culture systems, in Martini L, Ganong WF (eds): *Frontiers in Neuroendocrinology*. New York, Raven Press, 1980, vol 6.
67. Hökfelt T, Elde R, Fuxe K, et al: Aminergic and peptidergic pathways in the nervous system with special reference to the hypothalamus, in Reichlin S (ed): *The Hypothalamus*. New York, Raven Press, 1978.
68. Hökfelt T, Rehfeld JF, Skirboll L, et al: Evidence for coexistence of dopamine and CCK in meso-limbic neurones. *Nature* 285:476, 1980.
69. Horvath E, Kovacs K: Pathology of the pituitary gland, in Ezrin C, Horvath E, Kaufman B, et al (eds): *Pituitary Diseases*. Boca Raton, Fla., CRC Press Inc, 1980.
70. Hou S: Syndrome of inappropriate antidiuretic hormone secretion, in Reichlin S (ed): *The Neurohypophysis: Physiological and Clinical Aspects*. New York, Plenum Medical Book Co, 1984.
71. Hughes J, Smith TW, Kosterlitz HW, et al: Identification of two related pentapeptides from the brain with potent opiate agonist activity. *Nature* 258:577, 1975.
72. Ishii S: Association of luteinizing hormone–releasing factor with granules separated from equine hypophysial stalk. *Endocrinology* 86:207, 1970.
73. Itoh N, Obata K, Yanaihara N, et al: Human preprovasoactive intestinal polypeptide contains a novel PHI-27–like peptide, PHM-27. *Nature* 304:547, 1983.
74. Jackson IMD: Significance and function of neuropeptides in cerebrospinal fluid, in Wood JH (ed): *Neurobiology of Cerebrospinal Fluid*. New York, Plenum Medical Book Co, 1980.
75. Jackson IMD, Lechan RM: Thyrotropin-releasing hormone, in Krieger DT, Brownstein MJ, Martin JB (eds): *Brain Peptides*. New York, John Wiley & Sons Inc, 1983.
76. Joseph SA, Knigge KN: The endocrine hypothalamus: Recent anatomical studies, in Reichlin S (ed): *The Hypothalamus*. New York, Raven Press, 1978.
77. Kasting NW, Carr DB, Martin JB, et al: Changes in cerebrospinal fluid and plasma vasopressin in the febrile sheep. *Can J Physiol Pharmacol* 61:427, 1983.
78. Kasting NW, Mazurek MF, Martin JB: Endotoxin increases vasopressin release independently of known physiological stimuli. *Am J Physiol* 248:E420, 1985.
79. Kizer JS, Muth E, Jacobowitz DM: The effect of bilateral lesions of the ventral noradrenergic bundle on endocrine-induced changes of tyrosine hydroxylase in the rat median eminence. *Endocrinology* 98:886, 1976.
80. Kovacs K, Horvath E: Pituitary tumors: Pathologic aspects, in Tolis G, Labrie F, Martin JB, et al (eds): *Clinical Neuroendocrinology: A Pathophysiological Approach*. New York, Raven Press, 1979.
81. Kovacs K, Horvath E: Pathology of pituitary adenomas, in Givens JR (ed): *Hormone-Secreting Pituitary Tumors*. Chicago, Year Book Medical Publishers Inc, 1982.

82. Krieger DT: Brain peptides: What, where, and why? *Science* 222:975, 1983.
83. Krieger DT, Brownstein MJ, Martin JB (eds): *Brain Peptides*. New York, John Wiley & Sons Inc, 1983.
84. Krieger DT, Martin JB: Brain peptides. I. *N Engl J Med* 304:876, 1981.
85. Krieger DT, Martin JB: Brain peptides. II. *N Engl J Med* 304:944, 1981.
86. Land H, Schütz G, Schmale H, et al: Nucleotide sequence of cloned cDNA encoding bovine arginine vasopressin-neurophysin II precursor. *Nature* 295:299, 1983.
87. Lechan RM, Lin HD, Ling N, et al: Distribution of immunoreactive growth hormone–releasing factor (1-44) NH2 in the tuberoinfundibular system of the *Rhesus* monkey. *Brain Res* 309:55, 1984.
88. Lechan RM, Nestler JL, Jacobson S: The tuberoinfundibular system of the rat as demonstrated by immunohistochemical localization of retrogradely transported wheat germ agglutinin (WGA) from the median eminence. *Brain Res* 245:1, 1982.
89. Lechan RM, Nestler JL, Jacobson S, et al: The hypothalamic "tuberoinfundibular" system of the rat as demonstrated by horseradish peroxidase (HRP) microiontophoresis. *Brain Res* 195:13, 1980.
90. Lee CM, Emson PC, Iversen LL: Chromatographic behaviour and post-mortem stability of somatostatin in the rat and mouse brain. *Brain Res* 220:159, 1981.
91. Leeman SE, Aronin N, Ferris C: Substance P and neurotensin. *Recent Prog Horm Res* 38:93, 1982.
92. Ling N, Esch F, Böhlen P, et al: Isolation, primary structure, and synthesis of human hypothalamic somatocrinin: Growth hormone–releasing factor. *Proc Natl Acad Sci USA* 81:4302, 1984.
93. MacLeod RM: Regulation of prolactin secretion, in Martini L, Ganong WF (eds): *Frontiers in Neuroendocrinology*. New York, Raven Press, 1976, vol 4.
94. Mains RE, Eipper BA, Ling N: Common precursor to corticotropins and endorphins. *Proc Natl Acad Sci USA* 74:3014, 1977.
95. Manberg PJ, Youngblood WW, Nemeroff CB, et al: Regional distribution of neurotensin in human brain. *J Neurochem* 38:1777, 1982.
96. Marshall PE, Landis DMD, Zalneraitis EL: Immunocytochemical studies of substance P and leucine-enkephalin in Huntington's disease. *Brain Res* 289:11, 1983.
97. Martin JB: Huntington's disease: New approaches to an old problem. *Neurology* 34:1059, 1984.
98. Mauborgne A, Javoy-Agid F, Legrand JC, et al: Decrease of substance P–like immunoreactivity in the substantia nigra and pallidum of parkinsonian brains. *Brain Res* 268:167, 1983.
99. McKinney M, Davies P, Coyle JT: Somatostatin is not co-localized in cholinergic neurons innervating the rat cerebral cortex–hippocampal formation. *Brain Res* 243:169, 1982.
100. Mezey E, Palkovits M: Two-way transport in hypothalamo-hypophyseal system, in Ganong WF, Martini L (eds): *Frontiers in Neuroendocrinology*. New York, Raven Press, 1982, vol 7.
101. Miller M, Moses AM: Clinical states due to alteration of ADH release and action, in Moses AM, Share L (eds): *Neurohypophysis*. Basel, Switzerland, S Karger, 1977.
102. Moses AM: Diabetes insipidus and ADH regulation, in Krieger DT, Hughes JC (eds): *Neuroendocrinology: The Interrelationships of the Body's Two Major Integrative Systems—In Normal Physiology and in Clinical Disease*. Sunderland, Mass., Sinauer Associates Inc, 1980.
103. Moses AM: Clinical and laboratory features of central and nephrogenic diabetes insipidus and primary polydipsia, in Reichlin S (ed): *The Neurohypophysis: Physiological and Clinical Aspects*. New York, Plenum Medical Book Co, 1984.
104. Moss RL, Dyball REJ, Cross BA: Responses of antidromically identified supraoptic and paraventricular units to acetylcholine, noradrenaline and glutamate applied iontophoretically. *Brain Res* 35:573, 1971.
105. Mutt V: VIP, motilin, and secretin, in Krieger DT, Brownstein MJ, Martin JB (eds): *Brain Peptides*. New York, John Wiley & Sons Inc, 1983.
106. Nakanishi S, Inoue A, Kita T, et al: Nucleotide sequence of cloned cDNA for bovine corticotropin-β-lipotropin precursor. *Nature* 278:423, 1979.
107. Neill JD: Neuroendocrine regulation of prolactin secretion, in Martini L, Ganong WF (eds): *Frontiers in Neuroendocrinology*. New York, Raven Press, 1980, vol 6.
108. Nicoll RA, Schenker C, Leeman SE: Substance P as a transmitter candidate. *Annu Rev Neurosci* 3:227, 1980.
109. Nikitovitch-Winer M, Everett JW: Functional

restitution of pituitary grafts re-transplanted from kidney to median eminence. *Endocrinology* 63:916, 1958.
110. Nutt JG, Mroz EA, Leeman SE, et al: Substance P in human cerebrospinal fluid: Reductions in peripheral neuropathy and autonomic dysfunction. *Neurology* 30:1280, 1980.
111. Okon E, Koch Y: Localisation of gonadotropin-releasing and thyrotropin-releasing hormone in human brain by radioimmunoassay. *Nature* 263:345, 1976.
112. Page RB: Directional pituitary blood flow: A microcinephotographic study. *Endocrinology* 112:157, 1983.
113. Page RB, Bergland RM: The neurohypophyseal capillary bed: I. Anatomy and arterial supply. *Am J Anat* 148:345, 1977.
114. Palkovits M: Catecholamines in the hypothalamus: An anatomical review. *Neuroendocrinology* 33:123, 1981.
115. Palkovits M, Brownstein M, Saavedra JM, et al: Norepinephrine and dopamine content of hypothalamic nuclei of the rat. *Brain Res* 77:137, 1974.
116. Palkovits M, Kobayashi RM, Brown M, et al: Changes in hypothalamic, limbic and extrapyramidal somatostatin levels following various hypothalamic transections in rat. *Brain Res* 195:499, 1980.
117. Palkovits M, Saavedra JM, Jacobowitz DM, et al: Serotonergic innervation of the forebrain: Effect of lesions on serotonin and tryptophan hydroxylase levels. *Brain Res* 130:121, 1977.
118. Palkovits M, Záborsky L, Feminger A, et al: Noradrenergic innervation of the rat hypothalamus: Experimental biochemical and electron microscopic studies. *Brain Res* 191:161, 1980.
119. Patel YC, Rao K, Reichlin S: Somatostatin in human cerebrospinal fluid. *N Engl J Med* 296:529, 1977.
120. Pearse AG: The APUD concept and hormone production. *J Clin Endocrinol Metab* 9(2):211, July 1980.
121. Pelletier G: Immunohistochemical localization of hypothalamic hormones and other peptides in the central nervous system, in Collu R, Barbeau A, Ducharme JR, et al (eds): *Central Nervous System Effects of Hypothalamic Hormones and Other Peptides*. New York, Raven Press, 1979.
122. Perlow MJ, Reppert SM, Artman HA, et al: Oxytocin, vasopressin, and estrogen-stimulated neurophysin: Daily patterns of concentration in cerebrospinal fluid. *Science* 216:1416, 1982.
123. Perry EK, Blessed G, Tomlinson BE, et al: Neurochemical activities in human temporal lobe related to aging and Alzheimer-type changes. *Neurobiol Aging* 2:251, 1981.
124. Perry RH, Dockray GJ, Dimaline R, et al: Neuropeptides in Alzheimer's disease, depression and schizophrenia: A postmortem analysis of vasoactive intestinal peptide and cholecystokinin in cerebral cortex. *J Neurol Sci* 51:465, 1981.
125. Peters A, Miller M, Kimerer LM: Cholecystokinin-like immunoreactive neurons in rat cerebral cortex. *Neuroscience* 8:431, 1983.
126. Pickford M: The inhibitory effect of acetylcholine on water diuresis in the dog, and its pituitary transmission. *J Physiol* 95:226, 1939.
127. Popa G, Fielding U: A portal circulation from the pituitary to the hypothalamic region. *J Anat* 65:88, 1930.
128. Rehfeld JF, Kruse-Larsen C: Gastrin and cholecystokinin in human cerebrospinal fluid: Immunochemical determination of concentrations and molecular heterogeneity. *Brain Res* 155:19, 1978.
129. Reichlin S: Somatostatin, in Krieger DT, Brownstein MJ, Martin JB (eds): *Brain Peptides*. New York, John Wiley & Sons Inc, 1983.
130. Reichlin S: The neurohypophysis: Historical overview, in Reichlin S (ed): *The Neurohypophysis: Physiological and Clinical Aspects*. New York, Plenum Medical Book Co, 1984.
131. Renaud LP: Neurophysiological organization of the endocrine hypothalamus, in Reichlin S (ed): *The Hypothalamus*. New York, Raven Press, 1978.
132. Renaud LP: Neurophysiology and neuropharmacology of medial hypothalamic neurons and their extrahypothalamic connections, in Morgane PJ, Panksepp J (eds): *Handbook of the Hypothalamus*. New York, Marcel Dekker Inc, 1979, vol 1.
133. Rivier J, Spiess J, Thorner M, et al: Characterization of a growth hormone–releasing factor from a human pancreatic islet tumour. *Nature* 300:276, 1982.
134. Robertson GL: The regulation of vasopressin function in health and disease. *Recent Prog Horm Res* 33:333, 1977.
135. Robinson AG: Neurophysins, in Martini L, Besser GM (eds): *Clinical Neuroendocrinology*. New York, Academic Press Inc, 1977.
136. Robinson AG: The contribution of measured secretion of neurophysins to our understanding of neurohypophysial function, in Reichlin S

(ed): *The Neurohypophysis: Physiological and Clinical Aspects.* New York, Plenum Medical Book Co, 1984.
137. Rorstad OP, Martin JB, Terry LC: Somatostatin and the nervous system, in Barker JL, Smith TG Jr (eds): *The Role of Peptides in Neuronal Function.* New York, Marcel Dekker Inc, 1980.
138. Rossor MN, Emson PC, Mountjoy CQ, et al: Reduced amounts of immunoreactive somatostatin in the temporal cortex in senile dementia of Alzheimer type. *Neurosci Lett* 20:373, 1980.
139. Rossor M, Fahrenkrug J, Emson P, et al: Reduced cortical choline acetyltransferase activity in senile dementia of Alzheimer type is not accompanied by changes in vasoactive intestinal polypeptide. *Brain Res* 201:249, 1980.
140. Rossor MN, Hunt SP, Iversen LL, et al: Extrahypothalamic vasopressin is unchanged in Parkinson's disease and Huntington's disease. *Brain Res* 253:341, 1982.
141. Rossor MN, Iversen LL, Hawthorn J, et al: Extrahypothalamic vasopressin in human brain. *Brain Res* 214:349, 1981.
142. Rossor MN, Rehfeld JF, Emson PC, et al: Normal cortical concentration of cholecystokinin-like immunoreactivity with reduced choline acetyltransferase activity in senile dementia of Alzheimer type. *Life Sci* 29:405, 1981.
143. Rossor MN, Svendsen C, Hunt SP, et al: The substantia innominata in Alzheimer's disease: An histochemical and biochemical study of cholinergic marker enzymes. *Neurosci Lett* 28:217, 1982.
144. Roth J, LeRoith D, Schiloach J, et al: The evolutionary origins of hormones, neurotransmitters, and other extracellular chemical messengers. *N Engl J Med* 306:523, 1982.
145. Roth J, LeRoith D, Shiloach J, et al: Intercellular communication: An attempt at a unifying hypothesis. *Clin Res* 31:354, 1983.
146. Saavedra JM, Palkovits M, Brownstein MJ, et al: Serotonin distribution of the nuclei of the rat hypothalamus and preoptic region. *Brain Res* 77:157, 1974.
147. Sawchenko PE, Swanson LW: Immunohistochemical identification of neurons in the paraventricular nucleus of the hypothalamus that project to the medulla or to the spinal cord in the rat. *J Comp Neurol* 205:260, 1982.
148. Schally AV: Aspects of hypothalamic regulation of the pituitary gland: Its implications for the control of reproductive processes. *Science* 202:18, 1978.
149. Scharrer E, Scharrer B: Secretory cells within the hypothalamus. *Res Publ Assoc Res Nerv Ment Dis* 20:170, 1939.
150. Scharrer E, Scharrer B: Neuroendocrinology. New York, Columbia University Press, 1963.
151. Schmale H, Richter D: Immunological identification of a common precursor to arginine, vasopressin, and neurophysin II synthesized by in vitro translation of bovine hypothalamic mRNA. *Proc Natl Acad Sci USA* 78:766, 1981.
152. Scott DE, Kozlowski GP, Sheriden MN: Scanning electron microscopy in the ultrastructural analysis of the mammalian cerebral ventricular system. *Int Rev Cytol* 37:349, 1974.
153. Seidman CE, Duby AD, Choi E, et al: The structure of a rat preproatrial natriuretic factor as defined by a complementary DNA clone. *Science* 225:324, 1984.
154. Shambaugh GE III, Wilber JF, Montoya E, et al: Thyrotropin-releasing hormone (TRH): Measurements in human spinal fluid. *J Clin Endocrinol Metab* 41:131, 1975.
155. Share L: Vasopressin and cardiovascular regulation: Introduction. *Fed Proc* 43:78, 1984.
156. Snyder SH: Drug and neurotransmitter receptors in the brain. *Science* 224:22, 1984.
157. Sofroniew MV, Weindl A: Extrahypothalamic neurophysin-containing perikarya, fiber pathways and fiber clusters in the rat brain. *Endocrinology* 102:334, 1978.
158. Sørensen KV: Somatostatin: Localization and distribution in the cortex and the subcortical white matter of the human brain. *Neuroscience* 7:1227, 1982.
159. Sørensen KV, Christensen SE, Dupont E, et al: Low somatostatin content in cerebrospinal fluid in multiple sclerosis. *Acta Neurol Scand* 61:186, 1980.
160. Sørensen KV, Christensen SE, Hansen AP, et al: The origin of cerebrospinal fluid somatostatin: Hypothalamic or disperse central nervous system secretion? *Neuroendocrinology* 32:335, 1981.
161. Sourkes TL: Parkinson's disease and other disorders of the basal ganglia, in Siegel GJ, Albers RW, Agranoff BW, et al (eds): *Basic Neurochemistry,* ed 3. Boston, Little, Brown & Co Inc, 1981.
162. Spindel ER, Wurtman RJ, Bird ED: Increased TRH content of the basal ganglia in Huntington's disease. *N Engl J Med* 303:1235, 1980.
163. Spokes EGS: Neurochemical alterations in Huntington's chorea: A study of post-mortem brain tissue. *Brain* 103:179, 1980.

164. Struble RG, Cork LC, Whitehouse PJ, et al: Cholinergic innervation in neuritic plaques. *Science* 216:413, 1982.
165. Studler JM, Javoy-Agid F, Cesselin F, et al: CCK-8-immunoreactivity distribution in human brain: Selective decrease in the substantia nigra from parkinsonian patients. *Brain Res* 243:176, 1982.
166. Vale W, Spiess J, Rivier C, et al: Characterization of a 41-residue ovine hypothalamic peptide that stimulates secretion of corticotropin and β-endorphin. *Science* 213:1394, 1981.
167. Valverde-r C, Chieffo V, Reichlin S: Prolactin-releasing factor in porcine and rat hypothalamic tissue. *Endocrinology* 91:982, 1972.
168. Verney EB: Croonian lecture: The antidiuretic hormone and the factors which determine its release. *Proc R Soc Lond* 135:25, 1947.
169. Von Euler US, Gaddum JH: An unidentified depressor substance in certain tissue extracts. *J Physiol* 72:74, 1931.
170. Vorsattel JP, Myers RH, Stevens TJ, et al: Neuropathologic classification of Huntington's disease. *J Neuropathol Exp Neurol* (submitted 1985).
171. Werner S, Hulting AL, Hökfelt T, et al: Effect of the peptide PHI-27 on prolactin release in vitro. *Neuroendocrinology* 37:476, 1983.
172. Whitehouse PJ, Price DL, Struble RG, et al: Alzheimer's disease and senile dementia: Loss of neurons in the basal forebrain. *Science* 215:1237, 1982.
173. Wiegand SJ, Price JL: Cells of origin of the afferent fibers to the median eminence in the rat. *J Comp Neurol* 192:1, 1980.
174. Wislocki GB, King LS: The permeability of the hypophysis and hypothalamus to vital dyes, with a study of the hypophyseal vascular supply. *Am J Anat* 58:421, 1936.
175. Wood PL, Etienne P, Lal S, et al: Reduced lumbar CSF somatostatin levels of Alzheimer's disease. *Life Sci* 31:2073, 1982.
176. Wurtman RJ, Anton-Tay F: The mammalian pineal as a neuroendocrine transducer. *Recent Prog Horm Res* 25:493, 1969.
177. Wurtman RJ, Fernstrom JD: L-tryptophan, L-tyrosine, and the control of brain monoamine biosynthesis, in Snyder SH (ed): *Perspectives in Neuropharmacology: A Tribute to Julius Axelrod*. New York, Oxford University press Inc, 1972.
178. Zimmerman EA: Localization of hypothalamic hormones by immunocytochemical techniques, in Martini L, Ganong WF (eds): *Frontiers in Neuroendocrinology*. 4:25, 1976.
179. Zimmerman EA, Hou-Yu A, Nilaver G, et al: Anatomy of pituitary and extrapituitary vasopressin secretory systems, in Reichlin S (ed): *The Neurohypophysis: Physiological and Clinical Aspects*. New York, Plenum Medical Book Co, 1984.

CHAPTER 3

Pathology of the pituitary gland and sellar region

Normal histology
Normal electron microscopy
Immunologic staining
Frozen section diagnosis
Neoplastic disorders: pituitary origin
   Pituitary adenomas
      Prolactin cell adenoma
      Growth hormone cell adenoma
      Mixed prolactin cell–growth hormone cell adenomas
      Acidophilic stem cell adenomas
      Mammosomatotroph cell adenomas
      Corticotroph cell adenomas
      Gonadotroph cell adenomas
      Thyrotroph cell adenomas
      Plurihormonal adenomas
      Null cell adenomas
      Secondary changes in pituitary adenomas
        Hemorrhage and infarction
        Calcification
        Amyloid
        Bromocriptine-induced changes
   Invasive pituitary adenomas

   Ectopic pituitary adenomas
   Primary malignant tumors of the pituitary
   Granular cell tumors
   Craniopharyngiomas
Neoplastic disorders: nonpituitary origin
   Meningiomas
   Hypothalamic and optic gliomas
   Chordomas
   Dermoid and epidermoid cysts
   Germinomas and teratoid tumors
   Lipomas
   Other neoplasms
   Pituitary metastases
Non-neoplastic disorders
   Sellar and suprasellar cysts
   Aneurysms and other vascular malformations
Inflammatory disorders
   Pituitary abscess
   Sarcoidosis
   Histiocytosis X
   Lymphocytic hypophysitis

NORMAL HISTOLOGY

Using light microscopy and acidic and basic dyes, one can identify three types of cells in the anterior pituitary[14,55,131,213]: acidophilic, basophilic, and chromophobic cells, which comprise approximately 40%, 10%, and 50%, respectively, of the anterior pituitary cells.[204] The basophilic cells are also periodic acid–Schiff (PAS)-positive resulting from the presence of groups that can be oxidized to aldehyde by periodic acid. They contain either adrenocorticotropic hormone ([ACTH] corticotrophs), follicle-stimulating hormone–luteinizing hormone ([FSH-LH] gonadotrophs), or thyroid-stimulating hormone ([TSH] thyrotrophs). Corticotrophs and thyrotrophs are distributed mainly in a midline zone of the pars distalis known as the "mucoid wedge." Gonadotrophs are located at random throughout the anterior lobe. The acidophilic cells are PAS-negative and contain either growth hormone ([GH] somatotrophs) or prolactin ([PRL] lactotrophs). Somatotrophs predominate in the lateral "acidophilic wings" of the pars distalis. Lactotrophs are everywhere, predominating in the posteromedial and posterolateral edges, close to the posterior lobe. This regional division is somewhat artificial, and these cells are not completely restricted in their geographic distribution. The color in these cells is caused by staining of secretory granules, free hormone, or prehormone. Herlant's erythrosin[90] and Brookes' carmoisine[23] stains are useful in differentiating the two types of acidophilic cells. Both erythrosin and carmoisine were assumed to selectively stain secretory granules of prolactin cells. However, these techniques have become less valuable since the introduction of immunostaining techniques.

Chromophobic cells were initially thought to be inactive. However, electron microscopy, immunocytochemistry, and clinical correlation with chromophobic adenomas have shown that the majority of chromophobic adenomas are in fact endocrine active.[151] Using light microscopy, there is no absolute way to differentiate active from inactive chromophobic cells. All chromophobic cells contain secretory granules that are demonstrated by electron microscopy.

Aggregates of basophilic cells are frequently seen extending into the neurohypophysis from its border with the pars intermedia. These cells have been shown to be corticotrophs that produce ACTH, beta-lipotropin (β-LPH), and endorphin.

The pars intermedia is usually vestigial in the human and represented by a microscopic cleft lined by cuboid or columnar-ciliated or mucin-producing epithelial cells. Lymphocytes may be seen in this area. Some cells of the pars intermedia contain ACTH, melanocyte stimulating hormone (MSH), and other portions of the proopiocortin molecule as determined by the immunoperoxidase technique.[30]

The pars tuberalis is an extension of the pars distalis along the pituitary stalk. It is composed of gonadotrophs, corticotrophs, and thyrotrophs (primarily the former).[6]

Cells of the adenohypophysis are arranged in cords separated by a basement membrane with reticulin-rich connective tissue between cords and capillaries. Most adenohypophysial cells are in close proximity to capillaries that are lined by fenestrated endothelial cells, a relationship that may be important to the secretory process.[204]

NORMAL ELECTRON MICROSCOPY

Ultrastructural features of anterior pituitary cells are characteristic for different cells and add a new dimension in their recognition. By electron microscopy, it can be seen that cells of the pars distalis have round to oval nuclei with a single nucleolus.[57,94] There is a moderate amount of cytoplasm and a well-developed rough endoplasmic reticulum (RER) and Golgi apparatus. Of particular importance are the membrane-bound, dense-core secretory granules that are found in all cells. Some secretory granules have distinct ultrastructural features; these are, however, not sufficiently characteristic to permit the identification of hormones that the cells produce. Although the ultrastructural features can distinguish be-

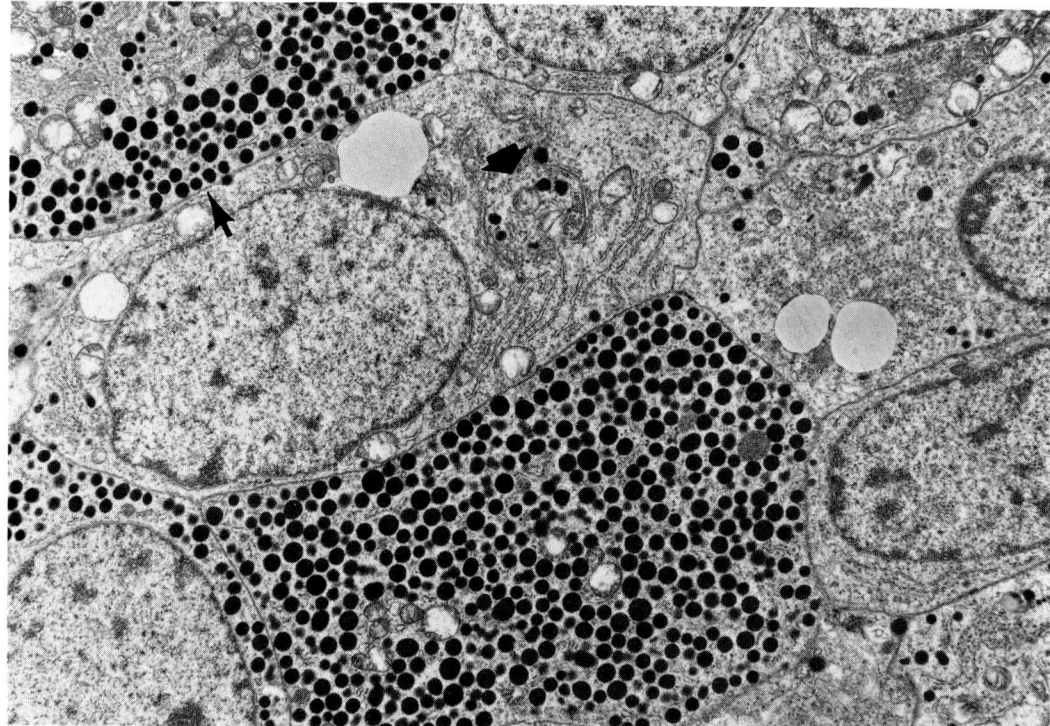

Fig. 3-1. Group of normal prolactin cells. Note well-developed lamellar RER, Golgi complex with developing granules (thick *arrow*) and granule extrusion (thin *arrow*). M × 8900.

tween resting cells and actively-secreting cells, the immunoperoxidase technique is more accurate and reliable in cell identification. Ultrastructural characteristics of each normal cell type are illustrated in Figs. 3-1 to 3-6.

IMMUNOLOGIC STAINING

Isolation and purification of the pituitary hormones have led to the development of antibodies directed against them. Various techniques have been developed to visualize cells containing a given hormone by coupling the appropriate antibody with microscopically visible substances. The most commonly used technique is the immunoperoxidase method in which sheep antirabbit globulin is coupled to peroxidase. The peroxidase is then visualized by a 3,3'diaminobenzidine. This technique is sensitive; it can be applied at light and electron microscopic levels, and it can be performed on formalin-fixed, paraffin-embedded material. Recently the avidin-biotin-peroxidase complex technique has been introduced; it appears to be more sensitive and eliminates nonspecific back-

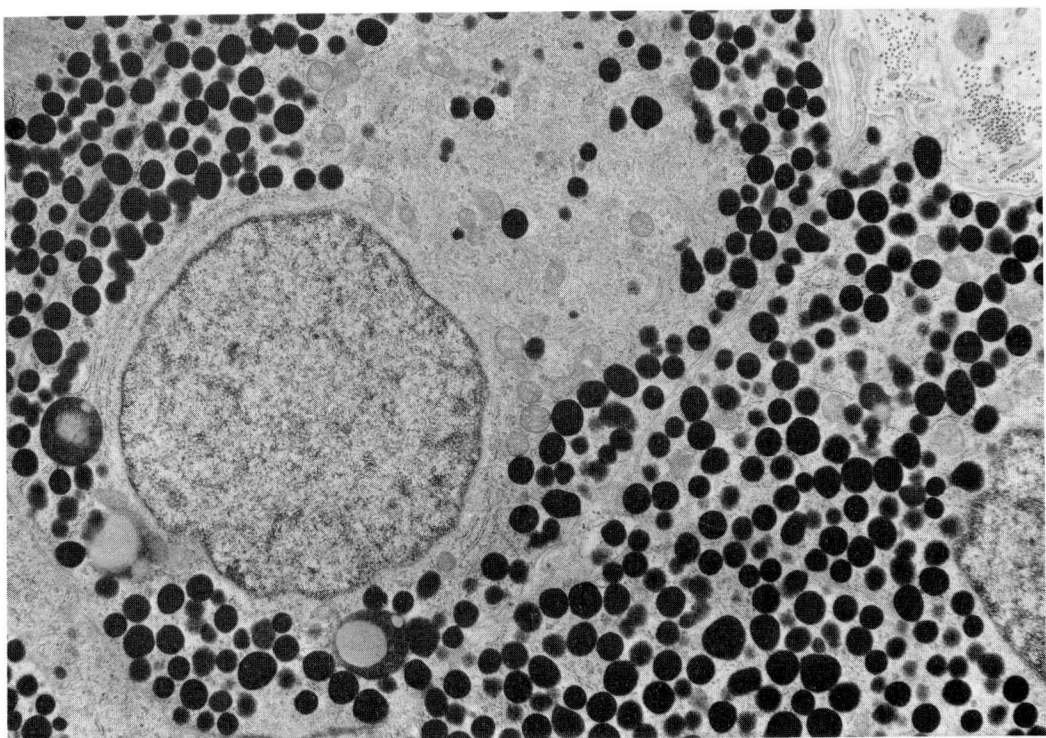

Fig. 3-2. Normal growth hormone cells containing spherical nucleus; well-organized RER; well-developed Golgi apparatus; and numerous large, dense, spherical, secretory granules. M × 10,700.

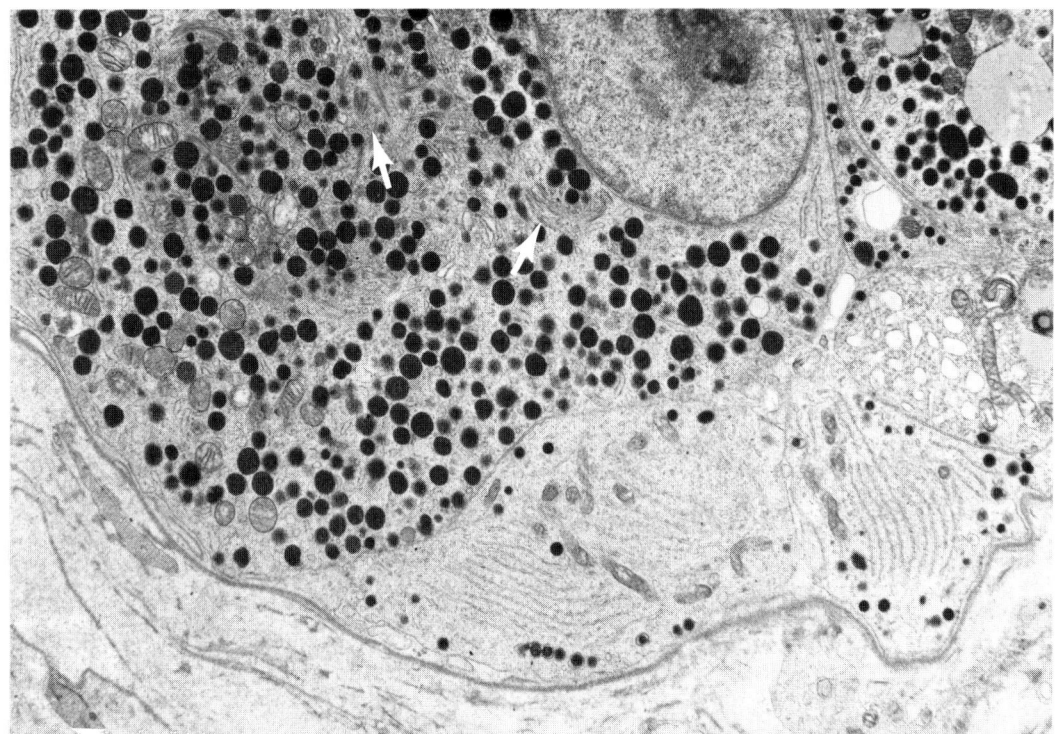

Fig. 3-3. Corticotroph cell. Secretory granules vary in electron density; some are irregular in shape. Note bundles of type I microfilaments *(arrow)*, ultrastructural marker of human corticotroph. M × 11,000.

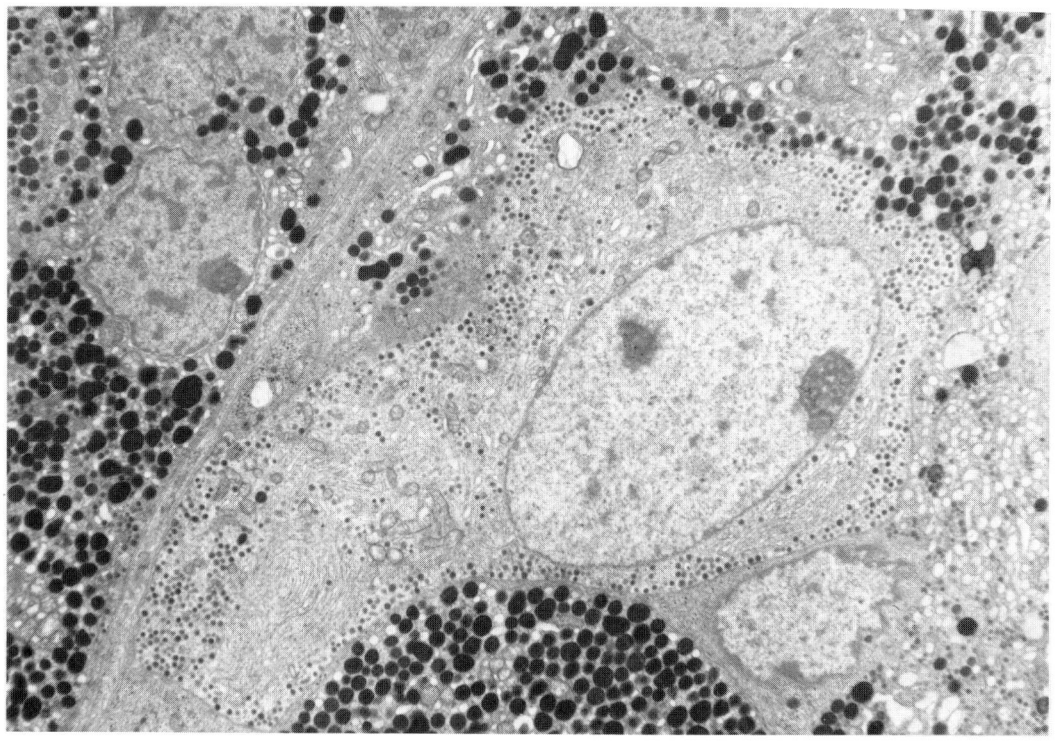

Fig. 3-4. Thyrotroph cell surrounded by growth hormone cells. Profiles of well-developed RER are slightly dilated; small secretory granules tend to accumulate at periphery of angular cell body. M × 5800.

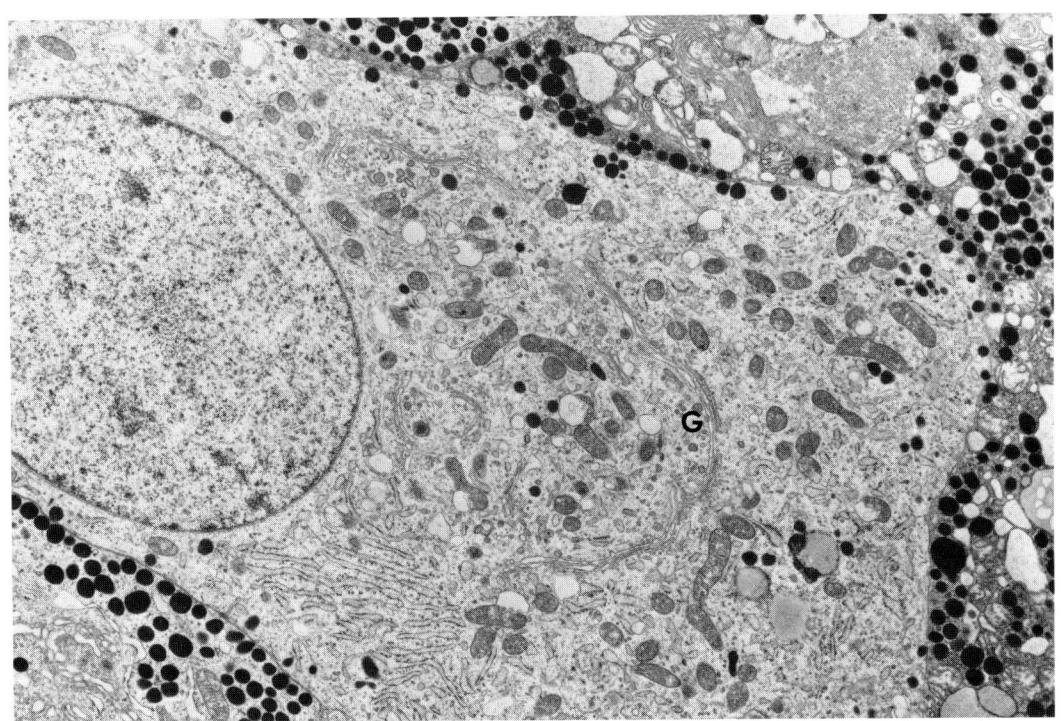

Fig. 3-5. Actively secreting gonadotroph cell in pituitary of previously ovariectomized woman. Evenly dilated, abundant RER contains fine granular substance of low electron density; prominent Golgi complex *(G)* harbors developing granules. M × 8900.

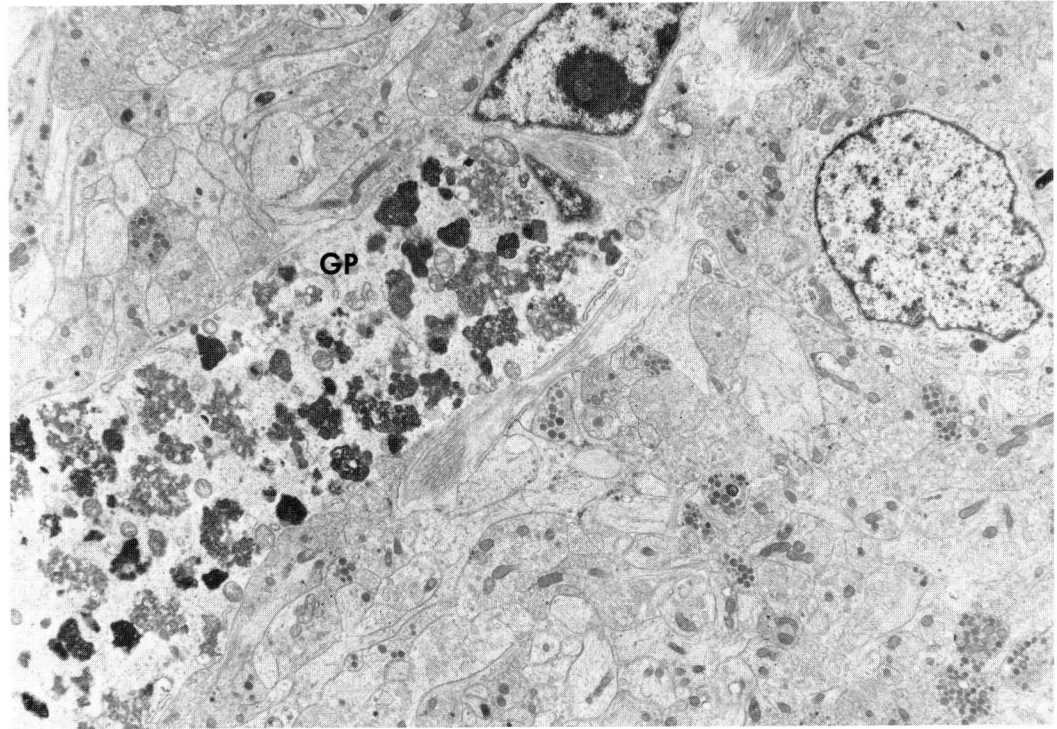

Fig. 3-6. Fine structural appearance of posterior lobe of human pituitary. Note part of granular pituicyte *(GP)*. M × 9380.

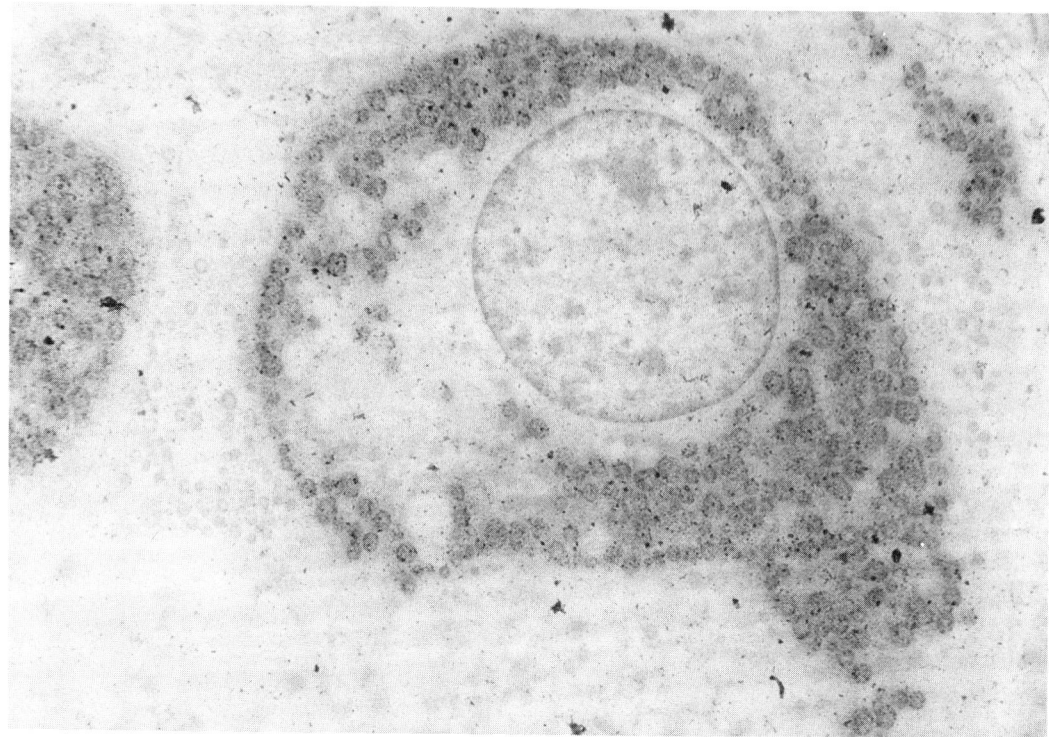

Fig. 3-7. Immunoreactive growth hormone is demonstrated in secretory granules of growth hormone cell by immunoelectron microscopy. M × 10,200.

ground staining better than the previously used immunoperoxidase technique.[102,103]

Immunologic staining is the most accurate method available for determining which hormones are present in normal or neoplastic pituitary cells and in assessing the cytogenesis of tumors (Fig. 3-7). Application of this method has emphasized the fact that traditional light microscopic staining methods are inaccurate in identifying the hormone content of normal and neoplastic pituitary cells. Many cells that are chromophobic by histochemical techniques will prove to contain prolactin, growth hormone, ACTH, or the glycoprotein hormones.

FROZEN SECTION DIAGNOSIS

Rapid frozen section determination of a surgical pathology specimen is often helpful to the neurosurgeon. The purpose is to identify the histology of the tissue removed and to supply this information to the operating surgeon so that the most appropriate operation can be achieved. Communication between the pathologist and surgeon before, during, or, at times, after the operation enhances the effectiveness of the procedure. Misleading results are often a result of sampling error, poor tissue preservation, or inadequate technique, including sectioning and staining.

The surgical specimen received by the pathologist is frequently only one to a few millimeters in width, especially if obtained transsphenoidally. It should be kept wet and placed on a cut piece of rubber such as a surgeon's glove and wrapped in a towel with an attached identification label. Much of the soft adenoma will be soaked up and lost or compressed if put on a piece of dry paper, towel or cotton pattie. The powder on surgical gloves produces an annoying artifact for the pathologist and should be rinsed off before use. After taking a small piece for electron microscopy, the specimen is ready to be frozen in a cryostat kept at $-20°$ C. A small stage or mount made up of an embedding medium for frozen sections is prepared on a chuck inside the cryostat and frozen. Sections are then cut to 3 or 4 microns thickness. A very sharp knife is important for cutting thin sections. The knife edge is wiped clean after each cut with 4- by 4-inch gauze sponges kept cold in the cryostat to prevent warming of the knife. The slides are then stained with hematoxylin and eosin (H & E) or toluidine blue (0.7% solution). The H & E stain is begun first, since it takes 3 minutes to complete, whereas the toluidine blue requires 1.5 minutes.

We believe that the frozen section diagnosis plays an important role in the operative procedure. This is especially true in cases where a microadenoma is not apparent and subtle changes of hyperplasia cannot be readily differentiated from normal gland. The frozen section report is also invaluable in cases in which other neoplasms or inflammatory disorders mimic a pituitary adenoma clinically and radiographically.

NEOPLASTIC DISORDERS: PITUITARY ORIGIN

The region of the pituitary gland and sella turcica include a variety of tissue types in close proximity. The intimate relationship of neural, endocrine, vascular, meningeal, and skeletal structures provides a myriad of pathologic possibilities in a small anatomic area. Many of these pathologic entities are listed as follows:

Neoplastic disorders
  Pituitary adenohypophysial origin
    Pituitary adenomas
    Carcinomas
  Pituitary nonadenohypophysial origin
    Sarcomas
    Granular cell tumors
    Craniopharyngiomas
  Nonpituitary origin
    Meningiomas
    Hypothalamic and optic gliomas
    Chordomas
    Dermoid and epidermoid cysts
    Teratomas and teratoid tumors
      including germinomas
    Lipomas
    Melanomas
    Paragangliomas
    Gangliocytomas

  Nonpituitary origin *(cont'd)*
    Chondromas
    Hemangioblastomas
    Olfactory neuroblastomas
    Lymphoproliferative disorders
    Tumors of skeletal origin
    Metastases
Non-neoplastic disorders
  Non-neoplastic cysts
    Rathke's pouch cysts
    Mucoceles
    Arachnoid cysts
    Aneurysms and other vascular
      malformations
  Inflammatory disorders
    Abscesses
    Sarcoidosis
    Histiocytosis X
    Lymphocytic hypophysitis

Pituitary adenomas

As with normal pituitary cells, classification of pituitary adenomas on the basis of their tinctorial affinity for acidic or basic dyes does not correlate with function. Traditionally, pituitary adenomas have been classified as acidophilic, basophilic, or chromophobic. Acidophilic adenomas were assumed to secrete growth hormone, causing acromegaly or gigantism. Basophilic adenomas were thought to secrete ACTH and cause Cushing's disease or Nelson's syndrome. The chromophobic adenomas were regarded as being hormonally inactive. This classification is of limited usefulness because it does not consider structure-function relationships or provide information on the cytogenesis or behavior of the tumors. To be of value, a morphologic classification of pituitary tumors requires the use of immunocytology and electron microscopy. Immunocytochemical studies will verify the presence of immunoreactive hormones in tumor cells. Using electron microscopy and special histochemical staining techniques, one can distinguish cytoplasmic granules in all chromophobic tumors.

A useful classification of pituitary tumors was developed by Horvath and Kovacs[93]:

> Prolactin cell adenomas
>   Sparsely granulated
>   Densely granulated
> Growth hormone cell adenomas
>   Sparsely granulated
>   Densely granulated
> Mixed prolactin cell–growth hormone cell adenomas
> Acidophilic stem cell adenomas
> Mammosomatotroph cell adenomas
> Corticotroph cell adenomas
>   Sparsely granulated
>   Densely granulated
> Gonadotroph cell adenomas
> Thyrotroph cell adenomas
> Plurihormonal adenomas
> Null cell adenomas
>   Oncocytomas

This scheme is based on the immunocytologic findings (i.e., presence of immunoreactive hormones stored in cell cytoplasm). It relies on the ultrastructural features of adenoma cells and attempts to identify the cell type from which the tumor derives. In addition, it aims to correlate the morphologic findings of the tumor with the clinical history of the patient, biochemical results, biologic behavior, and endocrine activity. In the following pages, their classification is described in some detail.

Prolactin cell adenoma. Prolactin cell adenomas (prolactinomas) occur in both sparsely granulated and densely granulated forms, the sparsely granulated variety being far more common. The densely granulated tumors are acidophilic by light microscopy and show positivity with Brookes' carmoisine or Herlant's erythrosin stains. The more common sparsely granulated prolactinomas are chromophobic as demonstrated by light microscopy. They are PAS- and lead hematoxylin–negative, and only a few cytoplasmic granules faintly stain with various acid dyes. Secretory granules can usually be identified by Herlant's erythrosin or Brookes' carmoisine techniques.

The immunoperoxidase technique is of great importance in establishing the diagnosis, since immunoreactive prolactin can be conclusively demonstrated.[121,124] Immunoperoxidase stains are strongly positive in the densely granulated prolactinomas. In the sparsely granulated prolactinomas, prolactin immunostaining is strong in the Golgi complexes despite the paucity of secretory granules.

By electron microscopy, the unusual densely granulated variant simulates the normal resting lactotroph (Fig. 3-8).* The adenoma cells are oval with oval nuclei and abundant cytoplasm. The rough endoplasmic reticulum is well developed, and Golgi complexes are prominent. The secretory granules are of a characteristic size and shape. They are oval or irregular, highly electron dense, and quite large, measuring up to 1200 nm in diameter with an average of 600 nm.

---

*See references 58,92,121,123,124,134, and 179.

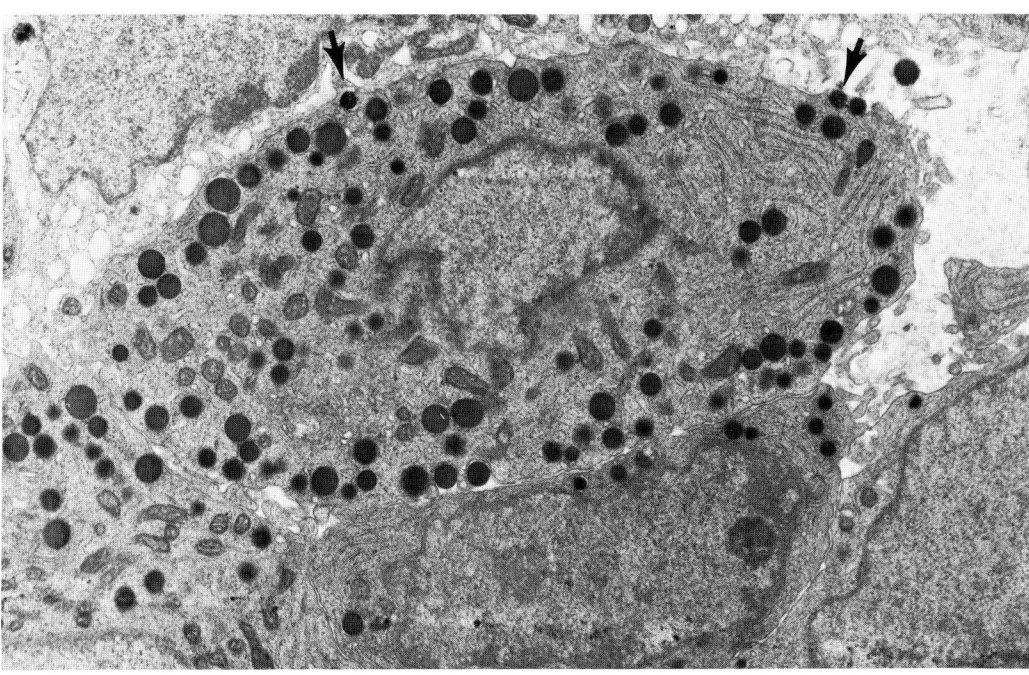

Fig. 3-8. Densely granulated prolactin cell adenoma. Relatively small, elongated cells with well-developed RER and Golgi complex, possess numerous large, dense secretory granules often engaged in exocytosis *(arrow)*. M × 7200.

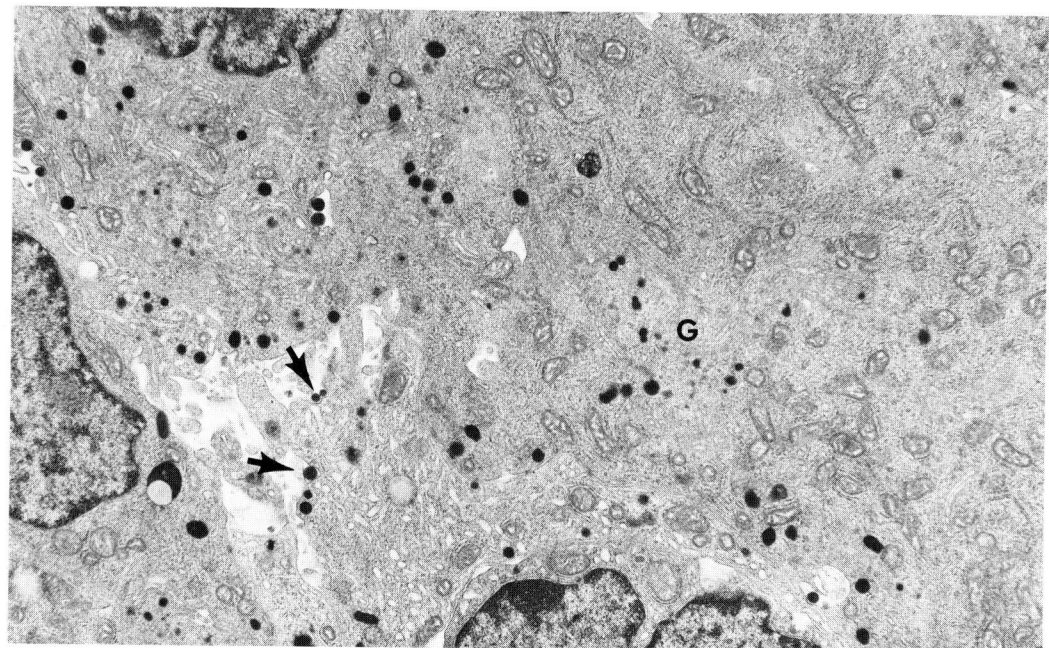

Fig. 3-9. Sparsely granulated prolactin cell adenoma consisting of irregular cells with abundant RER and prominent Golgi apparatus containing granules *(G)*. Secretory granules are sparse and rather small (150 to 250 nm). Note extrusion sites *(arrows)*. M × 11,000.

Electron microscopy of sparsely granulated prolactinomas discloses characteristic fine structural features (Fig. 3-9).* Adenoma cells are polyhedral with irregular nuclei, welldeveloped cytoplasm, and conspicuous Golgi complexes. The rough endoplasmic reticulum is prominent and frequently forms elaborate concentric whorls known as "Nebenkern" formations. The secretory granules are round, oval, or irregular and more sparse and much smaller than those seen in densely granulated prolactin-producing adenomas. They measure 150 to 500 nm in diameter with an average of 200 to 300 nm. Another diagnostic ultrastructural feature of this adenoma type is the presence of misplaced granule exocytoses.[92] In the normal pituitary, prolactin granule exocytosis occurs mainly at the vascular pole of the cell. Misplaced exocytoses, seen in this adenoma type and to a lesser extent in the densely granulated prolactinoma, occurs on the lateral side of the cells, away from capillaries and from intercellular extensions of the basement membranes. The cells of sparsely granulated prolactinomas show ultrastructural signs of high secretory activity and resemble cells found in the pituitary glands of women in late pregnancy and the early postpartum period, in the pituitary of lactating or estrogen-treated rats, and in the glands of men receiving estrogen therapy for carcinoma of the prostate.[106,144]

---

*See references 58,92,95,121,123,124,134,187, and 211.

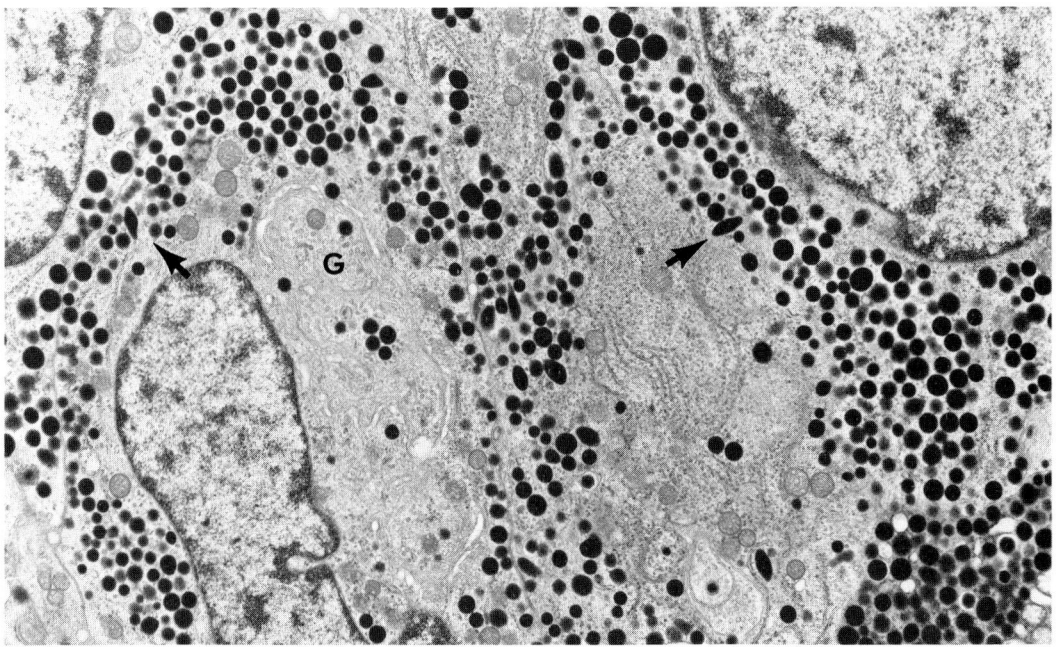

Fig. 3-10. Densely granulated growth hormone cell adenoma characterized by well-developed RER and Golgi complex *(G)* and numerous large, dense, spherical, secretory granules. Elongated, rhomboid granules *(arrows)* occur occasionally in this tumor type. M × 8700.

Growth hormone cell adenoma. As with the prolactinomas, growth hormone cell adenomas occur in both sparsely and densely granulated forms. Unlike the prolactinoma, however, the sparsely and densely granulated varieties occur with nearly equal frequency. The cells of densely granulated adenomas are acidophilic by light microscopy, and their cytoplasm stains positive with various acidic dyes such as eosin, phloxine, orange G, or light green. PAS and basic stains are uniformly negative. The sparsely granulated growth hormone cell adenomas are chromophobic by light microscopy. The cells are PAS- and lead hematoxylin–negative, and there is no staining with acidic dyes except for a few cytoplasmic granules, which may show positivity. The immunoperoxidase technique reveals the presence of growth hormone in the cytoplasm of the adenoma cells of each variety, confirming that these tumors are derived from growth hormone cells.[94,124]

Ultrastructurally, cells of densely granulated adenomas resemble nontumorous growth hormone cells with round, centrally located nuclei, well-developed cytoplasm, rough endoplasmic reticulum, and Golgi complexes. There are numerous spherical, electron-dense secretory granules measuring 300 to 600 nm (Fig. 3-10).*

---

*See references 92,118,124,133,134,203,205, and 216.

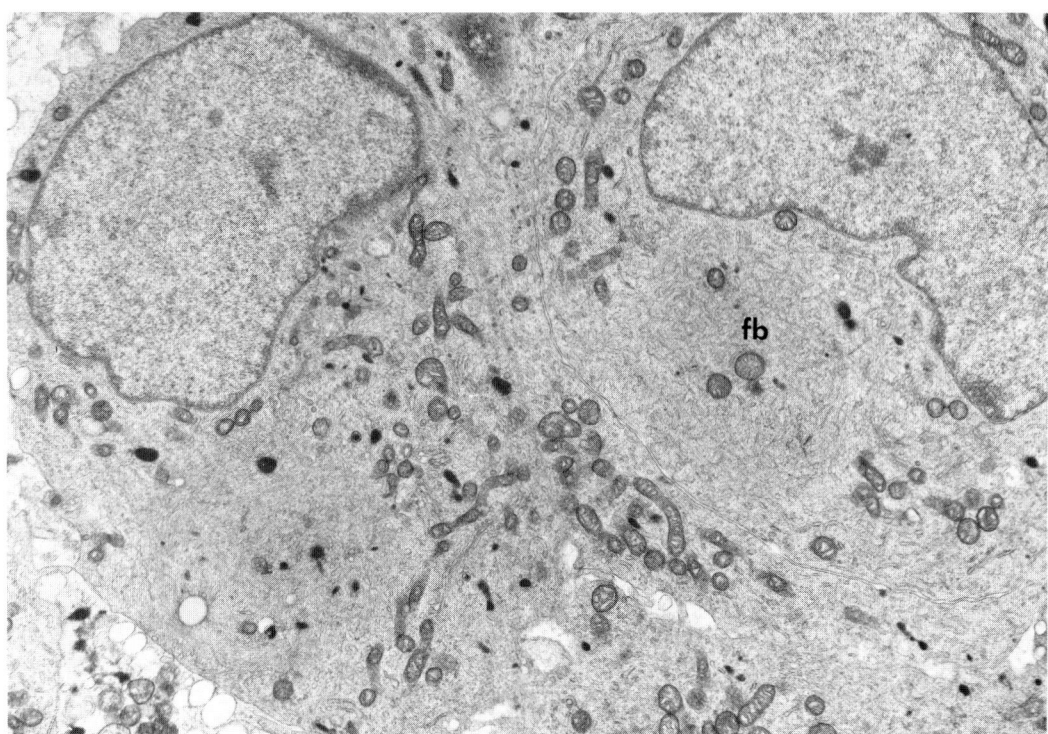

Fig. 3-11. Sparsely granulated growth hormone cell adenoma containing numerous fibrous bodies *(fb)*, located at concave side of crescent-shaped nucleus. Secretory granules are sparse and small. M × 9400.

Sparsely granulated adenomas differ from normal somatotrophs (Fig. 3-11). The cells vary in size, are irregular, and have irregular nuclei. There may be considerable cellular and nuclear pleomorphism.[94] The rough endoplasmic reticulum and Golgi complexes are well developed, and there may be marked abundance of the smooth endoplasmic reticulum. The secretory granules are small in number and size, measuring 100 to 300 nm. Some characteristic ultrastructural features of sparsely granulated growth hormone cell adenomas have been identified. The most distinctive is the appearance of paranuclear "fibrous bodies" located on the concave side of the indented nucleus and composed of 115 nm type II microfilaments.[129,216] These structures appear in mixed prolactin cell–growth hormone cell adenomas, acidophilic stem cell adenomas, and sparsely granulated growth hormone cell adenomas, indicating their reliability as a diagnostic feature of somatotropic adenoma cells. Intracytoplasmic supernumerary centrioles and cilia occur frequently in sparsely granulated growth hormone cell adenomas.[94,96] Tubular inclusions are found not in the adenoma cells but in the endothelial cells of blood vessels. Such inclusions in endothelial cells have been described in a variety of conditions (i.e., viral infections, autoimmune diseases, neoplasms including other adenomas). These inclusions are composed of a DNA core with a protein coat, but the presence of a virus has not been demonstrated and their significance is unknown.

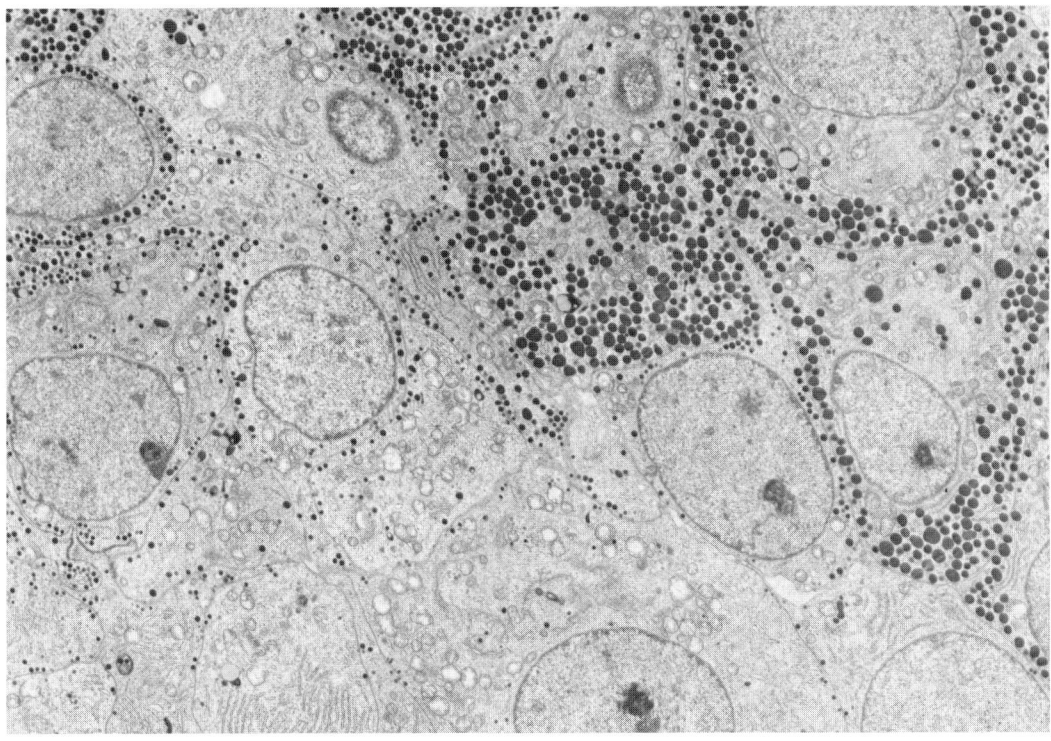

Fig. 3-12. Mixed pituitary adenoma consisting of densely granulated growth hormone cells *(upper right)* and sparsely granulated prolactin cells *(lower left)*. M × 4600.

Mixed prolactin cell–growth hormone cell adenomas. This is the only regularly occurring pituitary adenoma composed of two separate adenohypophysial cells. These tumors are composed of two distinct cell types: growth hormone cells and prolactin cells. They are associated with elevated growth hormone levels and acromegaly or gigantism. The serum prolactin levels may also be elevated with or without associated symptoms. These mixed tumors cannot be diagnosed clinically, since any pituitary tumor can cause hyperprolactinemia by interference with the synthesis, release, delivery, or action of prolactin-inhibiting factor (PIF). Therefore morphologic identity of both growth hormone and prolactin adenoma cells is essential to make the diagnosis.

By light microscopy, mixed adenomas range from acidophilic to chromophobic.* Variable positivity is seen with Brookes' carmoisine and Herlant's erythrosin stains. These tumors are PAS-negative. The immunoperoxidase technique demonstrates growth hormone in the cytoplasm of some adenoma cells and prolactin in others.

The ultrastructural features of the tumor cells are identical to those of the adenoma cells in growth hormone cell or prolactin cell adenomas (Fig. 3-12).

---

*See references 36,58,86,93,94, and 124.

Every combination of densely and sparsely granulated prolactin and growth hormone adenoma cells may be seen. Cells of the same cell type often form groups of variable size. The ultrastructural features of the growth hormone cells do not correlate with the growth hormone blood levels. However, elevated serum prolactin levels seem to be associated with those tumors that are sparsely granulated and have well-developed rough endoplasmic reticulum and prominent Golgi complexes. On the other hand, in patients with tumors composed of densely granulated prolactin cells, the serum prolactin levels are only slightly elevated or within the normal range.

Acidophilic stem cell adenomas. Unlike the mixed growth hormone-prolactin cell adenomas, which are composed of mature cells of both types, the acidophilic stem cell adenomas are made up of a single type of immature cell that has characteristics of both sparsely granulated growth hormone cells and prolactin cells.[58,99,122,124] These immature or "stem" cells are believed to be a precursor of the two types of acidophilic cells. The same cells have been identified in the normal pituitary gland. Patients that harbor such tumors usually do not have the clinical features of acromegaly and present as having nonfunctional lesions.

By light microscopy, the tumors are chromophobic, although in some cases occasional granules are seen by Herlant's erythrosin or Brookes' carmoisine methods. The adenoma cells are negative with acidic dyes and PAS. The immunoperoxidase technique reveals the presence of growth hormone or prolactin in the cytoplasm of some cells. Occasionally, both prolactin and growth hormone are seen in the same cells, further supporting the notion of a hybrid nature of the cells.

Some of the ultrastructural features of the tumor cells are characteristic of both growth hormone and prolactin cell adenomas (Fig. 3-13). Many cells possess cytoplasmic fibrous bodies and multiple centrioles seen in growth hormone cell adenomas plus misplaced exocytoses[92] characteristic of prolactin cell adenomas. The adenoma cells are elongated, are closely opposed, and have irregular nuclei. The Golgi apparatus is inconspicuous. The rough endoplasmic reticulum may be abundant in some cells and usually consists of dispersed short profiles. There may be an increased volume density of mitochondria indicating oncocytic transformation.[96] The secretory granules are sparse, spherical to irregular, electron dense, and measure 150 to 300 nm.

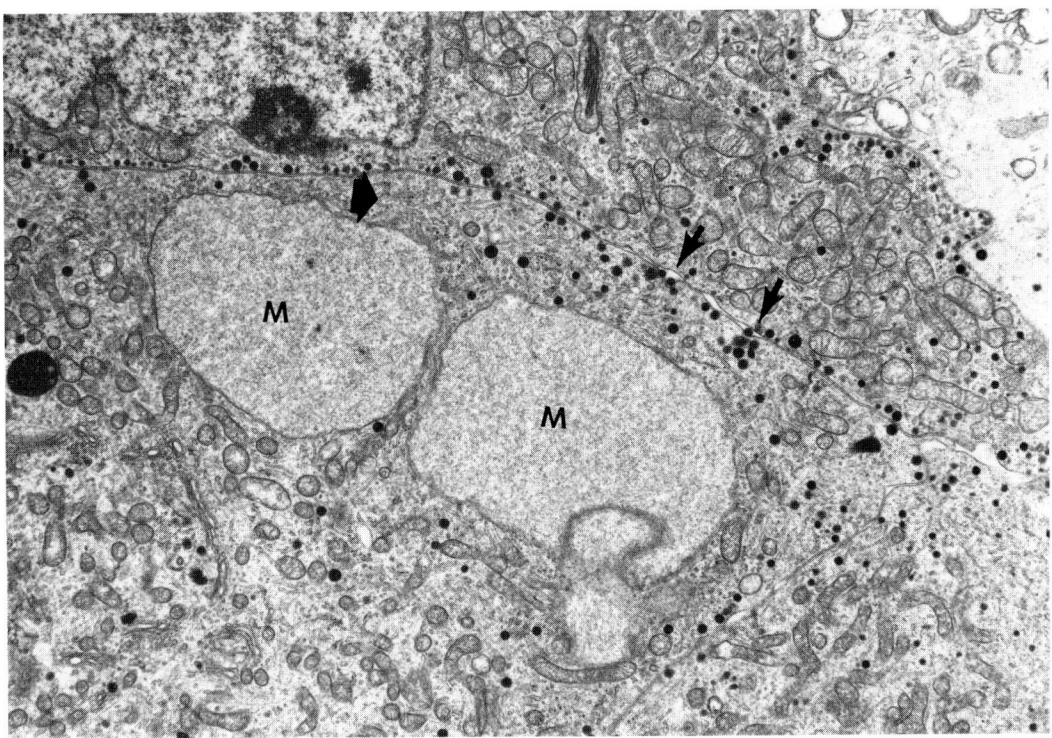

Fig. 3-13. Acidophil stem cell adenoma. Oncocytic tumor harbors several giant mitochondria *(M)*. Note smooth endoplasmic reticulum (SER) tubules under plasmalemma (thick *arrow*) and exocytoses (thin *arrows*). M × 6300.

Mammosomatotroph cell adenoma. Mammosomatotroph cell adenomas, like the mixed prolactin cell–growth hormone cell adenomas and the acidophil stem cell adenomas, are capable of producing both growth hormone and prolactin. Mammosomatotroph cell adenomas occur mostly in men and are invariably associated with acromegaly (or gigantism) and only slightly to moderately elevated serum prolactin levels. The majority are well-circumscribed intrasellar lesions that are well differentiated and slow growing. The clinical presentation and morphologic characteristics of mammosomatotroph cell adenomas have been described by Horvath et al.[97]

By light microscopy, the tumors are usually acidophilic and more rarely chromophobic. They are PAS-negative. The immunoperoxidase technique detects both growth hormone and prolactin within the same cells. Although GH is detected in all cases, the percentage of prolactin cells varies not only from case to case but also in different areas of the same cell.

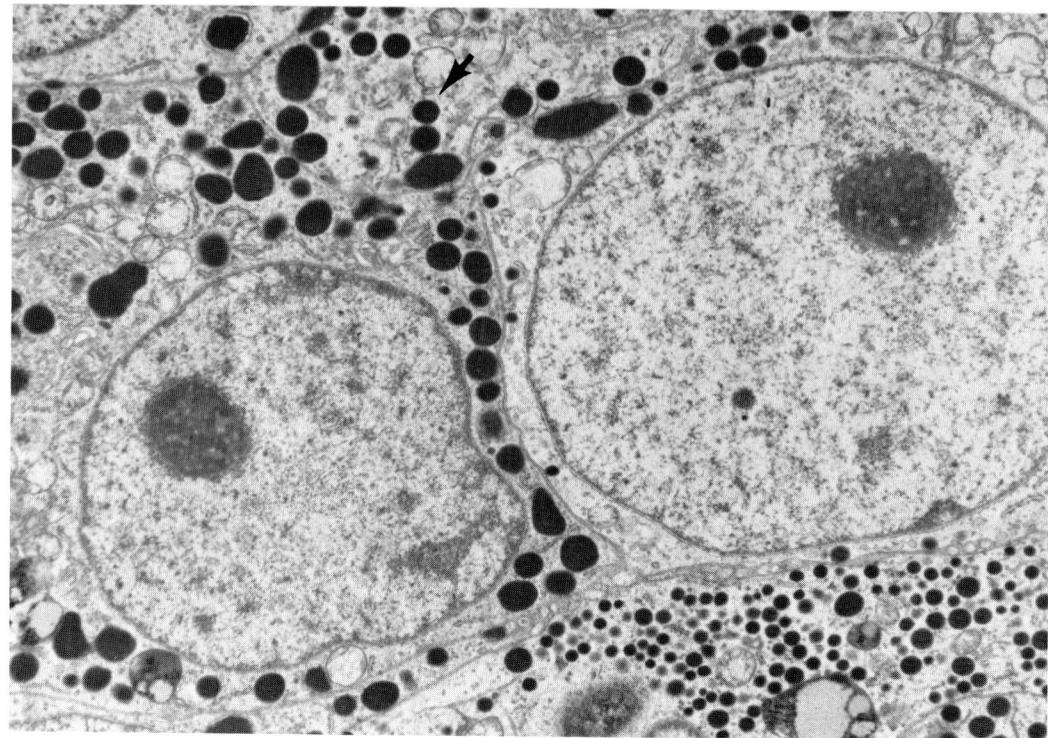

Fig. 3-14. Mammosomatotroph cell adenoma. Spherical and pleomorphic granules measure up to 2000 nm. Note large extruded secretory granule *(arrow)*. M × 10,400.

Electron microscopy reveals monomorphous tumors that are ultrastructurally similar to well-differentiated, densely granulated growth hormone cell adenomas (Fig. 3-14). This includes the presence of closely opposed polyhedral cells with uniform nuclei and spherical, dense nucleoli. Well-developed RER, large Golgi complexes, and a variable number of fibrous bodies are present.

The secretory granules range in size from 150 to 2000 nm and exhibit a morphologic heterogeneity. The majority are electron dense and have a limiting membrane similar to that seen in growth hormone cell adenomas and prolactin-producing adenomas. The others are larger, often with asymmetrically placed, mottled cores and irregular limiting membranes. A diagnostic marker of mammosomatotroph cell adenomas is the presence of extracellular deposits of electron-dense secretory material present in the intercellular space or at the perivascular surface of adenoma cells.

Corticotroph cell adenomas. Corticotroph cell adenomas may be associated with excessive production of ACTH, β-LPH, and endorphins, or they may be endocrinologically inactive ("silent" corticotroph cell adenomas). The active tumors are associated with Cushing's disease or Nelson's syndrome. The hormonally functional tumors associated with Cushing's disease are usually microadenomas and are more commonly found in the mucoid wedge. They are frequently purple and highly vascular. On rare occasions corticotroph cell adenomas are

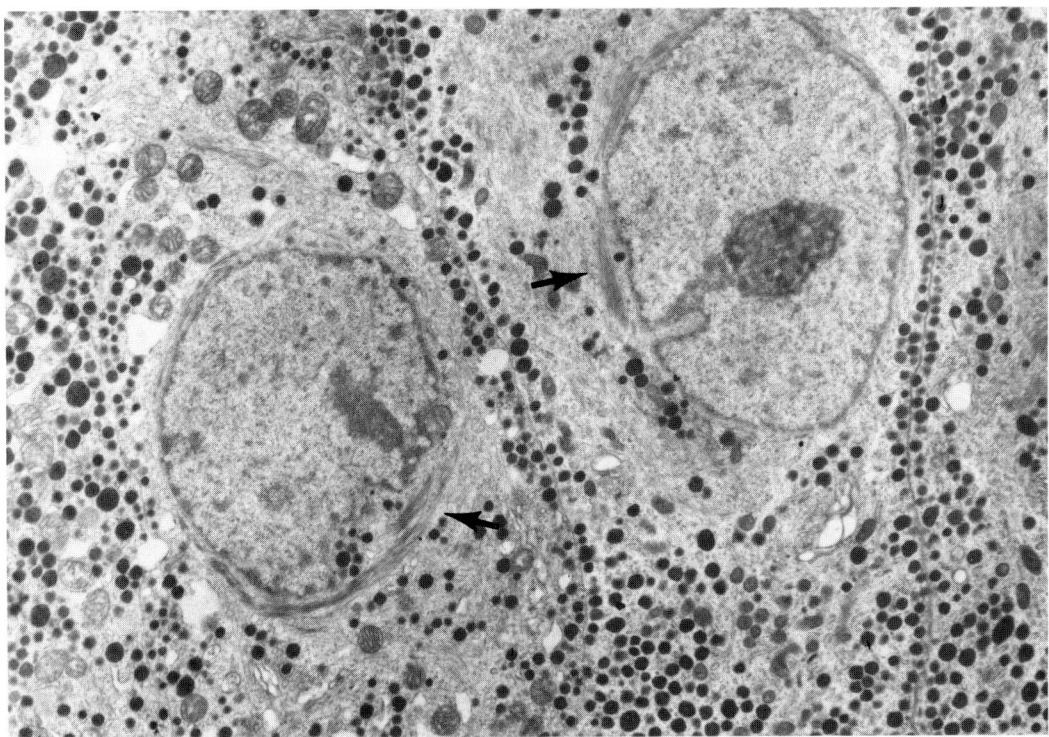

Fig. 3-15. Corticotroph cell adenoma. Secretory granules are spherical or irregular (dented or heart shaped) and vary in electron opacity. Note bundles of type I microfilaments (arrows). M × 9900.

found in the neurohypophysis, presumably arising from displaced basophils present in some posterior lobes. Tumors associated with Nelson's syndrome are often macroadenomas and frequently demonstrate local invasion.

By light microscopy, functioning corticotroph cell adenomas are basophilic, exhibiting PAS- and lead hematoxylin–positivity.* The tumor cells are negative with acid dyes such as eosin, phloxine, orange G, or light green. In some cases, however, tumor cells show positive cytoplasmic staining with Brookes' carmoisine technique. Silent corticotroph cell adenomas are either basophilic or chromophobic. The presence of ACTH, β-LPH, and endorphins in the cytoplasm is demonstrated by the immunoperoxidase technique.[218]

By electron microscopy, cells of active corticotroph cell adenomas closely resemble the normal corticotroph (Fig. 3-15).† They are angular and elongated with round or oval nuclei and electron-dense cytoplasm. The cells possess well-developed, rough endoplasmic reticulum and prominent Golgi complexes. The

---

*See references 163,164,191,192,195, and 196.
†See references 15,58,63,69,93,124,133,134,174, and 197.

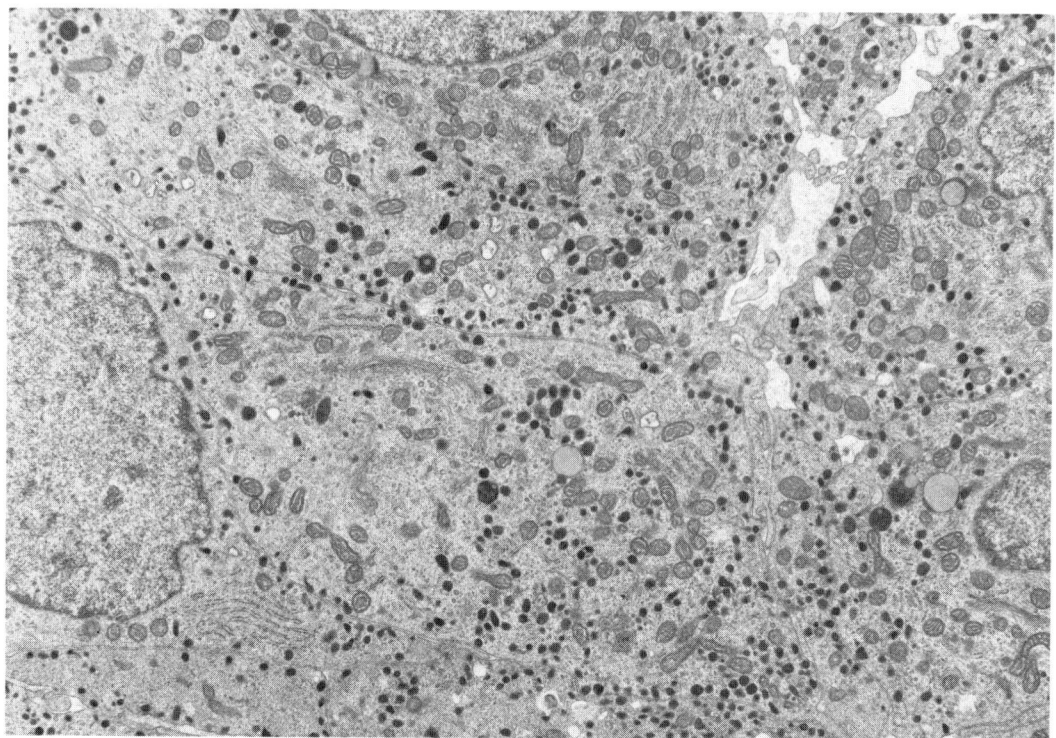

Fig. 3-16. "Silent" corticotroph cell adenoma unassociated with obvious endocrine abnormalities. Well-differentiated tumor has prominent RER and Golgi complexes. Several teardrop-shaped secretory granules are apparent. No microfilaments are noted. M × 9700.

secretory granules are spherical or slightly irregular and frequently line up along the cell membranes, although exocytoses are not seen. They are 250 to 700 nm in diameter and vary in electron density. In some cases the ultrastructural picture of silent corticotroph cell adenomas are indistinguishable from those of ACTH-secreting adenomas. Others, however, are significantly different[94] (Fig. 3-16).

Crooke's hyaline change is an alteration within the cytoplasm of corticotroph cells that occurs in association with hypercortisolism of any cause, either exogenous or endogenous (i.e., pharmacologic doses of corticosteroids, ACTH-secreting extrapituitary tumors in association with ectopic ACTH syndrome, adrenocortical tumors producing cortisol, Cushing's disease). These changes are absent or inconspicuous in Nelson's syndrome, in which there is no elevation of cortisol. The extent of Crooke's change induced by exogenous corticosteroids is independent of the dose or duration of corticosteroid therapy. Crooke's change is a cellular enlargement resulting from the accumulation of bundles of 70 nm (type I) microfilaments initially randomly scattered in the cytoplasm surrounding organelles then later orienting themselves in skeins and eventually displacing organelles (Figs. 3-17 and 3-18). Advanced Crooke's change may act as a "physiologic brake" on secretory granule secretion. As the cytoplasmic filaments replace the cytoplasm, the secretory granules are reduced in number.

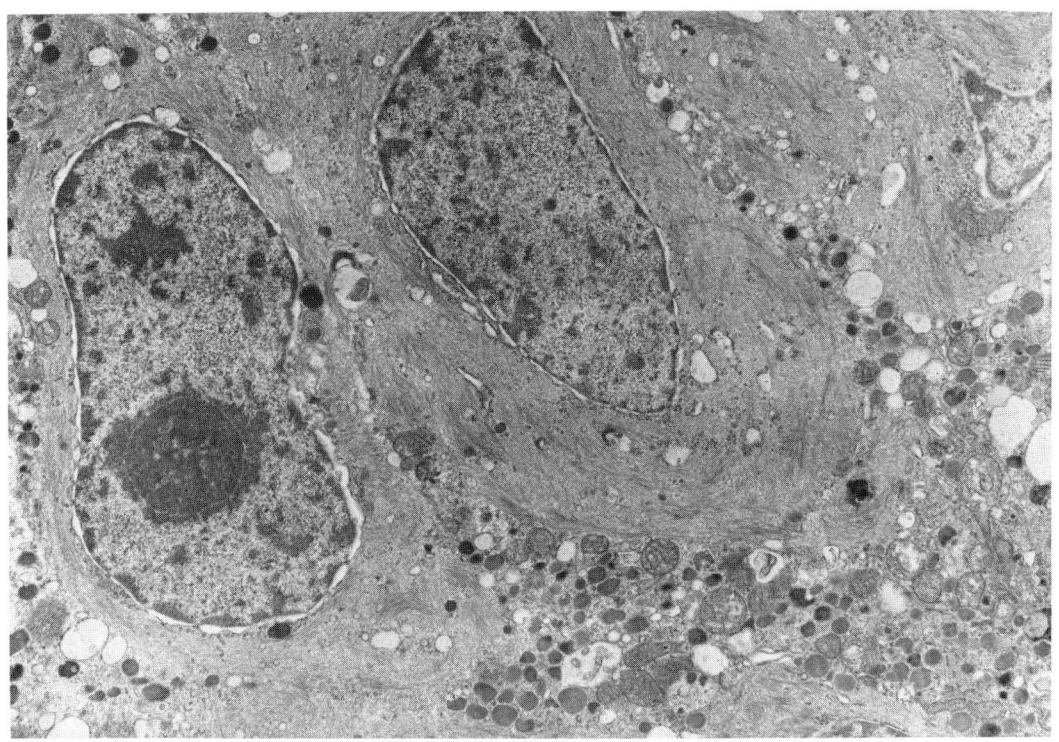

Fig. 3-17. Adenoma, associated with Cushing's disease, consisting of cells indistinguishable from Crooke's cells (i.e., corticotrophs showing massive accumulation of type I microfilaments ["Crooke's hyalin"]). M × 9900.

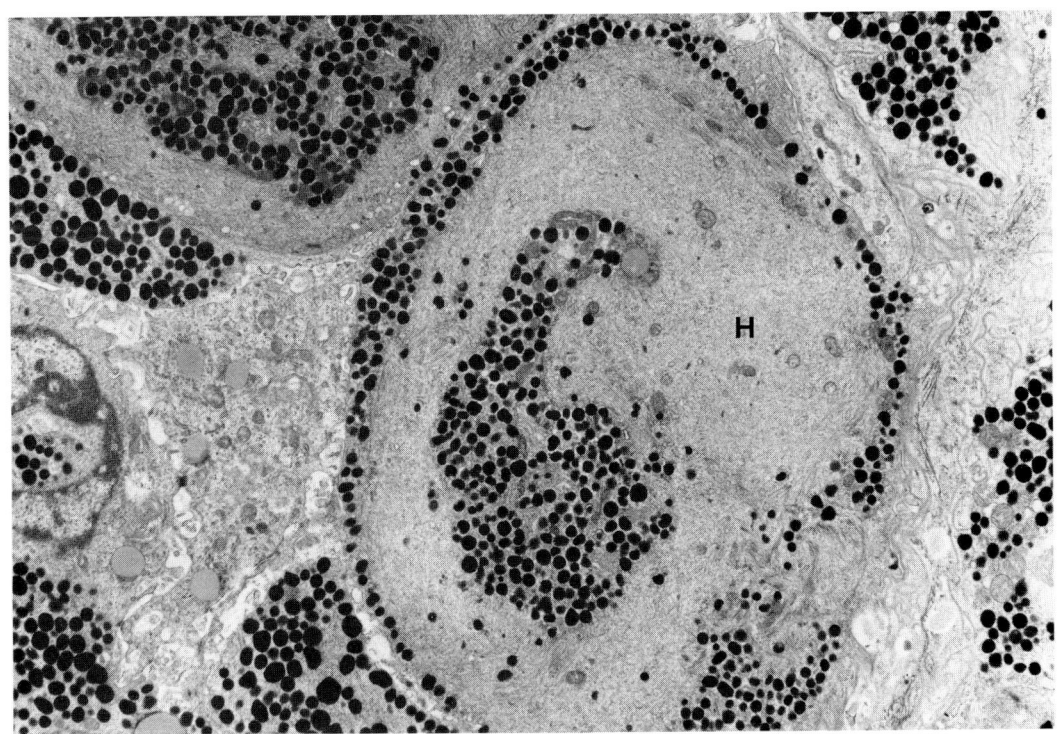

Fig. 3-18. Crooke's cells are suppressed corticotrophs. They are noticeable in nontumorous part of pituitary harboring corticotroph cell adenoma and show extensive accumulation of type I microfilaments ("Crooke's hyalin" [H]). M × 8900.

Gonadotroph cell adenomas. Gonadotroph cell adenomas are rare tumors that usually produce both FSH and LH, although FSH may be produced alone. This tumor occasionally develops in patients with long-standing hypogonadism.[127,240] Possibly related pathogenetically, experimental gonadectomy has been shown to induce hyperplasia of gonadotroph cells in the rat.

Most of these tumors have the same basic features.[43,65,130,225,240] By light microscopy, these tumors are chromophobic adenomas. No cytoplasmic staining occurs with acid dyes or lead hematoxylin. On occasion rare PAS-positive granules are identified.

The ultrastructural features of these tumors are often not characteristic enough to make a definitive diagnosis.[93,127,130,230] Therefore the immunoperoxidase technique is important in disclosing the cellular derivation of the tumor. The immunoperoxidase technique depends on the identification of the hormone-specific beta chain as the alpha subunits of FSH, LH, and TSH are immunologically similar and structurally identical. In gonadotroph cell adenomas, the immunoperoxidase technique demonstrates FSH and/or LH in the cytoplasm of the cells.

The fine structural features of these tumor cells sometimes resemble those of normal gonadotroph cells. In others, the tumors consist of immature, undifferentiated cells. The adenoma cells are small, elongated, and angular with oval nuclei. The rough endoplasmic reticulum is fairly well developed and composed

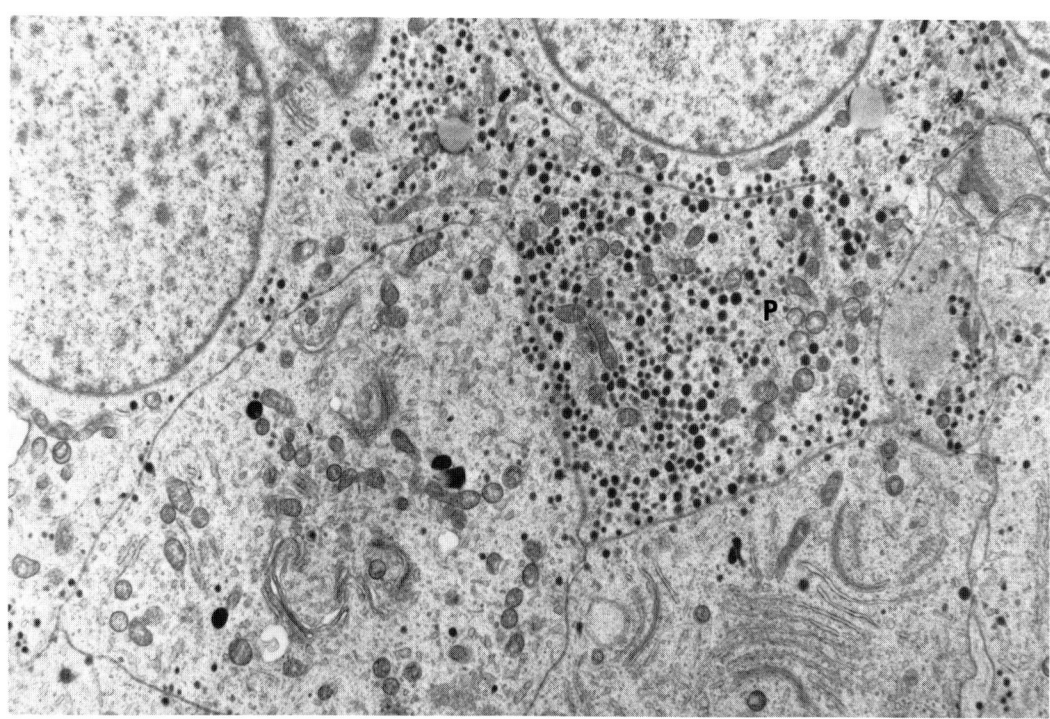

Fig. 3-19. Gonadotroph cell adenoma, male type. Middle-sized polyhedral cells contain moderately developed RER and Golgi apparatus; small secretory granules accumulate in cell processes *(P)*. M × 9800.

of parallel cisternae. There are conspicuous Golgi complexes and many microtubules. The secretory granules are sparse and spherical, measure 100 to 250 nm in diameter, and possess a prominent electron-lucent halo between the limiting membrane and the electron-dense core. They are peripherally lined up along the cell membranes, but no exocytoses are seen.

Horvath and Kovacs[95] have recently recognized a sex-linked dichotomy in the electron microscopic appearance of gonadotroph cell adenomas. They reported that by electron microscopy, gonadotroph adenomas in men had uncharacteristic features often similar to null cell adenomas with poorly or moderately developed cytoplasmic organelles (Fig. 3-19). In women, tumors were well differentiated with a highly distinctive vesicular dilatation of the Golgi complex (Fig. 3-20). By looking at these tumors, the sex of the patient can be recognized.

Thyrotroph cell adenomas. Thyrotroph cell adenomas are rare tumors of the pituitary gland that usually occur in patients with long-standing hypothyroidism. It has been suggested that the lack of negative feedback effect causes a sustained stimulation of TSH cells that may produce thyrotroph cell hyperplasia and eventually an adenoma. Furth and Clifton[66] induced thyrotroph cell tumors in hypothyroid animals, thus lending support to this notion. Following surgical or radiothyroidectomy and by the use of antithyroid drugs in experimental animals, these investigators were able to show progressive hyperplasia and nodularity

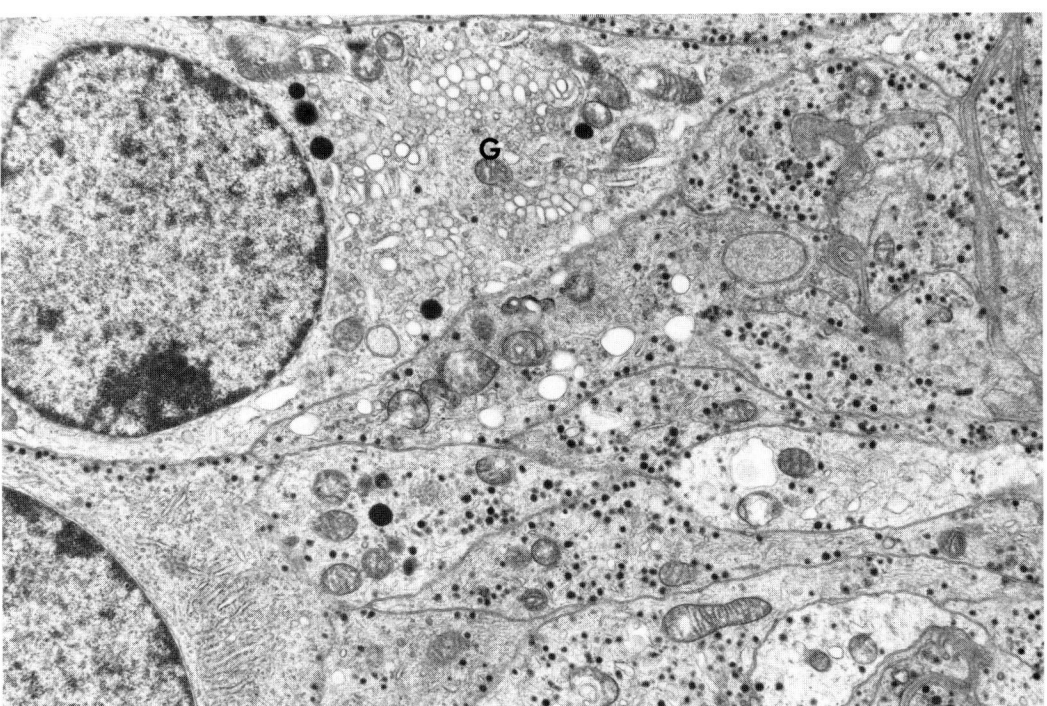

Fig. 3-20. Gonadotroph cell adenoma, female type. Well-differentiated tumor processes uniform nuclei; abundant, slightly dilated RER; and conspicuous Golgi complexes consisting of vesicular profiles ("honey-comb Golgi" *[G]*). Majority of small secretory granules (up to 150 nm) are abundant in long, thin cytoplasmic processes. M × 6600.

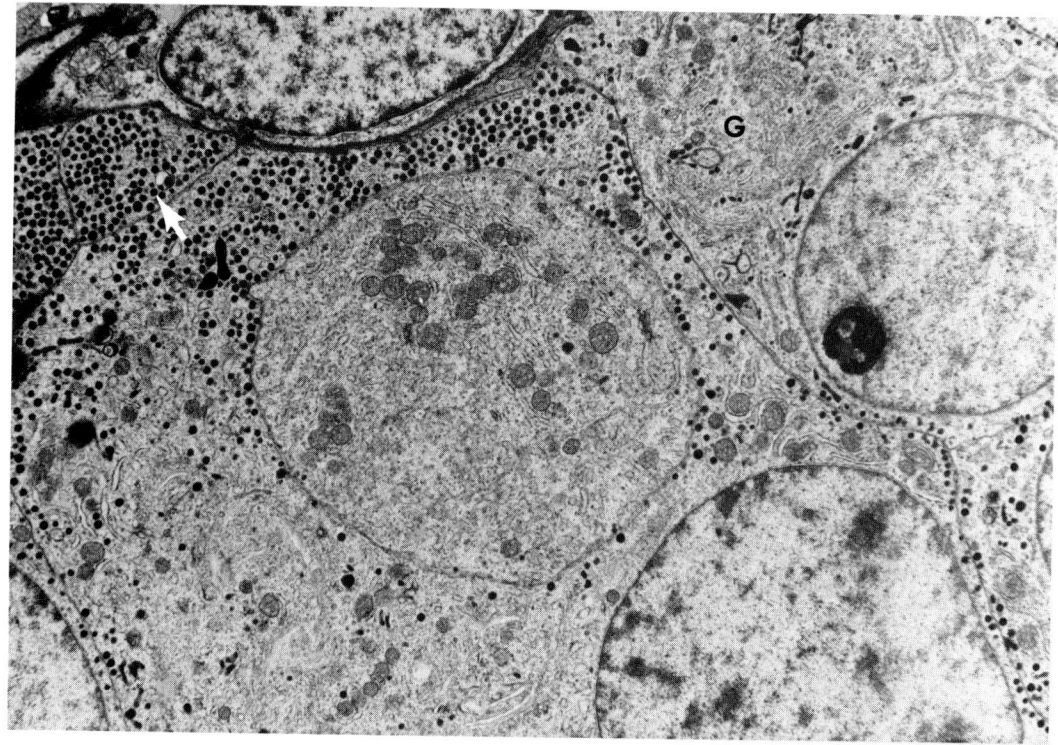

Fig. 3-21. Thyrotroph cell adenoma. Prominent RER exhibits slight, uniform dilation; Golgi complexes are well developed *(G)*. Small secretory granules (up to 200 nm) are more numerous in cytoplasmic processes *(arrow)* than in cell body. M × 10,200.

preceding the formation of thyrotroph adenomas, some of which had extrasellar extension. Rarely, hyperthyroidism may be caused by high blood levels of TSH associated with a thyrotroph cell adenoma.

By light microscopy, thyrotroph cell adenomas represent chromophobic tumors.* They have a few small PAS-positive, aldehyde fuchsin-positive, and aldehyde thionin-positive cytoplasmic granules. Although the immunoperoxidase technique may be positive for TSH, some tumors cannot be immunostained for obscure reasons.[198]

On electron microscopy, thyrotroph cell adenomas resemble gonadotroph cell adenomas (Fig. 3-21). The cells are elongated or angular with numerous cytoplasmic microtubules and irregular nuclei. The secretory granules are spherical, sparse in number, 100 to 200 nm in diameter, and often line up along the cell membrane. The secretory granules frequently have a prominent electron-lucent halo between the limiting membrane and electron-dense core.

In rare instances, thyrotroph adenomas are more well differentiated and are composed of larger cells, which resemble thyroidectomy cells.

Plurihormonal adenomas. Certain pituitary adenomas produce more than one adenohypophysial hormone. These tumors may be either monomorphous or plurimorphous.[150] In monomorphous adenomas, one cell population is identified,

---

*See references 58, 124, 137, 159, 180, and 198.

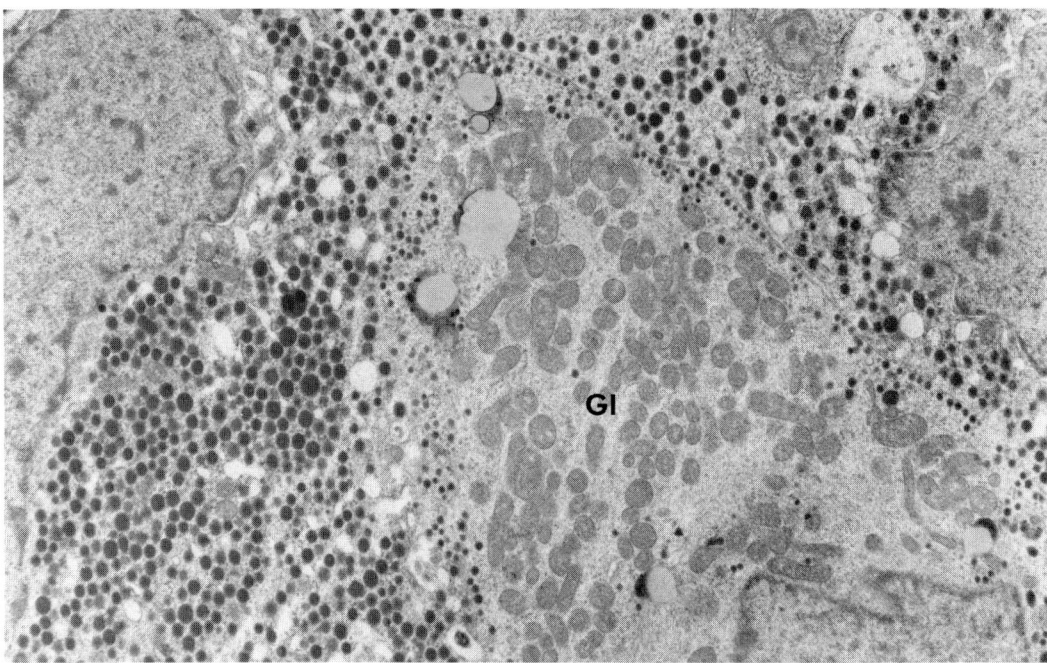

Fig. 3-22. Bimorphous adenoma, associated with acromegaly, containing immunoreactive growth hormone and alpha subunit. Centrally located cell *(Gl)* shows differentiation toward glycoprotein hormone-producing cell line. M × 9400.

which presumably produces the two or more hormones. In the plurimorphous adenomas, each different cell type contains only one or more hormones, most commonly growth hormone and TSH.[98] Rare occurrences of other plurihormonal adenomas harboring unusual combinations of adenohypophysial hormones have been reported.*

It is not unusual in pathologic examination to identify hormones within the pituitary tumors. Frequently, these hormones have no clinical correlation. This may result from the elaboration of tumor products that are immunoreactive but not bioactive. Alternatively, some of the detected hormones may not be secreted in excess, possibly as a result of an operational feedback mechanism.[98]

The cytogenesis of these plurihormonal adenomas is incompletely understood. The ultrastructurally monomorphous appearance of some less differentiated growth hormone-TSH–or prolactin-TSH–producing adenomas favors a theory of derivation from a common precursor cell.[98] Such a common immature progenitor cell with potential for divergent differentiation has not yet been identified. Plurimorphous tumors may simultaneously originate from two or more mature cell types or may result from differentiation of a common progenitor cell. It appears that those pituitary tumors that synthesize growth hormone and/or prolactin plus one or more glycoprotein hormones (usually TSH) show enough clinical and morphologic similarities to postulate a common cytogenesis.[98] The ultrastructural features of a plurihormonal adenoma are illustrated in Fig. 3-22.

---

*See references 51, 125, 128, 136, 150, and 202.

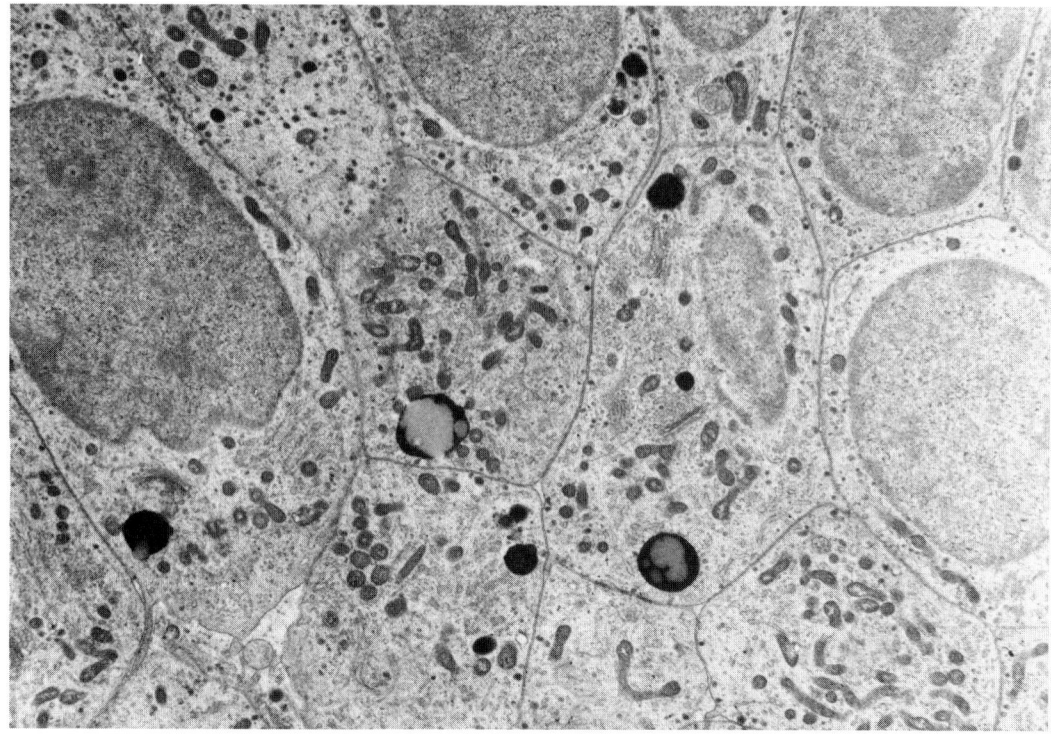

Fig. 3-23. Null cell adenoma consisting of small cells with poorly developed cytoplasmic organelles and small, very sparse secretory granules. M × 9800.

Null cell adenomas. About 25% of pituitary adenomas show no clinical, biochemical, and immunohistologic evidence of hormone production. The term *null cell adenoma* has been given to this group rather than the original term *undifferentiated cell adenoma* to avoid the implication of anaplasia rather than lack of secretory granule specificity and function. Because of their biochemical silence, these tumors can undergo prolonged growth and produce mass effects before their presence is recognized. They may cause hyperprolactinemia following an interference with the production and delivery of PIF. These tumors are much more common in the older population.

By light microscopy, null cell adenomas are chromophobic. However, oncocytic forms may exhibit a granular acidophilic appearance because of the affinity of mitochondria for acidic dyes. Stains with PAS and basic dyes are negative. The immunoperoxidase technique shows no hormone production. However, as mentioned previously, a few tumors may contain secretory granules positive for alpha subunit or other adenohypophysial hormones, suggesting that the tumors may have originated in hormone-producing cells of the pituitary and lost their endocrine potential through oncocytic transformation.

On electron microscopy, null cell adenomas are composed of closely opposed irregular cells with scant cytoplasm and pleomorphic nuclei (Fig. 3-23). The rough endoplasmic reticulum is inconspicuous and composed of scattered, short

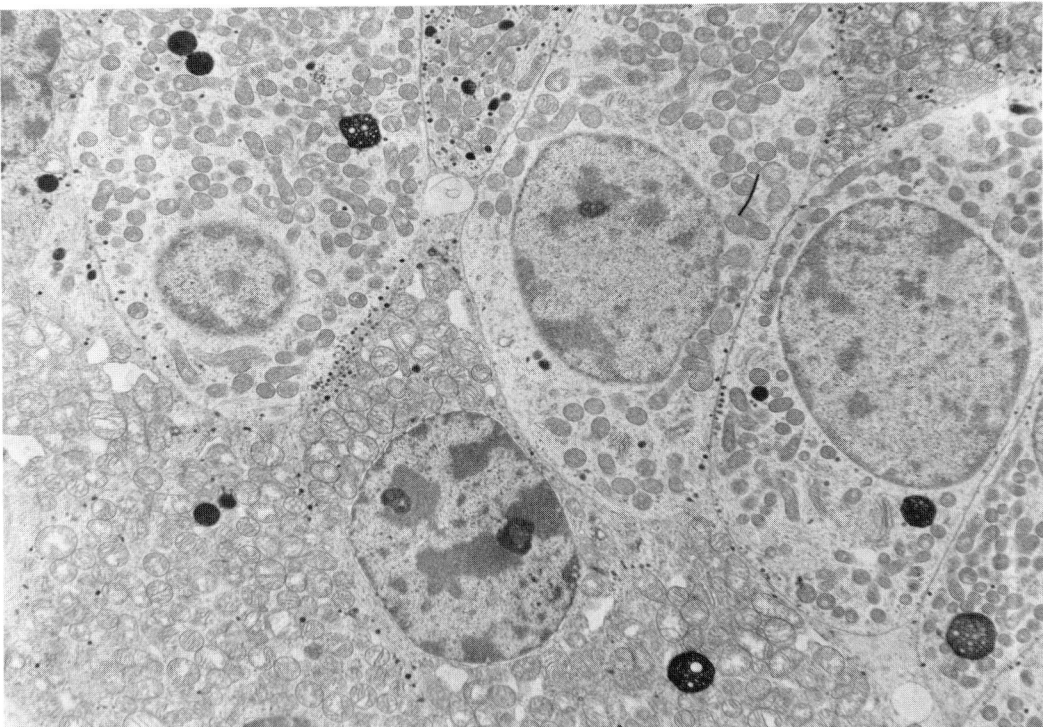

Fig. 3-24. Pituitary oncocytoma showing marked abundance of mitochondria obliterating other cytoplasmic organelles. M × 10,300.

stacks. Despite the paucity of the rough endoplasmic reticulum, the Golgi complexes may be prominent, and microtubules are abundant in many cells. Secretory granules are identified in all null cell adenomas by electron microscopy. They are spherical, measure 100 to 125 nm in diameter, and have an electron-dense core surrounded by an electron-lucent halo. Although they frequently line up along the cell membrane, no exocytoses are seen.

Although null cell adenomas do not produce any known hormone, it is unlikely that all these tumors represent a homogenous group. A spectrum of null cell adenomas exist, ranging from nononcocytic to oncocytic forms. Oncocytic transformation refers to an increase in the volume density of mitochondria within a cell, and such cells are called oncocytes (Fig. 3-24). Oncocytes are found in small numbers in the normal pituitary gland. Such an accumulation of mitochondria is known to occur in cells of the thyroid and parathyroid glands and in a variety of nonendocrine epithelial cells including the kidneys and salivary glands. Electron microscopy is necessary for the diagnosis of oncocytomas to identify the abundance of mitochondria (see Fig. 3-24).

Oncocytic transformation may become so extensive that the mitochondria obscure the other cytoplasmic organelles. Tumors composed of such cells are termed oncocytomas and comprise one third of null cell adenomas. The presence of alpha subunit or other adenohypophysial hormone is detectable in the cytoplasm

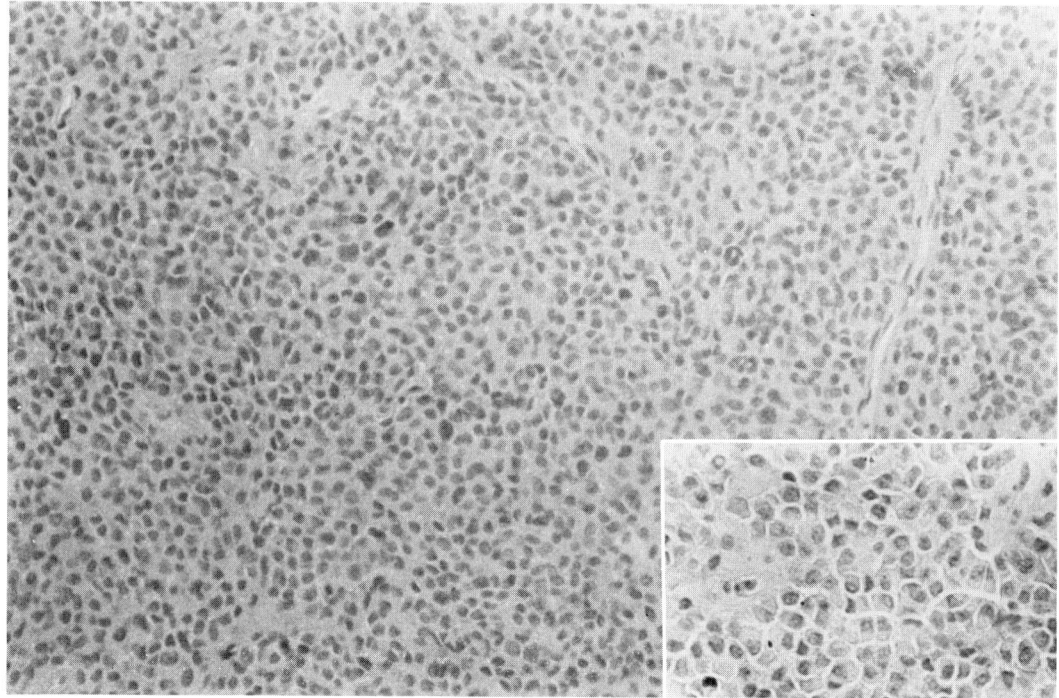

Fig. 3-25. Light microscopy of pituitary adenoma. Note absence of normal acinar structure and replacement with patternless sheet of cells. M × 150 (insert × 235).

of some oncocytomas. This suggests that oncocytic transformation may occur in hormone-active tumors as an irreversible abnormality. It has been shown that the proliferating or accumulating mitochondria involved in oncocytic transformation are defective and display insufficient oxidative phosphorylation.

The foregoing classification (which attempts to correlate clinical history, laboratory data, and morphologic analysis including electron microscopy and immunohistochemical techniques) has added greatly to our understanding of pituitary adenomas. It does require sophisticated morphologic techniques that may not be readily available. In addition, the exact significance of many of the subpopulations such as sparsely and densely granulated tumors and ultrastructural characteristics such as misplaced exocytoses, paranuclear fibrous bodies, or oncocytic changes is incompletely understood.

Of practical importance for histopathologic diagnosis is familiarity with the light microscopic appearances of pituitary adenomas (Figs. 3-25 and 3-26). Classification of the adenomas based on histomorphologic appearance (e.g., diffuse, papillary, sinusoidal) has no real value because of the absence of correlation with biologic behavior. However, these patterns of adenoma growth must be recognized as such.

It is often difficult to differentiate normal pituitary tissue from an adenoma, especially on a frozen section from a very small biopsy specimen. Abnormality

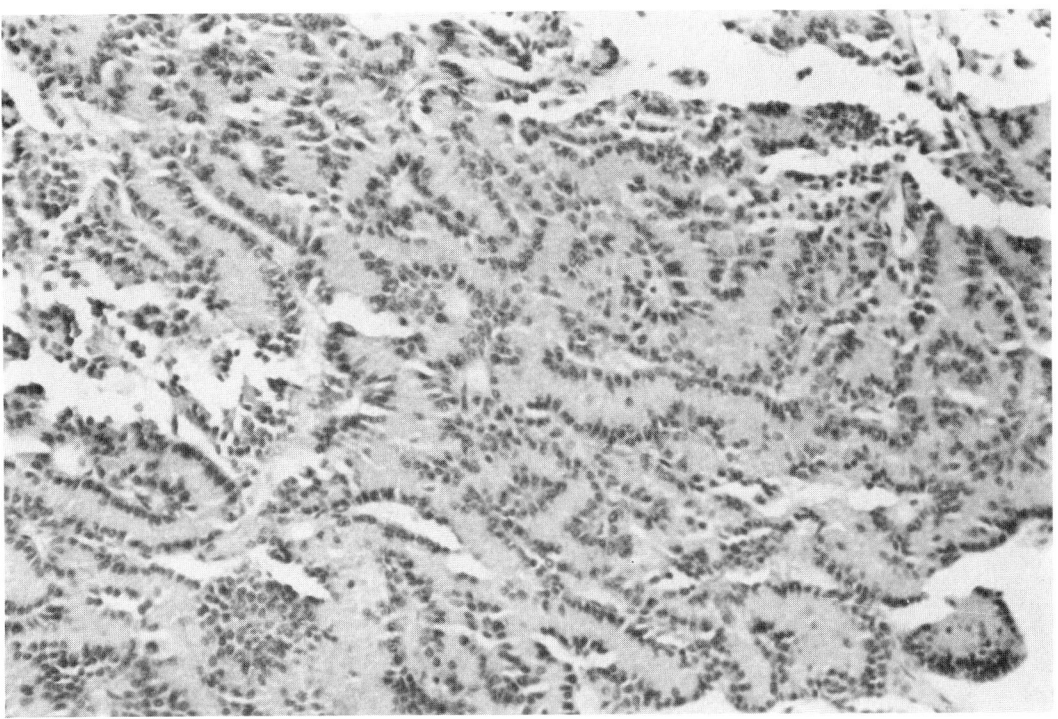

Fig. 3-26. Pituitary adenoma with papillary pattern. M × 150.

in tissue pattern is more important than cytologic appearances. In general, adenomas are randomly structured and monotonous without many conspicuous architectural features. A pituitary adenoma tends to lose the characteristic acinar pattern of the normal gland. The monotony is often relieved by delicate septae of connective tissue and perivascular halos. The normal pituitary has a well-developed stroma that is rich in reticulin, dividing the gland into cords and nests of cells. In contrast, pituitary adenomas have much less reticulin, accounting for their softer texture at surgery and for the increased number of cells in a touch-preparation of an adenoma compared to normal gland. Multinucleation and cellular pleomorphism are not uncommon in the adenoma but are not seen in the normal gland. Mitotic figures and anaplasia are rare. Features of compressed or distorted normal pituitary tissues include variation in cell size and secretory granule content with crowding of cells and an absence of multinucleation, nucleolar prominence, and mitotic activity.

Because of the diversity of appearances that adenomas of the adenohypophysis can take, they may mimic neoplasms of different cytogenesis. In our experience, malignant lymphomas and some meningiomas are most likely to create problems in misdiagnosis.

Secondary changes in pituitary adenomas

Hemorrhage and infarction. Pituitary apoplexy as a clinical entity is described in Chapter 4 and is a relatively unusual means of presentation of pituitary adenomas. Earle and Dillard[52] reported that approximately 1% of chromophobe adenomas present with pituitary apoplexy. Evidence of hemorrhage noted at the time of surgery or on the pathologic specimen, however, is not an uncommon occurrence. Such macroscopic and microscopic evidence of hemorrhage may be found 10% to 28% of the time.[157,160] We have encountered essentially total infarction of a pituitary adenoma on several occasions during transsphenoidal surgery. Careful pathologic examination of the specimen is often required to identify the neoplasm.

Calcification. Craniopharyngiomas frequently produce radiographically evident calcification, and its presence strongly suggest this diagnosis. Pituitary adenomas rarely have evidence of calcification on radiographic studies.[28,135] More often pituitary adenomas, especially prolactinomas, have microscopic deposits of calcification known as calcospherites. This process is believed to be a form of dystrophic calcification beginning in the cytoplasm of cells presumably undergoing degenerative changes.[204] Tumor size and patient age do not appear to have any influence on the tendency of adenomas to calcify.[204]

Amyloid. Amyloid deposition is occasionally encountered within the perivascular spaces and in the form of extracellular bodies. It occurs most often in prolactinomas and is of no known significance.

Bromocriptine-induced changes. Treatment of certain pituitary adenomas will produce rapidly reversible changes in the microscopic morphology of the tumor, whereas others are not affected by the drug.[11,185,228] Tindall et al have shown that in bromocriptine-responsive tumors there is a reduction of cytoplasmic volume as a result of reduction of ribosomes, rough endoplasmic reticulum, and Golgi complexes (Fig. 3-27).[11,228] The secretory granules were slightly increased in size. There was no evidence of lysosomal accumulation, necrosis, vascular damage, endothelial cell damage, platelet aggregation, or thrombosis. These findings indicate that bromocriptine may selectively inhibit protein and hormone synthesis in prolactin-secreting cells rather than have a direct cytotoxic or vascular effect.[11]

Invasive pituitary adenomas. Like many other endocrine neoplasms, the aggressiveness of pituitary adenomas cannot be reliably predicted by the histologic appearance of the tumor. Although they may appear quite benign under the microscope, certain pituitary adenomas may extend beyond the pituitary capsule and invade the dura of the cavernous sinus and cranial nerves; affect the sphenoid bone and sinus; or even infiltrate blood vessels, venous sinuses, or the brain.[143] These tumors are referred to as invasive pituitary adenomas. Although they grow in an infiltrating and destructive manner, metastases seldom develop.[143] Invasion of the cavernous sinus appears to be the most common extension of these tumors.[110,147] Based on an extensive review of the literature, Rovit and Duane[192] concluded that invasive behavior of pituitary adenomas occurred 2½ times more

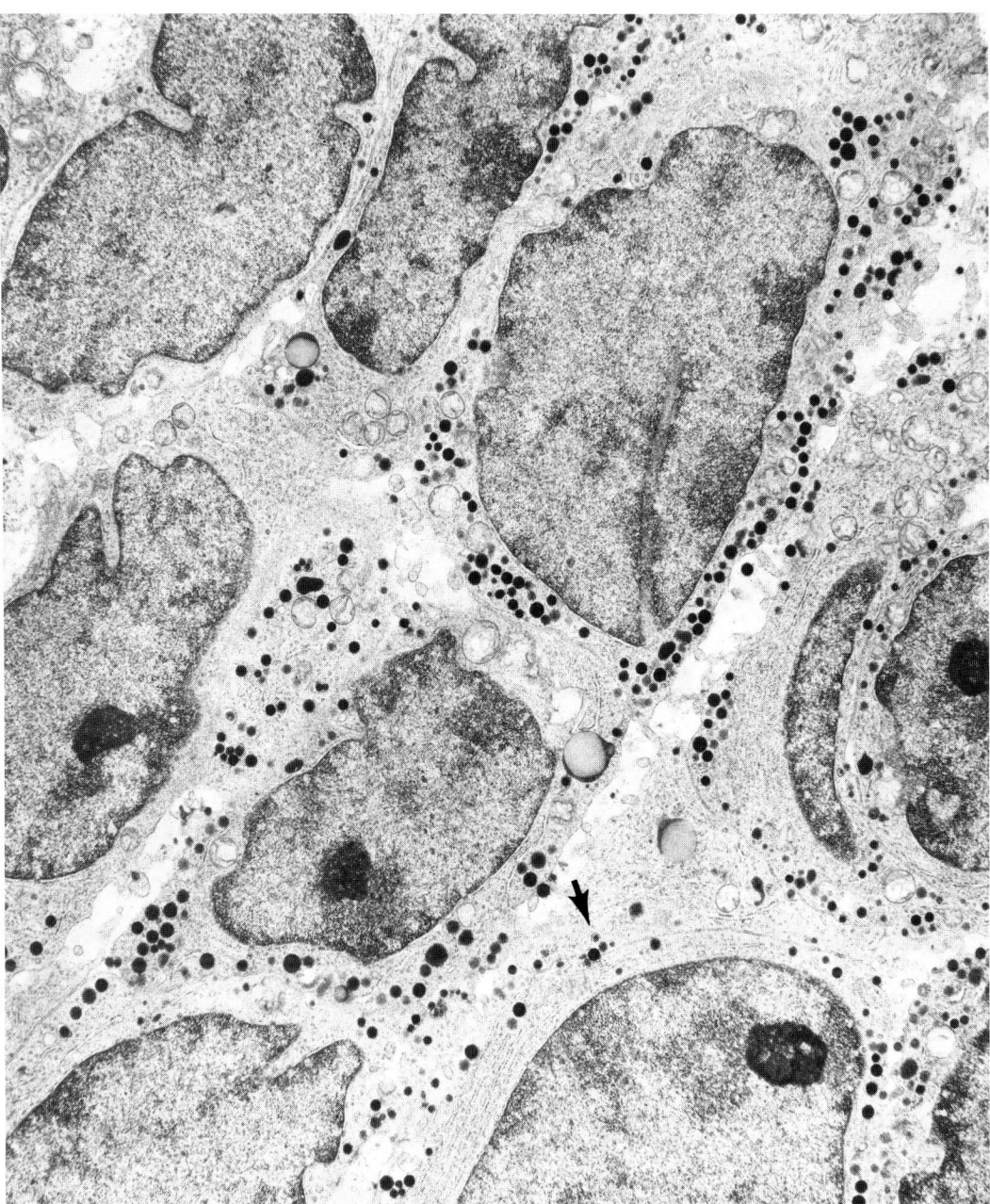

Fig. 3-27. Effect of bromocriptine on prolactin cell adenoma. Note irregular, cleaved nuclei with dark, clumped chromatin and smaller nucleoli. Cell size is decreased with marked involution of cytoplasm, loss of both RER and Golgi membranes. Occasional granule exocytoses still occur *(arrows)*. M × 9200.

frequently with ACTH-secreting chromophobes than in nonsecreting chromophobes.

Ectopic pituitary adenomas. Ectopic pituitary tumors have been reported to occur in various parts of the cranium.[19,115,190] The ectopic tissue could spread from a malignant pituitary tumor along the meninges or via the cerebrospinal fluid (CSF) or bloodstream.[148,168,169] This mechanism is not truly ectopic but metastatic. Dislodgement of adenoma cells during surgical treatment of a pituitary adenoma could be another mechanism for the development of an ectopic neoplasm. Alternatively, ectopic adenohypophysial tissue is known to occur in the sphenoid bone or roof of the pharynx.[155] These are nests of remnant cells along the path taken during embryonic development. On rare occasions an adenoma may arise from such tissue.[21,56] Suprasellar ectopic pituitary adenomas presumably arise from adenohypophysial cells of the pars tuberalis that normally extend above the diaphragm sella.[19,190]

Primary malignant tumors of the pituitary

Primary pituitary carcinoma is a distinctly rare lesion and may be impossible to diagnose by the histologic appearance alone. The presence of cellular pleomorphism, mitotic figures, and even local invasion are not conclusive evidence of malignancy, and an unequivocal diagnosis requires the demonstration of distant metastases. Both cerebrospinal and extracranial dissemination have been reported. Scheithauer[204] has reviewed these cases and compared the gross pathologic, radiographic, and clinical features of pituitary carcinoma producing cerebrospinal metastases with those presenting with extracranial dissemination. Patients with cerebrospinal metastases averaged 43 years of age (range 25 to 75 years), and average duration of disease was 8 years from onset of symptoms to death. Three fourths of these patients had endocrine inactive tumors; the remainder had acromegaly, except one with Cushing's disease. The average age of patients with extracranial metastases was 44 years (range 7 to 75 years) with an average survival of 2½ years from onset of symptoms to death. Half of these patients had Cushing's disease, and the remainder were endocrine inactive. The most common site of blood-borne metastasis was the liver with other sites including lung, bone, myocardium, and lymph nodes.

Carcinoma associated with only craniospinal metastases usually caused sellar expansion and had prominent extrasellar extension, whereas carcinoma with extracranial metastases usually produced little or no sellar enlargement but caused erosion or destruction of the sellar floor.[204]

Primary sarcomas are quite rare but have been reported in patients previously irradiated for pituitary adenomas.[82,183] These sarcomas are mainly fibrosarcomas, rarely osteosarcomas.

Granular cell tumors

Granular cell tumors, sometimes referred to as choristomas, are occasionally encountered as incidental autopsy findings identified in the neurohypophysis or infundibulum as small aggregates of plump, nonepithelial, polygonal cells with granular cytoplasm.[27,145] These so-called granular cell tumorettes occur in 6.8% to 17% of pituitary glands and may be multiple.[145] The tumorettes are usually asymptomatic and only cause insignificant displacement of glial cells (pituicytes) of the posterior lobe.[27] There is, however, a spectrum of enlargement to include masses that symptomatically compress the pituitary gland, optic chiasm, and/or hypothalamus. Although malignant forms have been reported, most are benign neoplasms and are hormonally inactive.[4]

Granular cell tumors of the pituitary are structurally identical to granular cell tumors found in other parts of the body, including the oral cavity, tongue, salivary glands, larynx, trachea, bronchi, gastrointestinal tract, urinary bladder, uterus, breast, and subcutaneous tissue. Neoplasms with similar morphology have been identified in the cerebral hemisphere, third ventricle, meninges of the spinal cord, and in spinal and cranial nerves.

The histogenesis of these tumors is uncertain. Many authors favor a Schwann cell or perineural cell origin,[9,67,68,220,229] but a variety of other possibilities have been proposed, including pituitary cells of the intermediate lobe, pituicytes of the posterior lobe (see Fig. 3-6), displaced basophilic rests, or macrophages.[27]

Grossly, the lesions are discrete, lobulated, rubbery masses lying in the intrasellar or suprasellar area. By light microscopy, the tumors are composed of polygonal nonepithelial cells that have abundant granular cytoplasm (Fig. 3-28).

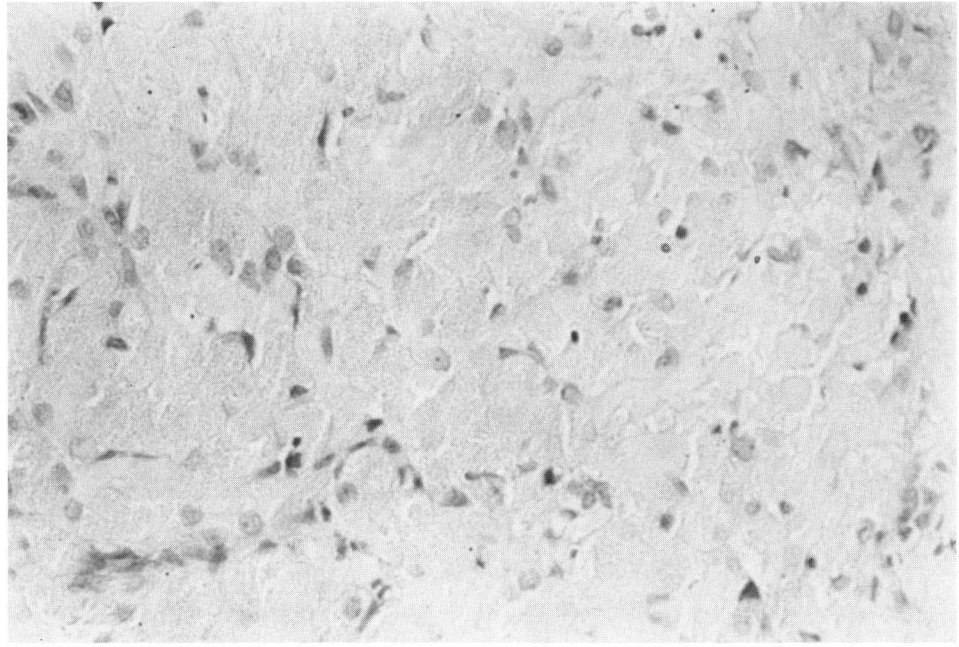

Fig. 3-28. Light microscopic appearance of granular cell tumor. M × 300.

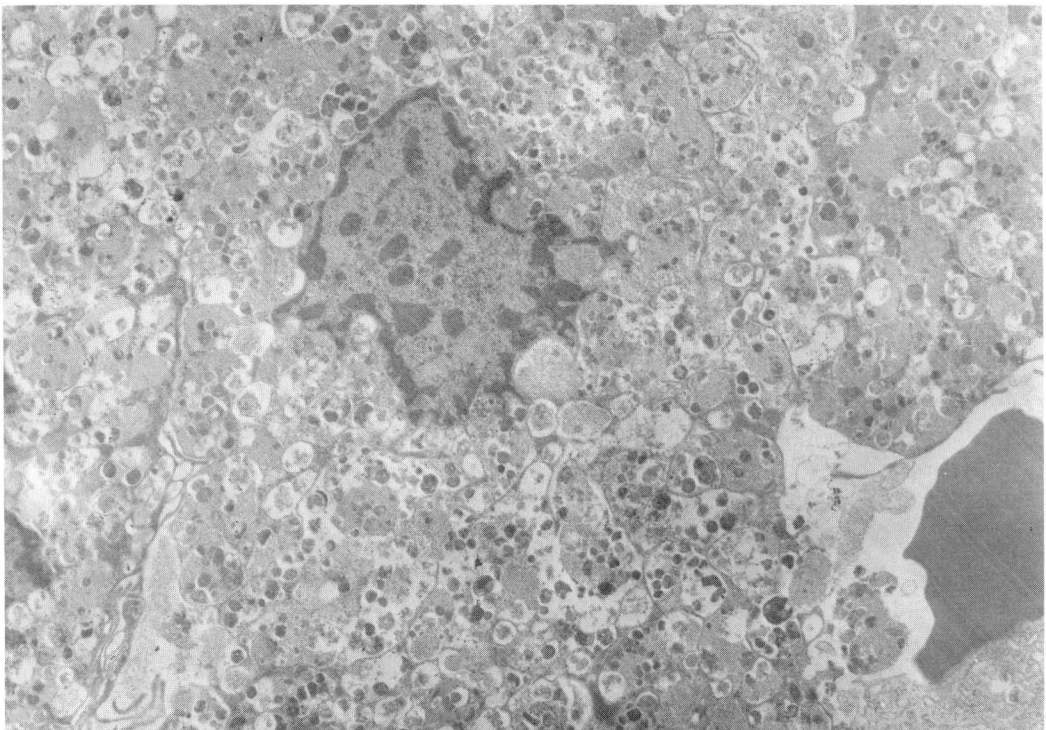

Fig. 3-29. Granular cell tumor found incidentally in posterior lobe at autopsy. M × 8400.

The granules are PAS-positive and diastase resistant. Ultrastructurally, the polygonal cells are 20 to 40 nm in diameter with granules composed of cytosegresomes of lysosomal origin (Fig. 3-29).[204]

Craniopharyngiomas

Craniopharyngiomas usually contain both a solid and cystic portion. The solid tissue is smooth, firm, and gray or pink. The cysts are filled with a brownish, muddy fluid containing suspended cholesterol crystals. The most common location of craniopharyngiomas is in the suprasellar space, but they may also be found in the intrasellar region or within the third ventricle. They vary considerably in size, usually ranging from 2 to 10 cm in diameter.[224] Craniopharyngiomas extend under the frontal or temporal lobes in approximately 2% of cases and into the posterior fossa in 1% of cases. The pituitary stalk is usually situated posterior to the tumor. These neoplasms are usually located beneath or anterior to the chiasm, but in one third of the cases they are located posterior to the chiasm.[70]

Approximately 10% to 20% of craniopharyngiomas are primarily intrasellar in location,[167,223] a situation related to a lower position of the primitive cells giving origin to the tumor. Hardy has commented that craniopharyngiomas associated with an enlarged sella can be assumed to have originated within the sella.[88,126] Although they have been reported to occur in the third ventricle, this location is

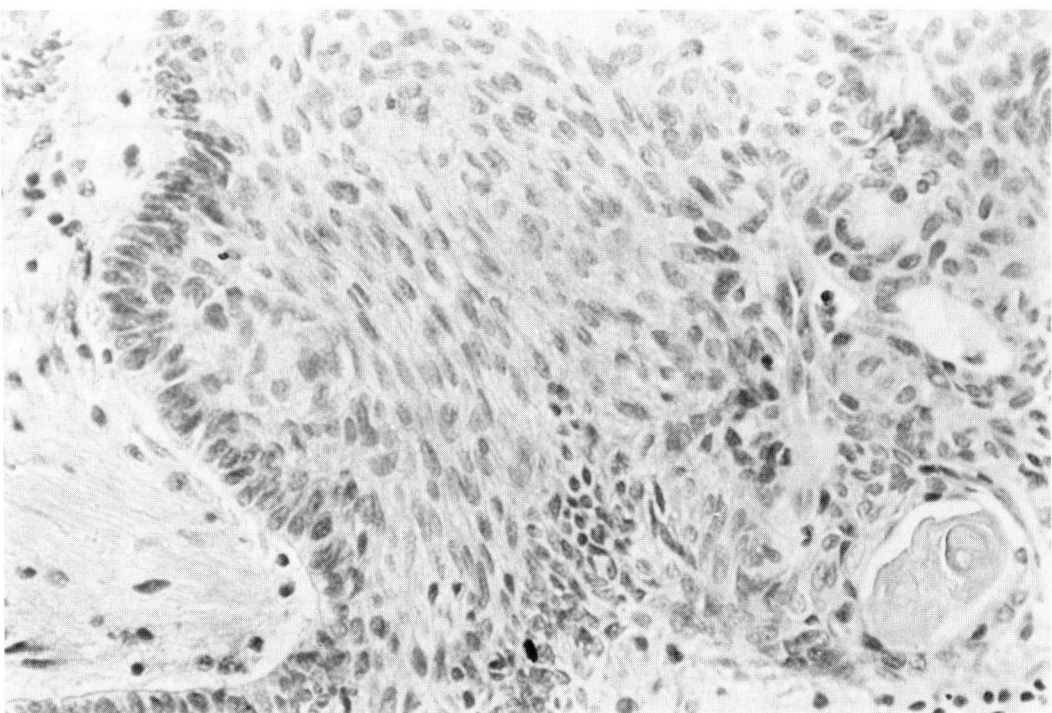

Fig. 3-30. Craniopharyngioma. Well-differentiated sheets of squamous epithelium. M × 300.

relatively rare.[154] In reality, the tumors probably originate beneath the hypothalamus; as they enlarge and extend upward, they displace a film of hypothalamus upward and only appear to arise within the third ventricle.[232]

Microscopically, craniopharyngiomas are well-differentiated tumors with strands or sheets of squamous epithelial cells separating varying sized cysts (Fig. 3-30). The epithelial cells have irregular nuclei with peripherally clumped chromatin and a moderate amount of cytoplasm that extends outward into cell processes and microvilli that interdigitate with neighboring cells or lie free in small cystic spaces. In some areas, fine fibrous strands attach to a narrow basal lamina. Larger, dense keratin fibers or calcium deposits are usually seen in the larger cystic cavities. Reactive astrocytes and phagocytic cells are commonly seen in areas adjacent to the tumor cells.[154]

Gliosis around the tumor is often marked and may pinch off small masses of craniopharyngioma cells, giving the erroneous impression of tumor infiltration and invasion.[194] There is usually an abundance of eosinophilic Rosenthal fibers included in the gliosis.

The characteristic electron microscopic features of craniopharyngiomas are illustrated in Figs. 3-31 and 3-32. These include the absence of secretory granules, the presence of junctional complexes, and bundles of intracytoplasmic tonofilaments.

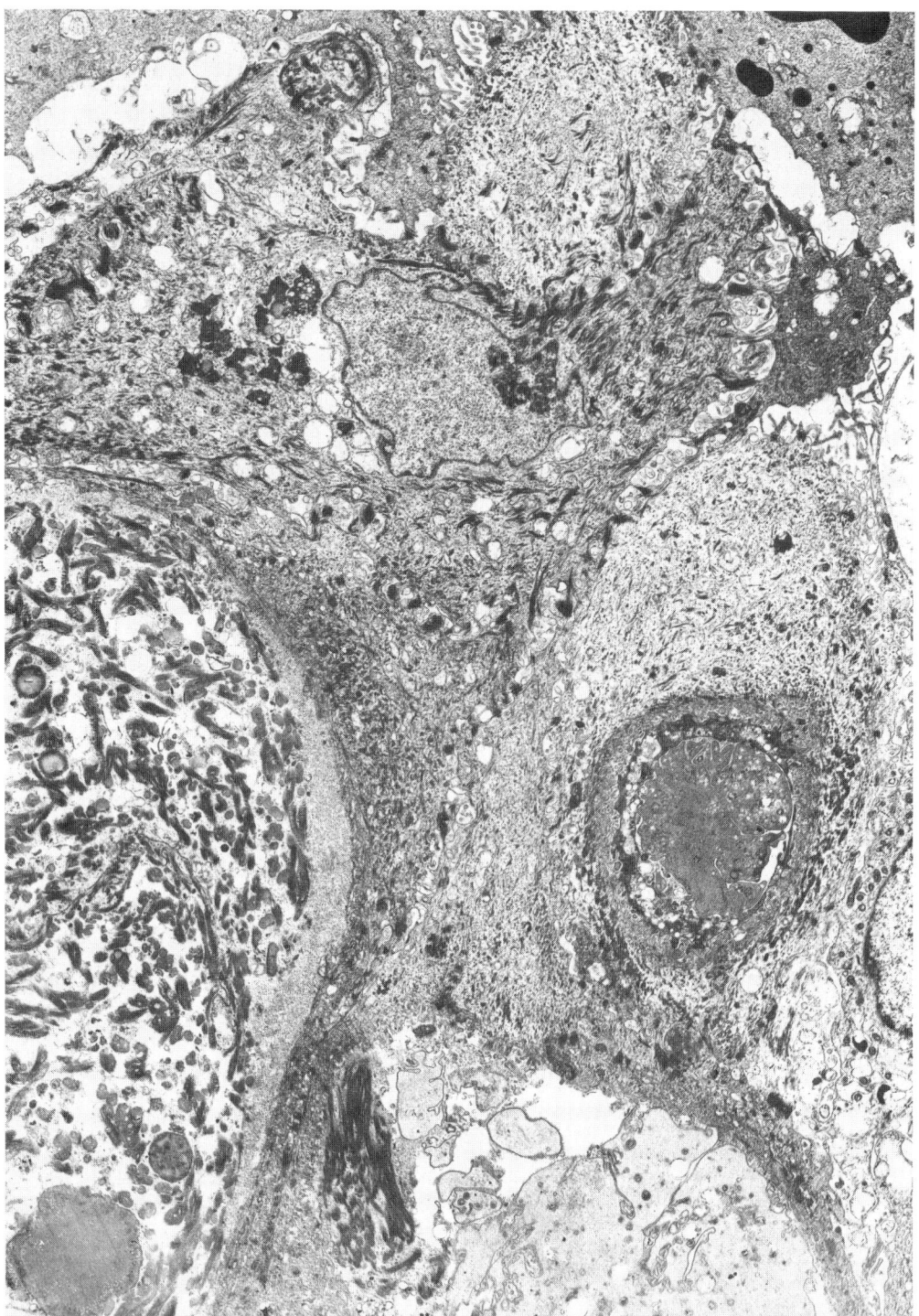

Fig. 3-31. Craniopharyngioma. Epithelial cells, joined by numerous desmosomes, contain thick bundles of tonofilaments. Note deposition of keratohyalin *(lower left)*. No secretory granules are seen. M × 6250.

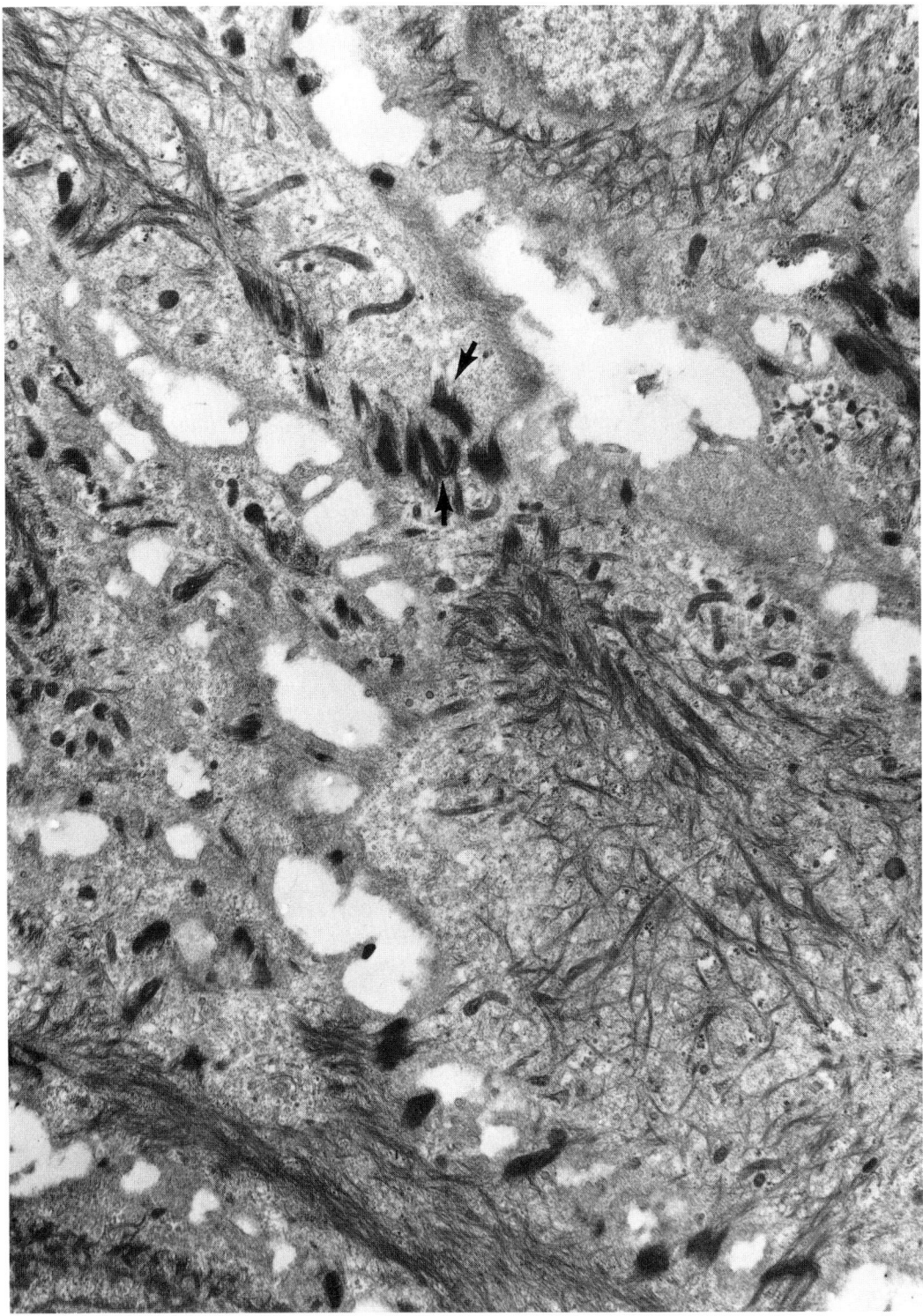

Fig. 3-32. Craniopharyngioma. Intricate network of tonofilaments and prominent desmosomes *(arrows)* are shown. M × 12,200.

Kahn[114] distinguishes between two types of craniopharyngioma: the childhood and the adult types. He describes the childhood form as a tumor with a distinct type of epithelium with palisading resembling that of embryonic dental and oral mucosa. Rounded masses of these cells in a connective tissue matrix are also seen and often contain nonviable cells, which undergo calcification.[143] The adult type is made up of squamous epithelium without palisading and with a less regular arrangement of the epithelial cells than occurs in the childhood type. The cells form islands and small cysts with no keratinization, no calcification, and very few mitoses. Although the childhood type is the most common and is usually seen in children and adolescents, it may be found in tumors occurring in all ages including the elderly adult.

Whether these differing histologic patterns clearly correlate with the different clinical courses often noted between adults and children is uncertain. According to some authors[143] the adult histologic type appears to have a better prognosis following partial surgical excision. Also there appear to be differences in clinical presentation, age of the patient, and the endocrine and radiologic findings.[143,147]

NEOPLASTIC DISORDERS: NONPITUITARY ORIGIN
Meningiomas

Meningiomas are extra-axial benign neoplasms arising from meningothelial cells that occur predominantly in the arachnoid villi.[27] Basal parapituitary meningiomas may take their dural origin from one of the following areas: tuberculum sella, medial sphenoid wing, olfactory groove, or optic nerve sheath. To this list Ojemann has added tumors arising from the floor of the anterior fossa over the roof of the orbit.[172] Intracranial meningiomas are most commonly diagnosed in the middle decades of life with a clear female predominance. An etiologic relationship of this neoplasm to prior trauma has been suggested,[38,231] especially by Cushing and Eisenhardt who recorded a definite history of prior head trauma in 33% of their 313 cases. No causal relationship, however, has ever been definitely established.

It has been shown that sex hormone receptors (estrogen and progesterone) are present in some meningiomas[48,182,207] and suggested that they play a role in the growth of these neoplasms.[116] Certain clinical observations support this idea, including: (1) the higher incidence of meningiomas in women among middle-aged persons and the lack of female prevalence at the extremes of life,[184] (2) the association between breast carcinoma and meningioma in the same patient,[116,209] and (3) the increased clinical manifestations (e.g., visual loss) of meningiomas during pregnancy and menstruation.[17] The best recognized examples of this last phenomenon are in meningiomas arising near the sella turcica (e.g., tuberculum sella, parasellar region, medial sphenoid ridge).[231] This is a result of the close proximity of the neoplasm to the optic nerves.

Grossly, meningiomas are firmly attached to the dura and usually appear nodular on the external surface. They have a tendency to excavate surrounding neural tissue without actually invading the brain. The majority of meningiomas

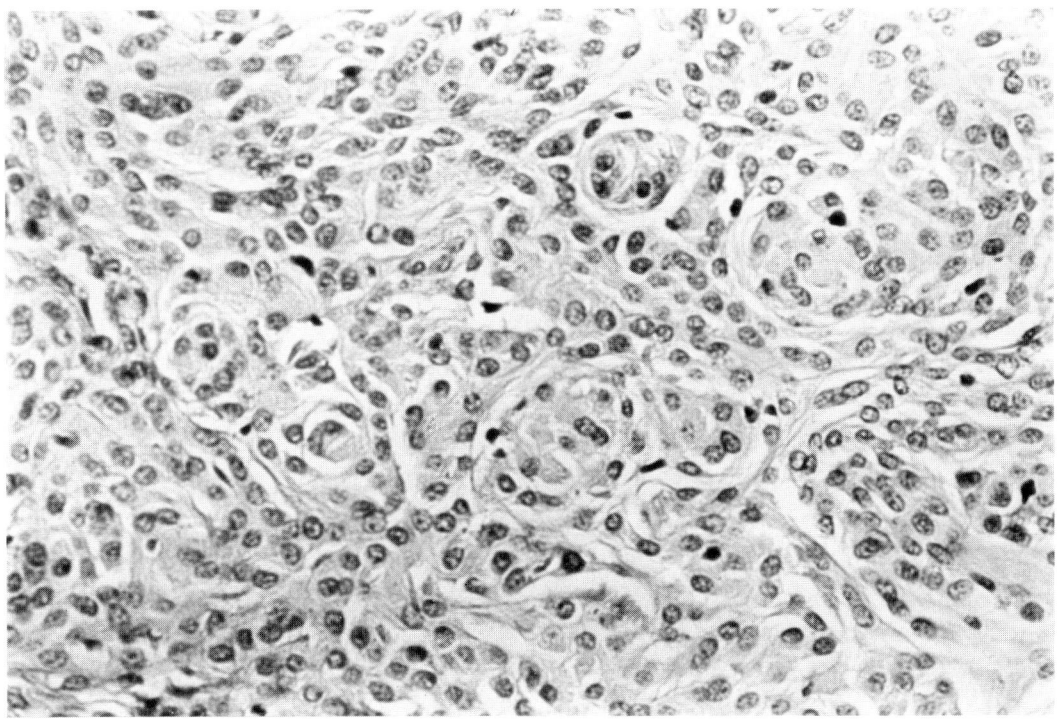

Fig. 3-33. Light microscopic appearance of meningothelial meningioma. Meningothelial cells are aggregated into whorls. M × 300.

are firm and tough and many develop calcified particles known as psammoma bodies that impart a hard, gritty character to the tumor.

A growth variant of meningiomas is the meningioma-en-plaque that not uncommonly occurs along the sphenoid ridge. These growths are not elevated above the level of the dura to a large degree but are prone to invade the underlying bone and produce hyperostosis. The bony thickening of hyperostosis is associated with invasion of the medullary spaces by tumor cells. The mechanism by which hyperostosis occurs is incompletely understood.

Many classifications of the microscopic appearance of meningiomas have been proposed, some quite complicated. The classic monograph of Cushing and Eisenhardt[38] lists nine major types and 20 subtypes. Even these authors admitted that much of this subdivision was of academic interest and of little prognostic significance. The pathologist, however, must be familiar with the various appearances of meningiomas. For practical purposes, we divide them into four types: syncytial (meningothelial), fibroblastic, transitional (psammomatous), and angioblastic.

The syncytial meningioma is formed by polygonal meningothelial cells aggregated into whorled sheets (Fig. 3-33). The individual cells have indistinct cell borders. The nuclei are relatively large and spherical and have pale nucleoplasm. Xanthoma cells may be present in large numbers and impart a yellowish tint to the tissue.

Fibroblastic meningiomas are composed of more elongated spindle cells forming interlacing bundles and sheets. The nuclei are narrow and occasionally tend to form palisades reminiscent of schwannomas. The transitional variant forms the typical whorls. Individual cells tend to be spindle shaped and contain fibroglial fibrils. The classification of angioblastic meningiomas has generated an ongoing debate that is beyond the scope of this book. "Angioblastic" refers to a neoplastic component of presumed endothelial, or pericytial, origin rather than from the stroma.[27] One type of angioblastic meningioma is pathologically identical to the hemangiopericytoma occurring elsewhere in the body. It consists of small cells with scanty cytoplasm and carrot-shaped nuclei. These tumors are highly cellular with an extensive reticulum network investing individual cells.

Hypothalamic and optic gliomas

Gliomas may develop within the hypothalamus or optic pathways to produce a suprasellar mass and pituitary dysfunction. All the common fibrillary astrocytic neoplasms (astrocytoma, anaplastic astrocytoma, and glioblastoma multiforme) may involve the region of the hypothalamus; a distinct type of astrocytic neoplasm, the pilocytic astrocytoma, characteristically arises in the walls of the third ventricle and the optic nerves. Although controversy exists over the preferred nomenclature, these tumors have a distinct morphology and clinical behavior. Clinically, there may be a long history of hypothalamic symptoms such as diabetes insipidus, obesity, bulimia, or emaciation resulting from the slow growth of these tumors. Two morphologic types of pilocytic astrocytomas have been described, the adult and juvenile pilocytic astrocytomas,[27,194] also called spongioblastoma (Fig. 3-34).[85,231,241]

The adult type is characteristically firm and discrete, although microscopic evidence of invasiveness is usually present. The neoplasm is predominantly composed of delicate, elongated, bipolar cells with areas where the cells are stellate and more randomly arranged. Rosenthal fibers (which are intracellular, intensely eosinophilic, elongated, or beaded bodies within the astrocytic cytoplasm) are frequently seen in these tumors. These fibers are believed to be the result of degeneration and are also seen in non-neoplastic disorders such as Alexander's disease, multiple sclerosis, and other disorders of the central nervous system.[91]

The juvenile variety of pilocytic astrocytomas is more common. The cells forming these tumors are similar to those described for the adult type but are more loosely arranged to produce a spongy, lobular, or microcystic pattern.[27] These areas are contiguous with more compact regions composed of strongly fibrillated cells that are often fusiform or polar.

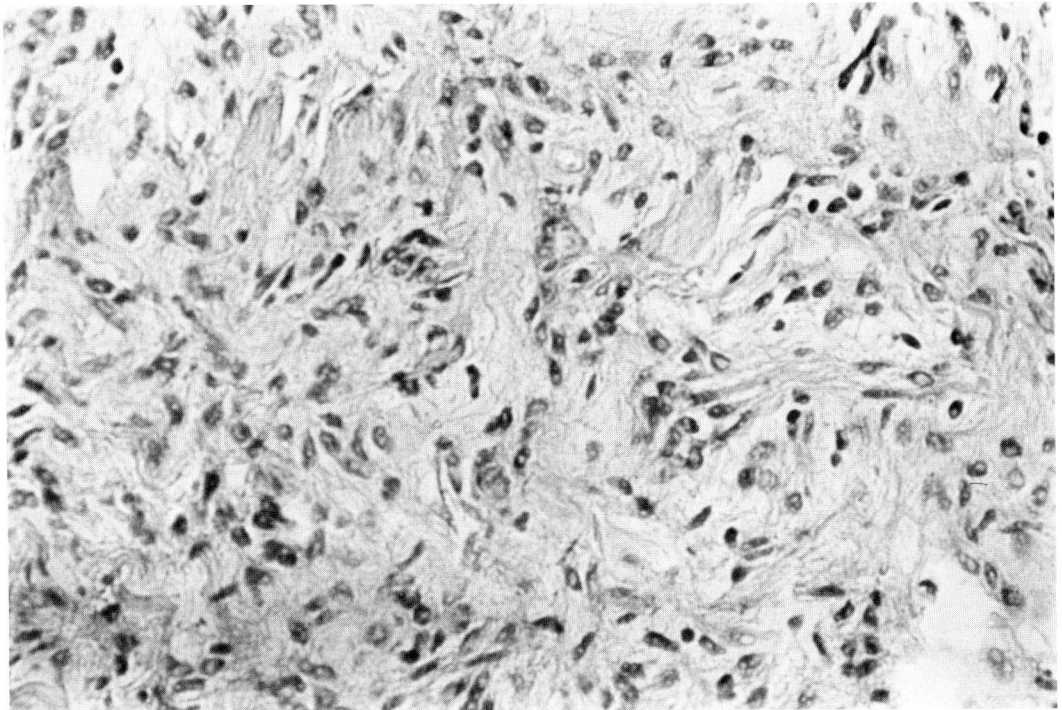

Fig. 3-34. Optic nerve glioma. M × 300.

The designation of spongioblastoma is controversial and is taken from the fusiform cells composing the tumors and the midline location of these tumors near the germinal epithelium, where spongioblasts originate.[27] A separate classification is justified on the basis of their benign behavior and characteristic location. Although the tumors are benign and slow growing, their location and adherence to vital structures limit life expectancy. Anaplastic degeneration may occur in the adult type more commonly than in the juvenile form.[101,238]

Gliomas of the optic nerves and chiasm produce visual loss, and those of the chiasm may cause hypothalamic and pituitary dysfunction. The optic nerve lesions most frequently occur in the first decade of life, often in association with von Recklinghausen's disease. A more aggressive variety may affect the chiasm of adults. Some believe the tumors of the optic nerve are quite benign with the biologic characteristics of a hamartoma,[100] whereas others regard them as having definite growth potential.[46,49,89,146,176]

Chordomas

Chordomas are slowly growing, destructive, and locally invasive tumors that originate from vestigial intraosseous remnants of the notochord. These tumors occur most commonly at the sacrococcygeal region and intracranially. The intracranial examples comprise about 40% of all chordomas and arise on the clivus at the spheno-occipital synchondrosis.[27] Rostral growth from this area with ac-

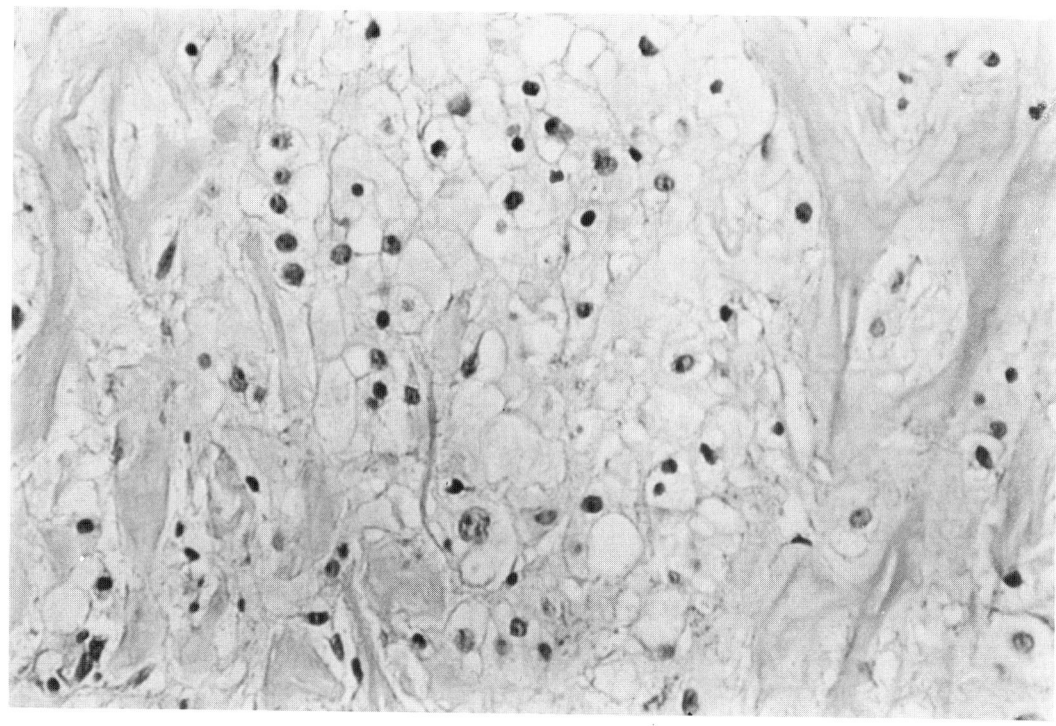

Fig. 3-35. Chordoma with various-sized clear cells separated by fibrous connective tissue. M × 300.

companying destruction of bone may involve the sella turcica, cavernous sinuses, optic pathways, and sphenoid sinus.

Grossly, chordomas are grayish, lobulated, and either soft or rather firm, frequently revealing areas of focal hemorrhages.

Microscopically, chordomas are composed of various-sized clear cells with a regular eosinophilic cytoplasm (Fig. 3-35). These cells are often organized into lobules or elongated cords separated by fibrous connective tissue. Many of the cells contain large intracytoplasmic vacuoles imparting a characteristic bubblelike appearance to the tumor termed "physaliphorous." The neoplastic cells contain and are surrounded by a variable amount of mucin.[27]

Although the cytologic features of chordomas are usually benign and mitoses are not found, the prognosis is poor because of the destructive and locally invasive characteristics of this neoplasm.

Dermoid and epidermoid cysts

Both dermoid and epidermoid cysts, also called "pearly" tumors, are believed to be formed as a result of the inclusion of epithelial elements at the time of closure of the neural tube between the third and fifth fetal week. Epidermoid cysts, or cholesteatomas, are lined by stratified squamous epithelium, whereas the lining of dermoids may also include skin appendages such as sweat glands, sebaceous glands, or hair follicles.

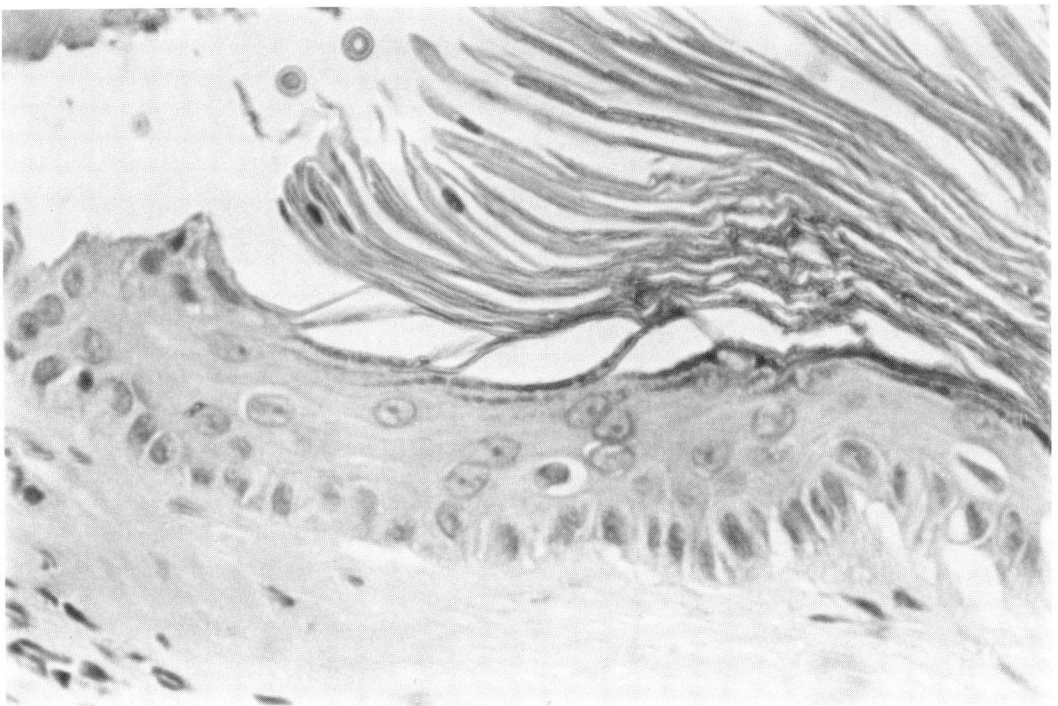

Fig. 3-36. Epidermoid. Note stratified squamous epithelium resting on an outer layer of connective tissue. M × 600.

Epidermoids occur more commonly in the intracranial cavity than dermoids. The epidermoid cysts are found most frequently in the cerebellopontine angle but also occur in the suprasellar and parasellar regions,[84] while intracranial dermoids are generally located in the posterior fossa as a midline cerebellar lesion.

These cysts present symptoms of a slowly enlarging mass. Leakage of cyst fluid from an epidermoid may produce a chemical meningitis, which may be recurrent.[27,84,212] Both dermoids and epidermoids appear as low density masses on the CT scan.

Grossly, dermoid cysts are well-defined, pink, sometimes lobulated masses in which calcification may be found. They contain sebaceous secretions and desquamated epithelium that is thick and yellowish.

Epidermoids are also well defined but have an irregular nodular surface that is thinner than that of the dermoid. Through the translucent capsule, the shiny white contents of the cyst can be seen and give the appearance from which the term *pearly tumor* is derived. The content of epidermoids is made up of desquamated epithelium that is soft, white, and flaky.

Microscopically, both dermoid and epidermoid cysts are lined by stratified squamous epithelium (Fig. 3-36). In dermoids, this epithelium also contains hair follicles and sebaceous and sweat glands. The epithelium of epidermoids lacks these appendages and rests on an outer layer of connective tissue. These tumors

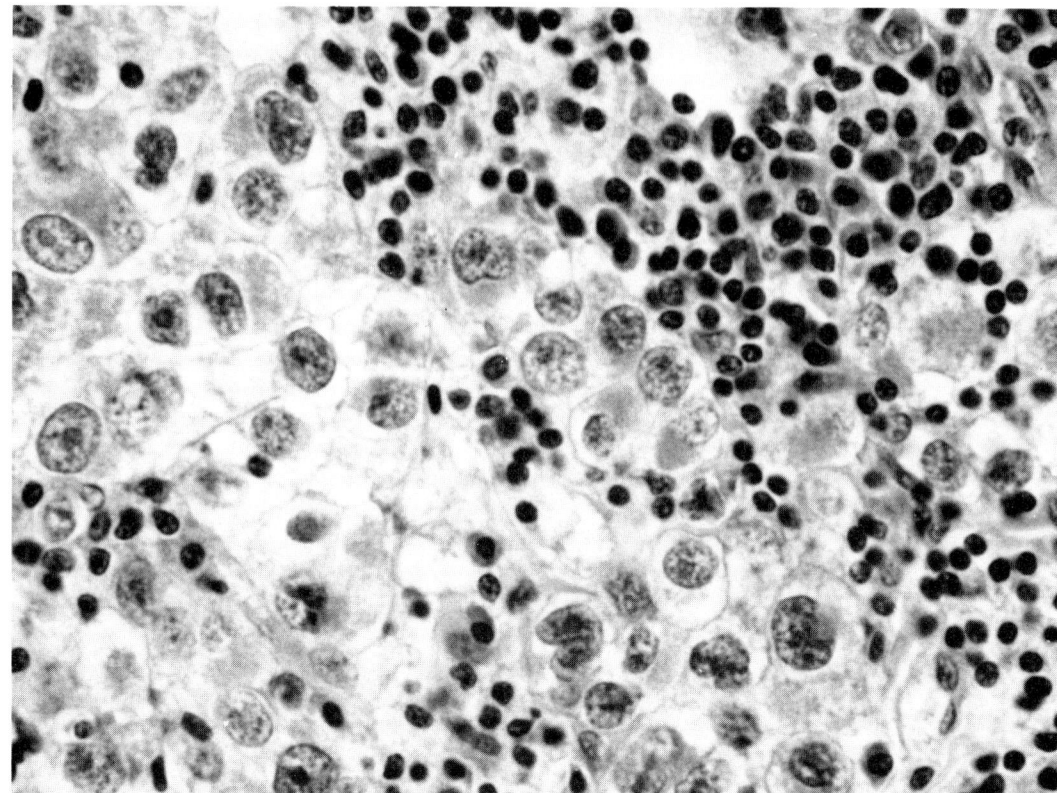

Fig. 3-37. Germinoma. Note two distinct cell types, large polygonal cells and small darkly staining lymphocytes. M × 700.

are both benign but will recur if incompletely removed. Malignant transformation of both dermoids and epidermoids has been noted but is quite rare.

Germinomas and teratoid tumors

Tumors of germ cell origin that occur in the gonads, mediastinum, and pineal region may also occur in the suprasellar or third ventricle areas, either in association with tumors of the pineal or as a solitary neoplasm (ectopic pinealoma). A primary intrasellar position has been reported but is quite rare.[73,75] Tumors of a germ cell origin in an intracranial location occur more commonly among the Japanese. They usually manifest themselves by production of diabetes insipidus, hypopituitarism, and loss of visual acuity. Hyperprolactinemia may result from interference with the action of PIF. Emaciation and precocious puberty may also occur.[193]

The most common of these germ cell tumors is the germinoma, which is histologically identical to the gonadal seminoma, dysgerminoma, and mediastinal germinoma. Grossly, these tumors are grayish, soft, and located in the suprasellar region adherent to the ventral surface of the brain and optic chiasm. Microscopically, the germinoma is composed of two distinct cell types: large polygonal or spherical cells and groups of small darkly staining lymphocytes (Fig. 3-37). The larger cells have conspicuous nuclei with large nucleoli and pale cytoplasm forming sheets and nests through which the smaller lymphocytes are interspersed. A feature of the hypothalamic germinoma is a marked hyperplastic neuroglial reaction surrounding the tumor.[193] Some germinomas contain human chorionic gonadotropin (HCG), which can be demonstrated by immunostaining and may cause elevated blood HCG levels. As with the testicular seminoma, the germinoma is regarded as being highly radiosensitive.

Other teratomatous tumors arising in the suprasellar region are all derived from totipotential cells and include the undifferentiated embryonal cell carcinoma, the teratoma (which is differentiated along embryonic lines), and the choriocarcinoma and yolk sac tumors (which differentiate along extraembryonic pathways). A given tumor may exhibit differentiation along different lines.

The primitive embryonal carcinoma is composed of anaplastic cuboid to columnar cells arranged in sheets and cords.[20,27,112] Some differentiation toward embryonic or extraembryonic elements may occur, producing cartilage or trophoblastic epithelium.[27] Alpha fetoprotein and human chorionic gonadotropin are produced by these tumors and may be detected in the serum and CSF.[3]

The teratoma is composed of three mature germinative layers. The microscopic appearance varies depending on the types of tissue elements derived from the three germ layers. There are often foci of squamous epithelium, cartilage, bone, and glandular elements.

The totipotential cells may rarely differentiate into extraembryonic tissues such as trophoblast or yolk sac to produce a choriocarcinoma or endodermal sinus tumor (yolk sac carcinoma), respectively.

Lipomas

Intracranial lipomas most commonly occur in the corpus callosum but have been described beneath the third ventricle or in the tuber cinereum, giving rise to hypothalamic disturbances.[234] Lipomas are believed to arise in the brain as a result of either metaplasia or heterotopic inclusion during embryonic development.[27]

Grossly, lipomas are yellow masses of fat that are well circumscribed and assume a variety of shapes. Microscopically, the tumors are composed of adipose cells with a variable amount of collagen interspersed. Various other tissues are occasionally found in lipomas, including Schwann cells,[26,194] hamartomatous blood vessels,[26,27] bone,[26,27,222] or cartilage.[26,206]

Other neoplasms

A variety of other neoplasms occur in the sella and parasellar area far less commonly than those entities already described. Indeed, some of these disorders are the subject of case reports only. A full description of the pathologic appearance of each of these unusual neoplasms is not warranted. Instead, we briefly discuss their existence and provide references for the interested reader.

Primary melanoma of the pituitary has been reported.[35,162,210] Acceptance as the primary tumor must depend on the exclusion of other possible primary extracranial sites. Because primary melanomas arising in the meninges are well documented,[31,74,193] it has been suggested that melanomas of the pituitary may arise from melanin-bearing cells of the diaphragm sella.[210] An origin from pigment-bearing cells of the neurohypophysis or adenohypophysis has also been proposed.[35,162] Copeland et al[35] hypothesized that a common origin of pituitary cells and melanocytes from neural crest derivatives could result in the heterotopic presence of melanocytes within the pituitary.

Bilbao et al[18] reported an intrasellar paraganglioma and suggested an origin from a nest of paraganglionic tissue included in the pituitary during development. As with melanocytes, paraganglionic tissue is derived from the neural crest, thus forming the basis for this theory.

Gangliocytomas may occur in the tuber cinereum and third ventricle or may present as intrasellar tumors.[7,81,109] The intrasellar neoplasms are believed to take origin from residual ganglionic cells known to be present in the fetal posterior lobe of the pituitary gland.[109] Some gangliocytomas may contain growth hormone–releasing factor (GHRF) and can be associated with acromegaly.[8]

Other rare intrasellar and parasellar tumors include chondromas,[41,142,177,200] hemangioblastomas,[39] schwannomas,[78] olfactory neuroblastomas,* lymphoproliferative disorders,† and tumors of skeletal origin.‡

Pituitary metastases

Both epithelial and hematopoietic neoplasms may metastasize to the pituitary gland. As many of these are asymptomatic, the reported incidence is dependent on how aggressively one searches for them.[1,120,189] Those primary tumors that most commonly metastasize to the pituitary in men are lung (62.9%), prostate (8.6%), and stomach (7.5%); whereas in women it is breast (66%), lung (13.2%), and stomach (7.5%).[226] The hematopoietic neoplasms that most commonly involve the pituitary are lymphoblastic leukemia (33.3%), non-Hodgkin's lymphoma (29%), and myeloblastic leukemia (21%).[25]

The pathologic picture is dependent on the particular primary tumor. With both carcinomas and hematopoietic neoplasms, the posterior pituitary is more frequently involved than the anterior pituitary (Fig. 3-38).[25,204,226] In these cases, the pituitary gland is usually grossly normal,[204] although large, symptomatic suprasellar extension is known to occur.[37,119,171]

---

*See references 72, 87, 108, 186, 188, and 208.
†See references 105, 113, 158, 173, and 221.
‡See references 2, 5, 32, 53, 60-62, 71, 149, 170, 181, 210, and 233.

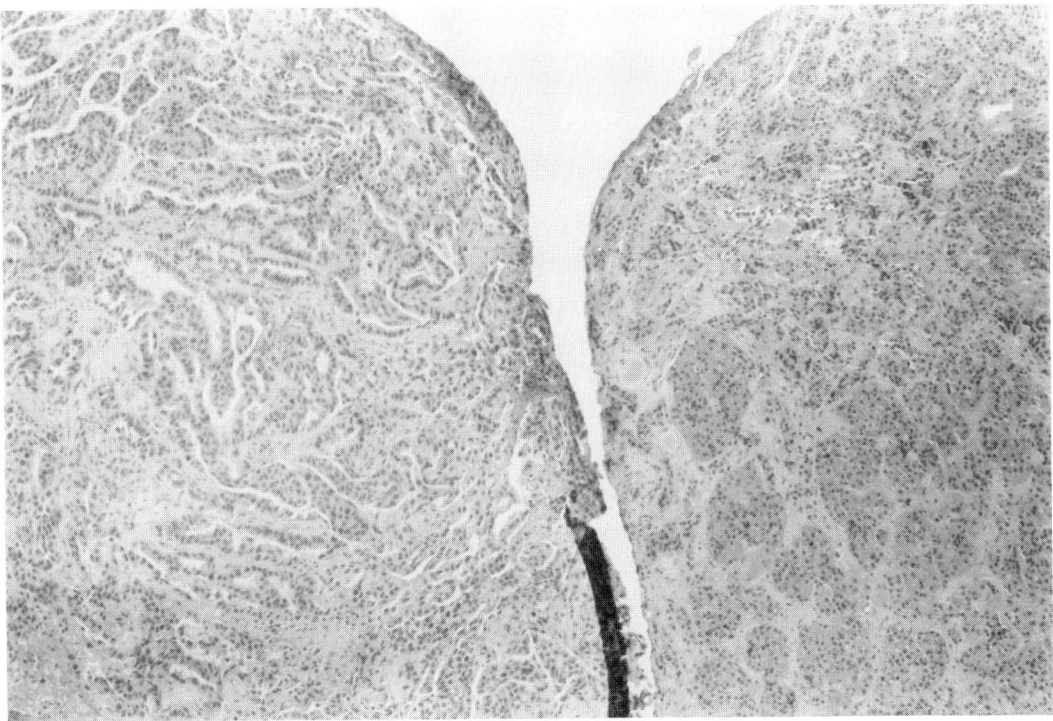

Fig. 3-38. Metastasis to posterior lobe of pituitary. Tumor within posterior lobe is on left-hand side with normal anterior lobe on right in this sagittal section of gland. M × 70.

NON-NEOPLASTIC DISORDERS
Sellar and suprasellar cysts

There are different types of cysts that may occur in the parasellar area. Like the craniopharyngioma and epidermoid cysts described earlier, Rathke's cleft cysts and mucoceles are lined by epithelial cells. Another type of cyst occurring in the sellar and suprasellar areas is the arachnoid cyst, which lacks an epithelial lining.

Rathke's cleft cysts are believed to form from remnants of Rathke's pouch, resulting from a persistence of the pouch between the developing anterior and intermediate lobes of the pituitary.[64,161] Some investigators have suggested that such cysts can be derived from neuroepithelium as well.[34,217] In support of this idea, Shuangshoti et al[217] emphasized that epithelial cysts of the pituitary region have a wide range of histologic features that were microscopically and histochemically indistinguishable from neuroepithelial (colloid) cysts. This may explain the mode of occurrence of Rathke's cleft cysts outside the sella turcica. Incidental cysts found in 13% to 23% of routine autopsies rarely exceed 7 mm in diameter.[13,153,214,215] Although unusual, Rathke's cleft cysts may enlarge and thus compress surrounding structures such as the pituitary gland, optic nerves or chiasm, hypothalamus, or third ventricle. They may also cause hyperprolactinemia.

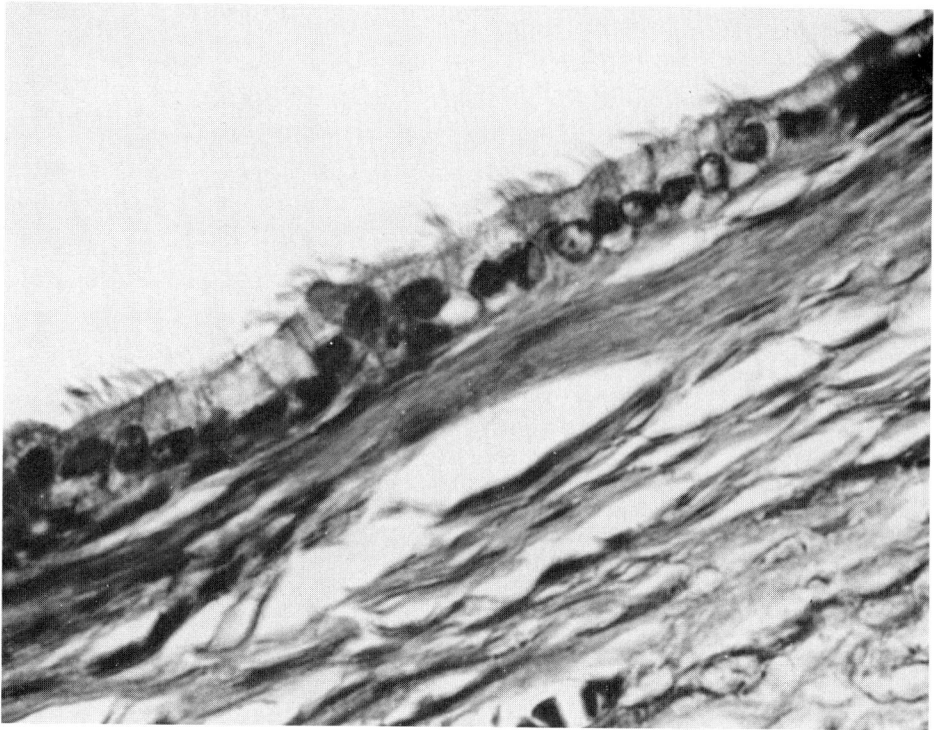

Fig. 3-39. Rathke's cleft cyst composed of single layer of ciliated columnar epithelium. M × 875.

The inner wall of a Rathke's cleft cyst is composed of a single layer of cuboid and/or columnar epithelium, many of which are ciliated (Fig. 3-39). They also contain mucus-secreting cells, which usually form a thick mucus content within the cyst. Accumulation of mucus has been cited as the cause of cyst enlargement to symptomatic size. The histologic description is variable. Rathke's cleft cysts lined by squamous epithelium have been described, and intrasellar and suprasellar epithelial cysts have shown histologic features of a craniopharyngioma. Fager and Carter[59] suggested that many Rathke's cleft cysts are misdiagnosed as craniopharyngiomas, a hypothesis supported by Banas' observation[10] that 4% of 160 intracranial masses diagnosed clinically and radiologically as craniopharyngiomas were histologically proved to be Rathke's cleft cysts.

Mucoceles are epithelial cysts that originate in the paranasal sinuses and are pathologically indistinguishable from Rathke's cleft cysts. This lesion may expand from a sinus with an occluded ostium and extend into the orbit or skull to compress the pituitary gland, optic nerves, or brain itself. The cysts are lined by ciliated, columnar, mucus-producing epithelium often identical to Rathke's cleft cysts. They do, however, frequently exhibit pressure atrophy of the epithelial cells, causing the cells to be more flattened. The differentiation of a mucocele from a Rathke's cleft cyst relies on the radiologic or gross observation of cyst extension from a paranasal sinus into the intracranial cavity.

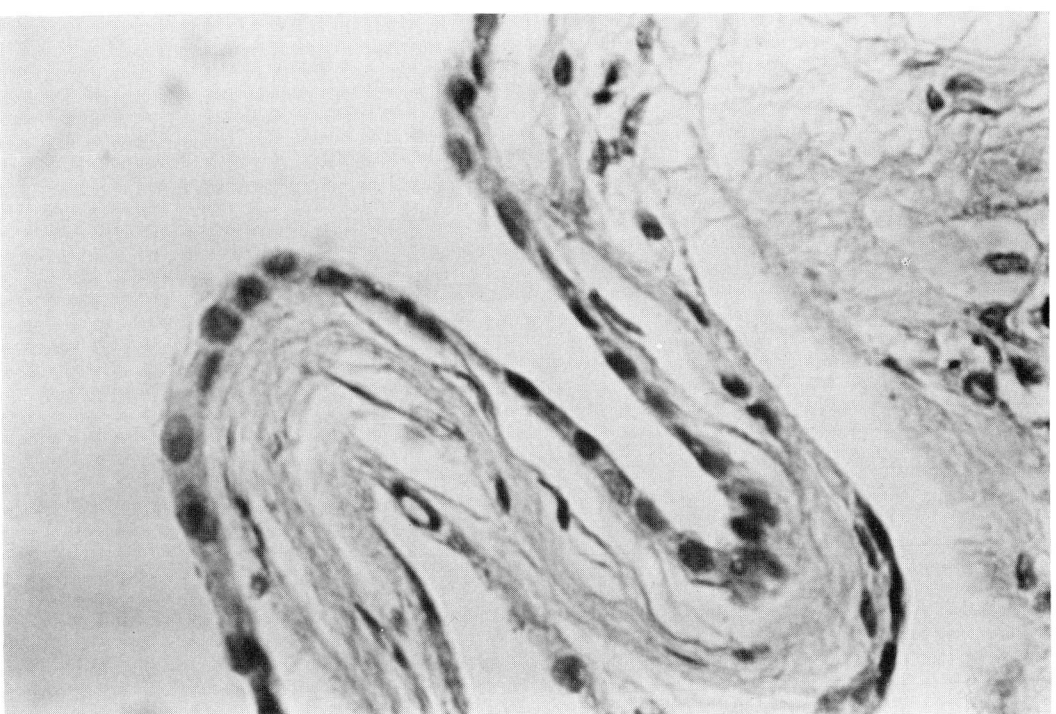

Fig. 3-40. Light microscopy of arachnoid cyst. M × 600.

Leptomeningeal or arachnoid cysts are distended areas of the subarachnoid space. They are filled with CSF and delineated on both inner and outer aspects by a delicate arachnoid membrane sparsely populated by meningothelial cells (Fig. 3-40). Enlargement is believed to occur either by an osmotic process or by a ball-valve phenomenon, where CSF intermittently gains entrance to the cyst without exit.

Aneurysms and other vascular malformations

An aneurysm, usually arising from the internal carotid artery, may occasionally simulate a pituitary tumor. By impinging on the pituitary stalk, the aneurysm may interfere with the delivery of PIF to the pituitary gland and result in hyperprolactinemia. Larger aneurysms may produce enough mass effect to result in hypopituitarism and mimic a nonfunctional pituitary adenoma.

A giant pituitary cavernous hemangioma has been reported as an incidental autopsy finding.[199] These lesions are considered by some to be congenital vascular malformations,[166] whereas others regard them as benign vascular neoplasms.[40,166,199,235] They usually occur in the brain parenchyma and are characterized by an aggregation of vascular sinusoids separated by fibrous septae without intervening glial tissue.

Dandy[40] also described a noncavernous angioma of the pituitary.

INFLAMMATORY DISORDERS

Pituitary abscess

An abscess of the pituitary is characterized pathologically by the presence of demarcated tissue destruction and an inflammatory reaction, which may be either acute or chronic. Cell necrosis and polymorphonuclear leukocytes characterize the histology. The abscess may be associated with the presence of a pituitary tumor.[47,141] This disorder is discussed more fully in Chapter 15.

Sarcoidosis

Sarcoidosis is a relatively common idiopathic granulomatous disease that may involve almost any organ system. Involvement of the nervous system occurs in approximately 5% of cases,[42,236] most commonly involving the peripheral and cranial nerves,[236] particularly the facial and optic nerves. Sarcoid lesions of the central nervous system are of two types. The more common is a granulomatous leptomeningitis with a predilection for the base of the brain, especially in the region of the hypothalamus and optic chiasm. Secondly, granulomas may occur in the brain or spinal cord parenchyma. Any level of the neuraxis may be affected to produce a wide variety of clinical manifestations.

In reported cases of hypothalamic involvement, presentations have included seizures, personality changes,[76] hypothermia,[22,111] diabetes insipidus,[239] obesity,[24] amenorrhea and galactorrhea,[24] and sleep derangement.[33] The lesions may simulate optic nerve gliomas and produce visual loss.[178] Hypopituitarism is said to be relatively uncommon but may be underestimated.[24,239] Hyperprolactinemia may occur with sarcoidosis. Angiotensin converting enzyme blood levels are elevated.

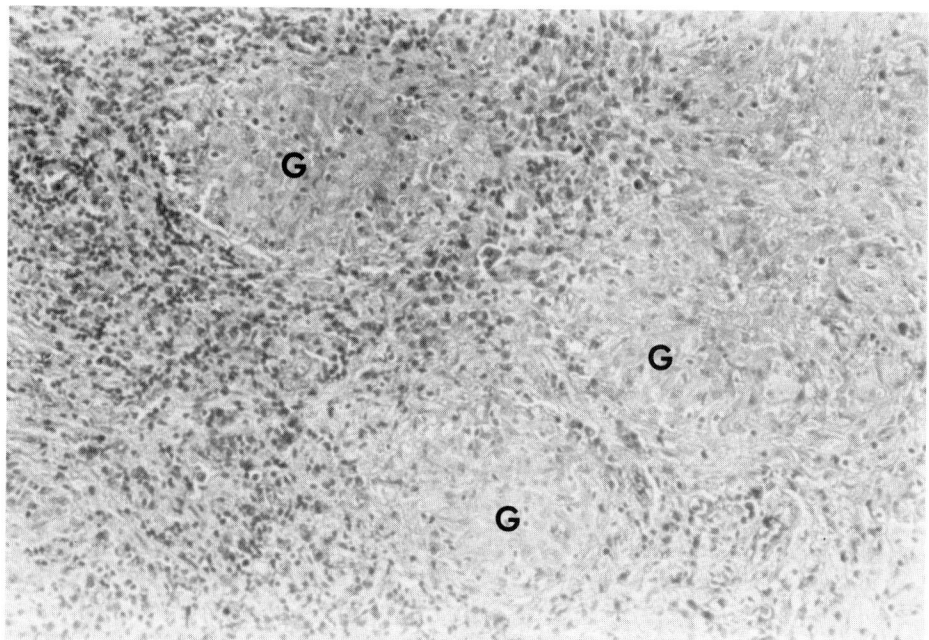

Fig. 3-41. Sarcoidosis. *G* marks noncaseating granulomas. M × 150.

Intracranial sarcoid varies in its gross appearance from meningeal thickening to well-circumscribed masses.[45,50,83,219] Microscopically, the lesions consist of accumulation of epithelioid cells, giant cells, macrophages, and fibroblasts forming noncaseating granulomas surrounded by lymphocytes (Fig. 3-41). The affinity of the sarcoid granuloma for cerebral vessels has been stressed.[50]

Histiocytosis X

Histiocytosis X refers to a group of histiocytic disorders ranging from the rather innocuous solitary eosinophilic granulomas of bone to deadly disseminated disorders of soft tissue. The nature of these disorders is incompletely understood. Although some have the pathologic and clinical appearance of an inflammatory disorder, others behave more like a neoplastic process. The solitary eosinophilic granuloma of the skull is almost always a self-limiting lesion that can be cured by excision.[80,140,152,175] A confident diagnosis can usually be made from the skull film, which reveals an osteolytic defect without peripheral sclerosis. They most commonly appear in younger patients between the ages of 2 and 20[139,140,152] and present as a slight mass with local tenderness. Grossly, they appear as soft, tan masses that have destroyed the full thickness of bone and are often adhered to but have not penetrated the dura. Microscopically, the lesion consists of a granulomatous reaction composed of large, pale histiocytes with foamy cytoplasm and smaller inflammatory cells, including lymphocytes, occasionally plasma cells, and eosinophils, which are most prominent (Fig. 3-42).

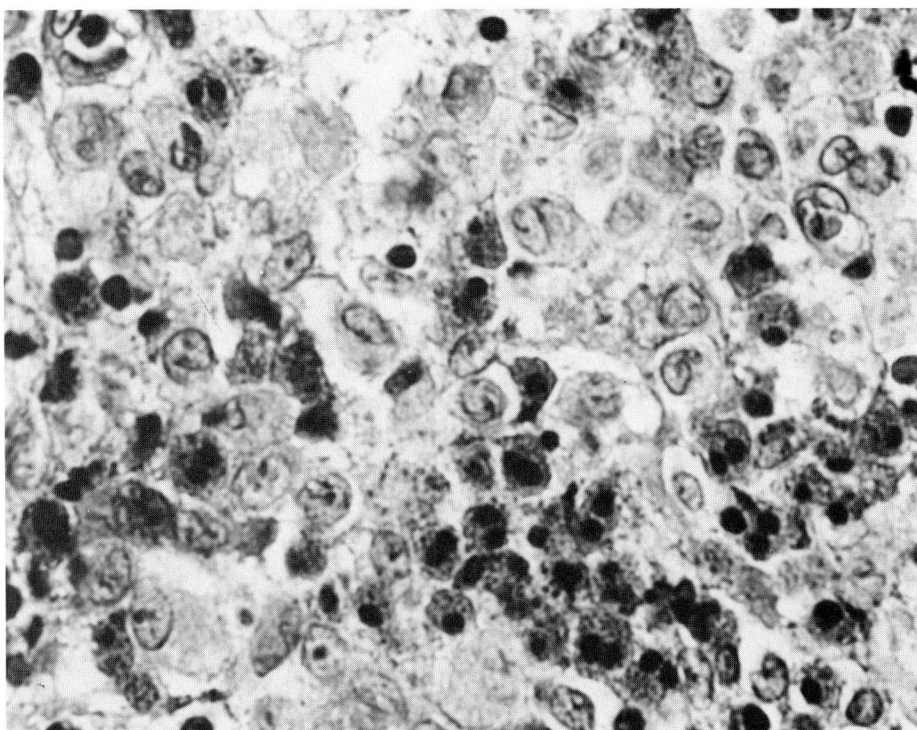

Fig. 3-42. Light microscopy of eosinophilic granuloma. M × 850.

By electron microscopy, the histiocytes that comprise the lesion have small processes and the cytoplasm contains lysosomes and a characteristic organelle known as the Langerhans', Birbeck's, or X granule.[12,165]

Beyond the solitary eosinophilic granuloma is the occurrence of disseminated histiocytosis X and much nosologic controversy. The entities of Hand-Schüller-Christian and Letterer-Siwe diseases are included in this latter category. The former refers to multifocal eosinophilic granuloma, which usually involves both the cranial vault and base of the skull, unlike the solitary lesions, which rarely involve the skull base. Lesions at the skull base may produce proptosis, growth retardation, and diabetes insipidus. The clinical presentation may include various forms of hypopituitarism. Localized masses involving primarily the infundibular region and hypothalamus have been described and produce other manifestations such as obesity and hypogonadism in addition to diabetes insipidus.[16,44,117,227] The isolated hypothalamic lesion is also referred to as Gagel's granuloma or Ayala's disease. The lesions of disseminated histiocytosis X and localized hypothalamic granulomas resemble those seen in isolated eosinophilic granuloma with Langerhans' granules and/or eosinophils. Various soft tissues may also be affected by multifocal eosinophilic granuloma, including skin, lymph nodes, liver, lung, spleen, and bone marrow.[29,107,156,165,237]

Letterer-Siwe disease refers to multiple histiolytic lesions primarily of the skin in a young patient, usually an infant.

Lymphocytic hypophysitis

Lymphocytic hypophysitis is believed to be an autoimmune disorder characterized by a destructive inflammatory process within the adenohypophysis that may result in varying degrees of hypopituitarism. In the cases reported in the literature, there was microscopically the presence of lymphoid nodules, a diffuse infiltrate of lymphocytes and plasma cells, interstitial fibrosis, and sparing of the posterior lobe.[54,77,79,104,132] Levine was able to produce an animal model of the disease in rats by injection of rat pituitary tissue and an immunologic adjuvant.[138]

Clinically, amenorrhea and galactorrhea may occur, and hyperprolactinemia may be noted. Hypopituitarism can also result. The disease occurs mainly in young women and is often associated with pregnancy or lactation. Thus, lymphocytic hypophysitis can mimic a prolactinoma.

REFERENCES

1. Abrams HL, Spiro R, Goldstein N: Metastases in carcinoma: Analysis of 1000 autopsied cases. *Cancer* 3:74, 1950.
2. Alexander MP, Goodkin DE, Poser CM: Solitary plasmacytoma producing cranial neuropathy. *Arch Neurol* 32:777, 1975.
3. Allen JC, Nisselbaum J, Epstein F, et al: Alpha fetoprotein and human chorionic gonadotropin determination in cerebrospinal fluid: An aid to the diagnosis and management of intracranial germ-cell tumors. *J Neurosurg* 51:368, 1979.
4. Al-Sarraf M, Loud AV, Vaitkevicius VK: Malignant granular cell tumor: Histochemical and electron microscopic study. *Arch Pathol* 91:550, 1971.
5. Amine ARC, Sugar O: Suprasellar osteogenic sarcoma following radiation for pituitary adenoma: Case report. *J Neurosurg* 44:88, 1976.
6. Asa SL, Horvath E, Kovacs K, et al: Cytology of the normal pituitary and pituitary tumors, in Odell WD, Nelson DH (eds): *Pituitary Tumors*. Mount Kisco, NY, Futura Publishing Co Inc, 1984.
7. Asa SL, Kovacs K, Tindall GT, et al: Cushing's disease associated with an intrasellar gangliocytoma producing corticotrophin-releasing factor. *Ann Intern Med* 101: 789, 1984.
8. Asa SL, Scheithauer BW, Bilbao JM, et al: A case for hypothalamic acromegaly: A clinicopathological study of six patients with hypothalamic gangliocytomas producing growth hormone–releasing factor. *J Clin Endocrinol Metab* 58:796, 1984.
9. Bangle R Jr: A morphological and histochemical study of the granular-cell myoblastoma. *Cancer* 5:950, 1952.
10. Banna M: Craniopharyngioma: Based on 160 cases. *Br J Radiol* 49:206, 1976.
11. Barrow DL, Tindall GT, Kovacs K, et al: Clinical and pathological effects of bromocriptine on prolactin secreting and other pituitary tumors. *J Neurosurg* 60:1, 1984.
12. Basset F, Escaig J, Le Crom M: A cytoplasmic membranous complex in histiocytosis X. *Cancer* 29:1380, 1972.
13. Bayoumi ML: Rathke's cleft and its cysts. *Edinburgh Med J* 55:745, 1948.
14. Benda C: Beiträge zur normalen und pathologischen: Histologie der menschlichen Hypophysis cerebri. *Berl Klin Wochenschr* 37:1205, 1900.
15. Bergland RM, Torack RM: An ultrastructural study of follicular cells in the human anterior pituitary. *Am J Pathol* 57:273, 1969.
16. Bernard JD, Aguilar MJ: Localized hypothalamic histiocytosis X: Report of a case. *Arch Neurol* 20:368, 1969.
17. Bickerstaff ER, Small JM, Guest IA: The relapsing course of certain meningiomas in relation to pregnancy and menstruation. *J Neurol Neurosurg Psychiatry* 21:89, 1958.
18. Bilbao JM, Horvath E, Kovacs K, et al: Intrasellar paraganglioma associated with hypopituitarism. *Arch Pathol Lab Med* 102:95, 1978.
19. Bonner RA, Mukai K, Oppenheimer JH: Two unusual variants of Nelson's syndrome. *J Clin Endocrinol Metab* 49:23, 1979.
20. Borit A: Embryonal carcinoma of the pineal region. *J Pathol* 97:165, 1969.
21. Borit A, Blanshard TP: Sphenoidal pituitary adenoma. *Hum Pathol* 10:93, 1979.
22. Branch EF, Burger PC, Brewer DL: Hypothermia in a case of hypothalamic infarction and sarcoidosis. *Arch Neurol* 25:245, 1971.
23. Brookes LD: A stain for differentiating two types of acidophil cells in the rat pituitary. *Stain Technol* 43:41, 1968.
24. Brust JCM, Rhee RS, Plank CR, et al: Sarcoidosis, galactorrhea, and amenorrhea: 2 autopsy cases, 1 with Chiari-Frommel syndrome. *Ann Neurol* 2:130, 1977.
25. Buchmann E, Schwesinger G: Hypophyse and Hämoblastosen. *Zentralbl Neurochir* 40:35, 1979.
26. Budka H: Intracranial lipomatous hamartomas (intracranial "lipomas"): A study of 13 cases including combinations with medulloblastoma, colloid and epidermoid cysts, angiomatosis and other malformations. *Acta Neuropathol* 28:205, 1974.
27. Burger PC, Vogel FS: *Surgical Pathology of the Nervous System and its Coverings*. New York, John Wiley & Sons Inc, 1976.
28. Camp JD: Significance of intracranial calcification in the roentgenologic diagnosis of intracranial neoplasms. *Radiology* 55:659, 1950.
29. Cancilla PA, Lahey ME, Carnes WH: Cutaneous lesions of Letterer-Siwe disease: Electron microscopic study. *Cancer* 20:1986, 1967.
30. Celio MR, Pasi A, Bürgisser E, et al: "Proopiocortin fragments" in normal human adult pituitary: Distribution and ultrastructural characterization of immunoreactive cells. *Acta Endocrinol* 95:27, 1980.
31. Christensen E: Two cases of primary intracranial melanoma. *Acta Chir Scand* 85:90, 1941.
32. Clarke E: Cranial and intracranial myelomas. *Brain* 77:61, 1954.
33. Colover J: Sarcoidosis with involvement of the nervous system. *Brain* 71:451, 1948.

34. Concha S, Hamilton BPM, Millan JC, et al: Symptomatic Rathke's cleft cyst with amyloid stroma. *J Neurol Neurosurg Psychiatry* 38:782, 1975.
35. Copeland DD, Sink JD, Seigler HF: Primary intracranial melanoma presenting as a suprasellar tumor. *Neurosurgery* 6:542, 1980.
36. Corenblum B, Sirek AMT, Horvath E, et al: Human mixed somatotrophic and lactotrophic pituitary adenomas. *J Clin Endocrinol Metab* 42:857, 1976.
37. Cox EV III: Chiasmal compression from metastatic cancer to the pituitary gland. *Surg Neurol* 11:49, 1979.
38. Cushing H, Eisenhardt L: *Meningiomas: Their Classification, Regional Behaviour, Life History and Surgical End Results*. Springfield, Ill., Charles C Thomas Publisher, 1938.
39. Dan NG, Smith DE: Pituitary hemangioblastoma in a patient with von Hippel–Lindau disease: Case report. *J Neurosurg* 42:232, 1975.
40. Dandy WE: Venous abnormalities and angiomas of the brain. *Arch Surg* 17:715, 1928.
41. de Divitiis E, Spaziante R, Cirillo S, et al: Primary sellar chondromas. *Surg Neurol* 11:229, 1979.
42. Delaney P: Neurologic manifestations in sarcoidosis: Review of the literature, with a report of 23 cases. *Ann Intern Med* 87:336, 1977.
43. Demura R, Kubo O, Demura H, et al: FSH and LH secreting pituitary adenoma. *J Clin Endocrinol Metab* 45:653, 1977.
44. Den Hartog JC, Guazzi GC, Vicente AN: Réticuloendothéliose cérébrale primitive (dite encéphalite granulomateuse) et granulome infundibulo-tubérien. *Rev Neurol* 102:20, 1960.
45. de Tribolet N, Zander E: Intracranial sarcoidosis presenting angiographically as a sub-dural hematoma. *Surg Neurol* 9:169, 1978.
46. Dodge HW Jr, Love JG, Craig WM, et al: Gliomas of the optic nerves. *Arch Neurol Psychiat* 79:607, 1958.
47. Domingue JN, Wilson CB: Pituitary abscesses: Report of seven cases and review of the literature. *J Neurosurg* 46:601, 1977.
48. Donnell MS, Meyer GA, Donegan WL: Estrogen receptor protein in intracranial meningiomas, *J Neurosurg* 50:499, 1979.
49. Dosoretz DE, Blitzer PH, Wang CC, et al: Mangement of glioma of the optic nerve and/or chiasm: An analysis of 20 cases. *Cancer* 45:1467, 1980.
50. Douglas AC, Maloney AFJ: Sarcoidosis of the central nervous system. *J Neurol Neurosurg Psychiatry* 36: 1024, 1973.
51. Duello TM, Halmi NS: Pituitary adenoma producing thyrotropin and prolactin: An immunocytochemical and electron microscopic study. *Virchows Arch* 376:255, 1977.
52. Earle KM, Dillard SH Jr: Pathology of adenomas of the pituitary gland, in Kohler PO, Ross GT (eds): *Diagnosis and Treatment of Pituitary Tumors*. Amsterdam, Excerpta Medica, 1973.
53. Echols DH: Giant cell tumor of the sphenoid bone: Report of a case. *J Neurosurg* 2:16, 1945.
54. Egloff B, Fischbacher W, von Goumoëns E: Lymphomatöse hypophysitis mit hypopyseninsuffizienz. *Schweiz Med Wochenschr* 99:1499, 1969.
55. Erdheim J: Zur normalen und pathologischen Histologie der Glandula Thyreoidea, Parathyreoida und Hypophysis. *Beitr Pathol Anat Allg Pathol* 33:158, 1903.
56. Erdheim J: Uber einen Hypophysentumor von ungewohnlichem. *Sitz Beitr Pathol Anat* 46:233, 1909.
57. Ezrin C, Horvath E, Kovacs K: Anatomy and cytology of the normal and abnormal pituitary gland, in De Groot LJ, Cahill GF, Odell WD, et al (eds): *Endocrinology*. New York, Grune & Stratton Inc, 1979, vol 1.
58. Ezrin C, Kovacs K, Horvath E: Hyperprolactinemia: Morphologic and clinical considerations. *Med Clin North Am* 62:393, 1978.
59. Fager CH, Carter H: Intrasellar epithelial cysts. *J Neurosurg* 24:77, 1966.
60. Faraci RP, Ketcham AS: Fibrous dysplasia of the sphenoid sinus in an adolescent male. *J Surg Oncol* 7:461, 1975.
61. Fernandez E, Colavita N, Moschini M, et al: "Fibrous dysplasia" of the skull with complete unilateral cranial nerve involvement: Case report. *J Neurosurg* 52:404, 1980.
62. Finney HL, Roberts TS: Fibrous dysplasia of the skull with progressive cranial nerve involvement. *Surg Neurol* 6:341, 1976.
63. Foncin JF, Billet R, LeBeau, J: A propos des tumeurs hypophysaires extensives a secretion corticotrope (etude ultrastructurale). *Ann Endocrinol* 33:449, 1972.
64. Frazier CH, Alpers BJ: Tumors of Rathke's cleft (hitherto called tumors of Rathke's pouch). *Arch Neurol Psychiatry* 32:973, 1934.
65. Friend JN, Judge DM, Sherman BM, et al: FSH-secreting pituitary adenomas: Stimulation and suppression studies in two patients. *J Clin Endocrinol Metab* 43:650, 1976.
66. Furth J, Clifton KH: Experimental pituitary tumours, in Harris GW, Donovan BT (eds): *The Pituitary Gland*. Berkeley, Calif., University of California Press, 1966, vol 2.

67. Fust JA, Custer RP: On the neurogenesis of so-called granular cell myoblastoma. *Am J Clin Pathol* 19:522, 1949.
68. Garancis JC, Komorowski RA, Kuzma JF: Granular cell myoblastoma. *Cancer* 25:542, 1970.
69. Garcia JH, Kalimo H, Givens JR: Human adenohypophysis in Nelson syndrome: Ultrastructural and clinical study. *Arch Pathol Lab Med* 100:253, 1976.
70. Garcia-Uria J: Surgical experience with craniopharyngioma in adults. *Surg Neurol* 9:11, 1978.
71. Geissinger JD, Siqueira EB, Ross ER: Giant cell tumors of the sphenoid bone. *J Neurosurg* 32:665, 1970.
72. Gerard-Marchant R, Micheau C: Microscopical diagnosis of olfactory esthesioneuromas: General review and report of five cases. *J Natl Cancer Inst* 35:75, 1965.
73. Ghatak NR, Hirano A, Zimmerman HM: Intrasellar germinomas: A form of ectopic pinealoma. *J Neurosurg* 31:670, 1969.
74. Gibson JB, Burrows D, Weir WP: Primary melanoma of the meninges. *J Pathol* 74:419, 1957.
75. Giuffrè R, Di Lorenzo N: Evolution of a primary intrasellar germinomatous teratoma into a choriocarcinoma: Case report. *J Neurosurg* 42:602, 1975.
76. Gjersøe A, Kjerulf-Jensen K: Hypothalamic lesions caused by Boeck's sarcoid. *J Clin Endocrinol* 10:1602, 1950.
77. Gleason TH, Stebbins PL, Shanahan MF: Lymphoid hypophysitis in a patient with hypoglycemic episodes. *Arch Pathol Lab Med* 102:46, 1978.
78. Goebel HH, Shimokawa K, Schaake T, et al: Schwannoma of the sellar region. *Acta Neurochir* 48:191, 1979.
79. Goudie RB, Pinkerton PH: Anterior hypophysitis and Hashimoto's disease in a young woman. *J Pathol* 83:584, 1962.
80. Green WT, Farber S: "Eosinophilic or solitary granuloma" of bone. *J Bone Joint Surg* 24:499, 1942.
81. Greenfield JG: The pathological examination of forty intracranial neoplasms. *Brain* 42:29, 1919.
82. Greenhouse AH: Pituitary sarcoma. *JAMA* 190:269, 1964.
83. Griggs RC, Markesbery WR, Condemi JJ: Cerebral mass due to sarcoidosis: Regression during corticosteroid therapy. *Neurology* 23:981, 1973.
84. Guidetti B, Gagliardi FM: Epidermoid and dermoid cysts: Clinical evaluation and late surgical results. *J Neurosurg* 47:12, 1977.
85. Gullotta F, Fliedner E: Spongioblastomas, astrocytomas and Rosenthal fibers: Ultrastructural, tissue culture and enzyme histochemical investigations. *Acta Neuropathol* 22:68, 1972.
86. Guyda H, Robert F, Colle E, et al: Histologic, ultrastructural and hormonal characterization of a pituitary tumor secreting both hGH and prolactin. *J Clin Endocrinol Metab* 36:531, 1973.
87. Hamilton AE, Rubinstein LJ, Poole GJ: Primary intracranial esthesioneuroblastoma (olfactory neuroblastoma). *J Neurosurg* 38:548, 1973.
88. Hardy J: Transsphenoidal hypophysectomy. *J Neurosurg* 34:582, 1971.
89. Heiskanen O, Raitta C, Torsti R: The management and prognosis of gliomas of the optic pathways in children. *Acta Neurochir* 43:193, 1978.
90. Herlant M: Etude critique de deux techniques nouvelles destinees a mettre en evidence les differentes categories cellulaires presentes dans la glande pituitaire. *Bull Microscopic Appl* 10:37, 1960.
91. Herndon RM, Rubinstein LJ, Freeman JM, et al: Light and electron microscopic observations on Rosenthal fibers in Alexander's disease and in multiple sclerosis. *J Neuropathol Exp Neurol* 29:524, 1970.
92. Horvath E, Kovacs K: Misplaced exocytosis. Distinct ultrastructural feature in some pituitary adenomas. *Arch Pathol* 97:221, 1974.
93. Horvath E, Kovacs K: Ultrastructural classification of pituitary adenomas. *Can J Neurol Sci* 3:9, 1976.
94. Horvath E, Kovacs K: Pathology of the pituitary gland, in Ezrin C, Horvath E, Kaufman B, et al (eds): *Pituitary Diseases*. Boca Raton, Fla., CRC Press Inc, 1980.
95. Horvath E, Kovacs K: Gonadotroph adenomas of the human pituitary: Sex-related fine-structural dichotomy: A histologic, immunocytochemical and electron microscopic study of 30 tumors. *Am J Pathol* 117:429, 1984.
96. Horvath E, Kovacs K, Ezrin C: Centrioles and cilia in non-tumorous anterior lobes and adenomas of the human pituitary. *Pathol Eur* 11:81, 1976.
97. Horvath E, Kovacs K, Killinger DW, et al: Mammosomatotroph cell adenoma of the human pituitary: A morphologic entity. *Virchows Arch* 398:277, 1983.
98. Horvath E, Kovacs K, Scheithauer BW, et al: Pituitary adenomas producing growth hormone, prolactin, and one or more glycoprotein hor-

mones: A histologic, immunohistochemical, and ultrastructural study of four surgically removed tumors. *Ultrastruct Pathol* 5:171, 1983.
99. Horvath E, Kovacs K, Singer W, et al: Acidophil Stem cell adenoma of the human pituitary. *Arch Pathol Lab Med* 101:594, 1977.
100. Hoyt WF, Baghdassarian SA: Optic glioma of childhood: Natural history and rationale for conservative management. *Br J Ophthalmol* 53:793, 1969.
101. Hoyt WF, Meshel LG, Lessell S, et al: Malignant optic glioma of adulthood. *Brain* 96:121, 1973.
102. Hsu S, Raine L, Fanger H: A comparative study of the peroxidase-antiperoxidase method and an avidin-biotin complex method for studying polypeptide hormones with radioimmunoassay antibodies. *Am J Clin Pathol* 75:734, 1981.
103. Hsu S, Raine L, Fanger H: The use of antiavidin antibody and avidin-biotin-peroxidase complex in immunoperoxidase technics. *Am J Clin Pathol* 75:816, 1981.
104. Hume R, Roberts GH: Hypophysitis and hypopituitarism: Report of a case. *Br Med J* 2:548, 1967.
105. Hunt WE, Bouroncle BA, Meagher JN: Neurologic complications of leukemias and lymphomas. *J Neurosurg* 16:135, 1959.
106. Hymer WC, McShan WH, Christiansen RG: Electron microscopic studies of anterior pituitary glands from lactating and estrogen-treated rats. *Endocrinology* 69:81, 1961.
107. Imamura M, Muroya K: Lymph node ultrastructure in Hand-Schüller-Christian disease. *Cancer* 27:956, 1971.
108. Jakumeit HD: Neuroblastoma of the olfactory nerve. *Acta Neurochir* 25:99, 1971.
109. Jakumeit HD, Zimmermann V, Guiot G: Intrasellar gangliocytomas: Report of four cases. *J Neurosurg* 40:626, 1974.
110. Jefferson G: *The Invasive Adenomas of the Anterior Pituitary*. The Sherrington Lectures. Liverpool, England, University of Liverpool Press, 1955, vol 3.
111. Jefferson M: Sarcoidosis of the nervous system. *Brain* 80:540, 1957.
112. Jellinger K: Primary intracranial germ cell tumours. *Acta Neuropathol* 25:291, 1973.
113. Jellinger K, Radaszkiewicz T: Involvement of the central nervous system in malignant lymphomas. *Virchows Arch* 370:345, 1976.
114. Kahn EA, Gosch HH, Seeger JF, et al: Forty-five years' experience with the craniopharyngiomas. *Surg Neurol* 1:5, 1973.
115. Kammer H, George R: Cushing's disease in a patient with an ectopic pituitary adenoma. *JAMA* 246:2722, 1981.
116. Kepes JJ: *Meningiomas, Biology, Pathology, and Differential Diagnosis*. New York, Masson Publishing USA Inc, 1982.
117. Kepes JJ, Kepes M: Predominantly cerebral forms of histiocytosis X: A reappraisal of "Gagel's hypothalamic granuloma," "granuloma infiltrans of the hypothalamus" and "Ayala's disease" with a report of four cases. *Acta Neuropathol* 14:77, 1969.
118. Kinnman JEG: *Acromegaly: An Ultrastructural Analysis of 51 Adenomas and a Clinical Study in 80 Patients Treated by Transanthrosphenoidal Operation*. Stockholm, Norstedt och SönersFörlag, 1973.
119. Kistler M, Pribram HW: Metastatic disease of the sella turcica. *AJR* 123:13, 1975.
120. Kovacs K: Metastatic cancer of the pituitary gland. *Oncology* 27:533, 1973.
121. Kovacs K: Morphology of prolactin-producing adenomas. *Clin Endocrinol* 6(suppl):715, 1977.
122. Kovacs K, Horvath E: Pathology of pituitary adenomas. *Bull Los Angeles Neurol Soc* 42:92, 1977.
123. Kovacs K, Horvath E, Corenblum B, et al: Pituitary chromophobe adenomas consisting of prolactin cells: A histologic, immunocytological and electron microscopic study. *Virchows Arch* 366:113, 1975.
124. Kovacs K, Horvath E, Ezrin C: Pituitary adenomas. *Pathol Annu* 12(pt 2):341, 1977.
125. Kovacs K, Horvath E, Ezrin C, et al: Adenoma of the human pituitary producing growth hormone and thyrotropin: A histologic, immunocytologic and fine-structural study. *Virchows Arch* 395:59, 1982.
126. Kovacs K, Horvath E, Kerenyi NA, et al: Light and electron microscopic features of a pituitary adenoma in Nelson's syndrome. *Adm J Clin Pathol* 65:337, 1976.
127. Kovacs K, Horvath E, Rewcastle NB, et al: Gonadotroph cell adenoma of the pituitary in a woman with long-standing hypogonadism. *Arch Gynecol* 229:57, 1980.
128. Kovacs K, Horvath E, Ryan N: Immunocytology of the human pituitary, in DeLellis RA (ed): *Diagnostic Immunohistochemistry*. New York, Masson Publishing USA Inc, 1981.
129. Kovacs K, Horvath E, Stratmann IE, et al: Cytoplasmic microfilaments in the anterior lobe of the human pituitary gland. *Acta Anat* 87:414, 1974.

130. Kovacs K, Horvath E, Van Loon GR, et al: Pituitary adenomas associated with elevated blood follicle-stimulating hormone levels: A histologic, immunocytologic, and electron microscopic study of two cases. *Fertil Steril* 29:622, 1978.
131. Kraus EJ: Zur Pathologie der basophilen Zellen der Hypophyse: Zugleich ein Beitrag zur Pathologie des Morbus Basedowi und Addisoni. *Virchows Arch* 247:421, 1923.
132. Lack EE: Lymphoid "hypophysitis" with end organ insufficiency. *Arch Pathol* 99:215, 1975.
133. Landolt AM: Ultrastructure of human sella tumors. *Acta Neurochir (suppl)* 22:1, 1975.
134. Landolt AM: Progress in pituitary adenoma biology: Results of research and clinical applications, in Krayerbühl H, Brihaye J, Loew F, et al (eds): *Advances and Technical Standards in Neurosurgery* (vol. 5). Wien: Springer-Verlag, 1978.
135. Landolt AM, Rothenbühler MS: Pituitary adenoma calcification. *Arch Pathol Lab Med* 101:22, 1977.
136. Lee AK, O-Briain DS, Beidelman B, et al: Thyrotropin-producing pituitary adenomas: An immunohistochemical and ultrastructural study. *Lab Invest* 46:48A, 1982.
137. Leong AS, Chawla JC, Teh EC: Pituitary thyrotropic tumour secondary to long-standing primary hypothyroidism. *Pathol Eur* 11:49, 1976.
138. Levine S: Allergic adenohypophysitis: New experimental disease of the pituitary gland. *Science* 158:1190, 1967.
139. Lichtenstein L: Histiocytosis X (eosinophilic granuloma of bone), Letterer-Siwe disease, and Schüller-Christian disease: Further observations of pathological and clinical importance. *J Bone Joint Surg* 46A:76, 1964.
140. Lieberman PH, Jones CR, Dargeon HWK, Begg CF: A reappraisal of eosinophilic granuloma of bone, Hand-Schüller-Christian syndrome and Letterer-Siwe syndrome. *Medicine* 48:375, 1969.
141. Lindholm J, Rasmussen P, Korsgaard O: Intrasellar or pituitary abscess. *J Neurosurg* 38:616, 1973.
142. List CF: Osteochondromas arising from the base of the skull. *Surg Gynecol Obstet* 76:480, 1943.
143. Lundberg PO, Drettner B, Hemmingsson A, et al: The invasive pituitary adenoma: A prolactin-producing tumor. *Arch Neurol* 34:742, 1977.
144. Lundin M, Schelin U: Light and electron microscopical studies on the pituitary in stilbol-treated rats. *Acta Pathol Microbiol Scand* 54:66, 1962.
145. Luse SA, Kernohan JW: Granular-cell tumors of the stalk and posterior lobe of the pituitary gland. *Cancer* 8:616, 1955.
146. MacCarty CS, Boyd AS Jr, Childs DS Jr: Tumors of the optic nerve and optic chiasm. *J Neurosurg* 33:439, 1970.
147. MacKay A, Hosobuchi Y: Treatment of intracavernous extensions of pituitary adenomas. *Surg Neurol* 10:377, 1978.
148. Martin NA, Hales M, Wilson CB: Cerebellar metastasis from a prolactinoma during treatment with bromocriptine: Case report. *J Neurosurg* 55:615, 1981.
149. Martins AN, Dean DF: Giant cell tumor of sphenoid bone: Malignant transformation following radiotherapy. *Surg Neurol* 2:105, 1974.
150. McComb DJ, Bayley TA, Horvath E, et al: Monomorphous plurihormonal adenoma of the human pituitary: A histologic, immunocytologic and ultrastructural study. *Cancer* 53:1538, 1984.
151. McCormick WF, Halmi NS: Absence of chromophobe adenomas from a large series of pituitary tumors. *Arch Pathol* 92:231, 1971.
152. McGavran MH, Spady HA: Eosinophilic granuloma of bone: A study of twenty-eight cases. *J Bone Joint Surg* 42A:979, 1960.
153. McGrath P: Cysts of sellar and pharyngeal hypophyses. *Pathology* 3:123, 1971.
154. McLone DG, Raimondi AJ, Naidich TP: Craniopharyngiomas. *Childs Brain* 9:188, 1982.
155. Melchionna RH, Moore RA: The pharyngeal pituitary gland. *Am J Pathol* 14:763, 1938.
156. Mihm MC Jr, Clark WH, Reed RJ: The histiocytic infiltrates of the skin. *Hum Pathol* 5:45, 1974.
157. Mohanty S, Tandon PN, Banerji AK, et al: Haemorrhage into pituitary adenomas. *J Neurol Neurosurg Psychiatry* 40:987, 1977.
158. Moore EW, Thomas LB, Shaw RK, et al: The central nervous system in acute leukemia: A postmortem study of 117 consecutive cases, with particular reference to hemorrhages, leukemic infiltrations, and the syndrome of meningeal leukemia. *Arch Intern Med* 105:451, 1960.
159. Mornex R, Tommasi M, Cure M, et al: Hyperthyroidie associee a un hypopituitarisme au cours de l'evolution d'une tumeur hypophysaire sécrétant TSH. *Ann Endocrinol* 33:390, 1972.
160. Muller W, Pia HW: Zur Klinik und Ätiologie

der Massenblutungen in Hypophysenadenome. *Dtschz Nervenheilkd* 170:326, 1953.
161. Naiken VS, Tellem M, Meranze DR: Pituitary cyst of Rathke's cleft origin with hypopituitarism. *J Neurosurg* 18:703, 1961.
162. Neilson JM, Moffat AD: Hypopituitarism caused by a melanoma of the pituitary gland. *J Clin Pathol* 16:144, 1963.
163. Nelson DH, Meakin JW, Thorn GW: ACTH-producing tumors following adrenalectomy for Cushing's syndrome. *Ann Intern Med* 52:560, 1960.
164. Nelson DH, Meakin JW, Dealy JB Jr, et al: ACTH-producing tumor of the pituitary gland. *N Engl J Med* 259:161, 1958.
165. Nezelof C, Frileux-Herbet F, Cronier-Sachot J: Disseminated histiocytosis X: Analysis of prognostic factors based on a retrospective study of 50 cases. *Cancer* 44:1824, 1979.
166. Noran HH: Intracranial vascular tumors and malformations. *Arch Pathol* 39:393, 1945.
167. Northfield DWC: Rathke-pouch tumours. *Brain* 80:293, 1957.
168. Ogilvy KM, Jakubowski J: Intracranial dissemination of pituitary adenomas. *J Neurol Neurosurg Psychiatry* 36:199, 1973.
169. Ogilvy KM, Jakubowski J, Shortland JR: Spinal subarachnoid spread of pituitary adenoma. *J Neurol Neurosurg Psychiatry* 37:1186, 1974.
170. Ohaegbulam SC, Gupta IM: Giant cell tumour of the sphenoid bone with dural extension. *J Neurol Neurosurg Psychiatry* 40:790, 1977.
171. Oi S, Ciric I, Mayer TK: Metastatic breast carcinoma in the pituitary gland. *No To Shinkei* 30:69, 1978.
172. Ojemann RG: Meningiomas of the basal parapituitary region: Technical considerations. *Clin Neurosurg* 27:233, 1979.
173. Okazaki H: Fundamentals of neuropathology. Tokyo, Igaku-Shoin Ltd, 1983.
174. Olivier L, Villa-Porcile E, Peillon F, et al: Etude en microscopie electronique des grains de secretion "basophiles" dans les cellules hypophysaires tumorales de la maladie de Cushing. *C R Soc Biol* 166:1591, 1972.
175. Otani S: A discussion on eosinophilic granuloma of bone, Letterer-Siwe disease and Schüller-Christian disease. *J Mt Sinai Hosp* 24:1079, 1957.
176. Oxenhandler DC, Sayers MP: The dilemma of childhood optic gliomas. *J Neurosurg* 48:34, 1978.
177. Paillas JE, Alliez B: Intrasellar chondromas: Case report. *Neurochirurgia* 17:136, 1974.
178. Papo I, Beltrami CA, Salvolini U, et al: Sarcoidosis simulating a glioma of the optic nerve. *Surg Neurol* 8:353, 1977.
179. Peake GT, McKeel DW, Jarett L, et al: Ultrastructural histologic and hormonal characterization of a prolactin-rich human pituitary tumor. *J Clin Endocrinol Metab* 29:1383, 1969.
180. Phifer RF, Spicer SS: Immunohistochemical and histologic demonstration of thyrotropic cells of the human adenohypophysis. *J Clin Endocrinol Metab* 36:1210, 1973.
181. Pitkethly DT, Kempe LG: Giant cell tumors of the sphenoid: Report of two cases. *J Neurosurg* 30:301, 1969.
182. Poisson M, Magdelenat H, Foncin JF, et al: Rècepteurs d'oestrogénes et de progestèrone dans les mèningiomes: Ètude de 22 cas. *Rev Neurol* 136:193, 1980.
183. Powell HC, Marshall LF, Ignelzi RJ: Post-irradiation pituitary sarcoma. *Acta Neuropathol* 39:165, 1977.
184. Quest DO: Meningiomas: An update. *Neurosurgery* 3:219, 1978.
185. Rengachary SS, Tomita T, Jefferies BF, et al: Structural changes in human pituitary tumor after bromocriptine therapy. *Neurosurgery* 10:242, 1982.
186. Riemenschneider PA, Prior JT: Neuroblastoma originating from olfactory epithelium (esthesioneuroblastoma). *AJR Rad Ther Nucl Med* 80:759, 1958.
187. Robert F, Hardy J: Prolactin-secreting adenomas: A light and electron microscopical study. *Arch Pathol* 99:625, 1975.
188. Robinson F, Solitare GB: Olfactory neuroblastoma: Neurosurgical implications of an intranasal tumor. *J Neurosurg* 25:133, 1966.
189. Roessmann U, Kaufman B, Friede RL: Metastatic lesions in the sella turcica and pituitary gland. *Cancer* 25:478, 1970.
190. Rothman LM, Sher J, Quencer RM, et al: Intracranial ectopic pituitary adenoma: Case report. *J Neurosurg* 44:96, 1976.
191. Rovit RL, Berry R: Cushing's syndrome and the hypophysis: A re-evaluation of pituitary tumors and hyperadrenalism. *J Neurosurg* 23:270, 1965.
192. Rovit RL, Duane TD: Cushing's syndrome and pituitary tumors: Pathophysiology and ocular manifestations of ACTH-secreting pituitary adenomas. *Am J Med* 46:416, 1969.
193. Rubinstein LJ: Tumors of the central nervous system, In *Atlas of Tumor Pathology*. Second Series, Fascicle 6. Washington, D.C., Armed Forces Institute of Pathology, 1972.

194. Russel DS, Rubinstein LJ: *Pathology of Tumours of the Nervous System*. Baltimore, Williams & Wilkins, 1971.
195. Russfield AB: Adenohypophysis, in Bloodworth JMB Jr (ed): *Endocrine Pathology*. Baltimore, Williams & Wilkins, 1968.
196. Ryan N, Kovacs K, Ezrin C: Staining of human pituitary glands with lead hematoxylin in comparison with other histochemical procedures, including the immunoenzyme technique. *Acta Histochem* 59:96, 1977.
197. Saeger W: Zur Ultrastruktur der Hypophysenadenome beim Cushing-Syndrom nach Adrenalektomie, *Virchows Arch* 361:39, 1973.
198. Samaan NA, Osborne BM, Mackay B, et al: Endocrine and morphologic studies of pituitary adenomas secondary to primary hypothyroidism, *J Clin Endocrinol Metab* 45:903, 1977.
199. Sansone ME, Liwnicz BH, Mandybur TI: Giant pituitary cavernous hemangioma: Case report. *J Neurosurg* 53:124, 1980.
200. Sarwar M, Swischuk LE, Schechter MM: Intracranial chondromas. *AJR* 127:973, 1976.
201. Sassin JF, Rosenberg RN: Neurological complications of fibrous dysplasia of the skull. *Arch Neurol* 18:363, 1968.
202. Scanarini M, Mingrino S: Pituitary adenomas secreting more than two hormones. *Acta Neuropathol* 48:67, 1979.
203. Schechter J: Electron microscopic studies of human pituitary tumors: II. Audiophilic adenomas. *Am J Anat* 138:387, 1973.
204. Scheithauer BW: Surgical pathology of the pituitary and sellar region, in Laws ER Jr, Randall RV, Kern DB, et al (eds): *Management of Pituitary Adenomas and Related Lesions with an Emphasis on Transsphenoidal Microsurgery*. East Norwalk, Conn., Appleton-Century-Crofts, 1982.
205. Schelin U: Chromophobe and acidophil adenomas of the human pituitary gland: A light and electron microscopic study. *Acta Pathol Microbiol Scand (Suppl)* 158:1, 1962.
206. Schmid AH: A lipoma of the cerebellum. *Acta Neuropathol* 26:75, 1973.
207. Schnegg JF, Gomez F, LeMarchand-Beraud T, de Tribolet N: Presence of sex steroid hormone receptors in meningioma tissue. *Surg Neurol* 15:415, 1981.
208. Schochet SS Jr, Peters B, O'Neal J, et al: Intracranial esthesioneuroblastoma: A light and electron microscopic study. *Acta Neuropathol* 31:181, 1975.
209. Schoenberg BS, Christine BW, Whisnant JP: Nervous system neoplasms and primary malignancies of other sites: The unique association between meningiomas and breast cancer. *Neurology* 25:705, 1975.
210. Scholtz CL, Siu K: Melanoma of the pituitary: Case report. *J Neurosurg* 45:101, 1976.
211. Schroffner WG: Prolactin-secreting pituitary tumor in early adolescence: Hormonal and electron microscopical studies. *Arch Intern Med* 136:1164, 1976.
212. Schwartz JF, Balentine JD: Recurrent meningitis due to an intracranial epidermoid. *Neurology* 28:124, 1978.
213. Severinghaus AE: Cellular changes in the anterior hypophysis with special reference to its secretory activities. *Physiol Rev* 17:556, 1937.
214. Shanklin WM: On the presence of cysts in the human pituitary. *Anat Rec* 104:379, 1949.
215. Shanklin WM: The incidence and distribution of cilia in the human pituitary with a description of micro-follicular cysts derived from Rathke's cleft. *Acta Anat* 11:361, 1951.
216. Shimizu T, Idhida Y, Takeda F: Electron microscopy of human pituitary adenomas: Correlation of the secretory granules with the experimentally and clinically evaluated hormone synthesis function of the adenoma tissue. *Neurol Med Chir* 18:107, 1978.
217. Shuangshoti S, Netsky MG, Nashold BS Jr: Epithelial cysts related to sella turcica: Proposed origin from neuroepithelium. *Arch Pathol* 90:444, 1970.
218. Singer W, Kovacs K, Ryan N, et al: Demonstration of immunoreactive alpha-endorphin in corticotroph cell adenomas of the human pituitary. *IRCS Med Sci* 52:3, 1974.
219. Skillicorn SA, Garrity RW: Intracranial Boeck's sarcoid-tumor resembling meningioma. *J Neurosurg* 12:407, 1955.
220. Sobel HJ, Marquet E, Schwarz R: Is schwannoma related to granular cell myoblastoma? *Arch Pathol* 95:396, 1973.
221. Sparling HJ Jr, Adams RD, Parker F Jr.: Involvement of the nervous system by malignant lymphoma. *Medicine* 26:285, 1947.
222. Sperling SJ, Alpers BJ: Lipoma and osteolipoma of the brain. *J Nerv Ment Dis* 83:13, 1936.
223. Svien HJ: Surgical experiences with craniopharyngiomas. *J Neurosurg* 23:148, 1965.
224. Svolos DG: Craniopharyngiomas: A study based on 108 verified cases. *Acta Chir Scand (Suppl)* 403:7, 1969.
225. Snyder PJ, Sterling FH: Hypersecretion of LH and FSH by a pituitary adenoma. *J Clin Endocrinol Metab* 42:544, 1976.

226. Teears RJ, Silverman EM: Clinicopathologic review of 88 cases of carcinoma metastatic to the pituitary gland. *Cancer* 36:216, 1975.
227. Tibbs PA, Challa V, Mortara RH: Isolated histiocytosis X of the hypothalamus: Case report. *J Neurosurg* 49: 929, 1978.
228. Tindall GT, Kovacs K, Horvath E, et al: Human prolactin-producing adenomas and bromocriptine: A histological, immunocytochemical, ultrastructural, and morphometric study. *J Clin Endocrinol Metab* 55:1178, 1982.
229. Tisher ER, Wechsler H: Granular cell myoblastoma—a misnomer: Electron microscopic and histochemical evidence concerning its Schwann cell deviation and nature (granular cell schwannoma). *Cancer* 15:936, 1962.
230. Trouillas J, Girod C, Sassolas G, et al: Human pituitary gonadotrophic adenoma: Histological, immunocytochemical, and ultrastructural and hormonal studies in eight cases. *J Pathol* 135:315, 1981.
231. Turner OA, Laird AT: Meningioma with traumatic etiology: Report of a case. *J Neurosurg* 24:96, 1966.
232. Van Den Bergh R, Brucher JM: L'abord transventriculaire dans les craniopharyngiomes du troisieme ventricule: Aspects neurochirurgicaux et neuro-pathologiques. *Neurochirurgie* 16:51, 1970.
233. Viale GL: Giant cell tumours of the sellar region. *Acta Neurochir* 38:259, 1977.
234. Vonderahe AR, Niemer WT: Intracranial lipoma: A report of four cases. *J Neuropathol Exp Neurol* 3:344, 1944.
235. White RJ, Wood MW, Kernohan JW: A study of fifty intracranial vascular tumors found incidentally at necropsy. *J Neuropathol Exp Neurol* 17:392, 1958.
236. Wiederholt WC, Siekert RG: Neurological manifestations of sarcoidosis. *Neurology* 15:1147, 1965.
237. Williams JW, Dorfman RF: Lymphadenopathy as the initial manifestation of histiocytosis X. *Am J Surg Pathol* 3:405, 1979.
238. Wilson WB, Feinsod M, Hoyt WF, et al: Malignant evaluation of childhood chiasmal pilocytic astrocytoma. *Neurology* 26:322, 1976.
239. Winnacker JL, Becker KL, Katz S: Endocrine aspects of sarcoidosis. *N Engl J Med* 278:427, 1968.
240. Woolf PD, Schenk EA: An FSH-producing pituitary tumor in a patient with hypogonadism. *J Clin Endocrinol Metab* 38:561, 1974.
241. Zülch KJ: Some remarks on spongioblastoma of the brain. *Acta Neurochir (Suppl)* 10:121, 1964.

CHAPTER 4

Clinical and endocrinologic evaluation of patients with pituitary tumors

Clinical features
   Mass effects
   Endocrinopathy
Neuro-ophthalmologic testing
Endocrinologic testing
   Assessment of pituitary hormone reserve
      Adrenal axis
      Thyroid axis
      Gonadal axis
      Prolactin
      Growth hormone
      Posterior pituitary
      Postoperative assessment
   Special endocrine testing
      Acromegaly
         Basal levels of growth hormone
         Growth hormone–glucose suppression test
         Somatomedin-C levels
         Thyrotropin-releasing hormone (TRH) test
         Growth hormone–releasing factor (GHRF) levels
      Cushing's syndrome (disease)
         Establishing diagnosis of Cushing's syndrome
         Identifying source of the disease
         Standard dexamethasone suppression test
         Determination of plasma adrenocorticotropin hormone (ACTH) levels
         Metyrapone test
         Radiologic studies
      Prolactinomas
Summary

Pituitary tumors produce two major types of clinical findings: mass effects, resulting from compression of neighborhood structures by gradual increase in the size of the adenoma; and endocrinopathy, resulting from excessive hormone secretion by the tumor. Knowledge of these clinical signs and symptoms is helpful in diagnosing pituitary tumors. Specific diagnosis, however, especially with hyperfunctional tumors, depends on a complete endocrine evaluation.

This chapter describes the clinical findings present in patients with proven or suspected pituitary tumors and methods for evaluating these patients. A complete, current, and practical protocol of endocrinologic testing is provided to assist the physician in assessing pituitary endocrine functions and in confirming the diagnosis of an endocrinopathy (e.g., acromegaly) in hypersecreting pituitary tumors, especially when the disorder is in an early stage and will usually indicate the etiologic locus of the disorder (e.g., Cushing's disease).

CLINICAL FEATURES
Mass effects

Mass effects (Table 4-1) result from compression of adjacent anatomic structures, primarily the optic chiasm and the normal pituitary gland, and are usually associated with nonfunctional pituitary tumors, although they may occasionally occur with functional tumors. Also other parasellar lesions, including

Table 4-1

Clinical findings resulting from mass effects in terms of anatomic structures involved

Clinical finding	Mass effect
Headache, usually constant; may be retro-orbital, bifrontal, and/or bitemporal	Stretching of dura or distortion of diaphragm sella
Visual field defects, usually bitemporal hemianopsia, loss of visual acuity	Compression or stretching of optic chiasm or tracts

Varying degrees of hypopituitarism
    Hypothyroidism—cold intolerance, weight gain, myxedema
    Hypoadrenalism—fatigability, orthostatic hypotension
    Hypogonadism—loss of libido, amenorrhea, infertility
    Diabetes insipidus (rare)—excessive thirst and urination, hypernatremia, lethargy
	Compromise of pituitary gland

Diplopia, ptosis, facial pain, proptosis (rare)	Compression of cranial nerves within cavernous sinus, tumor invasion of cavernous sinus
Headache, blindness, lethargy, coma	Compression of foramina of Monro with obstructive hydrocephalus
Pituitary apoplexy	Hemorrhage and/or infarction of adenoma
Seizures	Temporal lobe involvement

craniopharyngiomas, can cause mass effects that mimic those caused by a pituitary adenoma.

The clinical findings caused by mass effects include headache, visual impairment, hypopituitarism, extraocular palsies, facial pain, hydrocephalus, and those findings caused by pituitary apoplexy.

The most common objective manifestations of mass effects are visual: impairment of visual fields and loss of acuity.

The characteristic visual field defect caused by a pituitary tumor is a *bitemporal hemianopsia*. Examples of visual field defects are shown in Figs. 4-1 and 4-2. In a typical case, the superior temporal quadrants are affected initially, followed thereafter by the inferior temporal quadrants. In instances of progressive chiasmal compression from continued tumor growth, the inferior nasal followed by the superior nasal quadrants are subsequently involved, with resulting blindness. These defects are caused by involvement of the crossing and later the noncrossing fibers in the chiasm. Careful visual testing to small red isopters with targets presented bilaterally can provide important evidence for the presence of pituitary tumors. Deficits to red-color testing may precede detectable abnormalities to white or other targets. Also the use of smaller, less illuminated targets may bring out subtle visual field defects (see Fig. 4-1) that may otherwise be missed.

Another type of visual abnormality that frequently occurs in association with a pituitary adenoma is the *junctional scotoma* (see Fig. 4-2). Anatomically, lesions producing this visual field deficit are located at the optic nerve immediately adjacent to the chiasm. Involvement of the nerve accounts for the unilateral central scotoma, whereas involvement of the crossing inferior nasal fibers from the opposite optic nerve that loop forward in the involved optic nerve ("von Wilbrand's knee") accounts for the superior temporal quadrantanopsia in the contralateral eye.

The presence of optic disc pallor may represent ischemia of the optic nerve and may result in optic atrophy with associated visual impairment. Pallor may be difficult to recognize in early cases, and careful comparisons of each disc must be made. Papilledema, which results from either a large mass or, more commonly, increased intracranial pressure from obstruction of the third ventricle by a large extension of tumor, is a rare clinical finding in pituitary adenomas.

The pathophysiologic mechanism responsible for visual field impairment may be simple mechanical compression, ischemia, or a combination of these two mechanisms. Simple mechanical compression by the tumor and/or displacement of the optic nerve and chiasm against either the margins of the optic canals or the anterior cerebral arteries can account for the visual deficit. Notching of the chiasm by overlying arteries was reported by Rucker and Kernohan[33] in five patients with pituitary adenomas associated with bitemporal hemianopsia. Sunderland and Bradley[35] showed that the tensile strength of nerves is dependent on the endoneurial collagen. The optic nerves have collagenous septa to support the funiculi; whereas in the chiasm and optic tracts, the collagen is absent and the

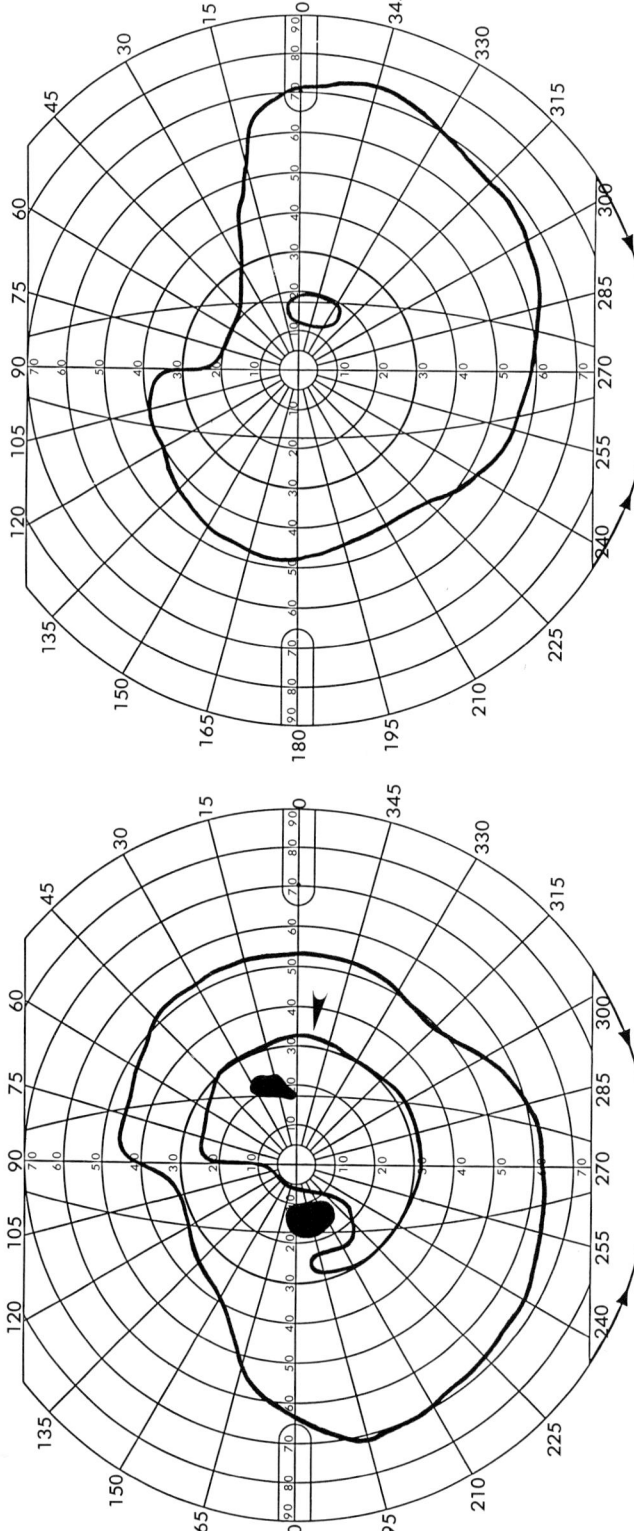

Fig. 4-1. Subtle bitemporal superior quadrantanopsia associated with a pituitary adenoma (Goldman perimeter). *Right,* I 4e size target outlined partial upper temporal quadrantanopsia. *Left,* same size target suggested upper temporal defect (large field). Using smaller target (I2e size, arrow), superior temporal quadrantanopsia was outlined. Visual acuity: 20/20, OU.

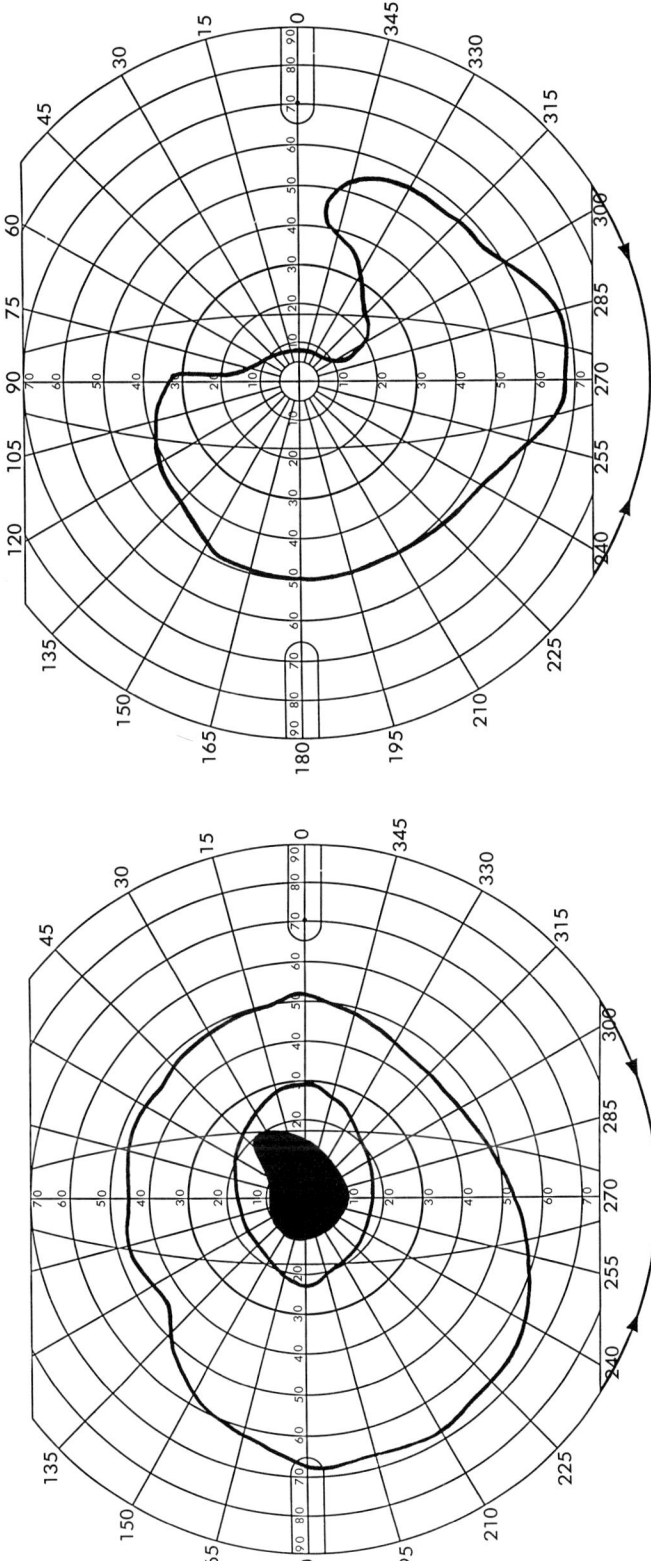

Fig. 4-2. Junctional scotoma in patient with pituitary adenoma. Left eye shows central (predominantly temporal) scotoma with preservation of peripheral visual field. Scotoma was detected using pinhead size but less illuminated target (I 3e). Visual acuity: OD: 20/20; OS: count fingers only. Right eye shows a superior temporal quadrantanopsia.

support consists of glial tissue. Because of this lack of collagen support for nerve fibers, it is postulated that the chiasm is more vulnerable to stretch injury.[29]

From surgical observations, Cushing and Walker[6] concluded that there must be a "physiologic block," which can be reversed relatively rapidly with removal of the mass. Assuming that the block would be a result of either mechanical distortion and/or ischemia, provided neither were long lasting in effect, they further postulated that it might interfere with the conduction of neural impulses at a subcellular level. These observations are consistent with the modern concept of axoplasmic transport, which entails a flow of substance from the nerve cell body to its axonal extensions. Compression of the chiasm by a pituitary tumor could impede this transport and cause failure of neural impulses to be transmitted. Feinsod et al,[10,11] who used visual evoked potentials (VEPs), perioperatively in two patients with tuberculum sella meningiomas and in one patient with a pituitary adenoma found that surgical removal of the tumor resulted in significant improvement in VEPs and vision. The visual improvement, which occurred in the early postoperative course and which correlated well with the restoration of VEPs to normal shortly after recovery from anesthesia, lends support to the theory of mechanical compression at a subcellular level.

The compression theory does not explain certain aspects of the chiasmal syndrome such as the relative resistance of the portion of the chiasm that would produce an altitudinal nasal field loss, which clinical experience has shown to be an uncommon finding. This finding implies that other mechanisms such as *ischemia* may play a role in the visual field loss associated with expanding pituitary tumors.

During the course of surgery for a pituitary tumor, Hughes[18] observed that the central portion of the chiasm was gray and fragmented but the lateral portions appeared normal, pink, and well vascularized. He interpreted these findings to be consistent with ischemia rather than mechanical compression as a cause for visual impairment.

Paralysis of the extraocular muscles, either partial or complete, is a relatively uncommon manifestation of pituitary adenomas. When present, the oculomotor nerve is the most commonly involved, followed next by the abducens and then the trochlear nerve.[26] The internal carotid artery offers some protection to the cranial nerves in the cavernous sinus from expanding adenomas, but occasionally the nerves are compressed against the edge of the dura at their entry into the sinus.[36] *Proptosis* is a very rare clinical finding of pituitary adenomas and can occur following tumor invasion of the cavernous sinus with resultant vascular congestion.[42]

The *headache* associated with pituitary tumors is usually bilateral and localized to the frontotemporal region. Headaches are seen in approximately one third of patients with pituitary tumors and have no special distinguishing features. The headache in most cases is believed to be caused by stretching of the diaphragm sella, which is innervated by the first division of the fifth cranial nerve. On rare occasions, severe headaches related to the tumor may disappear over a short period of time. In these cases, it is postulated that the tumor has extended through the diaphragm sella with relief of pressure on the latter structure.

Compression of the normal gland and/or the pituitary stalk by the tumor can result in varying degrees of *pituitary endocrine deficiency,* or *hypopituitarism.* Usually, however, tumors reach a relatively large size before compromising pituitary function. *Diabetes insipidus,* resulting from impairment of antidiuretic hormone (ADH) production or release, rarely occurs with pituitary adenomas, even those lesions that reach considerable size. This clinical finding is more likely to occur in association with a craniopharyngioma. Both hypopituitarism and diabetes insipidus resulting from a pituitary tumor and/or craniopharyngioma are discussed in more detail in Chapter 15 and to some extent in Chapter 11.

Pituitary apoplexy refers to the abrupt onset of signs and symptoms that occur as a result of rapid enlargement of a pituitary adenoma caused by hemorrhage and infarction with resultant swelling. Although pathologic evidence of either macroscopic or microscopic hemorrhage occurs in 1.5% to 27.7% of chromophobe adenomas, the term *pituitary apoplexy* should be reserved for those cases in which there is a sudden onset of neurologic symptoms.[25,41] Although Wakai et al[41] found evidence of hemorrhage in 16.6% of 560 cases of pituitary adenomas, less than half of the 16.6% had clinical findings suggestive of pituitary apoplexy. It is estimated that approximately 1% of pituitary adenomas present clinically with apoplexy.[8,31] Spontaneous hemorrhage or infarction may occur in a nonadenomatous pituitary but is much less common.

Outgrowth of the vascular supply by a pituitary tumor has been cited as the underlying pathologic mechanism responsible for pituitary apoplexy.[2,25] Another mechanism might be compression of the nutrient vessels by the adenoma with resulting vascular stasis causing thrombosis, ischemic necrosis, and hemorrhage. Once infarction has occurred, much or all of the adenoma becomes hemorrhagic and rapidly swells. The sudden increase in volume and tension causes compression of neighboring structures such as the optic apparatus, cranial nerves within the cavernous sinus, carotid arteries, and hypothalamus. The excellent pathologic study by Brougham, Heusner, and Adams[2] supports the contention that both hemorrhage and infarction occur as a consequence of rapid tumor growth. Other investigators have found no correlation between adenoma size and pituitary apoplexy.[41] Earlier reports in the literature suggested that the adenomas associated with acromegaly[2,19,37] or Cushing's disease[31,32] were more commonly associated with pituitary apoplexy. However, a review of the more recent literature shows that there is no evidence for such a consistent predilection.[9,41]

The patient with pituitary apoplexy may be previously asymptomatic or have symptoms of a pre-existing pituitary adenoma. Onset of neurologic signs and symptoms are sudden or subacute and include headache, nausea, vomiting, photophobia, nuchal rigidity, loss of vision, diplopia, findings of acute adrenal insufficiency, and alterations in level of consciousness. The constellation of presenting signs and symptoms may mimic the clinical findings seen with subarachnoid hemorrhage caused by the spontaneous rupture of an intracranial aneurysm.

Although hemorrhage and/or infarction often occur in a previously undiagnosed adenoma, David et al[7] report that at least 30% of patients have a preexisting endocrinopathy. Several reports have suggested factors believed to precipitate pituitary apoplexy. For instance, occurrence during preoperative irradiation therapy for an adenoma is recognized[9,42] and the syndrome has been reported to occur during bromocriptine therapy.[41] Other factors thought to be of etiologic importance or at least reported in association with the condition are pregnancy, head trauma,[40] anticoagulation,[1,28] lumbar puncture,[7] myelography,[7] and angiography.[9]

Endocrinopathy

Three commonly encountered clinical syndromes that result from a hormone-secreting pituitary adenoma, in order of frequency, are (1) the amenorrhea-galactorrhea syndrome (hyperprolactinemia), (2) acromegaly (excess growth hormone [GH]), and (3) Cushing's disease (excess adrenocorticotropic hormone [ACTH] with hypercortisolism). Pituitary tumors that produce excessive levels of thyrotropin and gonadotropin have been described but are very rare.[5,14,16] Nelson's syndrome is a result of a pituitary adenoma that develops in a patient who has undergone bilateral adrenalectomy for Cushing's disease.[27] The tumors associated with Nelson's syndrome are usually biologically aggressive lesions. Current opinion seems to hold that the pituitary tumor was present before the adrenalectomy and caused the Cushing's disease. The hypersecretion syndromes and associated hormonal and clinical features are listed in Table 4-2. There have

Table 4-2

Clinical features associated with hypersecreting pituitary tumors

Syndrome	Hormonal excess	Clinical features
Acromegaly	GH	Enlargement of hands and feet (thickened heel pad); distortion of facial features (prognathism); peripheral nerve entrapment syndromes; gigantism (when prepubertal)
Cushing's disease	ACTH	Centripetal obesity ("moon" facies, "buffalo hump," supraclavicular fat pad); purple striae; ecchymoses; hirsutism; psychiatric disturbance; hypertension; glucose intolerance
Nelson's syndrome	ACTH	Hyperpigmentation
Amenorrhea-galactorrhea syndrome	PRL	Amenorrhea or oligomenorrhea; variable galactorrhea
Thyroid-stimulating hormone (TSH)–secreting adenoma (rare)	TSH	Features of hyperthyroidism (weight loss, tachycardia, tremor, heat intolerance)
Luteinizing hormone (LH)– and/or follicle-stimulating hormone (FSH)–secreting adenoma (rare)	LH, FSH	No specific clinical features known

been rare reports of pituitary tumors secreting more than one hormone,[5,44] and in these cases the clinical features are mixed.

Occasionally, an adenoma causing an endocrinopathy will also produce mass effects. For instance, a patient with the amenorrhea-galactorrhea syndrome as a result of a prolactinoma may exhibit a bitemporal hemianopsia, or a patient with acromegaly may have headaches and impaired pituitary endocrine function. Usually, adenomas causing Cushing's disease are small, and signs of mass effects are rarely seen in association with this tumor.

Patients harboring pituitary tumors that secrete excessive quantities of prolactin (hyperprolactinemia), the so-called prolactinoma, have few distinctive clinical features. Women give a history of amenorrhea ranging from months to several years and may or may not have spontaneous galactorrhea. The discharge from the nipples is usually a thin, white, milky fluid that may require minimal nipple manipulation for its appearance. Galactorrhea is rare in men with prolactinomas. Impotence and hypogonadism in males have been ascribed to the hyperprolactinemia.

The appearance of patients with well-established Cushing's disease and acromegaly is so characteristic that the experienced clinician will have little trouble in recognizing either of these entities. However, difficulty in positive recognition may arise in the early stages of both diseases. The clinical features of Cushing's disease (see also Chapter 7) include the characteristic facies, centripetal obesity, hypertension, thin skin, purple striae, ecchymoses, osteoporosis, amenorrhea and hirsutism (in women), glucose intolerance, and emotional disorders. The centripetal obesity is a very typical finding.

The distinctive clinical features of acromegaly include overgrowth of head, hands, and feet (especially thickening of the heel pads); prognathism; arthritic manifestations; acroparesthesia (including carpal tunnel syndrome); impairment of glucose tolerance (with clinically manifest diabetes mellitus in 10% to 15% of cases); cardiomyopathy; and hyperhidrosis. The overgrowth of the facial features produces an unmistakable picture. The fingers and toes are significantly widened.

NEURO-OPHTHALMOLOGIC TESTING

Quantitative visual field testing using a Goldman perimeter is ideal but may be impractical or even impossible in certain situations. For example, some patients may be too ill to be moved to the testing area, and children and aphasic or demented subjects cannot comply with the examiner's instructions. Obviously, in these patients, minor impairment of visual acuity and the presence of small visual field defects are virtually impossible to determine with accuracy.

Nevertheless, there are other techniques available for evaluating visual fields; although they are less objective than perimetry, they may be the only effective method of testing this parameter in these clinical situations. One method for visual field testing consists of placing two similarly colored objects in different visual fields and testing each eye separately. One of the colored objects is placed in the temporal field and the other in the nasal field, and the patient is instructed to maintain fixation on the examiner's nose. The patient is then asked if one object appears brighter or duller in reference to the other. The object in the intact hemifield will usually be described as either brighter or richer in hue. Once visual field defects are suspected, further testing is performed. This includes determination of the point of transition, that is, the point where the stimulus that appears darker becomes as bright as the companion stimulus when the object is moved from one visual field to another. Areas of duller perception should always be explored by moving the test stimulus slowly into the zones of brighter experience. In this manner, one may detect hemianopic, quadrantic, and cecocentral visual field defects.

One of the most objective tests for evaluating the visual system is testing for an afferent pupillary defect or the Marcus Gunn pupil. The test is performed by first shining a bright light in one eye, observing the speed and extent of pupillary contraction, and then quickly moving the light to the other eye and making the same observations. Dilatation of a pupil directly exposed to light is referred to as a Marcus Gunn sign. The presence of this sign indicates a lesion in the prechiasmal portion of the ipsilateral optic nerve.

ENDOCRINOLOGIC TESTING

For practical purposes, these tests are divided into *baseline* assessment of pituitary hormone reserve, tests that are obtained in all patients with pituitary tumors, both functional and nonfunctional; and *special* endocrine tests that are obtained in certain endocrinopathies (e.g., Cushing's disease, acromegaly).

Assessment of pituitary hormone reserve

Determination of the adequacy of anterior and posterior pituitary function in patients known to have pituitary tumors is important to identify clinically significant hormone deficiency states caused by the tumor itself and re-evaluate patients after pituitary surgery or irradiation to detect hormone deficiencies that occur as a result of treatment. Although it is possible to evaluate many different aspects of "pituitary function," a selective approach to testing specific functions is appropriate. Deficiencies of adrenal, thyroid, and gonadal hormones may be subtle or mild but should be assessed, since replacement therapy is usually indicated. Deficiency of ADH (vasopressin) severe enough to cause diabetes insipidus is usually quite apparent, and simple screening tests are often adequate. It is not necessary to evaluate adult patients routinely for growth hormone or prolactin reserves, since deficiencies of these hormones are not clinically important. The extent of evaluation should be tailored to the individual circumstances.

Although assays for anterior and posterior pituitary hormones are widely available, the sensitivity of most of these assays does not permit one to distinguish an abnormally low value from the lower range of normal. Assessment of a particular aspect of pituitary function should include clinical assessment for signs and symptoms of hormone deficiencies and laboratory tests of target gland function

Table 4-3
Evaluation of pituitary hormone reserve

	Screening	Further study
Adrenal	AM cortisol, cosyntropin stimulation	ITT, metyrapone, corticotropin-releasing factor (CRF)
Thyroid	T_4 (total or free)	Thyrotropin-releasing hormone (TRH) stimulation
Gonadal	LH, FSH, testosterone (men), estradiol (women)	Gonadotropin-releasing hormone (GnRH) stimulation, clomiphene
Prolactin	Baseline prolactin	Not recommended
Growth hormone	Not recommended in adults	ITT, arginine, glucagon, growth hormone–releasing factor (GHRF)
ADH	Urine volume, serum electrolytes	Water deprivation test, hypertonic saline infusion

(e.g., thyroxine, cortisol, etc.). Measurement of pituitary hormones under conditions designed to stimulate their release should be performed in selected instances. A scheme for testing is shown in Table 4-3.

Adrenal axis. Some physicians consider a normal AM serum or plasma cortisol a satisfactory indication of an intact hypothalamic-pituitary-adrenal axis; others prefer to use a simple provocative test, the cosyntropin-stimulating test. This is done by obtaining a baseline blood sample for cortisol, giving 250 mcg of cosyntropin (a potent preparation of ACTH) IM or IV, and repeating samples for cortisol at 30 and/or 60 minutes. A normal response is a plasma cortisol rise of more than 7 mcg/dl and a peak value of over 20 mcg/dl.

Sensitive tests of the entire axis such as the insulin tolerance test (ITT, insulin-induced hypoglycemia) or the metyrapone test may occasionally be abnormal in patients who have normal AM cortisol levels and normal response to cosyntropin, with no signs of adrenal insufficiency. Although an abnormality on one of these sensitive tests suggests some diminution of ACTH reserve, the clinical significance of such impairment is not clear. These tests should be reserved for patients in whom there is some clinical suspicion of adrenal insufficiency or where an AM cortisol or response to cosyntropin has been found to be abnormal. Standard protocols for performance and interpretation of these tests have been published. These tests involve some patient risk and discomfort and should only be performed by an experienced physician.

Measurement of ACTH in blood, either baseline or after stimulation with insulin or metyrapone, is not generally helpful. With more experience, ACTH measurement after administration of corticotropin-releasing factor (CRF) may become the first-line test of pituitary ACTH reserve.

Thyroid axis. If serum thyroxine (total or free) is clearly normal, the hypothalamic-pituitary-thyroid axis may be assumed to be intact. If hypothyroidism is suspected clinically, if serum T_4 is low or borderline, or if more precise testing of this axis is indicated, a thyrotropin-releasing hormone (TRH) stimulation test should be done. This is accomplished by drawing a baseline blood sample for determination of TSH, giving 500 mcg of TRH IV, and obtaining additional samples for TSH at 30 and 60 minutes after injection. A normal response is a peak serum TSH of twice the baseline value at 30 minutes. An impaired TSH response to TRH in a patient with a low serum T_4 indicates a pituitary abnormality, whereas a delayed TSH peak (at 45 or 60 minutes) indicates hypothalamic dysfunction. A blunted TSH response is also seen in patients with hyperthyroidism. The significance of a blunted TSH response in a patient with a normal serum T_4 and no clinical evidence of thyroid dysfunction is not clear.

Gonadal axis. The history and physical examination are helpful in evaluating the pituitary-gonadal axis, particularly in women in the reproductive age range. A baseline laboratory assessment should include measurement of serum gonadotropins (LH and FSH) and sex steroids (estradiol in women, testosterone in men). Provocative tests of LH and FSH after stimulation with gonadotropin-releasing hormone (GnRH or luteinizing hormone–releasing hormone [LHRH]) or clomiphene are only useful in selected cases. These tests have not proved to be reliable in differentiating pituitary disorders from hypothalamic dysfunction.

Prolactin. Prolactin should be measured in all patients with hormonally "silent" or "nonsecretory" tumors; many such patients will be found to have elevated values resulting from secretion of prolactin by the tumor or from pressure of the tumor on the hypothalamus or pituitary stalk. Although prolactin normally rises in response to TRH and other agents, such tests of prolactin reserve have little clinical value.

Growth hormone. Routine measurement of growth hormone as a test of pituitary reserve is not useful. Provocative tests (ITT, arginine infusion, glucagon stimulation, growth-hormone releasing factor [GHRH]) may reveal growth hormone deficiency, but, as is the case with prolactin, growth hormone deficiency in adults is not clinically significant.

Posterior pituitary. Deficiency of ADH usually has striking clinical manifestations—polyuria and polydipsia, with urine output over 2.5 liters a day (often 5 liters or more and sometimes as much as 15 to 20 liters a day). The history will usually reveal nocturia and urinary frequency. If there is a suspicion of diabetes insipidus, a 24-hour urine collection can be done to determine volume, with further tests of ADH done if volume is excessive. Serum electrolytes should be measured but are generally normal except when diabetes insipidus is severe, when thirst is impaired, or when access to water is limited.

Detailed evaluation of ADH may be done with an indirect test (water deprivation, to demonstrate normal urinary concentration) or a direct test (hypertonic saline infusion, measuring plasma ADH response to an osmotic stimulus). Determination of serum and urine osmolality is not generally useful except in the context of one of these tests or in a patient with abnormal serum electrolytes or elevated urine output. Further discussion of diabetes insipidus is found in Chapter 15.

Postoperative assessment. The optimal time for retesting endocrine function is not known. The protocol that has been used at Emory University Hospital follows.

Urine output and specific gravity, fluid balance, and serum electrolytes are monitored at least daily. It is usually not difficult to determine whether or not diabetes insipidus is present, but it may be difficult to determine whether the condition is temporary or permanent. "Stress" steroid coverage with hydrocortisone is administered immediately before, during, and following surgery. If adrenal function was normal before surgery, steroid coverage is stopped on day 2 or 3, and an AM cortisol is drawn 24 hours later. If the plasma cortisol is ≤5 μg/dl, ACTH deficiency is likely, and steroid coverage is reinstituted. If the plasma cortisol is >5 μg/dl, hypothalamic-pituitary-adrenal function is probably normal; confirmation of this with an ITT or metyrapone test on day 6 to 8 is desirable, especially if the plasma cortisol is borderline (5 to 10 μg/dl). From 6 to 8 days after pituitary surgery, T_4, LH, FSH, and testosterone (in men) or estradiol (in women) are measured. If prolactin was elevated before surgery, it should be measured again at this time, and any stimulation tests that are indicated (e.g., TRH test, ITT, metyrapone test) are performed.

Special endocrine testing

Additional endocrine tests that are obtained in certain endocrinopathies include the following:

> Acromegaly
> > Growth hormone levels
> > Somatomedin-C levels
> > Glucose suppression
> > TRH test
> > GHRF levels
>
> Cushing's syndrome (disease)
> > Urinary free cortisol
> > Dexamethasone suppression, low-/high-dose
> > Metyrapone test
> > ACTH levels
>
> Prolactinoma
> > Serum prolactin levels × 2
> > Chlorpromazine (CPZ) test
> > TRH test

In these situations testing is useful in making a positive diagnosis of the specific endocrinopathy, in identifying the source of the disorder (i.e., the pituitary in Cushing's syndrome), and in evaluating the effectiveness of a given therapy. Recommended tests for each of the endocrinopathies follow.

Acromegaly. In addition to the baseline endocrine studies just cited, in patients with suspected or proven acromegaly, special studies include basal levels of growth hormone, GH-glucose suppression test, determination of somatomedin-C levels, TRH stimulation test, and GHRF levels.

Basal levels of growth hormone. Basal levels of growth hormone should be drawn in a fasting, rested state. False positives can be caused by exercise and stress, especially in estrogenized women, and by hypoglycemia.

Growth hormone—glucose suppression test. Basal levels of growth hormone are elevated (i.e., >10 ng/ml) in about 90% to 95% of patients with acromegaly. When 100 g of glucose is orally administered to a normal individual, serum growth hormone levels fall to less than 5 ng/ml when measured 2 hours later. In patients with acromegaly, the elevated levels of growth hormone will not suppress to the 5 ng/ml level during the 2 hours following a glucose load. In some cases of acromegaly, a paradoxic rise in the growth hormone levels occurs.

Somatomedin-C levels. The effect of growth hormone on peripheral tissues is mediated through the somatomedins, a group of polypeptides with insulin-like activity, which are produced in the liver.[30,39] Clemmons et al[3] found that somatomedin-C levels determined by radioimmunoassay appeared to provide a reliable means for confirming the diagnosis of acromegaly. In their study, the mean fasting serum somatomedin-C concentration was 6.8 U/ml (range, 2.6 to 21.7) for acromegalic subjects as compared with 0.67 U/ml (range, 0.31 to 1.4) for normal subjects. Other studies have not found such a strong correlation.[34] Somatomedin-C levels do seem to correlate well with symptoms indicative of excess growth hormone. The determination of somatomedin-C levels is useful in patients who are suspected of having acromegaly but who do not have significantly elevated basal growth hormone levels. Somatomedin-C levels may also be an indicator of response to treatment,[3] but Stonesifer et al[34] compared somatomedin-C levels with subjective clinical response and growth hormone levels and found no apparent advantage of somatomedin-C determinations over growth hormone in evaluating the response of patients treated for acromegaly.

Thyrotropin-releasing hormone (TRH) test. Although the TRH test is not essential in establishing the laboratory diagnosis of acromegaly, it has potential value in assessing the effectiveness of treatment. A significant rise in serum growth hormone follows the administration of TRH in acromegalic patients as opposed to no significant change in growth hormone in normal subjects. This laboratory finding may have predictive value in terms of long-term cures following surgery (see Chapter 6). Patients who appear to be cured immediately after surgery but who show an abnormal growth hormone response to TRH seem to be at greater risk for recurrence than patients who show normal responses following an operation. For more discussion of this issue, the reader is referred to Chapter 6, especially the section on results of surgical treatment.

Growth hormone–releasing factor (GHRF) levels. Circulating GHRF levels in acromegaly are generally below the sensitivity of present radioimmunoassays, but are measurable by bioassays. This is also true of levels in normal patients. As the assays become more sensitive, there may be other indications for this test, but at present the only indication is to diagnose acromegaly caused by tumors producing ectopic GHRF.

Cushing's syndrome (disease). As with acromegaly, baseline endocrine studies as outlined previously are obtained in patients with Cushing's syndrome in addition to the following special studies.

There are two important phases in the special endocrine evaluation of patients with Cushing's syndrome. These include establishing the diagnosis of hypercortisolism and identifying the source of the disease. Although establishing the diagnosis of hypercortisolism by endocrine testing usually is not difficult, determining the *source* of the disease (i.e., ectopic versus pituitary versus adrenal) is more involved and in some cases not easy to achieve.

Establishing diagnosis of Cushing's syndrome. Measurement of *free cortisol* in a 24-hour urine sample, *urinary free cortisol* (UFC), in the unstressed patient is an excellent assessment of cortisol production. An elevation of UFC, especially greater than twice the upper limit of normal, is strongly suggestive of Cushing's syndrome. For most patients, a 24-hour urine sample can be accurately collected on an outpatient basis. Elevated UFC can also be caused by depression and alcoholism.

Another useful screening test for Cushing's syndrome is the overnight dexamethasone suppression test. A dose of 1 mg of dexamethasone is administered at bedtime and plasma cortisol determined the following morning. If plasma cortisol does not fall to <5 µg/dl, the diagnosis of Cushing's syndrome is very likely. However, failure to show suppression may be seen in patients who are under stress; in patients who fail to take their medication; when plasma cortisol-binding globulin is increased, as with phenytoin (Dilantin) therapy; in about 50% of patients with depression; and when dexamethasone is rapidly metabolized, as with anticonvulsant therapy. *Normal* suppression nearly excludes Cushing's syndrome. The determination of UFC in a 24-hour urine sample coupled with the overnight dexamethasone suppression test forms a very powerful screening study that can be done on outpatients to establish hypercortisolism.

Plasma cortisol levels in normal subjects follow the circadian rhythm of ACTH secretion. The values are relatively high early in the waking day, become low as time for sleep approaches, and reach a nadir during the middle of sleep. Patients with Cushing's syndrome tend to lose the normal circadian rhythm and have relatively high values at all hours.[23] In Cushing's syndrome, plasma cortisol concentrations usually range from 15 to 25 µg/dl regardless of time of day whereas in normal subjects morning values range from 12 to 25 µg/dl and late evening values from 1 to 8 µg/dl. There is considerably more overlap in morning values between normal subjects and patients with Cushing's syndrome than with late evening values, which are more diagnostic.

Identifying the source of the disease. Once the diagnosis of hypercortisolism (Cushing's syndrome) is suggested, more specialized tests are used to determine the cause. The most common cause is a partially autonomous, ACTH-secreting pituitary adenoma (Cushing's disease), which accounts for about 60% of cases.[22] A primary adrenal disease, either an adrenal adenoma or adrenal carcinoma, accounts for about 25% of cases. An ectopic source of ACTH is found in about

15% of cases, usually from one of the following neoplasms: small cell carcinoma of the lung, bronchial or intestinal carcinoid, thymoma, pancreatic islet cell tumor, medullary carcinoma of the thyroid, or pheochromocytoma. These three major causes of Cushing's syndrome—pituitary, adrenal, or ectopic ACTH—can be distinguished on the basis of biochemical and morphologic studies. However, the etiologic diagnosis of Cushing's syndrome remains one of the most difficult in endocrinology.

The major tests used in the differential diagnosis of Cushing's syndrome are (1) dexamethasone suppression test,[21] (2) ACTH levels, especially in conjunction with CRF stimulation, (3) metyrapone test, and (4) radiologic studies (e.g., computed tomography (CT) of sella, adrenal glands). A summary of typical laboratory findings in various types of Cushing's syndrome/disease is shown in Table 4-4.

Table 4-4
Typical laboratory findings in various types of Cushing's syndrome

Tests	Normal subjects	Cushing's disease pituitary origin	Ectopic ACTH syndrome	Adrenal tumor
Plasma cortisol	10-25 μg/dl Rhythmic	High Nonrhythmic	High Nonrhythmic	High Nonrhythmic
Urinary free cortisol	Normal	Increased	Increased	Increased
Response to low-dose dexamethasone				
Urinary 17-OHCS	Decreased	No change	No change	No change
Plasma cortisol	Decreased	No change	No change	No change
Response to high-dose dexamethasone				
Urinary 17-OHCS	Decreased	Decreased	No change	No change
Plasma cortisol	Decreased	Decreased	No change	No change
Response to metyrapone				
Urinary 17-OHCS	Increased	Increased	No change	No change (rarely increased)

Modified from Liddle GW: Pathogenesis of glucocorticoid disorders. *Am J Med* 53:638, 1972.

Standard dexamethasone suppression test. Originally developed by Liddle, this test consists of evaluating response of urinary excretion of 17 hydroxycorticosteroids (17-OHCS) to stepwise increases in dexamethasone.[21] Serial 24-hour urine collections are done for 6 days. The first 2 days are basal collections. The next 2 days the patient takes 0.5 mg dexamethasone (low-dose) every 6 hours for 48 hours, and the final two days the patient takes 2 mg dexamethasone (high-dose) every 6 hours for 48 hours. All collections are corrected to creatinine excretion and expressed as mg 17-OHCS/g creatinine/24 hours. Basal values greater than 7 mg/g creatinine/24 hours are elevated. Normals suppress on low-dose dexamethasone to less than 50% of basal or less than 4 mg/g creatinine/24 hours on the second day of collection. Patients with Cushing's disease fail to suppress on low-dose dexamethasone but suppress to less than 50% of basal levels on high-dose dexamethasone (Table 4-4). Patients with primary adrenal disease or ectopic ACTH production fail to suppress to either low- or high-dose dexamethasone. This test is very sensitive and specific when done in the standard fashion. Major factors can confuse interpretation, especially alterations in dexamethasone metabolism and periodic hormonogenesis, which can be found with all three causes of Cushing's syndrome.

Determination of plasma ACTH levels. Plasma ACTH levels are elevated in patients with Cushing's disease and in patients with an ectopic source of ACTH (see Table 4-4). Apart from the finding that the levels are usually higher in the ectopic syndrome, plasma ACTH levels, which are determined by radioimmunoassay, do not provide definitive information for separating patients with Cushing's disease from those with the ectopic ACTH syndrome. Patients with adrenal tumors have low plasma ACTH levels. One drawback is that the plasma ACTH assay is technically difficult and lacks the standardization of some of the other diagnostic procedures. Also normal values for plasma ACTH may be present in a significant number of patients with proven Cushing's disease. However, the assay assumes more importance when venous blood is obtained from an organ or tissue suspected as being the site of abnormal ACTH secretion. For instance, selective venous sampling for ACTH in blood from the petrosal sinus, which contains the venous effluent from the pituitary, may be useful in the diagnostic evaluation of Cushing's syndrome. Pituitary hormones enter the systemic circulation through multiple small venous effluents into the cavernous sinus, which in turn drains posteriorly into the inferior and superior petrosal sinuses and ultimately into the internal jugular vein.[15] Thus blood samples obtained from the petrosal sinus should provide a reasonably accurate measurement of ACTH production in the pituitary gland. Plasma levels of ACTH from the inferior petrosal sinus have been found to be at least two-fold higher than simultaneous peripheral levels in patients with pituitary dependent Cushing's disease.[4,12,20] Blood obtained at the level of the jugular bulb is mixed with blood drained from different areas of the brain and therefore is less useful diagnostically.[12] It also appears that pituitary venous drainage is lateralized and that ACTH levels in blood from each of the two inferior petrosal sinuses may differ.[24] One may therefore miss an elevated ACTH level if only one petrosal sinus is sampled. Furthermore, this lateralization of drainage may be useful to the surgeon in predicting the side of the pituitary gland in which the tumor will be found. Measurement of ACTH levels before and after CRF stimulation is a good method to determine the putative role of the pituitary and to lateralize an adenoma within the gland. Ectopic sources of ACTH do not seem responsive to CRF, especially based on petrosal sinus sampling.

Metyrapone test. Metyrapone blocks the final steps in cortisol biosynthesis by inhibiting activity of the adrenal enzyme, 11-β-hydroxylase. This block results in a fall in plasma cortisol levels, which, through its feedback mechanism, stimulates increased secretion of pituitary ACTH in normal subjects. The latter is reflected by a prompt rise in the urinary 17-OHCS level because the excretory product of 11-deoxycortisol (which responds to increased ACTH secretion) possesses the same side chain on ring D of the steroid molecule as cortisol's end products.[43] Patients with Cushing's disease normally have a two- to four-fold increase over basal urinary 17-OHCS levels as opposed to patients with either adrenal tumors or an ectopic source, who typically fail to show a response (see Table 4-4). The reason for this response in Cushing's disease is that although secretion of ACTH is inappropriate for a given plasma level of cortisol, it is not completely autonomous and is responsive to negative feedback by cortisol or other glucocorticoids such as dexamethasone. Thus inhibition of cortisol biosynthesis by metyrapone in patients with Cushing's disease results in increased ACTH secretion. A functioning adrenal adenoma or carcinoma suppresses pituitary ACTH, and thus no increase in urinary steroid will occur in response to the drug. In performing the test, metyrapone is administered orally in a dosage of 750 mg every 4 hours for 24 hours, and urinary 17-OHCS is measured basally, the same day as metyrapone, and the day after. A two-fold rise above basal values is a positive response. No increase in 17-OHCS excretion is strongly against pituitary dependent Cushing's syndrome. However, a positive response does not rule out an adrenal-based process or ectopic source of ACTH.

Radiologic studies. When the diagnosis of hypercortisolism is confirmed, morphologic studies can be used to corroborate the biochemical data and provide preoperative information to the surgeon. A CT scan of the sella should be done although most ACTH-secreting pituitary adenomas are not visualized. An abdominal CT can evaluate the adrenal glands for symmetry and hyperplasia and other organs such as the pancreas for evidence of tumors. Symmetry of the adrenals suggests an ACTH-mediated process, whereas unilateral enlargement suggests a primary adrenal source. A chest x-ray examination or CT scan should be done to exclude lung nodules or an enlarged mediastinum, which might indicate an ectopic source of ACTH. Further studies can be done if these prove equivocal such as adrenal vein catheterization, angiography, and iodocholesterol scan.

Because of the potential for difficulty in interpretation of tests, we believe all patients with suspected Cushing's disease should have a full endocrine workup, preferably at the center where surgery might be performed. This should include (1) basal UFC and 17-OHCS levels, (2) standard dexamethasone suppression test with both low- and high-dose dexamethasone, (3) ACTH levels—basal and during dexamethasone suppression, (4) metyrapone test, and (5) morphologic studies with at least CT scans of the sella and adrenals.

Table 4-4 shows typical laboratory values in normal subjects and in patients with various types of Cushing's syndrome/disease under basal conditions and in response to various treatments.

Prolactinomas. In patients with suspected or proven prolactinomas, the baseline studies as outlined previously are obtained; in addition, we believe that at least two separate determinations of fasting AM serum prolactin values should be obtained. For practical purposes, serum prolactin levels >150 ng/ml are diagnostic of a prolactin-secreting pituitary tumor (prolactinoma). Values <150 ng/ml and certainly values between 20 and 100 ng/ml can be caused by several other conditions including hypothyroidism and ingestion of certain drugs. Pituitary or suprasellar lesions (including nonfunctional pituitary tumors) that interfere with the normal delivery of prolactin inhibiting factor (PIF) to the adenohypophysis can cause hyperprolactinemia. Usually, the serum prolactin values are less than 100 ng/ml. Pituitary or suprasellar lesions that cause elevated serum prolactin in this manner are referred to as "pseudoprolactinomas."

Special studies in patients with suspected prolactinomas include chlorpromazine (CPZ) stimulation test[38] and TRH stimulation test.[17] CPZ is a dopamine antagonist—the mechanism of action being through inhibition of PIF, thus allowing the normal adenohypophysis to secrete an unrestrained release of prolactin for a limited period of time. Thus in normal subjects the administration of CPZ is followed by a two- or three-fold increase in serum prolactin. The test is performed in fasting patients following a baseline serum prolactin determination with repeat determinations at 1, 2, 3, and 4 hours after the administration of 50 mg of CPZ.[38] In patients with pituitary tumors, the normal post-CPZ elevation of serum prolactin is blunted, and in many patients, no significant change in values over baseline measurements occurs. The test has limited application in evaluating patients with suspected prolactinomas mainly because of its lack of specificity for pituitary tumors. The CPZ test is positive in other conditions that cause hyperprolactinemia. The administration of 50 mg of CPZ also produces marked lethargy in many patients. These patients have a tendency to fall if they attempt to stand or walk during the period of maximal drug action. For these reasons (lethargy and nonspecificity), it is not a widely used test. Perhaps the major value of the test would be to compare pretreatment with posttreatment (especially postsurgical) values to determine whether the treatment restored a normal prolactin reserve response.

The TRH test also evaluates normal prolactin reserve but through a different mechanism of action than CPZ. TRH causes a release not only of TSH from the adenohypophysis but also stimulates the release of prolactin. In the normal fasting subject, the administration of TRH is followed by a marked increase in the level of serum prolactin, whereas in patients with pituitary tumors, the response is blunted or flat. The test is performed in the fasting state; after obtaining baseline values, the patient is given 500 mcg TRH, and values of serum prolactin are determined at 15, 30, 45, and 60 minutes. This test, although not specific for pituitary tumors, is positive in the majority of patients with this lesion. Frantz[13] found that 15 of 16 patients with prolactin secreting tumors in his series showed an abnormal response to TRH administration. However, the criticism expressed previously related to the diagnostic value of the CPZ test can also be made for the TRH test. Like the CPZ test, the TRH test is nonspecific for pituitary tumors and probably not required in the routine investigation of patients with suspected prolactinomas. As with the CPZ test, the main value of the TRH test would be to evaluate whether surgery restored the prolactin secretory mechanisms to normal. In this respect, the TRH test may be a more valuable procedure than the CPZ administration and probably has a higher percentage of accuracy.

SUMMARY

The clinical features of pituitary and other parasellar lesions consist of mass effects and/or endocrinopathy. The most common manifestations of mass effect are visual, but other findings include headache, extraocular palsies, hypothalamic impairment, seizures, and pituitary apoplexy. The common endocrinopathies are the amenorrhea-galactorrhea syndrome resulting from hyperprolactinemia, acromegaly, and Cushing's disease. Current clinical and endocrinologic evaluation will identify the majority of these disorders.

REFERENCES

1. Barron KD, Fergusson G: Intracranial hemorrhage as a complication of anticoagulant therapy. *Neurology* 9:447, 1959.
2. Brougham M, Heusner AP, Adams RD: Acute degenerative changes in adenomas of the pituitary body—with special reference to pituitary apoplexy. *J Neurosurg* 7:421, 1950.
3. Clemmons DR, Van Wyk JJ, Ridgway EC, et al: Evaluation of acromegaly by radioimmunoassay of somatomedin-C. *N Engl J Med* 301:1138, 1979.
4. Corrigan DF, Schaaf M, Whaley RA, et al: Selective venous sampling to differentiate ectopic ACTH secretion from pituitary Cushing's syndrome. *N Engl J Med* 296:861, 1977.
5. Cunningham GR, Huckins C: An FSH and prolactin-secreting pituitary tumor: Pituitary dynamics and testicular histology. *J Clin Endocrinol Metab* 44:248, 1977.
6. Cushing H, Walker CB: Fourth paper. Distortions of the visual fields in cases of brain tumour: Chiasmal lesions, with especial reference to bitemporal hemianopsia. *Brain* 37:341, 1915.
7. David NJ, Gargano FP, Glaser JS: Pituitary apoplexy in clinical perspective, in Glaser JS, Smith JL (eds): *Neuro-Ophthalmology.* St Louis, The CV Mosby Co, 1975.
8. Earle KM, Dillard SH Jr: Pathology of adenomas of the pituitary gland, in Kohler PO, Ross GT (eds): *Diagnosis and Treatment of Pituitary Tumors.* Amsterdam, Excerpta Medica, 1973.
9. Ebersold MJ, Laws ER, Scheithauer BW, et al: Pituitary apoplexy treated by transsphenoidal surgery: A clinicopathological and immunocytochemical study. *J Neurosurg* 58:315, 1983.
10. Feinsod M, Auerbach E: The electroretinogram and the visual evoked potential in two patients with tuberculum sellae meningioma before and after decompression of the optic nerve. *Ophthalmologica* 163:360, 1971.
11. Feinsod M, Selhorst JB, Hoyt WF, et al: Monitoring optic nerve function during craniotomy. *J Neurosurg* 44:29, 1976.
12. Findling JW, Aron DC, Tyrrell JB, et al: Selective venous sampling for ACTH in Cushing's syndrome: Differentiation between Cushing's disease and ectopic ACTH syndrome. *Ann Intern Med* 94:647, 1981.
13. Frantz AG: Prolactin. *N Engl J Med* 298:201, 1978.
14. Friend JN, Judge DM, Sherman BM, et al: FSH-secreting pituitary adenomas: Stimulation and suppression studies in two patients. *J Clin Endocrinol Metab* 43:650, 1976.
15. Green HT: The venous drainage of the human hypophysis cerebri. *Am J Anat* 100:435, 1957.
16. Hamilton CP, Adams LC, Maloof F: Hyperthyroidism due to thyrotropin-producing pituitary chromophobe adenoma. *N Engl J Med* 283:1077, 1970.
17. Hershman JM: Clinical application of thyrotropin-releasing hormone. *N Engl J Med* 290:886, 1974.
18. Hughes B: Blood supply of the optic nerves and chiasma and its clinical significance. *Br J Ophthalmol* 42:106, 1958.
19. Jacobi JD, Fishman LM, Daroff RB: Pituitary apoplexy in acromegaly followed by partial pituitary insufficiency. *Arch Intern Med* 134:559, 1974.
20. Kley HK, Stolze T, Krüskemper HL: Jugular-

vein sampling of ACTH, letter. *N Engl J Med* 297:731, 1977.
21. Liddle GW: Tests of pituitary-adrenal suppressibility in the diagnosis of Cushing's syndrome. *J Clin Endocrinol Metab* 20:1539, 1960.
22. Liddle GW: Pathogenesis of glucocorticoid disorders. *Am J Med* 53:638, 1972.
23. Lindsay AE, Migeon CJ, Nugent CA, et al: The diagnostic value of plasma and urinary 17-hydroxycorticosteroid determinations in Cushing's syndrome. *Am J Med* 20:15, 1956.
24. Manni A, Latshaw RF, Page R, et al: Simultaneous bilateral venous sampling for adrenocorticotropin in pituitary-dependent Cushing's disease: Evidence for lateralization of pituitary venous drainage. *J Clin Endocrinol Metab* 57:1070, 1983.
25. Mohanty S, Tandon PN, Banerji AK, et al: Haemorrhage into pituitary adenomas. *J Neurol Neurosurg Psychiatry* 40:987, 1977.
26. Neetens A, Selosse P: Oculomotor anomalies in sellar and parasellar pathology. *Ophthalmologica* 175:80, 1977.
27. Nelson DH, Meakin JW, Thorn GW: ACTH-producing pituitary tumors following adrenalectomy for Cushing's syndrome. *Ann Intern Med* 52:560, 1960.
28. Nourizadeh AR, Pitts FW: Hemorrhage into pituitary adenoma during anticoagulant therapy. *JAMA* 193:623, 1965.
29. O'Connell JEA: The anatomy of the optic chiasm and heteronymous hemianopia. *J Neurol Neurosurg Psychiatry* 36:710, 1973.
30. Phillips LS, Vassilopoulou-Sellin R: Somatomedins: First of two parts. *N Engl J Med* 302:371, 1980.
31. Rovit RL, Duane TD: Cushing's syndrome and pituitary tumors: Pathophysiology and ocular manifestations of ACTH-secreting pituitary adenomas. *Am J Med* 46:416, 1969.
32. Rovit RL, Fein JM: Pituitary apoplexy: A review and reappraisal. *J Neurosurg* 37:280, 1972.
33. Rucker CW, Kernohan JW: Notching of the optic chiasm by overlying arteries in pituitary tumors. *Arch Ophthalmol* 51:161, 1954.
34. Stonesifer LD, Jordan RM, Kohler PO: Somatomedin C in treated acromegaly: Poor correlation with growth hormone and clinical response. *J Clin Endocrinol Metab* 53:931, 1981.
35. Sunderland S, Bradley KC: Stress-strain phenomena in human peripheral nerve trunks. *Brain* 84:102, 1961.
36. Symonds C: Ocular palsy as the presenting symptom of pituitary adenoma. *Bull Johns Hopkins Hosp* 111:72, 1962.
37. Taylor Al, Finster JL, Raskin P, et al: Pituitary apoplexy in acromegaly. *J Clin Endocrinol Metab* 28:1784, 1968.
38. Tolis G, Goldstein M, Friesen HG: Functional evaluation of prolactin secretion in patients with hypothalamic pituitary disorders. *J Clin Invest* 52:783, 1973.
39. Van Wyk JJ, Underwood LE: Relation between growth hormone and somatomedin. *Annu Rev Med* 26:427, 1975.
40. VanWagenen WP: Haemorrhage into a pituitary tumor following trauma. *Ann Surg* 95:625, 1932.
41. Wakai S, Fukushima T, Teramoto A, et al: Pituitary apoplexy: Its incidence and clinical significance. *J Neurosurg* 55:187, 1981.
42. Weinberger LM, Adler FH, Grant FC: Primary pituitary adenoma and the syndrome of the cavernous sinus: A clinical and anatomic study. *Arch Ophthalmol* 24:1197, 1940.
43. Weiss ER, Rayyis SS, Nelson DH, et al: Evaluation of stimulation and suppression tests in the etiological diagnosis of Cushing's syndrome. *Ann Intern Med* 71:941, 1969.
44. Zimmerman EA, Defendini R, Frantz AG: Prolactin and growth hormone in patients with pituitary adenomas: A correlative study of hormone in tumor and plasma by immunoperoxidase technique and redioimmunoassay. *J Clin Endocrinol Metab* 38:577, 1974.

CHAPTER 5
Neuroradiology

Neuroradiologic studies
  Skull films
    Assessment of size and configuration of the sella turcica
      Volumetric increase
      Increase in linear measurements
    Gross abnormalities in the sellar and parasellar area
    Extent of pneumatization of the sphenoid sinuses
  Sellar polytomography
  Computed tomography
  Cerebral angiography
  Digital intravenous angiography
  Metrizamide cisternography
  Cavernous sinus venography and petrosal sinus sampling
  Magnetic resonance imaging
Radiologic findings in specific pathologic disorders
  Pituitary adenomas
  Craniopharyngiomas
  Meningiomas
  Hypothalamic and optic gliomas
  Chordomas
  Non-neoplastic cysts
  Aneurysms
  Pituitary abscesses
  Sarcoidosis
  Histiocytosis X
  "Empty sella" syndrome

Over the past several years, significant advances have been made in neuroimaging techniques that have influenced the diagnostic workup of patients with lesions in the vicinity of the pituitary gland. In general, current neurodiagnostic procedures are more comfortable for the patients, carry less risk, and the data provided by modern studies are superior and more meaningful than that afforded by older techniques such as pneumoencephalography (PEG).

In this chapter, the focus is on those neuroimaging techniques that are believed to be appropriate and useful for the current diagnostic evaluation of patients with lesions in or around the sella turcica, including pituitary tumors. Each procedure will be described, many will be illustrated, and the indication(s) for each in the current diagnostic protocol of patients with intrasellar and parasellar lesions will be provided. Older techniques, which in our opinion are no longer indicated in the routine diagnostic workup, will be mentioned briefly only in a historic perspective.

NEURORADIOLOGIC STUDIES
Skull films

A single lateral skull x-ray film is obtained in all patients who are undergoing evaluation for sellar or parasellar lesions. In the past, it was customary to obtain multiple films in different planes (e.g., submentovertex, anteroposterior [AP]). However, relatively little useful information can be gathered from plain x-ray examinations other than the lateral projection. Since other more definitive diagnostic procedures are now available, it is often no longer practical or necessary to obtain these other views.

A normal film is shown in Fig. 5-1. The important bony elements that make up the sellar and parasellar area should each be identified and assessed for normality. The lateral skull x-ray film can provide much useful information, including (1) an assessment of the size and configuration of the sella turcica and skull; (2) detection of gross abnormalities, including calcification in the sellar and/or suprasellar region; (3) determination of the extent of pneumatization of the sphenoid sinus; and (4) an indication of any unusual bony anatomic feature(s) that may be useful to the surgeon.

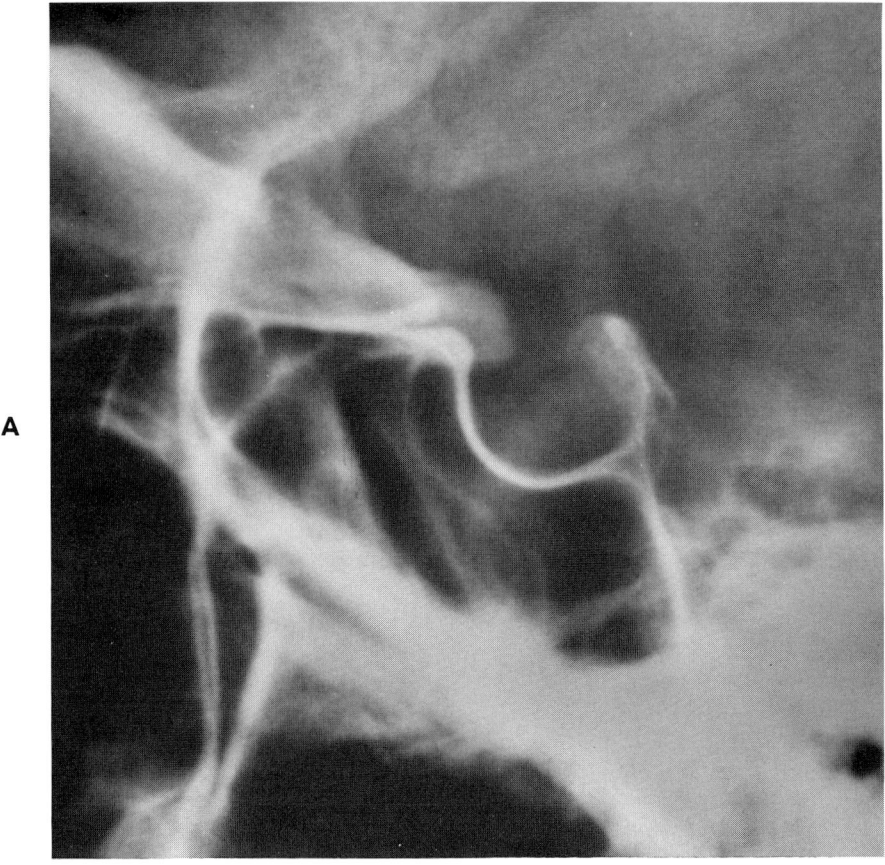
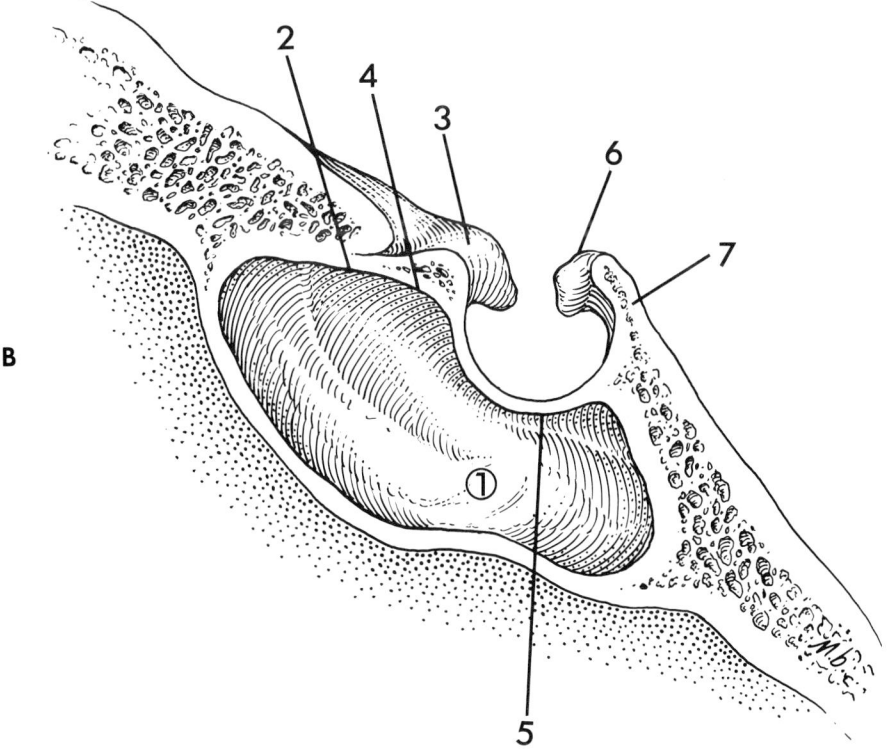

Fig. 5-1. A, Normal lateral x-ray of the sella. **B,** Illustration of anatomic components: *1*, Sphenoid sinus; *2*, planum sphenoidale; *3*, anterior clinoid; *4*, tuberculum sellae; *5*, lamina dura; *6*, posterior clinoid; *7*, dorsum sella.

148 *Disorders of the pituitary*

In obtaining the film, it is essential that a true lateral projection be obtained as indicated by the superimposition of the two anterior clinoid processes. Obliquity of the lateral x-ray film resulting from rotation may occasionally give an erroneous impression of a sellar floor being depressed on one side producing a "false" double floor (Fig. 5-2). The false double floor may also be seen in skull films that are nonrotated, true lateral views. In this case, the appearance of the double floor is probably produced by uneven development of the sphenoid sinuses[36] (Fig. 5-3). This sellar contour may also result from the groove caused by the intracavernous carotid artery.

Assessment of size and configuration of the sella turcica. There are two methods for determining whether the sella is abnormally enlarged: volumetric increase and increase in linear measurements.

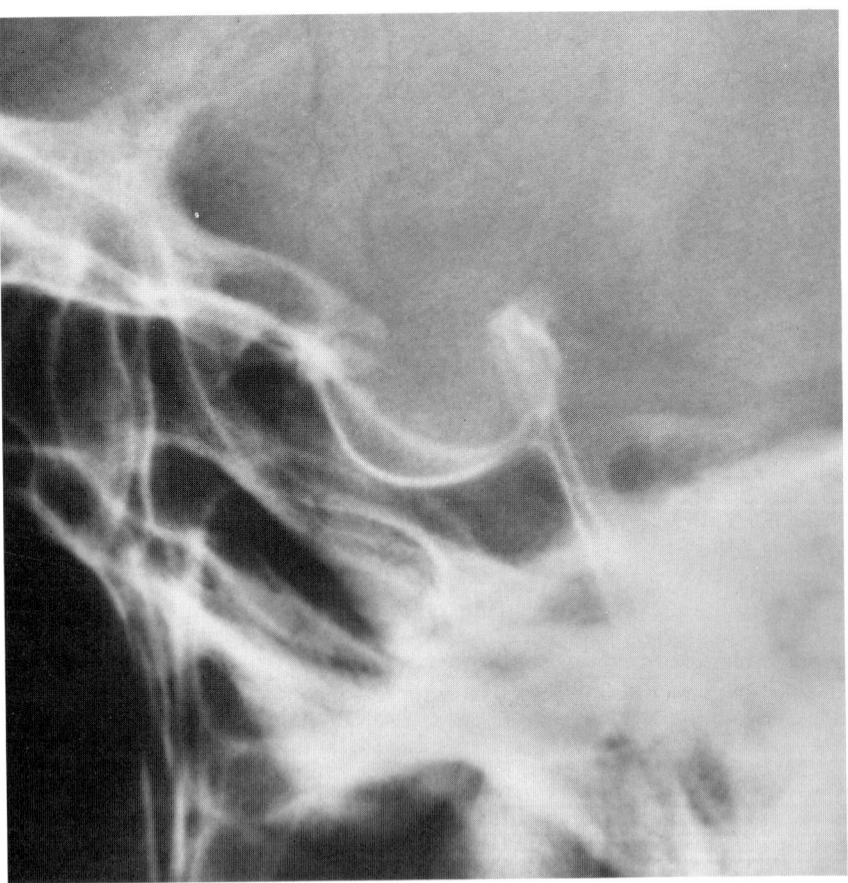

Fig. 5-2. False double floor caused by rotation of skull.

Volumetric increase. Di Chiro[10] has suggested that it is possible to calculate the volume of the sella by applying the following mathematic formula:

$$\text{Volume (in cm)}^2 = \frac{\frac{1}{2}(\text{Length} \times \text{Width} \times \text{Height [in mm]})}{1000}$$

In a study of adult sellae evaluated with this formula, the mean value was 594 cm^2 and the maximal value was 1092 cm^2.[10] Although this method represents a means for attempting to quantify an abnormal increase in the size of the sella, most clinicians and radiologists have not found it to be practical.

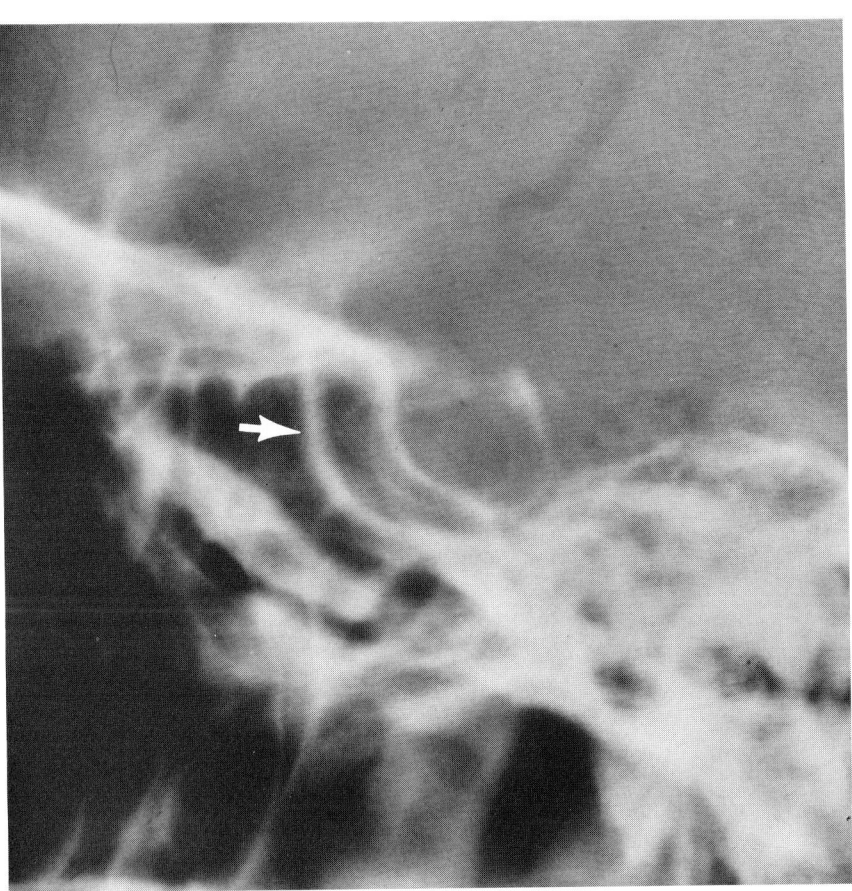

Fig. 5-3. False double floor caused by transversely oriented sphenoid sinus septae (arrow).

Increase in linear measurements. Taveras and Wood[36] described a relatively simple means for determining an increase in sella size. As illustrated in Fig. 5-4, their method is based on making three measurements that include horizontal diameter, vertical diameter (depth), and width. The width, which requires an AP film is probably the least important of the three measurements. The AP diameter is measured from the most anterior to the most posterior margin of the sella and should not exceed 17 mm. The depth is measured from the lowest point of the pituitary fossa to a line extending from the top of the dorsum sellae to the tuberculum sella. The upper limit of normal for this measurement is 13 mm, and the width of the sella should not exceed 15 mm. These measurements are relatively generous, and experience has shown that they are usually abnormal only when there is gross distortion of the sella from either a relatively large tumor or in cases of the "empty sella" syndrome (ESS). Although this method for determining an abnormal increase in sella size can be applied in suspicious cases, in actual practice, an experienced radiologist can determine from a review of a lateral skull film whether the sella is abnormally large without the necessity of using either volumetric or linear measurements.

Gross abnormalities in the sellar and parasellar area. In addition to pathologic enlargement of the sella, gross abnormalities include erosion of the sellar floor, thinning of the dorsum sella, loss of the lamina dura forming the floor of the sella, soft tissue densities within the sphenoid sinus, and suprasellar or intrasellar calcification. These pathologic alterations may be caused by pituitary

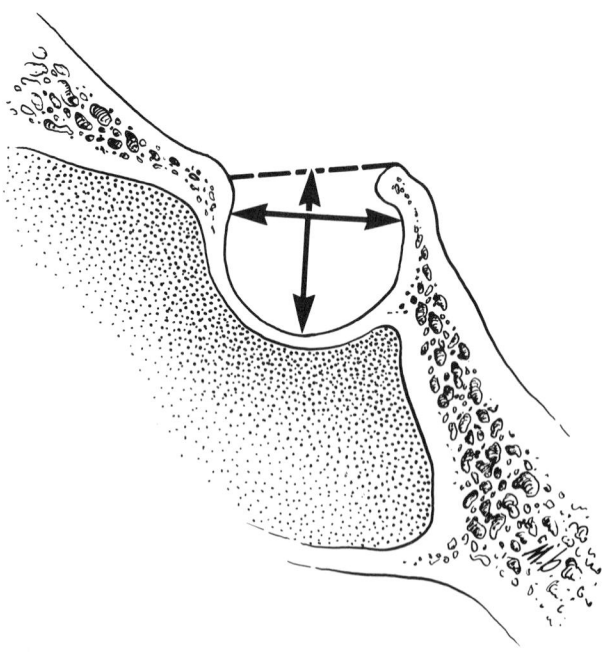

Fig. 5-4. Taveras and Wood method for measuring AP diameter and depth (vertical plane) of sella.

adenomas. Other lesions (e.g., tuberculum sellae meningioma, aneurysm, craniopharyngioma, clivus chordoma) can produce parasellar bony changes such as localized hyperostosis and destruction or may contain areas of calcification that can be detected on plain skull films.

Extent of pneumatization of the sphenoid sinuses. Lateral skull x-ray films are valuable to the surgeon planning a transsphenoidal operation by determining the extent of pneumatization of the sphenoid sinuses and the thickness of the floor of the sella turcica. The degree of pneumatization varies among individuals, and it can influence significantly the technical aspects of a transsphenoidal operation. Based on the extent of pneumatization, the sphenoid sinus can be divided into one of three groups: sellar, presellar and conchal. These three types are illustrated in Fig. 5-5.

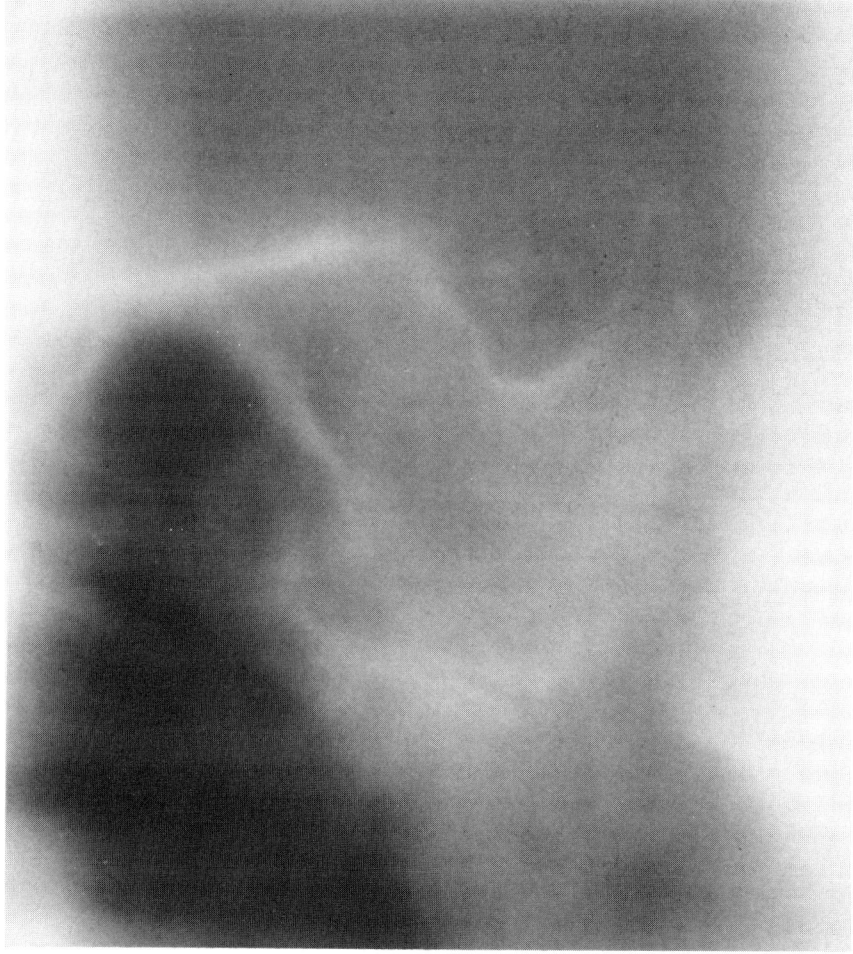

Fig. 5-5. Types of sphenoid sinuses based on degree of pneumatization.

Continued.

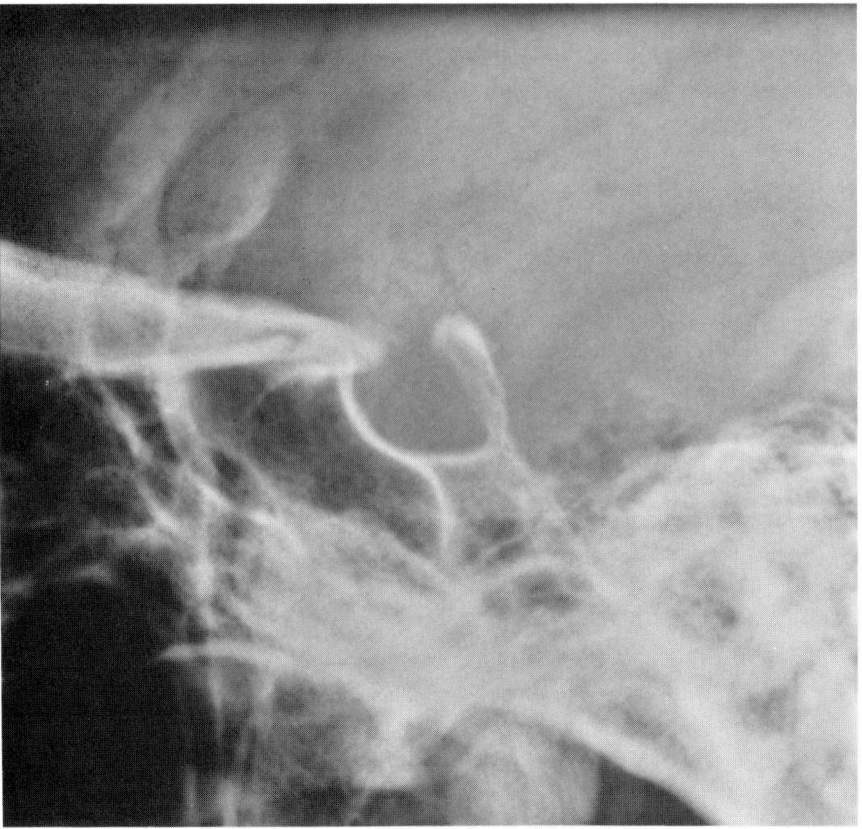

Fig. 5-5, cont'd. Types of sphenoid sinuses based on degree of pneumatization.

The sellar type of sphenoid sinus is well pneumatized, and the sellar floor bulges distinctively into the sinus. When viewed from within the sphenoid sinus by the surgeon, the floor of the sella can be recognized without difficulty. The anterior wall of the sella turcica usually measures less than 1 mm in thickness.

The presellar type of sphenoid sinus does not penetrate beyond a plane perpendicular to the sphenoid plane through the tuberculum sella, a line easily located on the skull film. In this type of sphenoid, the anterior wall of the sella turcica does not bulge into the sphenoid sinus.

The conchal type of sphenoid sinus does not reach into the body of the sphenoid bone. It is small and separated from the sella turcica by a cancellous wall approximately 10 mm thick. It is more likely to be encountered in young children and simply represents a situation in which the sinus has not reached a mature or more pneumatized state. Of the three types of sphenoid sinuses, Hamberger et al found that the sellar type of sphenoid sinus was most common, occurring bilaterally in 59% and on at least one side in 86%. Both sphenoid sinuses were of the presellar type in 11% and of the conchal type in 3%.[15]

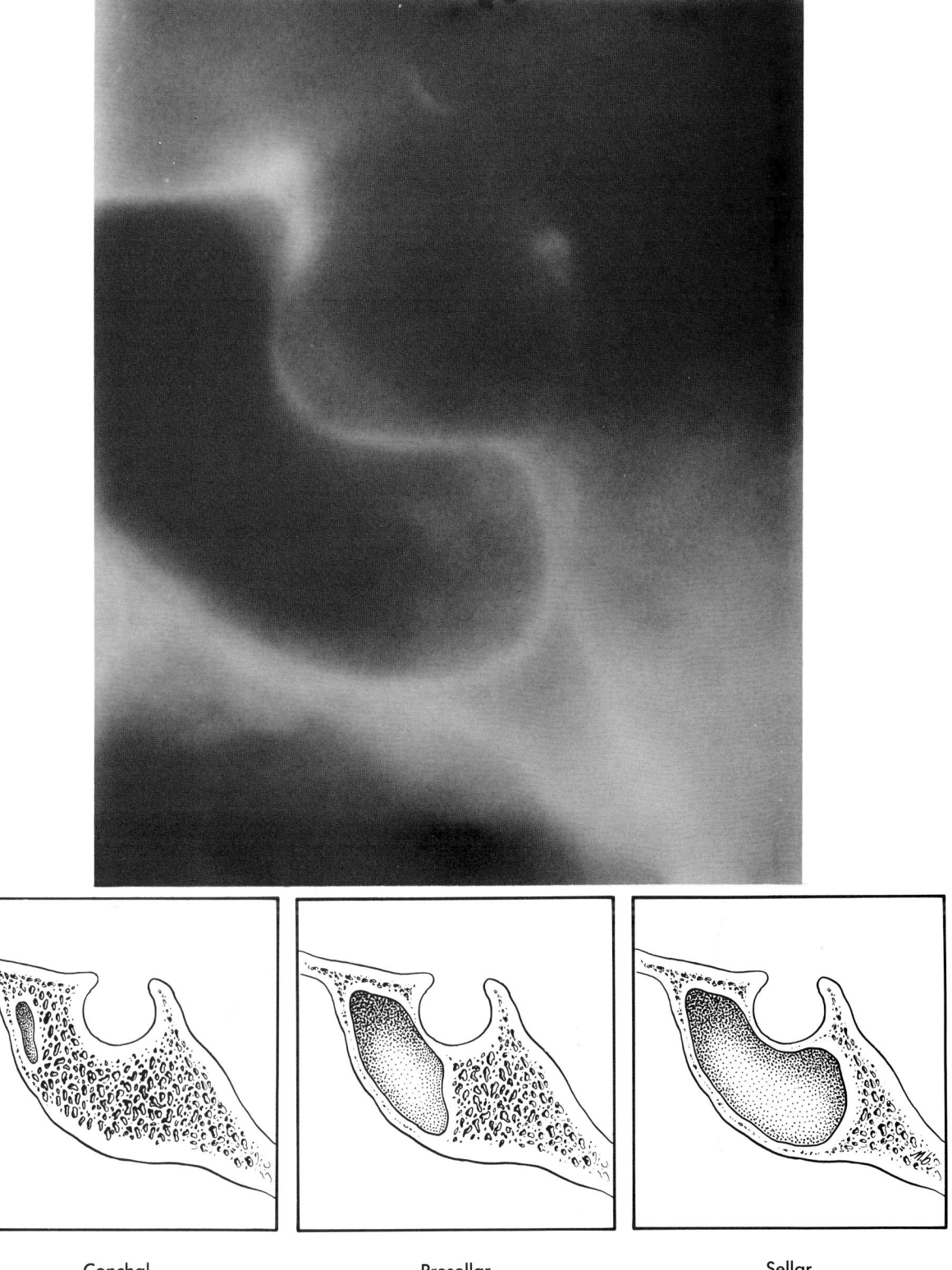

Conchal Presellar Sellar

Fig. 5-5, cont'd. Types of sphenoid sinuses based on degree of pneumatization.

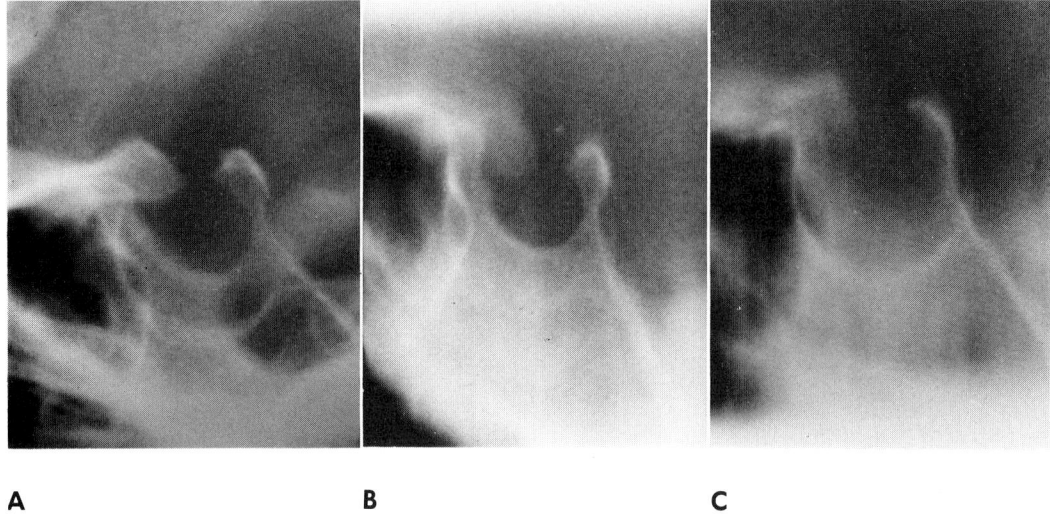

Fig. 5-6. Polytomography of double-floored sella. **A,** Lateral skull x-ray showing double floor. **B** and **C,** Polytome cuts through different areas of sella to better define anatomy.

Sellar polytomography

Polytomography is a special radiographic technique that provides a more detailed and accurate study of a given anatomic area than can be obtained from routine x-ray examinations. When used to evaluate the sella, polytomography will usually detect small bony changes (i.e., focal bulge or erosion of the sellar floor) caused by microadenomas and bony destruction caused by larger tumors that may not be visible on plain films. An example of the fine detail obtained by tomography is shown in Fig. 5-6.

Before the availability of high-resolution computed tomographic (CT) scanners, polytomography was a vital part of the neuroradiologic examination of patients undergoing an evaluation for suspected pituitary tumors. During the course of a routine examination, multiple films were obtained usually at 1 mm intervals in the lateral plane and at 2 mm intervals in an AP plane. In fact, so many films were obtained that the amount of local irradiation received was a major problem. The exposure was such that during a single examination a patient could receive locally as much as 6 to 10 rad.

Computed tomography

Currently, high-resolution computed tomography (CT) of the sella turcica is the most valuable diagnostic radiologic procedure available for evaluating pituitary and parapituitary tumors and thus is recommended as a routine examination in all patients undergoing investigation for such lesions. For pituitary tumors, the scan is obtained in the coronal plane both with and without intravenous contrast

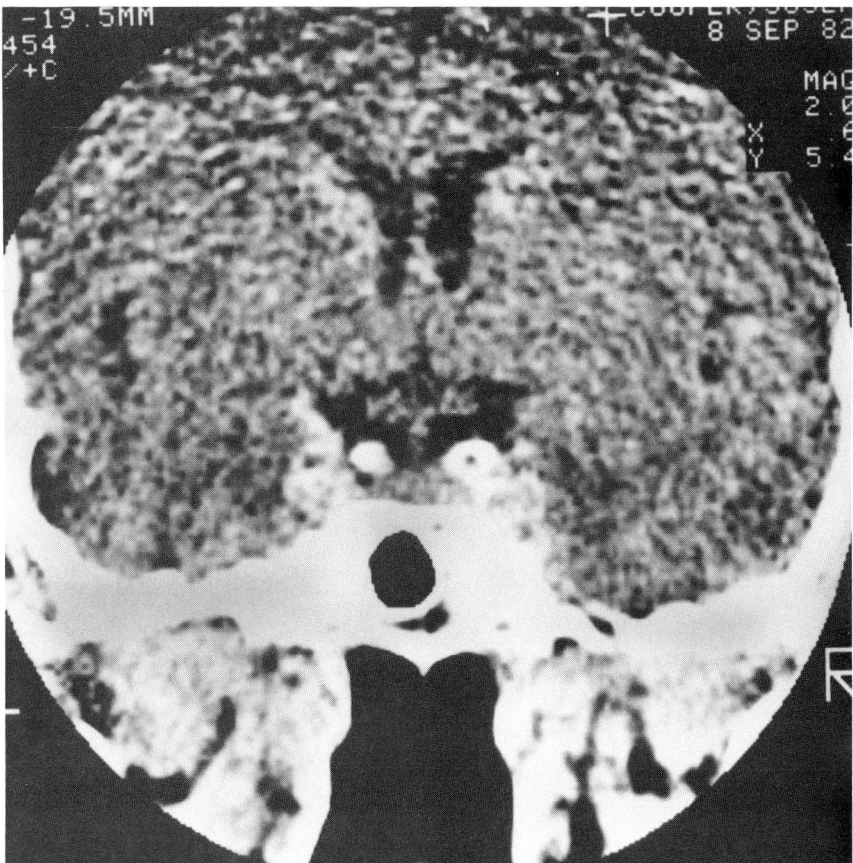

Fig. 5-7. High-resolution coronal CT scan of normal pituitary gland.

administration. It is important that the patient be positioned in the scanner so that several thin section cuts (1.5 mm) are obtained, starting at the dorsum sella and advancing anteriorly through the sella turcica to the tuberculum. Previous dental work can interfere with the quality of the scan unless the CT cuts are oriented so that the teeth are left out of the field of scanning. A lateral scout view on the CT allows one to choose the plane of the CT cuts. Maintaining the required head and neck position for the time necessary to obtain the scan can be uncomfortable for the patient. If direct coronal scans are not feasible, serial axial cuts may be obtained, and coronal and sagittal computer images may then be reconstructed.

Because the pituitary gland does not have a blood-brain barrier, opacification by intravenous contrast is virtually instantaneous.[13] The normal gland usually enhances homogenously. Differentiation of the cavernous sinuses can be achieved with rapid sequence (''dynamic'') scanning (Fig. 5-7). Although coronal scans are the only views required for most pituitary adenomas, some other suprasellar and parasellar lesions are evaluated more adequately by axial scans. Sagittal reconstructions will often demonstrate the relationship of a suprasellar mass to the optic chiasm.

Occasionally, a patient will give a history of a previous reaction to the use of contrast media. If the reaction was a serious anaphylactic response (i.e., vascular collapse, respiratory distress), it is our recommendation that contrast media should not be administered. If the reaction was not serious and consisted of itching or hives, for example, it is, in our opinion, appropriate to proceed with the contrast examination. We generally administer diphenhydramine (50 mg) and cimetidine (300 mg) orally, 1 hour before the administration of the contrast media for the H_1 and H_2 antihistamine effects, respectively. Four to six mg of dexamethasone is given intravenously at the same time, and a physician should be readily available during the examination.

Cerebral angiography

In the past, cerebral angiography was used to (1) determine the extent of suprasellar and/or parasellar extension of a pituitary tumor, (2) exclude the presence of an aneurysm, (3) determine whether major blood vessels (i.e., internal carotid) were involved by tumor, and (4) detect tumor blushes in vascular parasellar tumors such as a meningioma.

Cerebral angiography is performed via a modified Seldinger percutaneous femoral technique.[31] Magnification and subtraction techniques are helpful in detecting some of the subtle abnormalities associated with pituitary and parasellar neoplasms.

Digital intravenous angiography

Digital intravenous angiography (DIVA) is a technique that allows the visualization of small amounts of intra-arterial contrast following its intravenous injection. The basic DIVA system consists of five major components[26]: (1) a high-flux x-ray generation source, (2) a large field, high-quality x-ray image intensifier; (3) a precision digital video camera; (4) an analog-digital processing computer with storage facilities; and (5) a digital image store with mapping memory.

Although DIVA is not as accurate as conventional angiography in a definitive preoperative evaluation of intracranial vascular lesions, it can often be of diagnostic value and avoid the arterial puncture of conventional angiography.

If the purpose of arterial visualization is to rule out the presence of an intracranial aneurysm simulating a pituitary or parapituitary neoplasm, DIVA can provide this information. A normal DIVA is shown in Fig. 5-8.

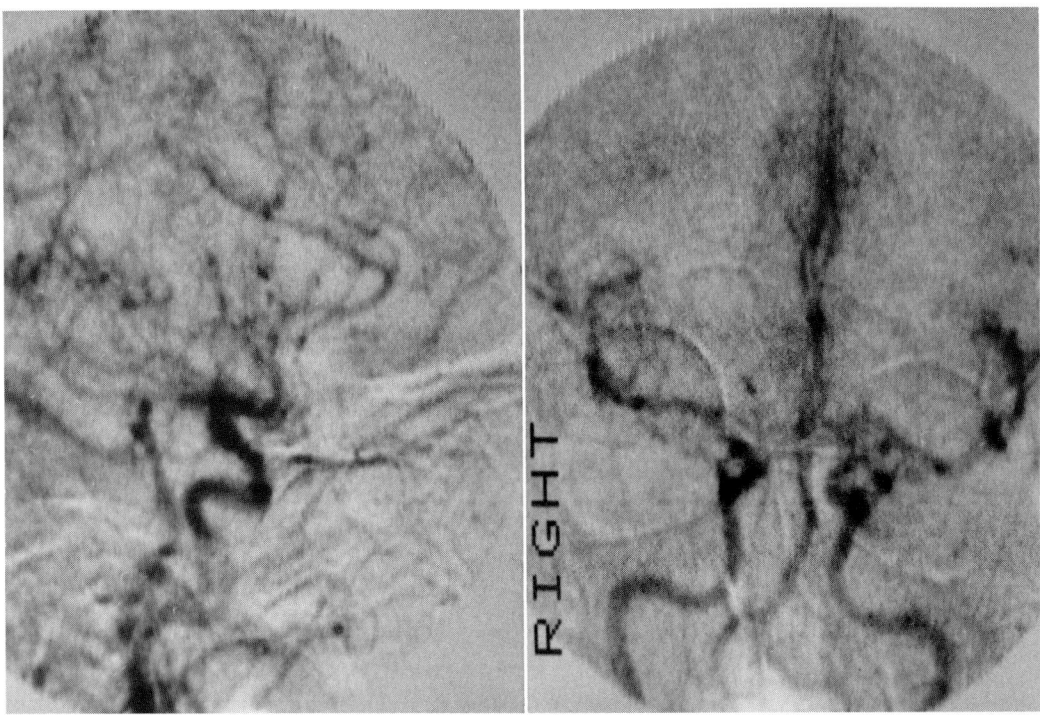

Fig. 5-8. Normal lateral and AP DIVA.

158 *Disorders of the pituitary*

Metrizamide cisternography

Metrizamide cisternography is a special procedure that combines the intrathecal administration of metrizamide (Amipaque) with CT scanning. It is not a routine test and is recommended only in specific situations in which more detailed visualization of the suprasellar or other basilar cisterns is required to illustrate anatomic relationships. Specific clinical situations in which it is often indicated include (1) an ESS in which the CT is not confirmatory, (2) small- to moderate-sized suprasellar lesions (e.g., craniopharyngiomas, optic gliomas, hypothalamic tumors) associated with a normal-sized sella turcica, and (3) cerebrospinal fluid rhinorrhea.

The technique of metrizamide cisternography involves a lumbar puncture using a #22 g needle. After satisfactory placement of the needle tip in the

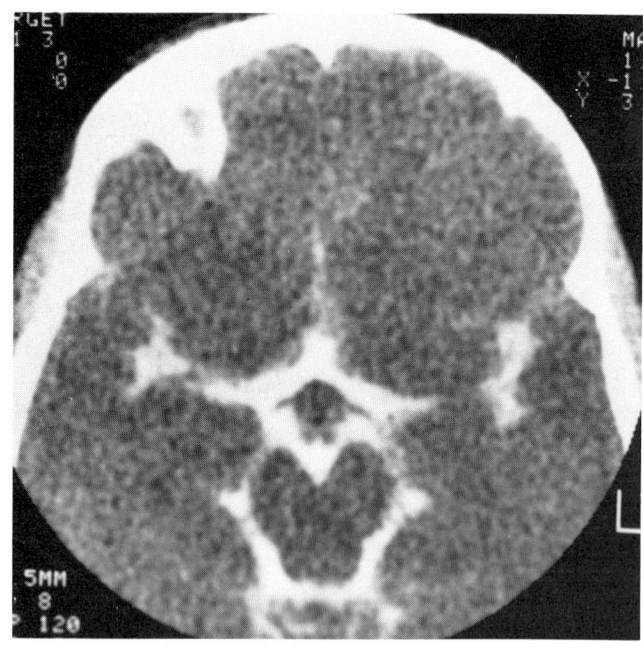

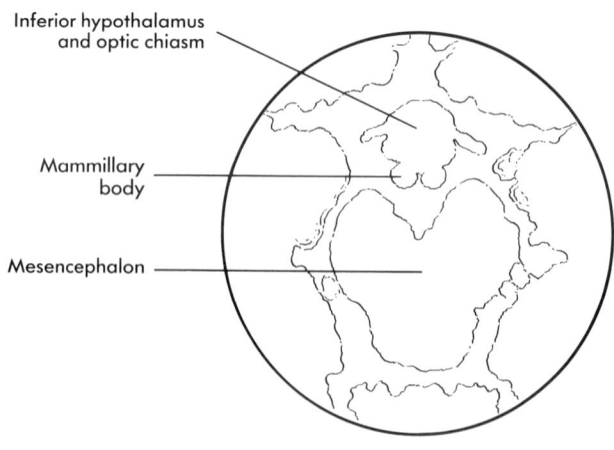

Fig. 5-9. Normal metrizamide cisternogram (axial view). **A,** Section through optic chiasm and mammillary bodies.

subarachnoid space, 5 cc of metrizamide (190 mg/cc) is injected slowly. The contrast media is gravitated into the basilar cisterns by placing the patient in a 60 degree Trendelenberg position for 2 minutes. CT scans are then obtained using serial sections 5 mm thick in both the sagittal and coronal planes. An example of a normal metrizamide cisternogram is shown in Fig. 5-9.

Serious reactions may be associated with metrizamide cisternography and include seizures, encephalopathy, and cortical blindness. These complications are usually dosage related and have been rare in our experience. However, because of the potential severity of these complications, the clinician should use this procedure only when it is believed that the information will have a significant bearing on therapeutic decision making. Additionally, as low a dosage of metrizamide as possible should be administered.

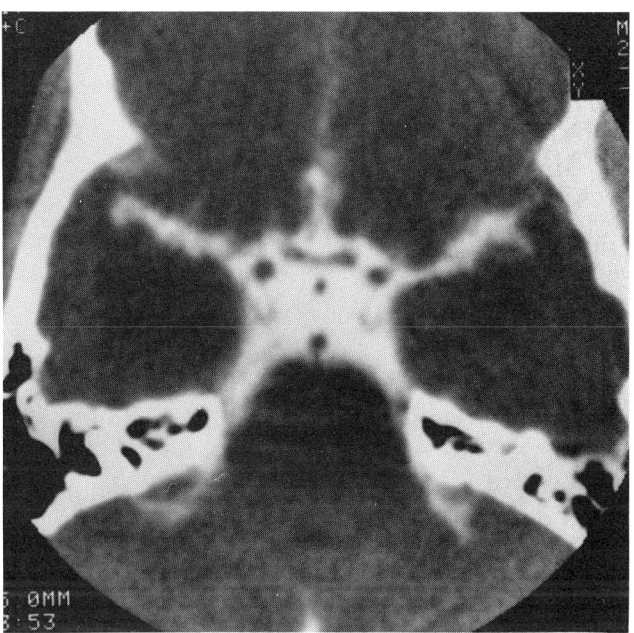

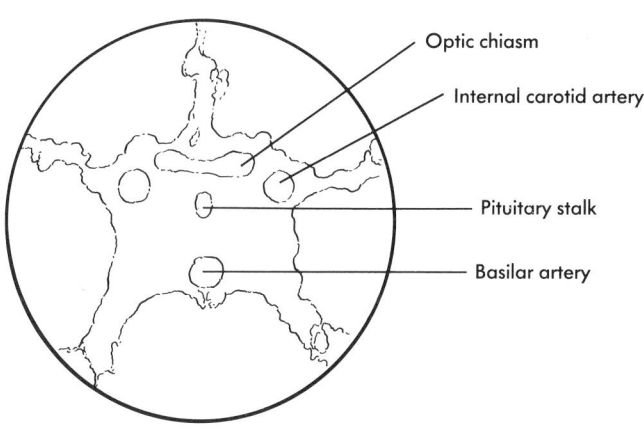

Fig. 5-9, cont'd. B, Section at slightly higher level.

Pneumoencephalography

PEG was used in the past to determine the relationship of a suprasellar mass to the optic nerves, diagnose suprasellar diverticula, and establish the presence of an empty sella. In current practice, high-resolution CT scanning usually provides more precise anatomic information about suprasellar masses and intrasellar masses with suprasellar extension than PEG. The presence of an empty sella and relationship of suprasellar masses to the optic chiasm and/or nerves is better determined by metrizamide cisternography. Consequently, PEG, which is a very painful procedure, is no longer indicated in the evaluation of these patients.

Cavernous sinus venography and petrosal sinus sampling

Cavernous sinus venography and petrosal sinus sampling are procedures used only in special circumstances during the workup of certain pituitary adenomas. Cavernous sinus venography has been used to demonstrate the lateral extension of a pituitary tumor[28] and diagnose the presence of pituitary microadenomas.[32,37] This angiographic procedure will occasionally confirm the presence of cavernous sinus invasion in small- or moderate-sized tumors—information that can have a significant bearing on therapeutic decisions.

The technique of visualizing the cavernous sinuses can be accomplished by retrograde filling of this structure by injecting either the orbital veins or the inferior petrosal sinus. Theron et al[37] believe that injection of the latter provides better visualization of the cavernous and intercavernous sinuses. Fig. 5-10 illustrates variations in the normal patterns of drainage of the inferior petrosal sinuses observed during cavernous sinus venography.

In addition to the injection of contrast media for visualization of the cavernous sinus, catheterization of the inferior petrosal sinuses provides an opportunity to sample the venous blood draining directly out of the pituitary.[11] This technique has been used in patients with Cushing's disease in an effort to demonstrate that the highest levels of adrenocorticotropic hormone (ACTH) are originating in the pituitary—information that would confirm that a pituitary microadenoma rather than an ectopic source is responsible for the elevated ACTH secretion. Differences in the ACTH level between the two petrosal sinuses may aid in determining within which side of the gland the adenoma resides.

Petrosal sinus sampling may theoretically prove useful in patients with hyperprolactinemia who may have a microprolactinoma. In diagnostically difficult cases, significant elevation of prolactin in the petrosal sinus as compared to peripheral blood may lend confirmatory support to the diagnosis of pituitary microadenoma in these cases. However, this supposition needs to be tested in a significant number of patients before coming to any conclusion about its diagnostic value in microprolactinomas.

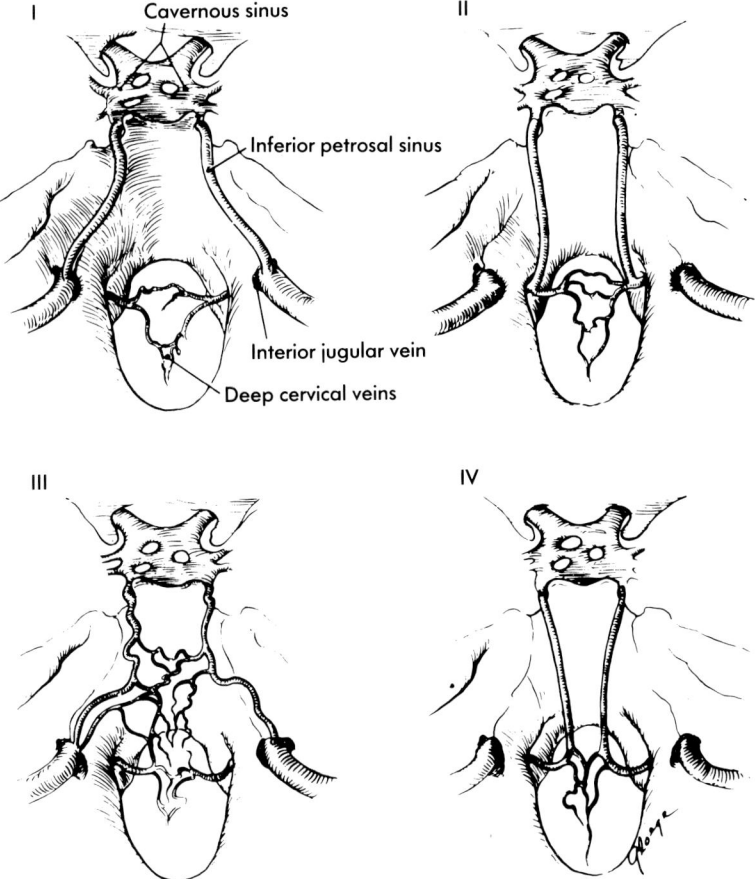

Fig. 5-10. Variations in normal patterns of drainage of inferior petrosal sinuses.
From Rand RW, Hanafee WN: Cavernous sinus venography and stereotaxic cryohypophysectomy, *J Neurosurg* 26:521, 1967.

Magnetic resonance imaging

Magnetic resonance imaging (MRI) is a recent technique of neuroimaging that uses the principles of nuclear magnetic resonance (NMR). At the time of this writing, sufficient experience with MRI has not been accrued to determine the role of this technique in the diagnostic evaluation of patients with pituitary and parasellar tumors. To play a major role, MRI will have to provide important information that currently is beyond the capability of high-resolution CT scanners. The inherent ability of MRI to differentiate small tissue differences makes it potentially advantageous in pituitary gland evaluation. The insensitivity to bone may be an advantage by ignoring the sella and imaging only soft tissue. On the other hand, focal bone changes will not be well visualized.

162 *Disorders of the pituitary*

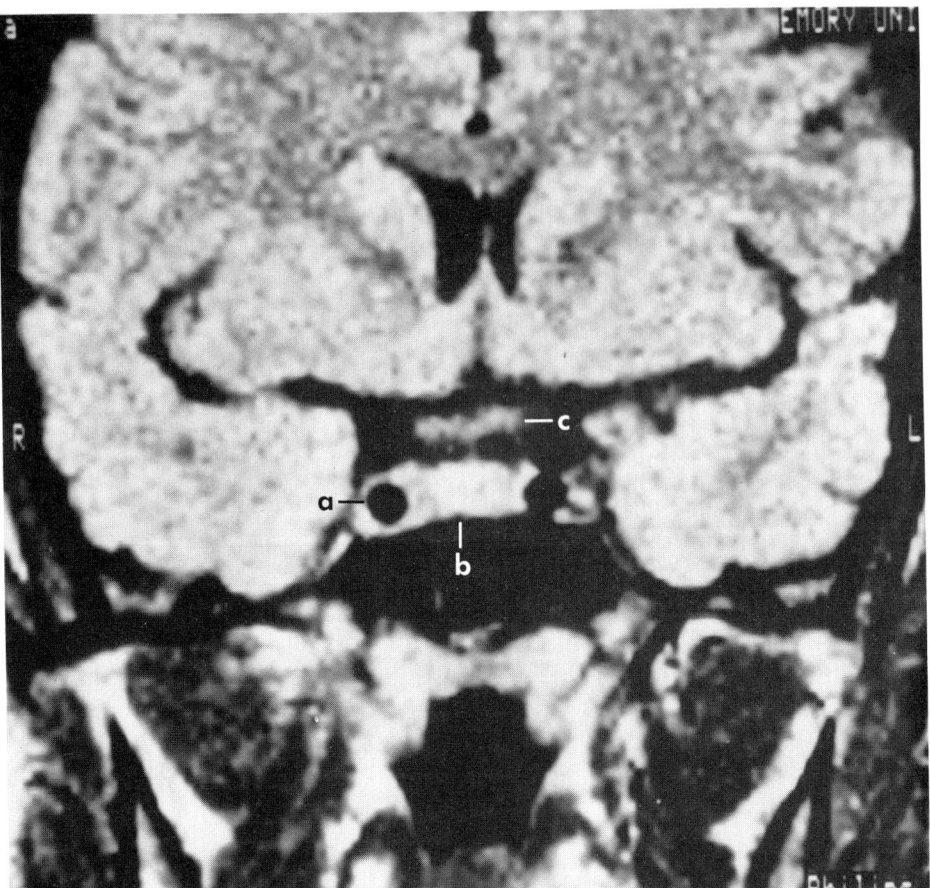

Fig. 5-11. Coronal MRI of normal pituitary gland and related structures. TE 50 ms and TR 1500 ms. First echo shows *a*, internal carotid artery; *b*, pituitary gland; *c*, optic chiasm.

In the coronal plane the pituitary gland most frequently appears rectangular. The lateral margins are defined by the carotid arteries, which appear as circular low-intensity signals in the cavernous sinus and supraclinoid region[17] (Fig. 5-11). The superior margin of the pituitary is outlined by the low signal of cerebrospinal fluid (CSF) within the suprasellar cistern. The low or absent signal of the bony lamina dura and air within the sphenoid sinus form the inferior margin of the gland.

Because CSF is characterized by a long T1 relaxation time and thus a low intensity on partial saturation sequences, there is a sharp delineation of the CSF-pituitary interface.[17] Therefore the exact height and configuration of the pituitary gland can be identified.

RADIOLOGIC FINDINGS IN SPECIFIC PATHOLOGIC DISORDERS

Pituitary adenomas

The major use of plain skull films in the evaluation of pituitary adenomas is to assess the extent of pneumatization of the sphenoid sinus and determine the size and configuration of the sella turcica—important information for the surgeon in planning transsphenoidal surgery. The plain skull film of a patient harboring a pituitary adenoma may be normal or have one of a variety of abnormalities, including erosion of the sellar floor, thinning of the lamina dura, soft tissue densities within the sphenoid sinus, and pathologic calcifications. Some of these abnormalities are illustrated in Fig. 5-12.

The diagnostic accuracy of polytomography in the detection of microadenomas varied among different reports. This was not surprising as investigators were often reporting different sizes and types of tumors, variables that would be expected to affect the success rate of detecting radiologic sella abnormalities. For instance, in 100 proven microadenomas (<10 mm) (and with preoperative serum prolactin levels <200 ng/ml) associated with hyperprolactinemia in our series,[12] sella polytomography was abnormal in only 56%; whereas in a series of 140 microadenomas studied with polytomography by Robertson and Newton[29] abnormalities of the sella were demonstrated in all but three patients. Interestingly, in this latter series, 50% of the patients had a normal sella on plain skull films. It should be emphasized that most investigators have not achieved the high success rate with polytomography reported by Robertson and Newton.

Polytomography is discussed primarily to put this once-important radiologic examination in historic perspective. In recent years, it has been replaced in the diagnostic evaluation of patients with pituitary tumors by the high-resolution CT scanner. Thus polytomography is *no* longer a recommended procedure in these patients.

At first glance, it would appear that CT is the ideal procedure for the diagnosis of pituitary adenomas. The capabilities of high-resolution CT are such that the diagnosis of a macroadenoma (tumors that are >1 cm in greatest diameter) should rarely, if ever, be missed, provided a good quality, properly performed CT scan is obtained.

Based on experience to date, however, problems in diagnosing microadenomas (<1 cm) will occasionally be encountered. There are two aspects to this problem: the "false negative" scan in the patient who has a completely normal CT scan but who subsequently is proven (by surgery) to have a microadenoma and the "false positive" scan in the patient who shows CT abnormalities but who does not have a microadenoma or other abnormality of the pituitary gland on surgical exploration.

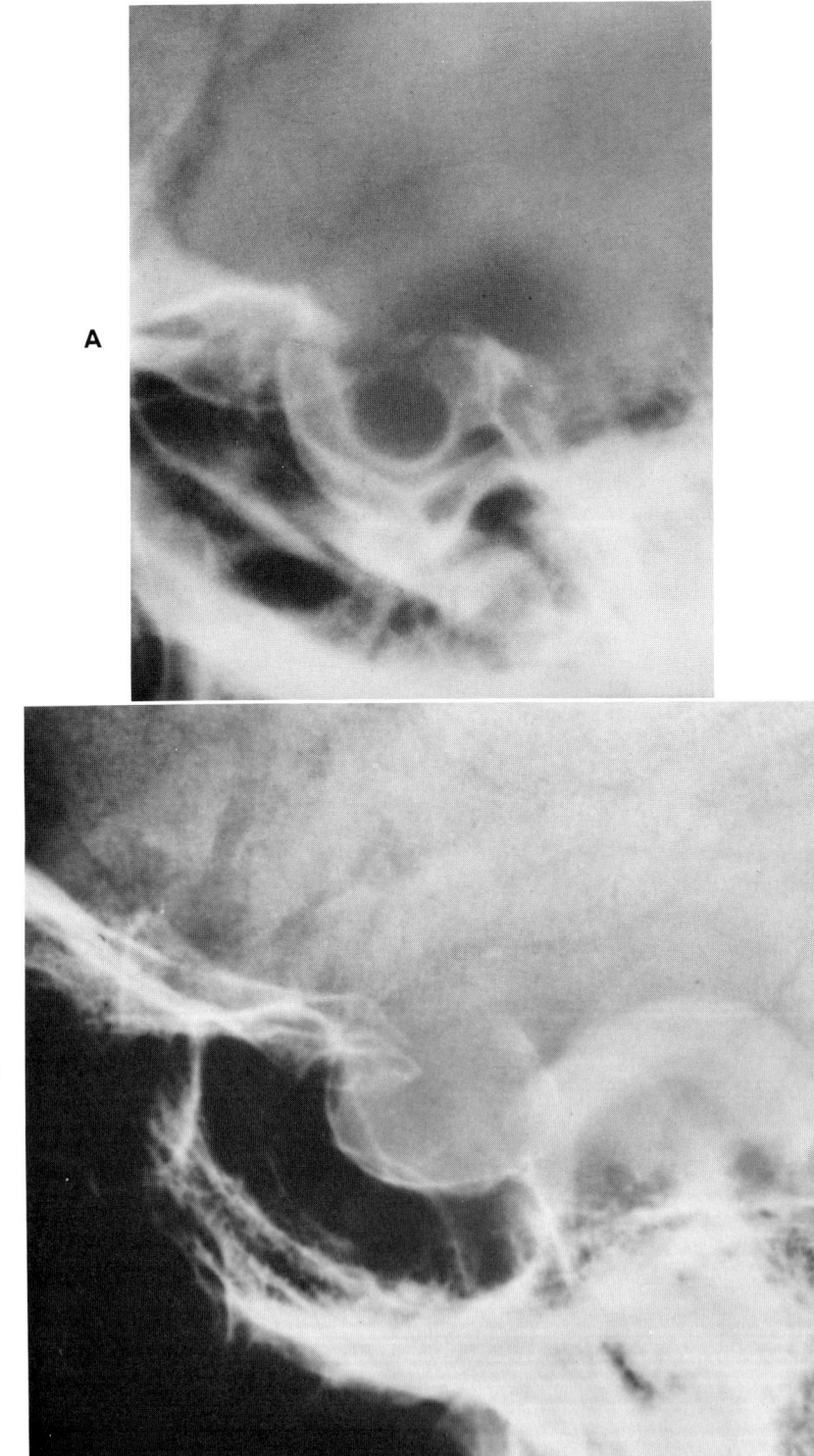

Fig. 5-12. Skull film abnormalities with pituitary tumors. **A,** Double-floored sella with microadenoma. **B,** Enlarged and partly eroded sella resulting from moderate-sized adenoma.

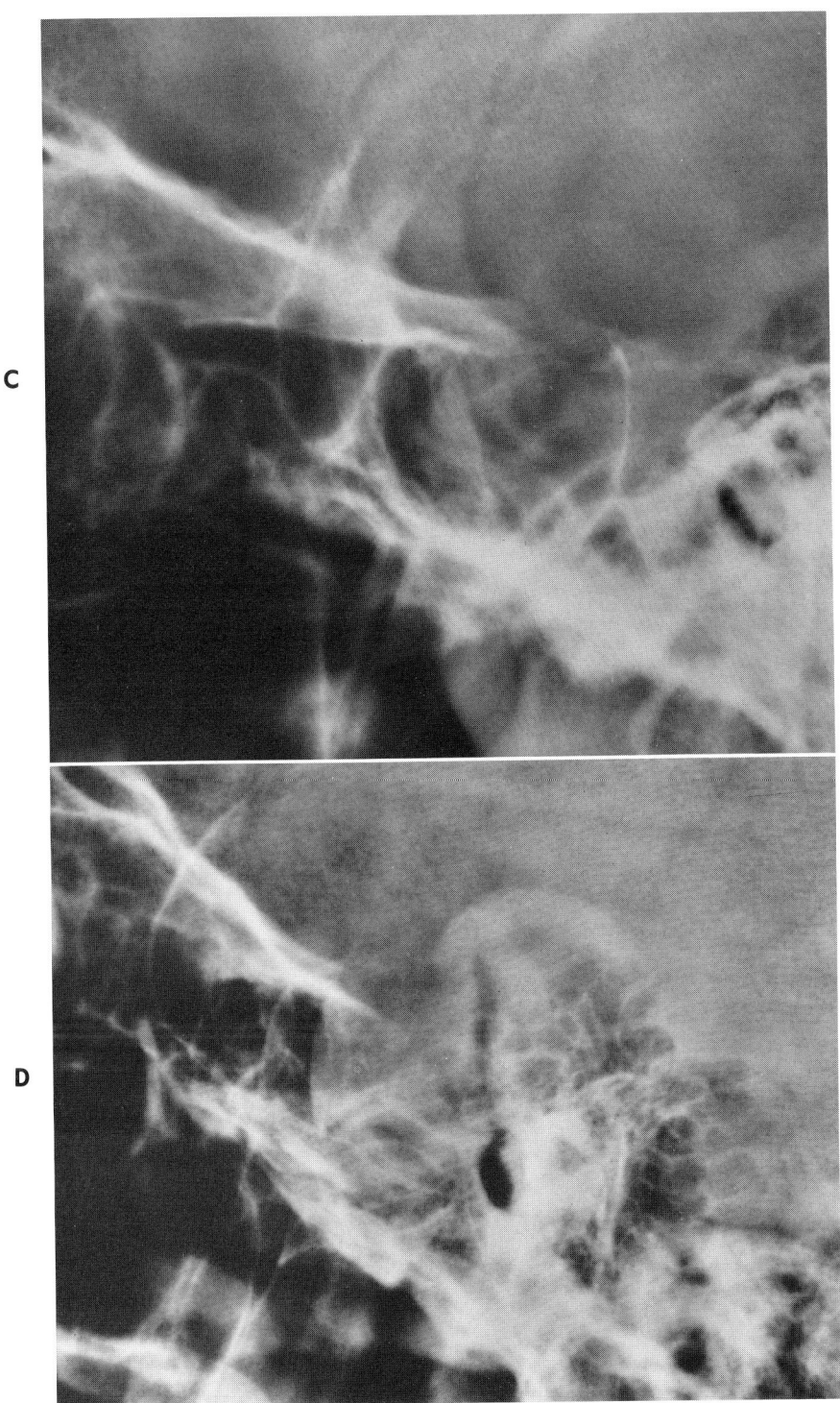

Fig. 5-12, cont'd. C, Marked sellar enlargement and erosion caused by large adenoma. **D,** "Ghost" sella as a result of large invasive adenoma.

166 *Disorders of the pituitary*

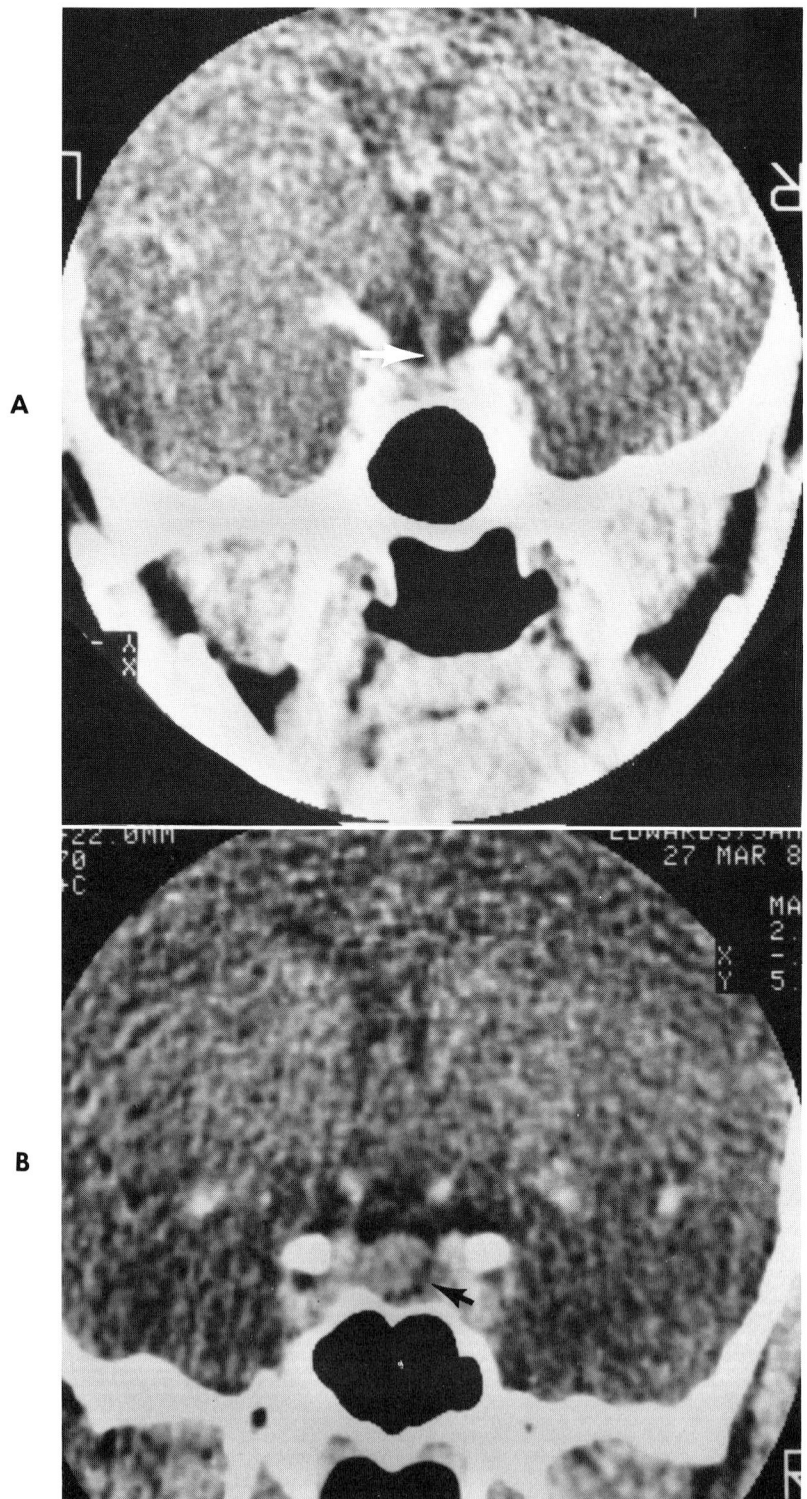

Fig. 5-13. CT abnormalities caused by pituitary adenomas. **A,** Stalk shifted to right (arrow) and gland size at upper limits of normal in patient with surgically proven microadenoma. **B,** Convex diaphragm with intrasellar low-density area (arrow).

Abnormalities produced by pituitary tumors on a high-resolution CT scanner include an increase in size of the pituitary gland, areas of low density within the pituitary gland, calcifications, convexity or elevation of the diaphragm sella, shift of the pituitary stalk, and erosion of the sella floor. Illustrations of CT characteristics of pituitary adenomas are shown in Fig. 5-13.

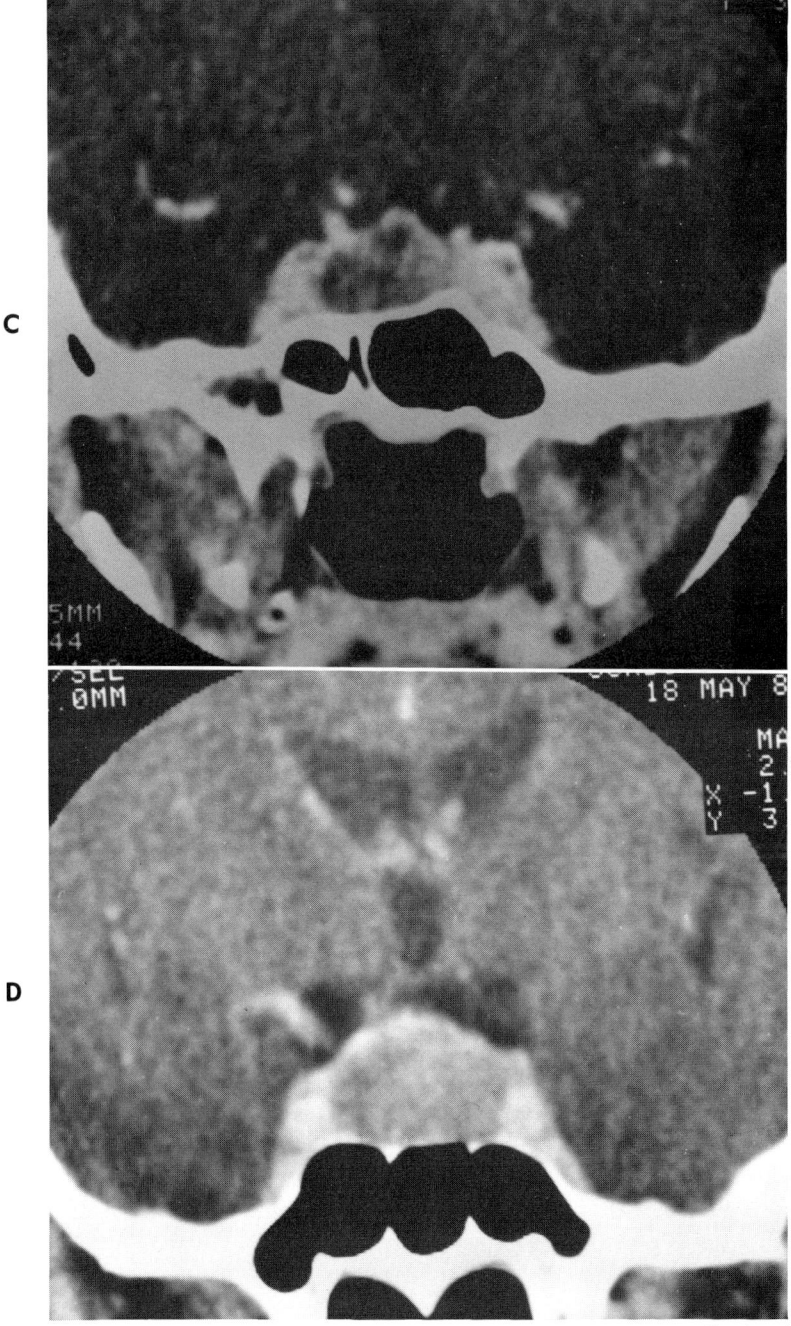

Continued.

Fig. 5-13, cont'd. C and **D**, Moderate-sized tumors.

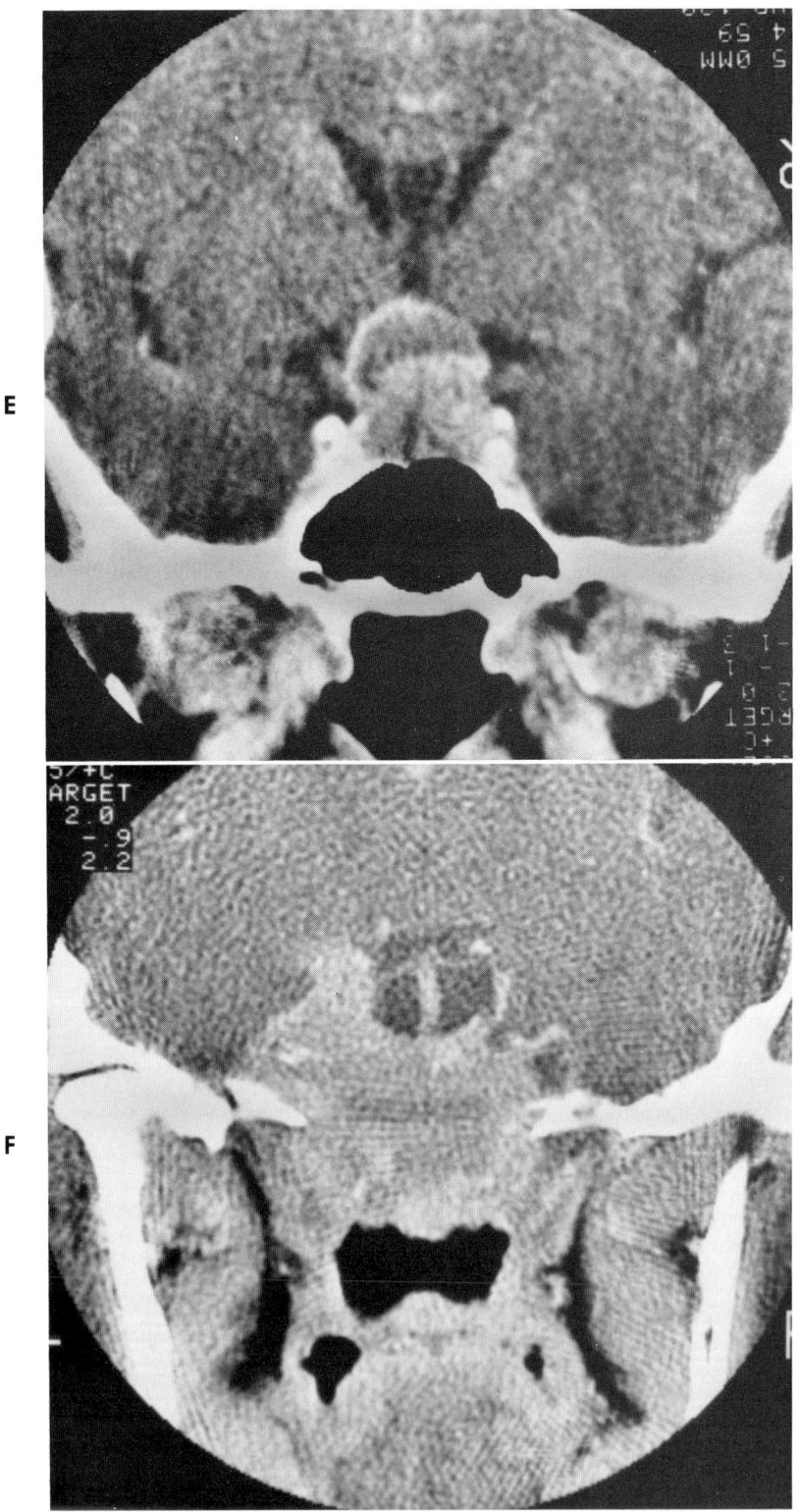

Fig. 5-13, cont'd. E, Significant suprasellar extension with impingement on floor of third ventricle. **F,** Grossly invasive tumor.

A few comments should be made about these abnormalities. Various CT studies suggest that there is considerable variability in the size and shape of the normal gland, especially in women. An early CT study indicated that the height of the normal pituitary is less than 6.7 mm in normal women and less than 5 mm in men.[35] A more recent report by Swartz et al[34] performed on normal, reproductive age, female volunteers found a mean gland height of 7.1 mm, with a standard deviation of 1.1 mm and range of 5.4 to 9.7 mm. Fifty-six percent of the glands were flat or upwardly concave, but 44% were upwardly convex. In this same study, 36% of these normal patients demonstrated focal "defects" of unknown origin. We consider a gland >8 mm in height to be abnormal. Other investigators consider a 7 to 10 mm gland as borderline enlarged and >10 mm definitely abnormal.[13] Although pituitary tumors produce elevation of the diaphragm, an upwardly convex diaphragm can be seen in normal subjects.[34] However, asymmetric protrusion of the diaphragm is unusual in normal subjects.[13] The normal pituitary stalk is invariably midline, and a shift is indicative of a pathologic condition.

The incidence of the "false negative" scan may be as high as 20% to 25% in patients subsequently proven to have microadenomas at surgery. For instance, Davis et al[9] retrospectively correlated CT and surgical findings in 51 patients seen at our institution with the preoperative diagnosis of prolactin-secreting pituitary microadenomas. The scans were evaluated for gland height, presence of focal lesions, sellar floor erosion, displacement of the infundibulum, and shape of the diaphragm sella. Thirty-nine of the patients had microadenomas at surgery, and 12 did not (nine hyperplasia, two normal, and one benign cyst). A laterally placed pituitary infundibulum was present only in patients with microadenomas but was present in just five of the 39. All other criteria evaluated were present in patients with microadenomas and in some who had no tumor. The presence of a focal lesion was a statistically significant indicator for microadenoma as 19 of the 21 cases with focal lesions had proven microadenomas. CT scan was the primary radiologic study in 100 cases of Cushing's disease studied by Boggan, Tyrrell, and Wilson.[3] In their series, 30% of the patients showed no radiologic abnormalities.

The incidence of the "false positive" CT scan is difficult to estimate. As mentioned previously, Swartz et al[34] found that 44% of normal subjects had a clearly elevated diaphragm sella and 36% had focal defects within the intrasellar contents (Fig. 5-14). In assessing the data of Swartz et al, one has to take into account the fact that approximately 10% (range from 8% to 15%) of all adults are estimated to have incidental pituitary microadenomas.*

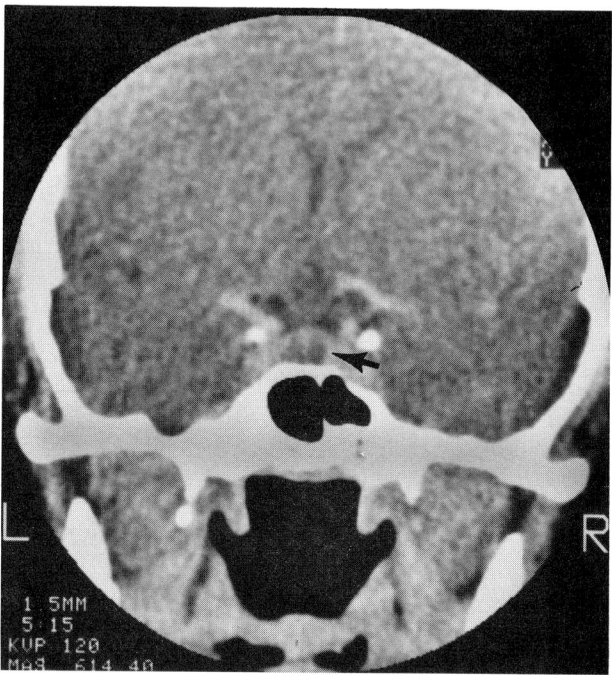

Fig. 5-14. False positive CT scan. Elevated diaphragm and low-density area (arrow). Careful surgical exploration revealed no abnormality.

In addition to confirming the presence of a pituitary tumor, the CT scan also provides an accurate depiction of the size, shape, and extent of the lesion—important data that helps the physician determine the most appropriate therapeutic option to recommend to the patient. Despite the high degree of resolution provided, CT scans have not been able to reliably determine invasion of the cavernous sinus by pituitary adenomas. This type of information, which may influence therapeutic decision making, may be provided by cavernous sinus venography (Fig. 5-15). However, when the sinus is grossly involved by tumor, this fact can be documented on the CT scan by determining the position of the intracavernous portion of the internal carotid artery in relation to the tumor on the contrast-enhanced scan. An example of an adenoma that showed gross involvement of the cavernous sinuses with tumor encirclement of the internal carotid is shown in Fig. 9-1.

---

*See references 6,8,16,18,23,27, and 33.

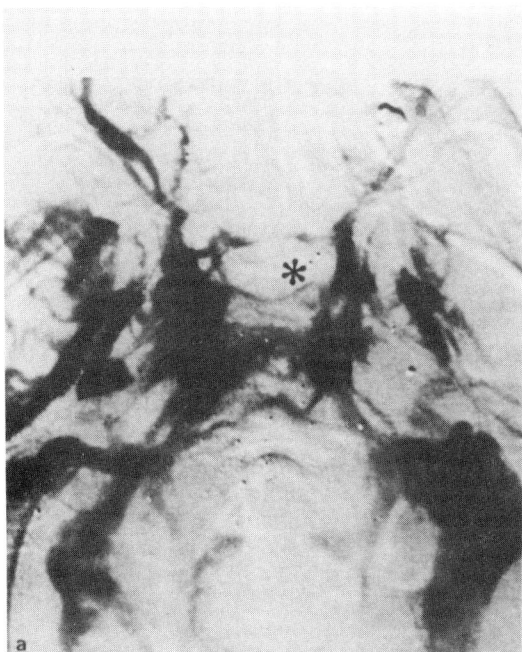

Fig. 5-15. Abnormal cavernous sinus venogram. Adenoma (*) compresses medial aspect of cavernous sinus.

From Rand RW, Hanafee WN: Cavernous sinus venography and stereotaxic cryohypophysectomy, *J Neurosurg* 26:521, 1967.

Currently, the only recommended use of angiography in the radiologic evaluation of a pituitary tumor is to exclude the possibility that the "pituitary tumor" being investigated is not an aneurysm with intrasellar extension. The clinical situation in which an aneurysm might masquerade as a pituitary tumor is in an adult with a nonfunctional tumor causing mass effects. The one exception in the hyperfunctional tumor group is a patient with a pituitary tumor with moderate hyperprolactinemia (i.e., serum prolactin, 25 to 150 ng/ml). Although this finding could be presumed to be a result of a prolactinoma, it is just as likely to be found in patients with a "pseudoprolactinoma," in which case the elevated prolactin values are a result of stalk compression, which can result from any mass lesion, including an aneurysm. Abnormalities that may be seen on angiography in patients with large pituitary tumors include lateral displacement of the intracavernous carotid arteries on the AP films and opening of the carotid siphon in patients with suprasellar extension. A vascular blush is rarely seen[19] and should alert one to the possible presence of a meningioma.

From a practical standpoint, DIVA will provide adequate intracranial arterial visualization to exclude the diagnosis of an intrasellar aneurysm and thus has virtually replaced conventional cerebral angiography in the diagnostic workup of patients with pituitary tumors.

The neuroradiologic evaluation of patients with suspected pituitary tumors is not a fixed, static process. With continued refinement in imaging techniques, the diagnostic protocol continues to be revised and updated. Yet to be determined but almost certain to play a significant role in the diagnostic workup, is MRI; its role should become clearer in the next few years.

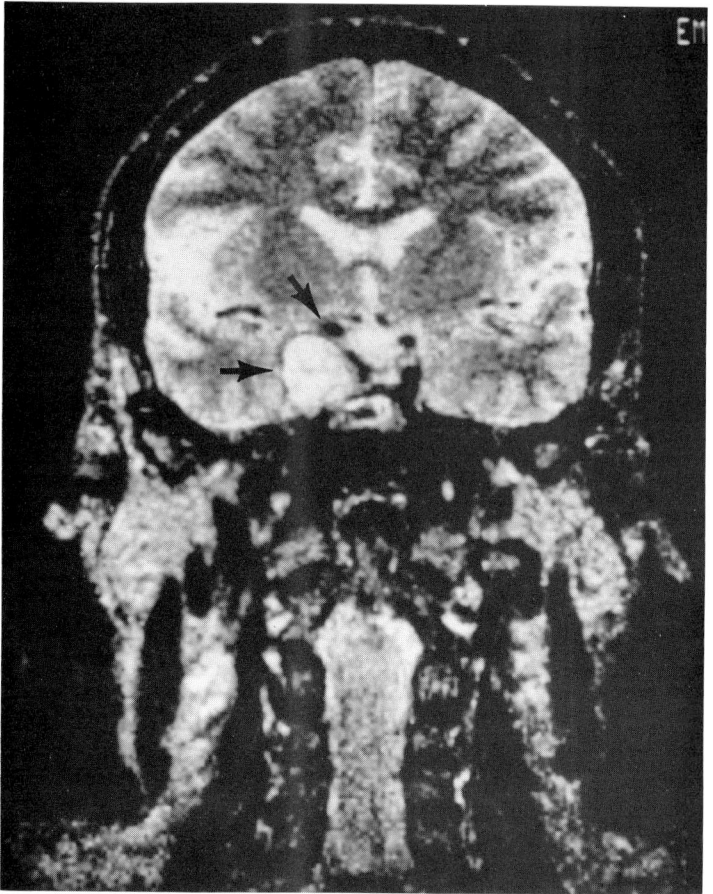

Fig. 5-16. Coronal MRI of recurrent pituitary tumor with extension into middle fossa. TE 50 ms and TR 1750 ms. Second echo demonstrates mass with long T2 (lower arrow) situated lateral to internal carotid artery (upper arrow).

The two parameters that determine an abnormal pituitary gland on MRI are size and configuration and the tissue characterization.[17] The normal pituitary gland has a signal intensity on the partial saturation sequence approximately equal to that of the brainstem and exhibits no increase in T2 values on T2 weighted sequences. Pituitary adenomas are seen on MRI as hypointense (longer T1 value) or hyperintense (shorter T1 value) on the partial saturation sequences and as an increased intensity (increased T2 value) on the spin-echo T2 weighted sequences[17] (Fig. 5-16).

One area in which MRI may prove helpful is in determining whether or not the cavernous sinus is invaded by tumor. Although gross invasion can be detected with coronal CT, at present the instrument will not determine minimal invasion; perhaps MRI can make this important diagnosis. It also appears that MRI may be able to detect some of the small microadenomas, many of which are currently missed on high-resolution CT scanners (Fig. 5-17).

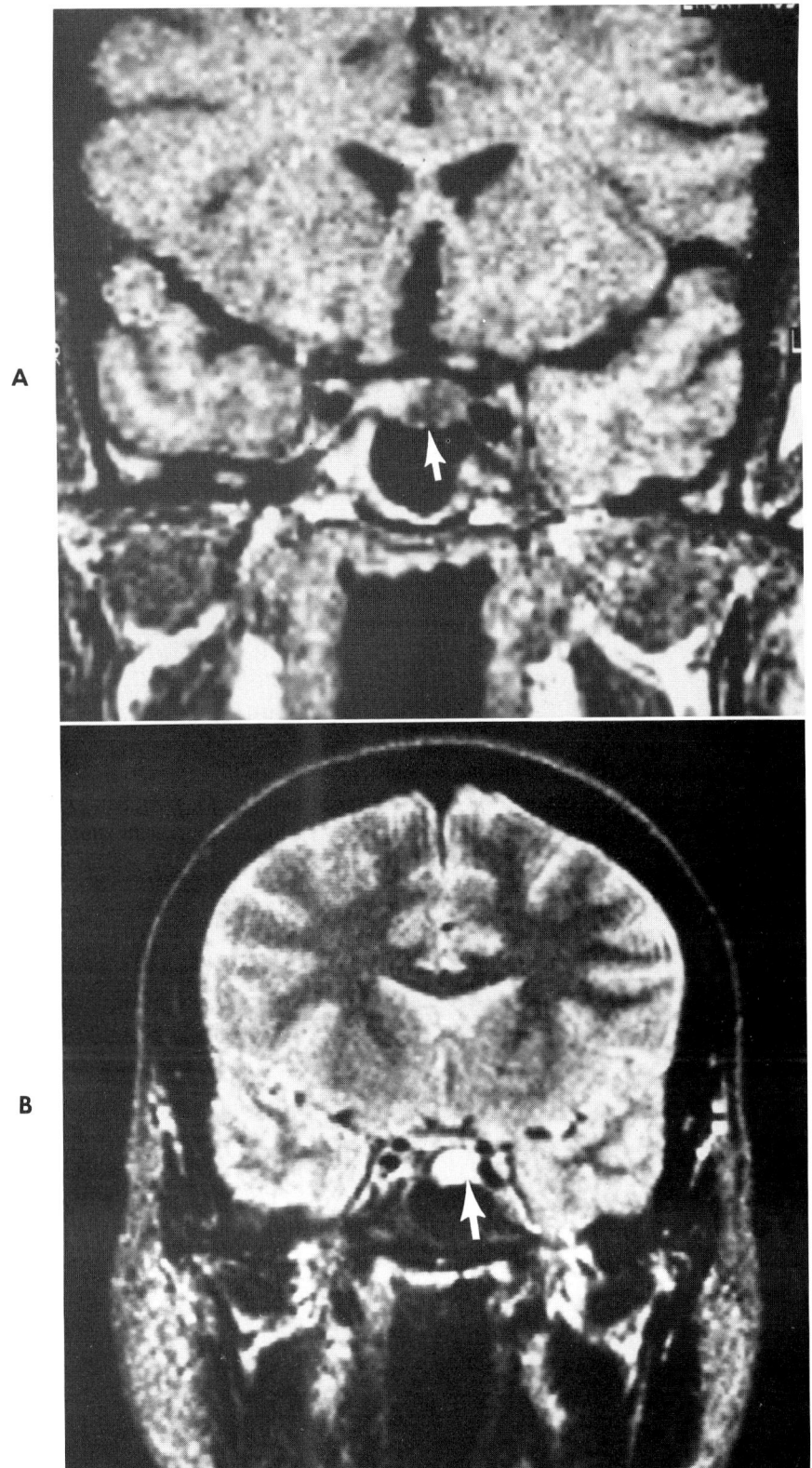

Fig. 5-17. Coronal MRI of microprolactinoma in patient that had negative coronal CT scan. **A,** TE 30 ms and TR 500 ms. First echo shows long T1 on left side of gland (arrow). **B,** TE 50 ms and TR 2000 ms. Second echo shows area of increased T2 on left side of sella (arrow). Note how different echos change tissue intensities.

In our opinion, all patients with suspected pituitary tumors should have a lateral skull x-ray examination and a high-resolution coronal CT scan made both with and without contrast enhancement. These studies are the only neuroradiologic procedures indicated in patients with acromegaly; Cushing's disease, in whom endocrine tests implicate the pituitary as the source of the elevated ACTH; and the amenorrhea-galactorrhea syndrome, in whom the level of serum prolactin is >150 ng/ml.

Additionally, DIVA is indicated in patients with nonfunctional pituitary tumors causing mass effects and pituitary tumors associated with hyperprolactinemia, in whom levels of serum prolactin are <150 ng/ml when the possibility of the lesion being an intracranial aneurysm exists.

The use of other tests requires individualized decision making. For instance, in patients with Cushing's disease, in whom the CT is negative and in whom endocrine testing has left some uncertainty, petrosal sinus blood sampling of ACTH levels may serve to confirm the pituitary as the site of the microadenoma. Also in a patient in whom cavernous sinus invasion is suspected, cavernous sinus venography may serve to confirm the sinus invasion, thus having an influence on choice of therapy.

Craniopharyngiomas

Plain skull films are helpful in the diagnosis of craniopharyngiomas. It is estimated that over 60% of adults and 90% of children with craniopharyngiomas have abnormal skull films, with calcification in the tumor being the most prominent and common abnormality (Fig 5-18). Other radiologic abnormalities (which may include enlargement and/or erosion of the sella turcica, split sutures, digital skull markings, and enlargement of the optic foramen) are seen in about half the patients. The presence or absence of sellar enlargement may influence the planned surgical approach. The sellar erosive changes may be the only abnormality seen on either plain radiography or tomography. These consist of erosion and loss of bony substance of the tuberculum sella, planum sphenoidale, or dorsum sella.[24]

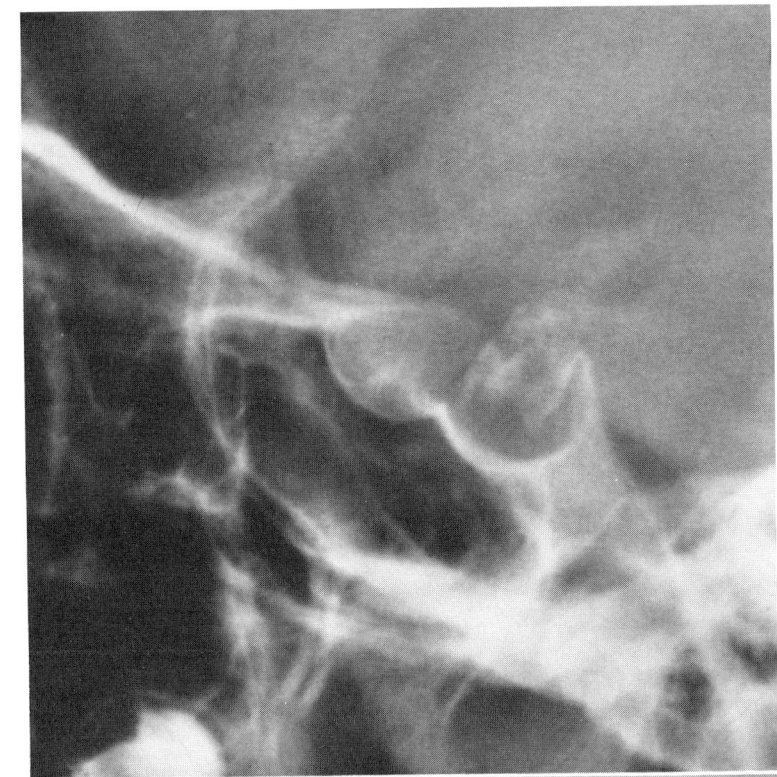

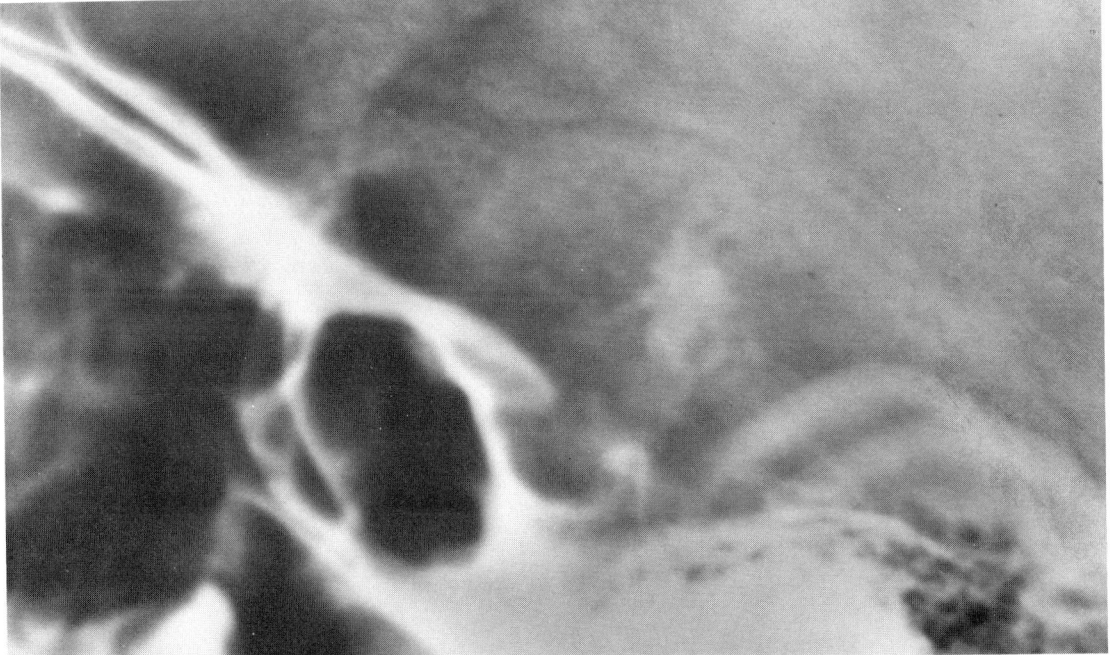

Fig. 5-18. Skull film—craniopharyngioma. **A,** Intrasellar calcification with enlargement of chiasmatic sulcus resembling J-shaped sella. **B,** Suprasellar calcification resulting from craniopharyngioma.

The CT scan is currently the definitive neuroradiologic study in the diagnostic workup of a craniopharyngioma. Although it can be expected to have nearly a 100% sensitivity, specificity will be lower as a craniopharyngioma cannot always be differentiated from other suprasellar masses by CT. CT provides valuable information regarding the extent of both the solid and cystic portions of the tumor and its anatomic relationship to adjacent normal structures. Also alterations in the sella and surrounding bony structures, size and configuration of the ventricles, and the presence and extent of calcification can be determined with CT. Examples of these CT abnormalities in craniopharyngiomas are shown in Fig. 5-19.

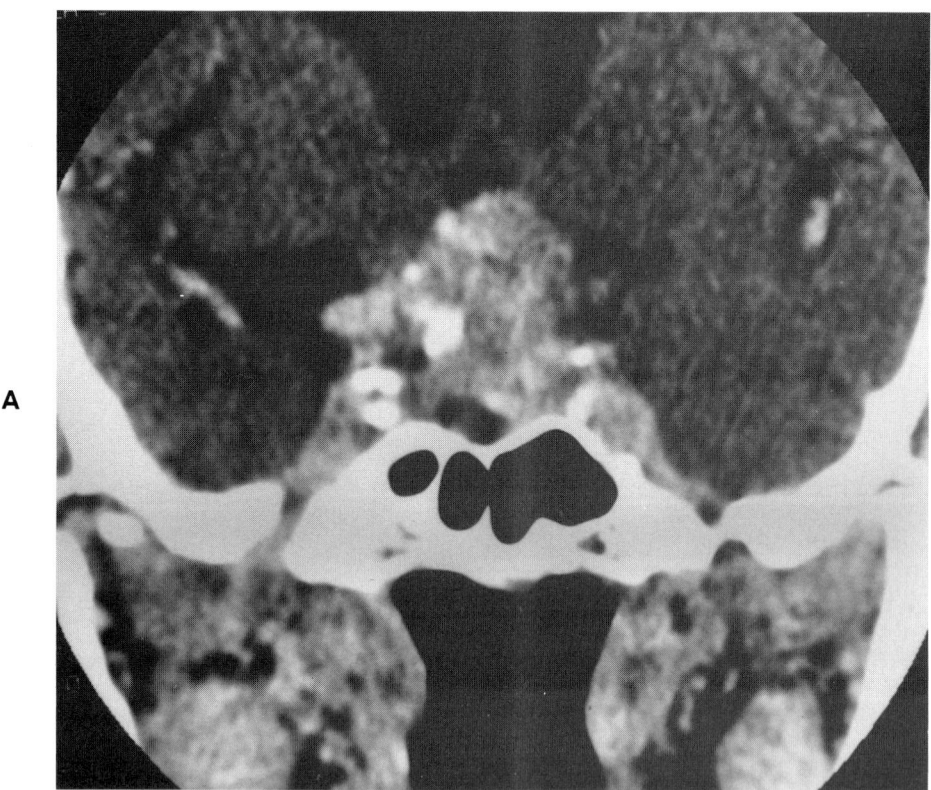

Fig. 5-19. CT—craniopharyngioma. **A,** Coronal enhanced CT scan showing large enhancing and calcified suprasellar mass. **B,** Axial enhanced CT showing enhancing suprasellar mass (arrow) invading third ventricle.

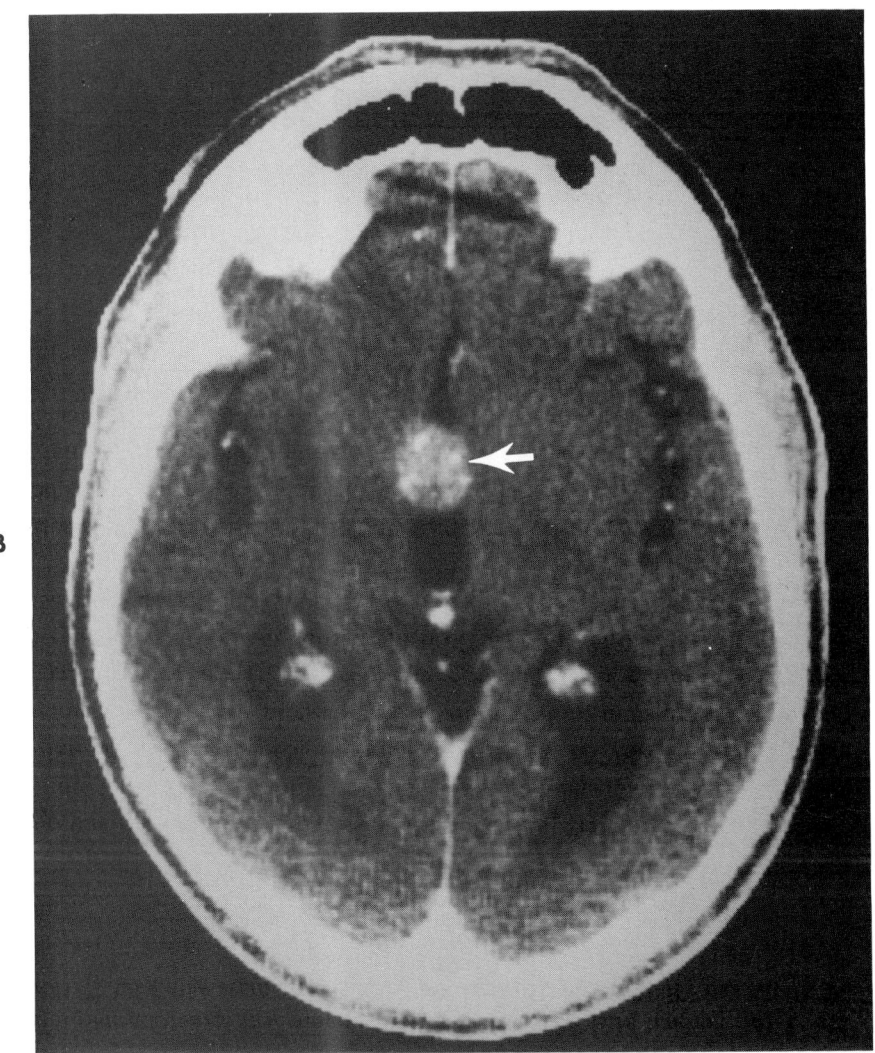

Fig. 5-19, cont'd. For legend see opposite page.

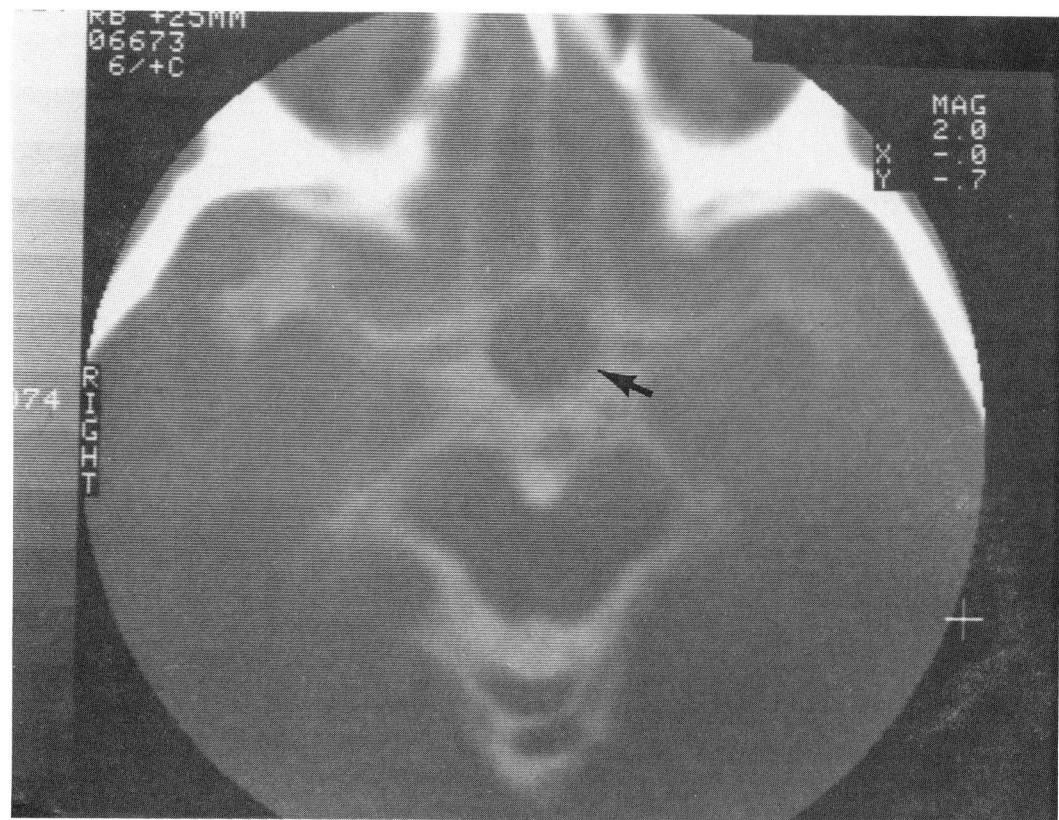

Fig. 5-20. Metrizamide cisternogram—craniopharyngioma. Axial CT slice through suprasellar cistern with metrizamide outlining suprasellar mass (arrow).

Metrizamide cisternography is not a routine diagnostic procedure in patients with a suspected craniopharyngioma but rather is reserved for those cases with clinical and/or radiologic evidence of either a suprasellar or parasellar lesion, in which a high-resolution CT scan does not clearly define the lesion (particularly the presence of an intrasellar component), its extent, and its relationship to the optic chiasm. An example of a case is shown in Fig. 5-20.

Although not a routine procedure, conventional cerebral angiography may be performed in patients with suprasellar lesions if there is any doubt about the pathologic nature from a review of the skull films and CT scan and if determination of the degree of vascularity of the tumor is felt to be necessary. Cerebral angiography will frequently demonstrate abnormalities such as stretched or displaced vessels, but one rarely visualizes neovascularity or a tumor blush.[1,24]

In our opinion, DIVA does not provide diagnostic quality imaging in these lesions and thus lacks the diagnostic accuracy to merit recommendation. However, if the angiogram is performed to differentiate a suprasellar tumor from an intracranial aneurysm, DIVA will suffice and spare the patient an arterial injection.

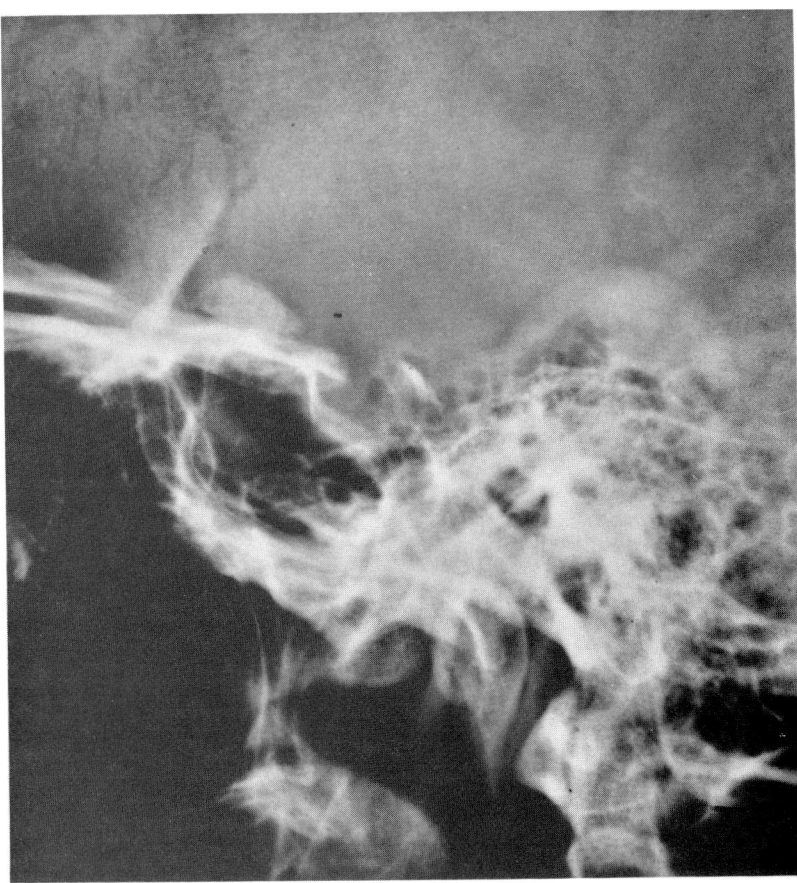

Fig. 5-21. Skull film—meningioma. Lateral skull film shows abnormal calcification over tuberculum sella in patient with meningioma.

Meningiomas

Plain skull film findings that are highly suggestive of a meningioma include the following: (1) well-defined areas of speckled calcification (resulting from calcified psammoma bodies) [Occasionally, a meningioma will be densely calcified.]; (2) enlargement of calvarial grooves of the meningeal arteries providing blood to the tumor; and (3) reactive hyperostosis of the tuberculum sella, planum sphenoidale, or sphenoid ridge (Fig. 5-21). More rarely, meningiomas cause only bony destruction.

180 *Disorders of the pituitary*

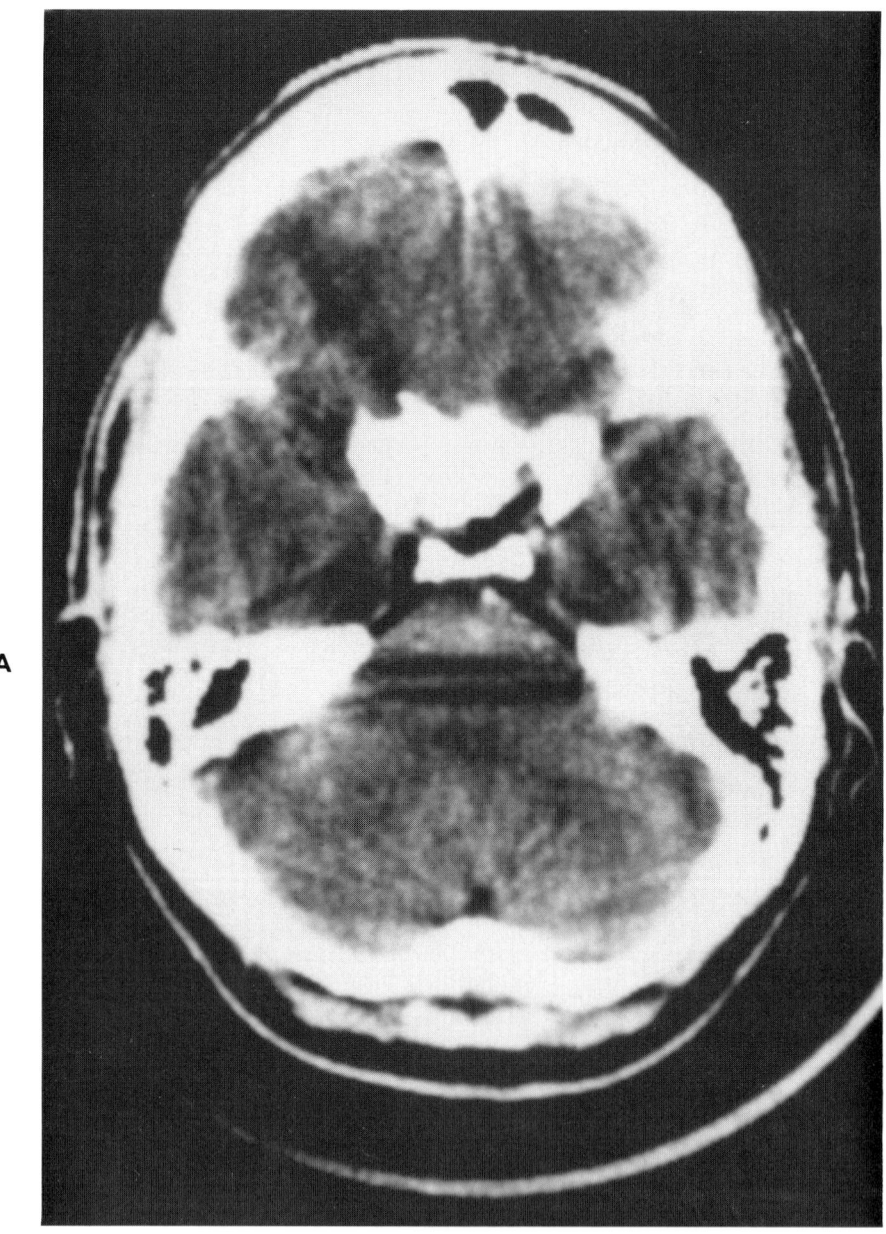

Fig. 5-22. CT—meningioma. **A,** Axial enhanced CT reveals densely enhancing mass in region of tuberculum sella. **B,** Higher cut shows extension of tumor into suprasellar region. This is same patient shown in Fig. 5-21.

The CT appearance of a meningioma is quite characteristic and diagnostic in over 95% of cases, making CT the neurodiagnostic procedure of choice (Fig. 5-22). The bony changes associated with meningiomas such as invasion or hyperostosis are well seen with CT. On a noncontrasted CT, the meningioma will frequently be visible as an area of increased density, occasionally with scattered focal areas of calcification. In many cases, meningiomas may be isodense with brain and rarely may be cystic. After the infusion of contrast, there is typically a marked homogenous enhancement of the tumor. The amount of edema sur-

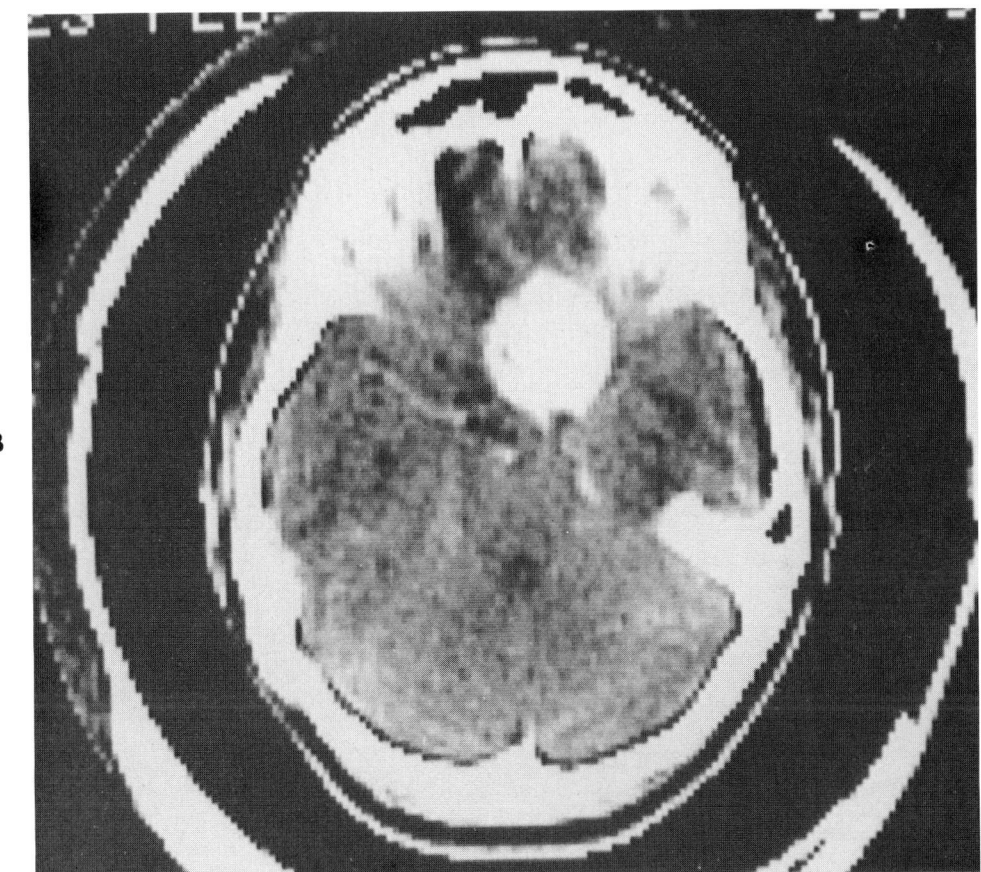

Fig. 5-22, cont'd. For legend see opposite page.

rounding a meningioma is variable. There may be little or no edema, whereas in some cases there is massive edema, producing significant shifts of intracranial structures.

Although the presence of a meningioma can usually be determined by the typical location and CT appearance, many surgeons desire an angiogram to evaluate both the vascular supply and involvement of major vessels by the tumor. Meningiomas typically derive their vascular supply from meningeal vessels and have a characteristic tumor blush that remains throughout the venous phase of the arteriogram (Fig. 5-23). Parasellar meningiomas are frequently supplied by the small meningeal vessels that arise from the cavernous portion of the carotid artery. The meningohypophysial trunk may be demonstrably enlarged on the angiogram. Depending on the location of the tumor, the carotid siphon may be either opened or closed, and the supraclinoid artery may be displaced either medially or laterally.

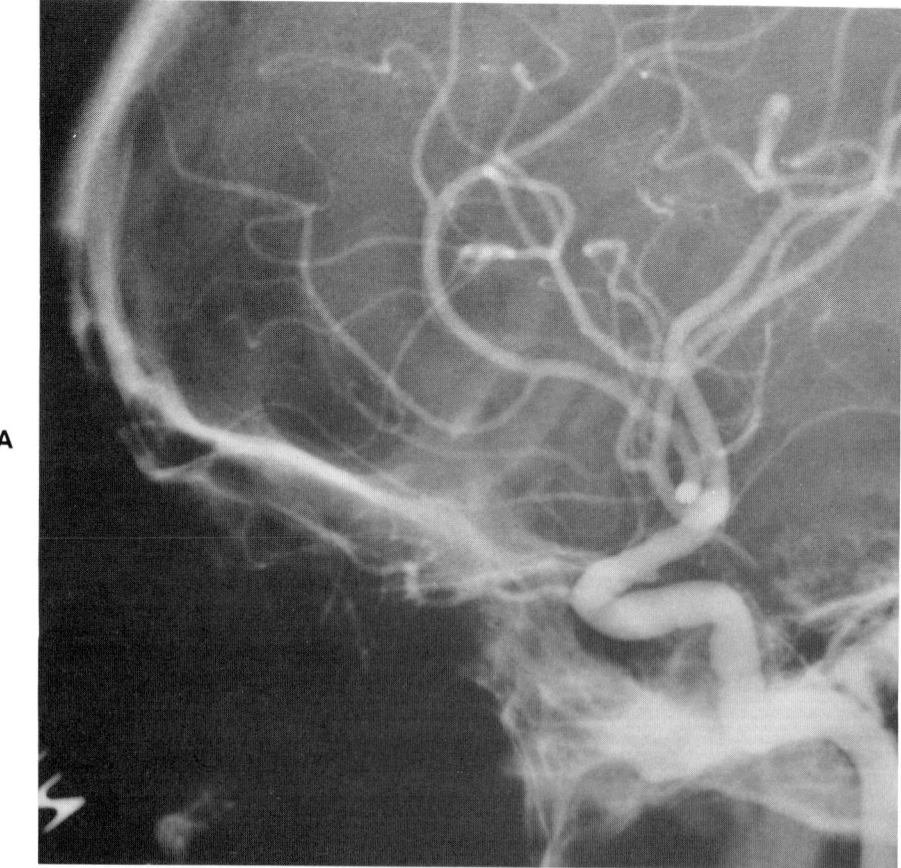

Fig. 5-23. Angiogram—meningioma. **A,** Arterial phase of lateral internal carotid injection shows suprasellar carotid displaced posteriorly. **B,** Venous phase of external carotid injection illustrates tumor blush.

DIVA is a useful method for determining the preoperative extent and vascularity of meningiomas.[25] It is an outstanding technique for assessing the patency of intracranial venous sinuses. Meningiomas fed primarily by the external carotid artery are not visualized as well by DIVA as by selective external carotid artery catheterization.[25] However, CT combined with DIVA will provide the surgeon with all necessary preoperative information in the majority of meningiomas.

Metrizamide cisternography would rarely be of value in the neuroradiologic evaluation of a meningioma.

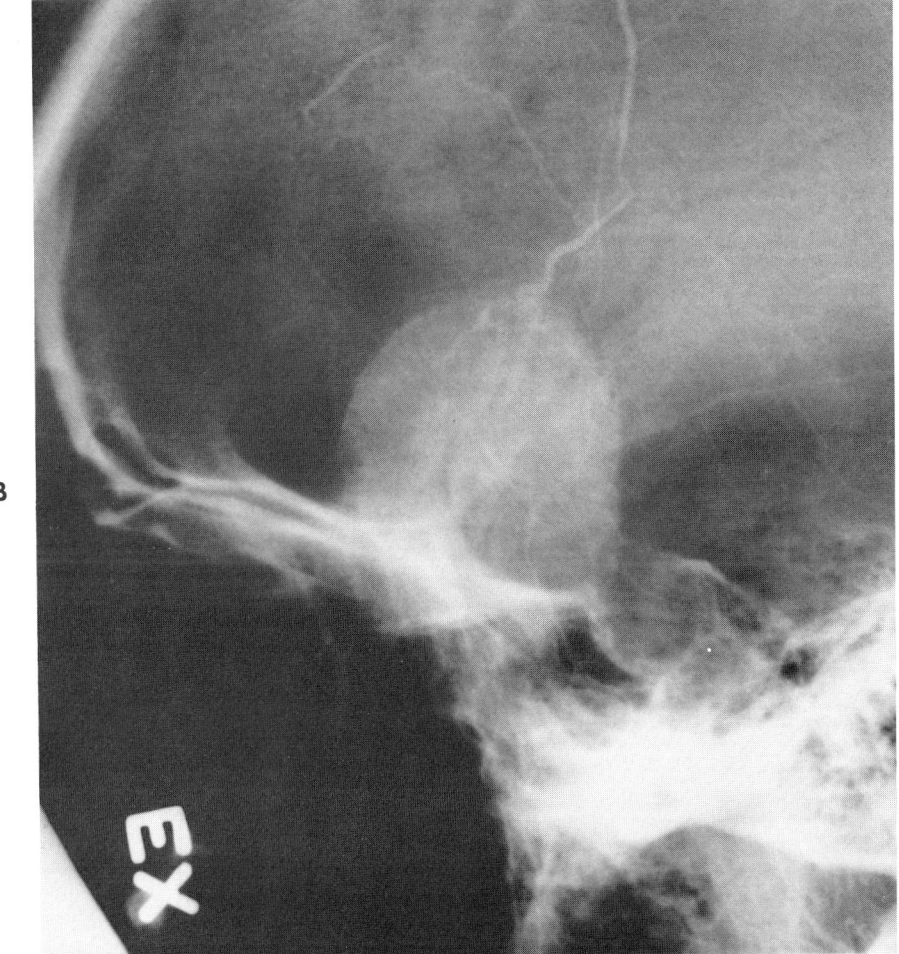

Fig 5-23, cont'd. For legend see opposite page.

184 *Disorders of the pituitary*

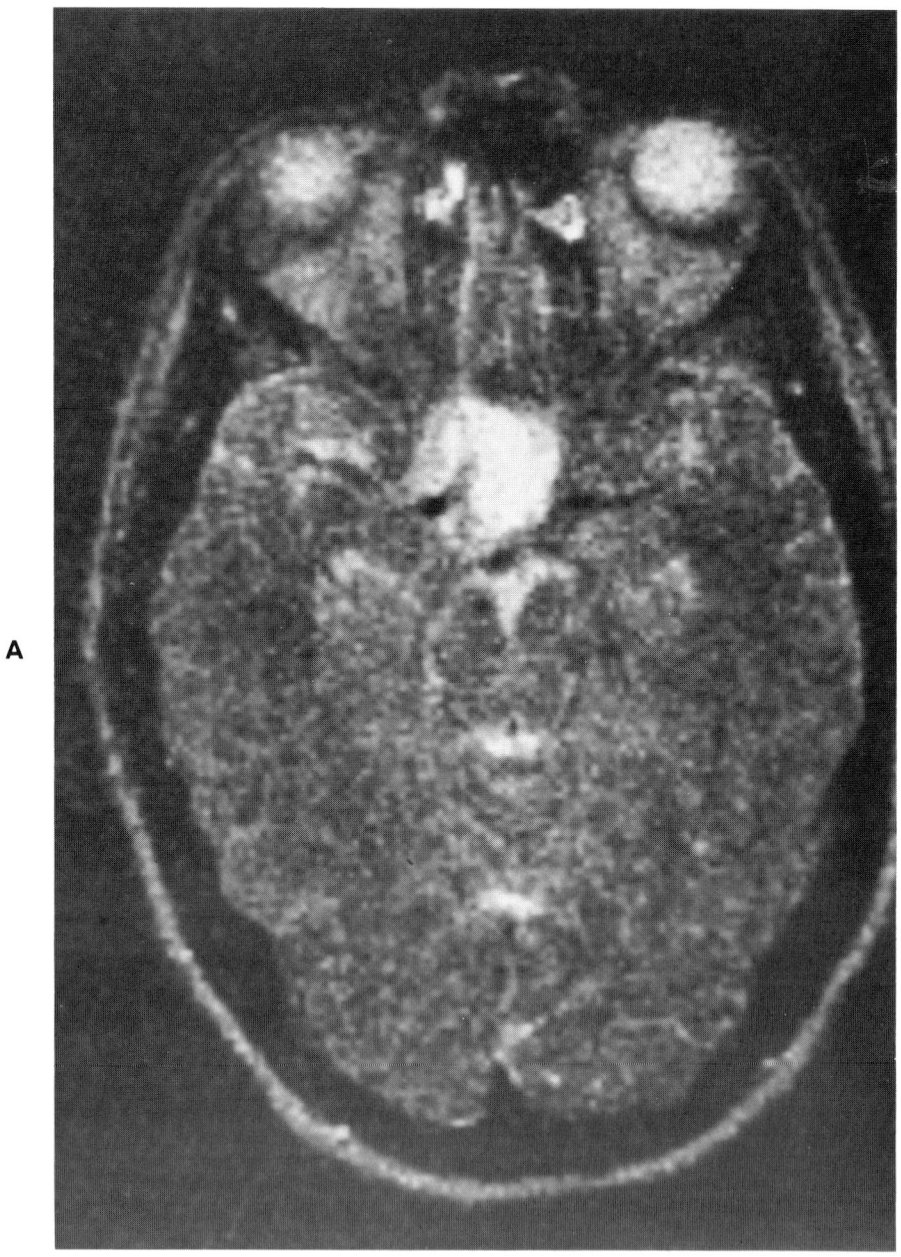

Fig. 5-24. MRI-hypothalamic glioma. **A,** Axial MRI. TE 50 ms and TR 500 ms. Fourth echo shows area of long T2 involving hypothalamus and suprasellar region.

Hypothalamic and optic gliomas

Plain skull films will either be negative or show subtle bony erosive changes in the dorsum sella, tuberculum, or anterior clinoid. Optic gliomas will usually produce enlargement of the ipsilateral optic canal that will be apparent on plain films or tomography. The latter is no longer indicated in the evaluation of these disorders, since CT is a superior test with less radiation.

CT will reveal a suprasellar mass that enhances with contrast. The area of abnormal tissue characterization seen on MRI shows the pathological condition and its relationship to surrounding structures in various planes (Fig. 5-24). Either of these lesions may produce hydrocephalus by obliterating the third ventricle.

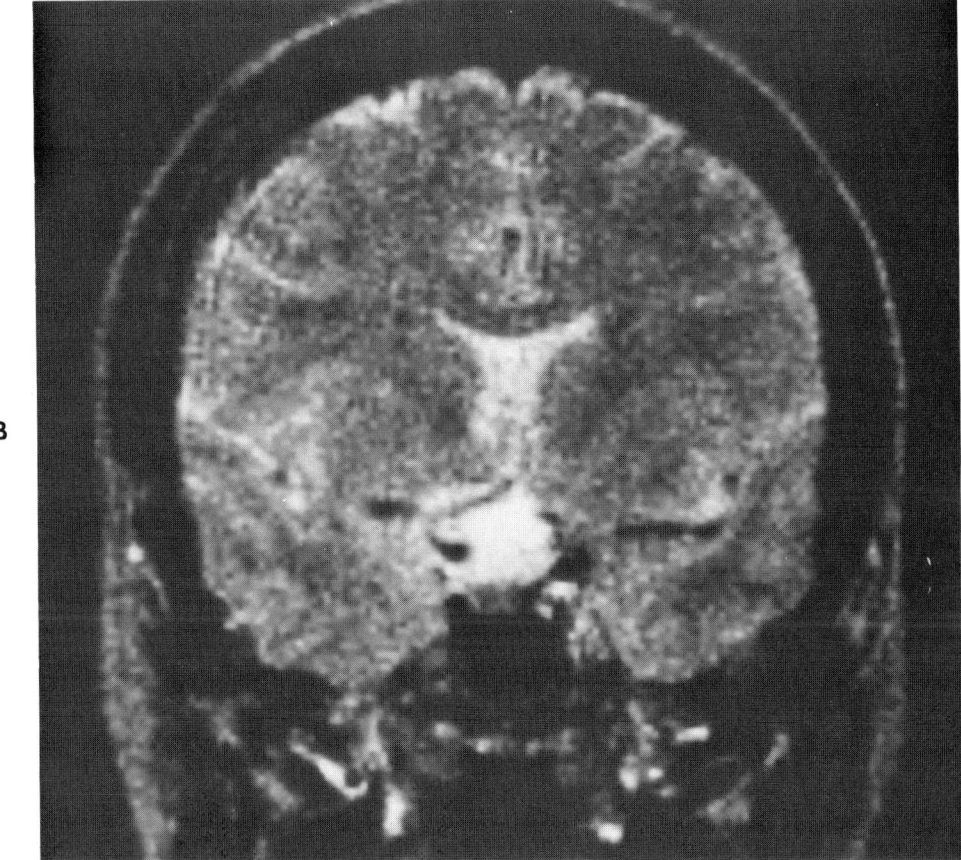

Fig. 5-24, cont'd. B, Coronal MRI. TE 50 ms and TR 1000 ms. Third echo demonstrates lesion.

Continued.

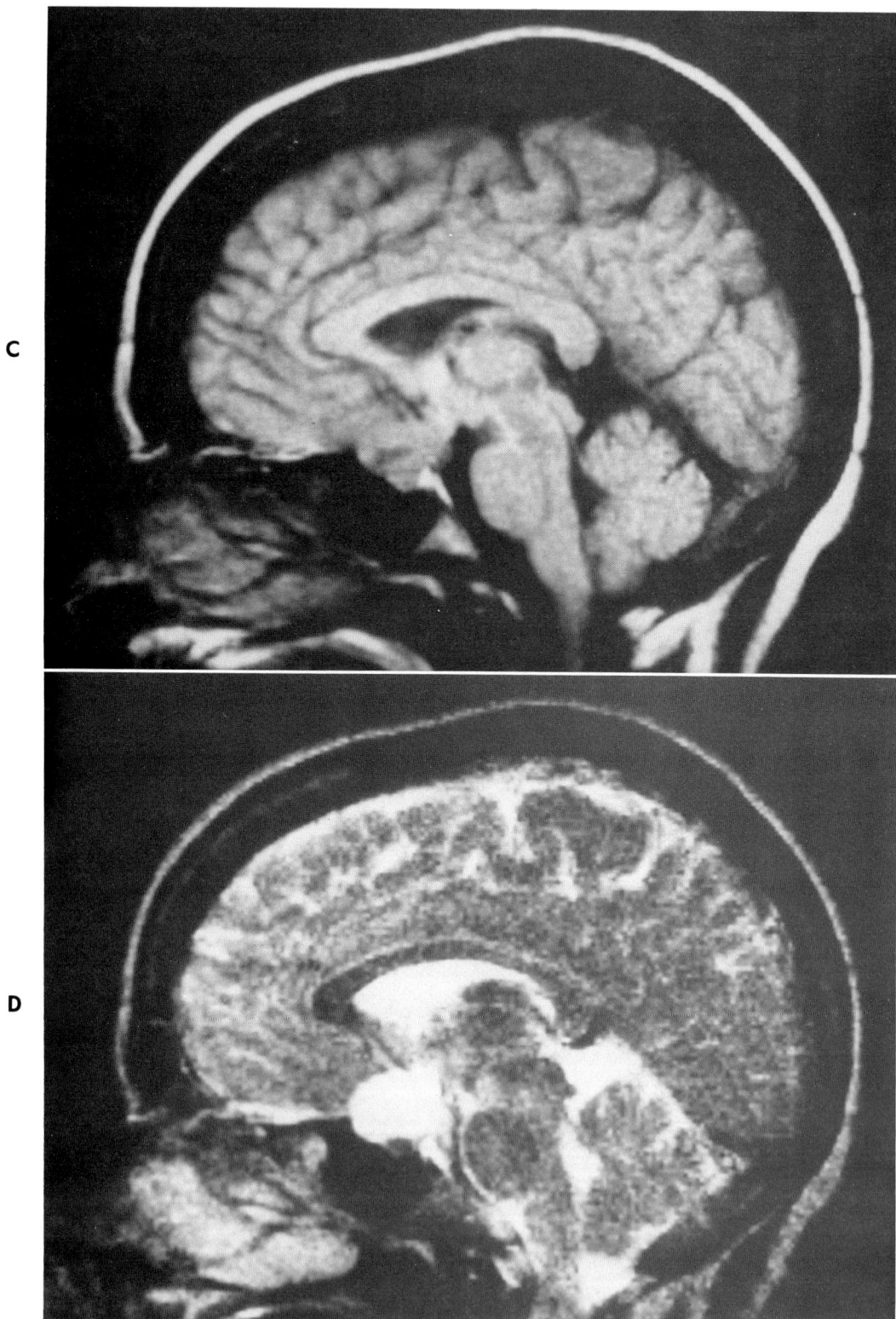

Fig. 5-24, cont'd. C, Sagittal MRI. TE 50 ms and TR 700 ms. First echo demonstrates mass in hypothalamic area with intensity similar to normal brain. **D,** Sagittal MRI. TE 50 ms and TR 700 ms. Fourth echo better delineates area of long T2 involving hypothalamus and suprasellar region. Note how different echos bring out certain pathological findings better than others.

In the case of an optic nerve or chiasmatic glioma, there is usually demonstrable enlargement of the optic nerve or chiasm. These gliomas frequently invade the hypothalamus, making the site of origin difficult to determine. Metrizamide cisternography is occasionally useful in determining the relationship of these lesions to the optic nerve and chiasm (Fig. 5-25). MRI also demonstrates this relationship well (see Fig. 10-4).

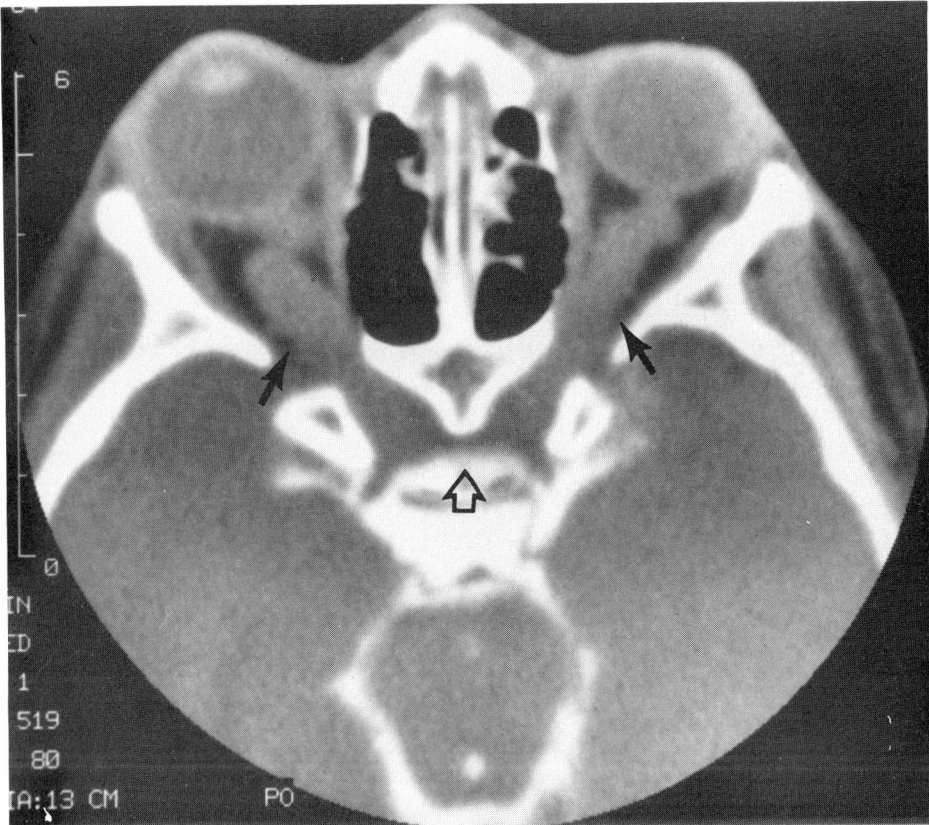

Fig. 5-25. CT metrizamide cisternogram—bilateral optic nerve gliomas. Axial section through bilaterally enlarged optic nerves (solid arrows). Metrizamide outlines normal, uninvolved optic chiasm (open arrow).

188 *Disorders of the pituitary*

Chordomas

Chordomas usually arise intracranially in the midline at the clivus, dorsum sella, or spheno-occipital synchondrosis. On plain skull films, one may see calcification of the mass and bony erosion of the clivus (Fig. 5-26). CT usually reveals a midline calcified mass with extensive bony destruction (Fig. 5-27). MRI clearly demonstrates some of these lesions (see Fig. 10-5).

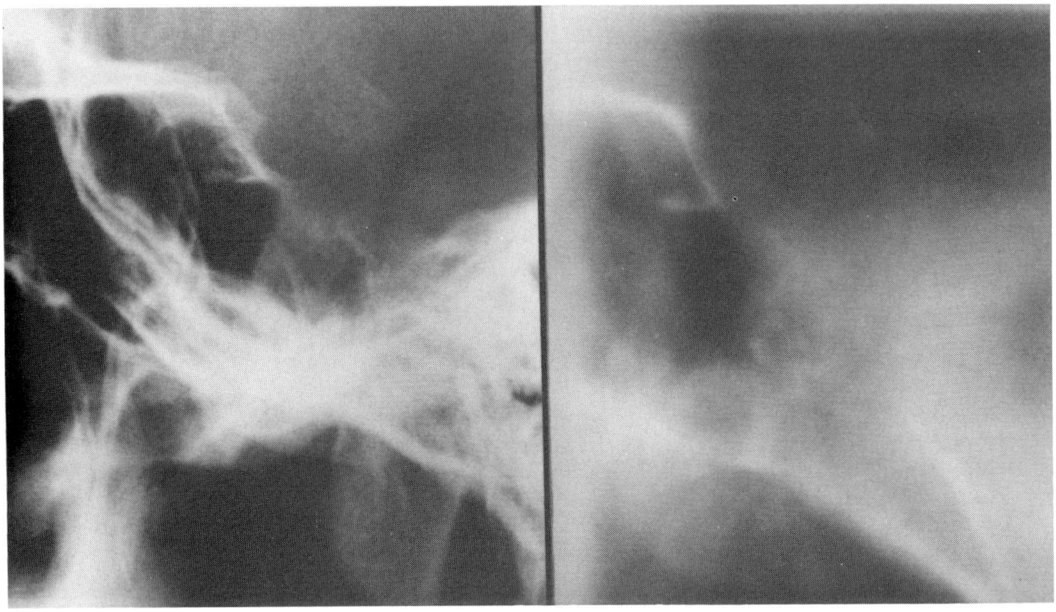

Fig. 5-26. Skull film, tomogram—chordoma. **A,** Skull film shows erosion of posterior clinoid, dorsum sella, clivus, and floor of sella caused by a chordoma. **B,** Tomogram provides fine detail of similar findings plus extension of soft tissue into sphenoid sinus.

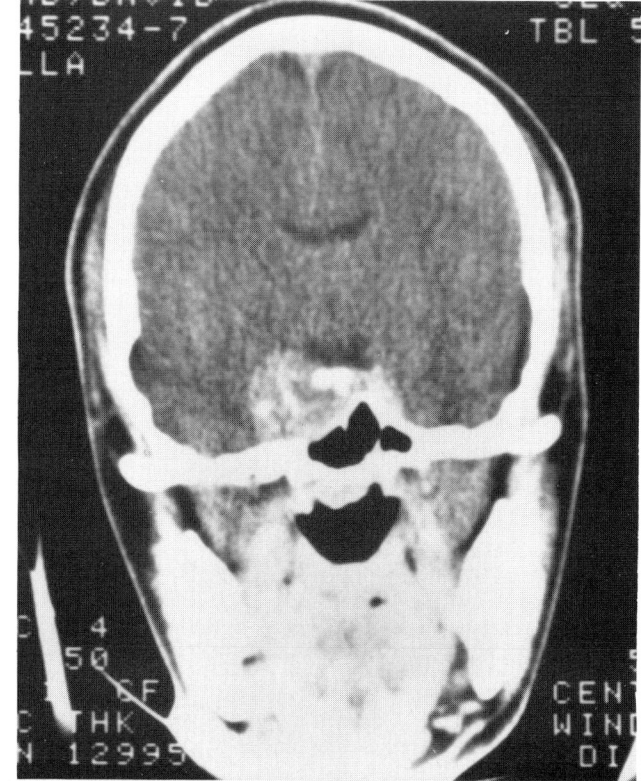
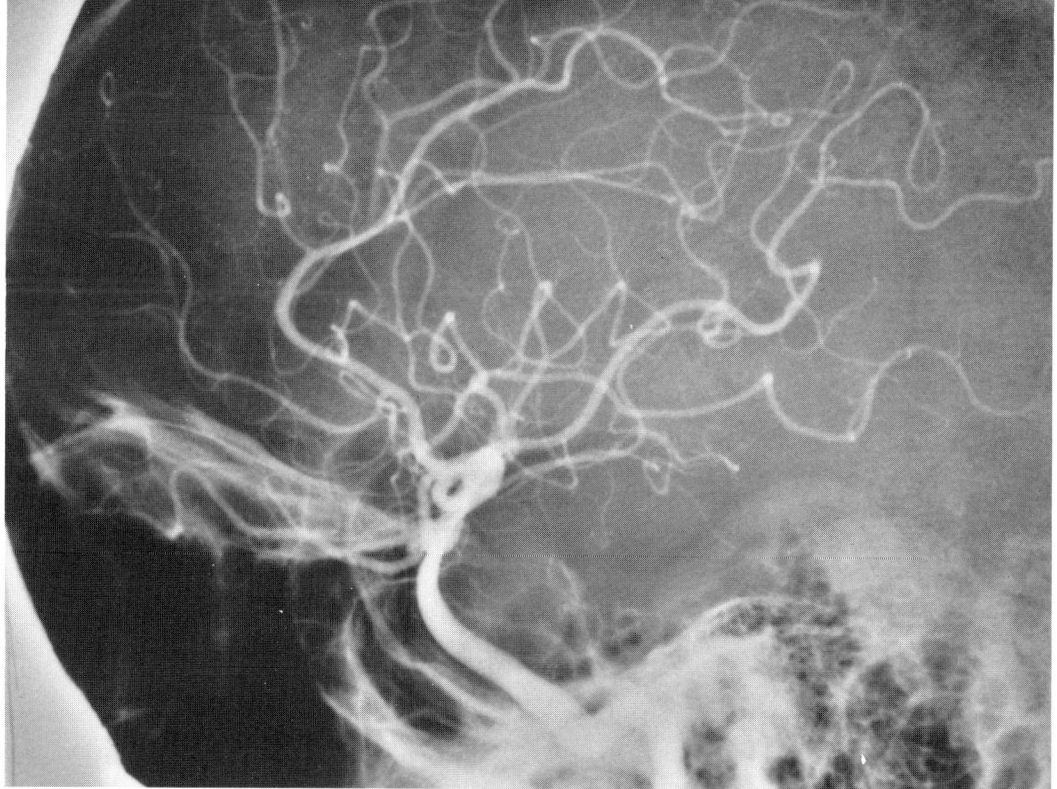

Fig. 5-27. CT and arteriogram—chordoma. **A,** Coronal enhanced CT scan shows enhancing, calcified parasellar mass eroding base of skull. **B,** Lateral internal carotid arteriogram shows erosion of clivus with anterior displacement of carotid artery.

Non-neoplastic cysts

Included in this category of pathological conditions are Rathke's pouch cysts, mucoceles, and arachnoid cysts. Any of these lesions can produce sellar erosion and enlargement on plain skull films. CT or polytomography may be necessary to demonstrate a defect in the posterior wall of a frontal or other paranasal sinus associated with a mucocele.

The typical CT appearance of a Rathke's pouch cyst is an intrasellar, non-calcified, cystic mass with or without suprasellar extension that does not enhance with contrast media. We have recently treated three of these lesions, all of which were entirely suprasellar and associated with a normal sella turcica. Metrizamide cisternography was helpful in determining the absence of an intrasellar extension of the lesions (Fig. 5-28).

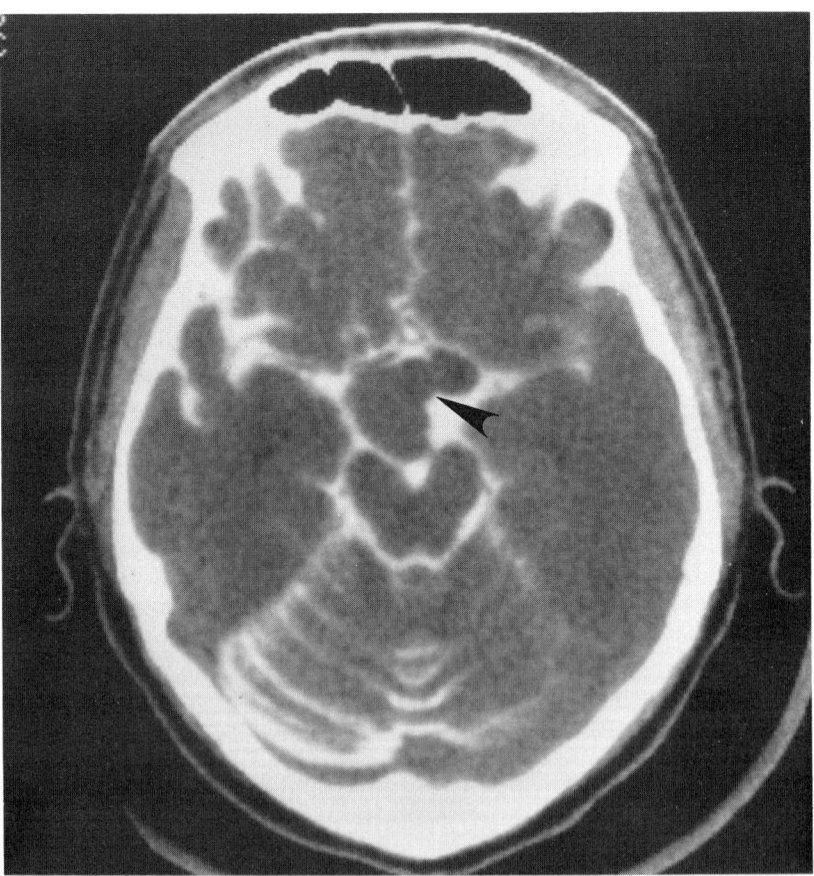

Fig. 5-28. CT—metrizamide cisternogram—Rathke's cleft cyst. Axial cut through suprasellar cistern. Arrow points to large eccentric suprasellar mass outlined by metrizamide.

Arachnoid cysts appear as a low-density cystic structure in the suprasellar region that may obliterate the third ventricle and produce hydrocephalus (Fig. 5-29). Metrizamide cisternography will usually demonstrate the size and extent of the cyst as well as its relationship to surrounding structures.

Angiography is of little value in the workup of these lesions and only reveals an avascular mass.

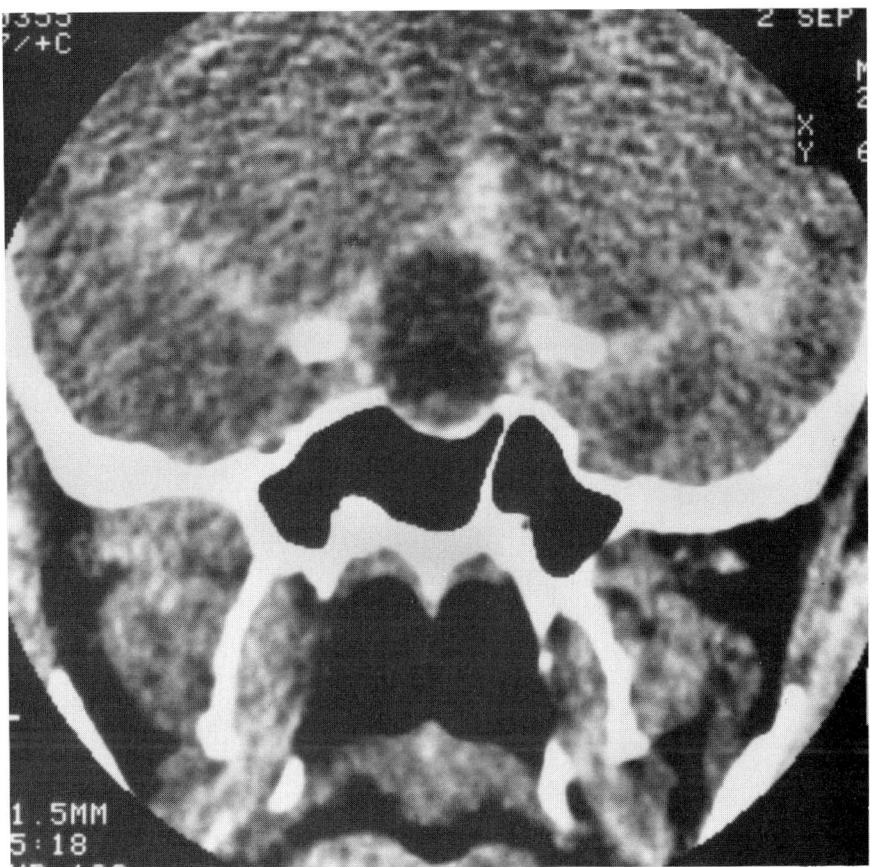

Fig. 5-29. CT—metrizamide cisternogram—arachnoid cyst. Coronal CT scan demonstrates intrasellar and suprasellar low-density area. Metrizamide outlines cyst and fails to enter sella, thus excluding presence of empty sella.

Aneurysms

Plain films may demonstrate sellar region changes caused by pressure effects (Fig. 5-30), including erosion of the sphenoid bone, anterior clinoid, and sellar floor (producing a double floor). In some cases, one will see calcification of the artery in the suprasellar or juxtasellar region.

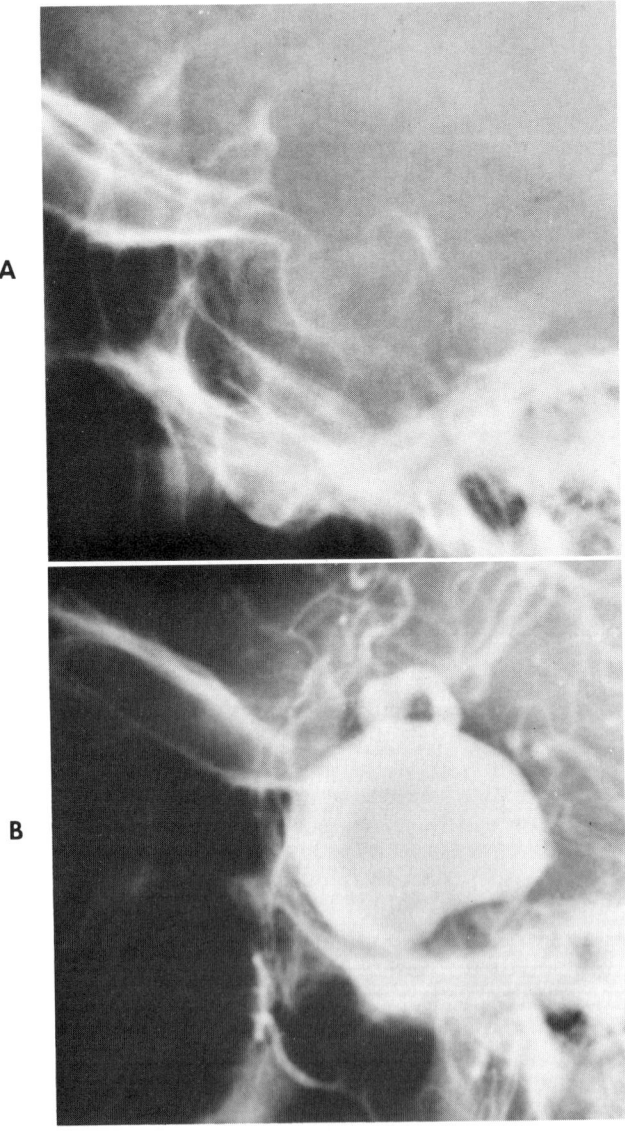

Fig. 5-30. Skull film and arteriogram—aneurysm. **A,** Lateral skull film shows enlarged sella with erosion of clinoids, dorsum sella, and thinning of sellar floor. **B,** Lateral internal carotid arteriogram reveals giant parasellar aneurysm.

Aneurysms are seen on CT as round mass lesions of increased density (Fig. 5-31, *A*). In addition to the expected enhancement on contrasted CT scans, there is frequently a change in the size and shape. The enhancement is usually homogenous immediately after the administration of contrast. However, if the scan is delayed, there can be irregular enhancement that can be mistaken for a sellar region tumor.[5,22]

Cerebral angiography remains the definitive diagnostic procedure for intracranial aneurysms (Fig. 5-31, *B*).

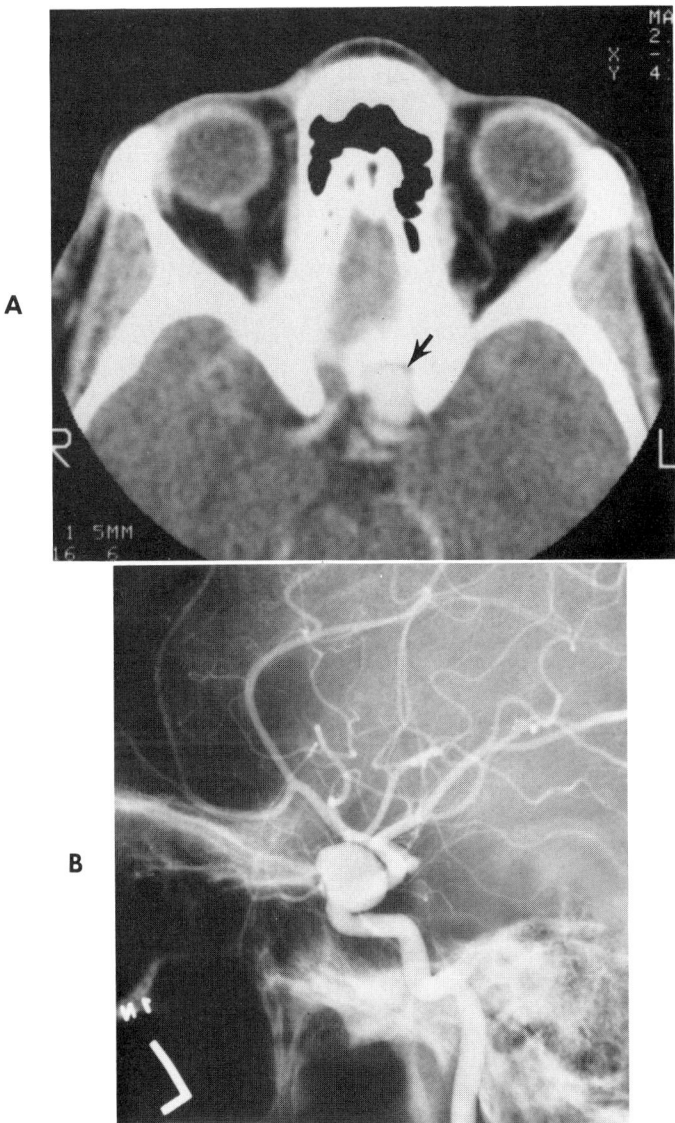

Fig. 5-31. CT and arteriogram—aneurysm. **A,** Enhanced axial CT demonstrates enhancing parasellar mass. **B,** Internal carotid arteriogram shows aneurysm.

Pituitary abscesses

A pituitary abscess may be found in the presence of a pituitary adenoma, in which case the sella may be enlarged or may reveal any of the plain film and CT findings associated with such tumors. Fig. 5-32 shows the CT appearance of a pituitary abscess with marked enhancement of the intrasellar and suprasellar mass.

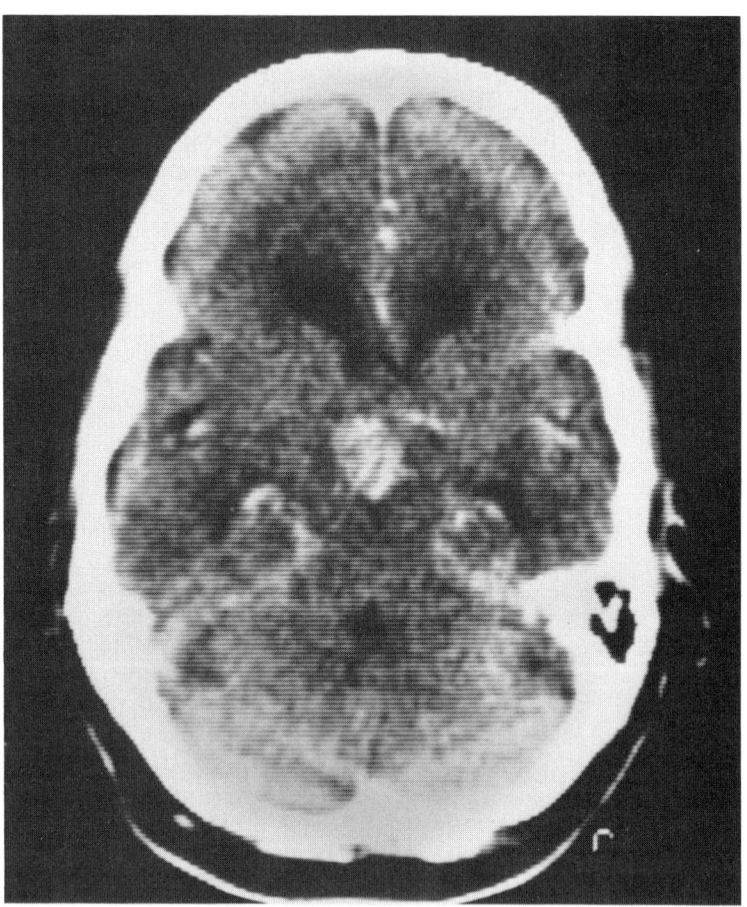

Fig. 5-32. CT—pituitary abscess. Axial CT scan demonstrates enhancing suprasellar mass proven at surgery to be a pituitary abscess.

Sarcoidosis

Plain skull films may demonstrate lytic skull lesions of sarcoidosis, usually without marginal sclerosis.[30] Other abnormalities include sellar enlargement, suprasellar calcification, and reactive bone formation.[4,14]

CT may reveal only nonspecific findings of hydrocephalus; enhancement of the basilar cisterns caused by granulomatous leptomeningitis; intracranial masses in the region of the optic nerve and/or chiasm, pituitary infundibulum, or hypothalamus.[4] These masses usually enhance homogenously after the administration of contrast (Fig. 5-33).

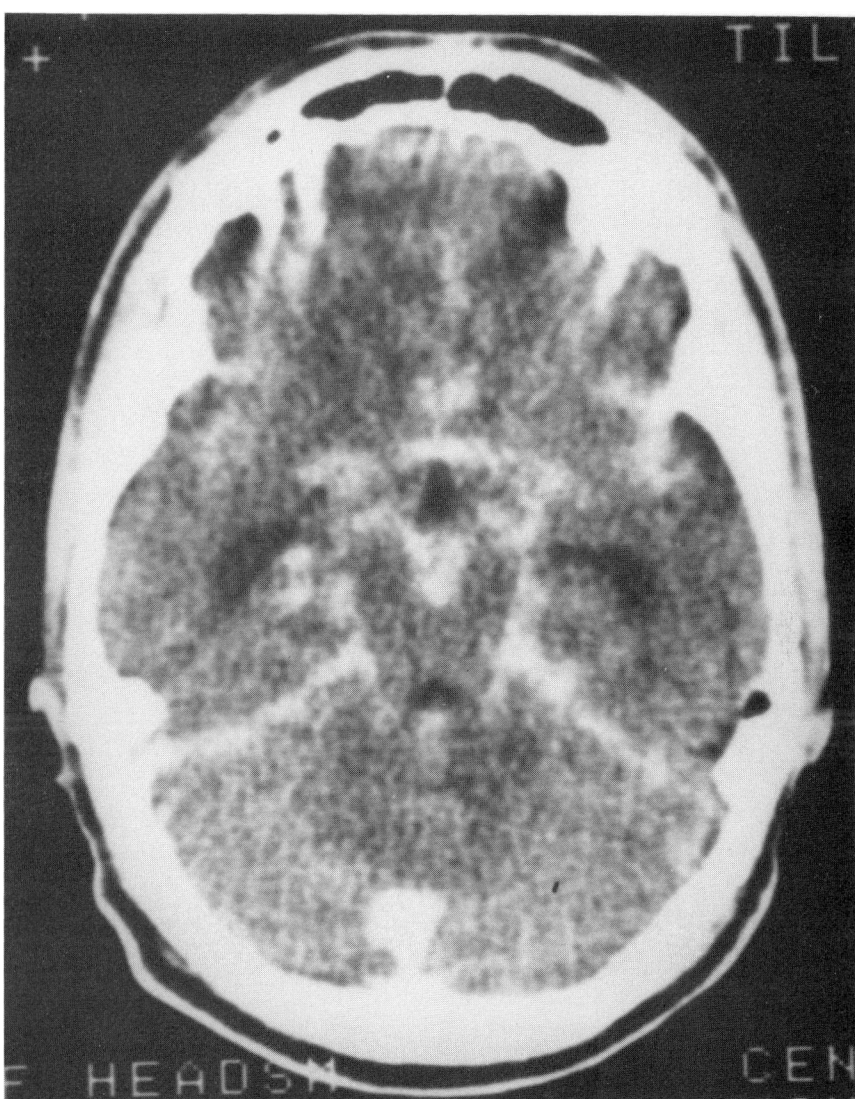

Fig. 5-33. CT—sarcoidosis. Contrast enhanced axial CT shows marked enhancement of basilar cisterns in this patient with known sarcoidosis and pituitary dysfunction.

Metrizamide cisternography may be helpful in determining the relationship of a sarcoid mass to the optic chiasm and/or nerve.

Angiography has been reported to illustrate a sarcoid angiitis.[21] However, this diagnostic study is usually not necessary in the evaluation of neurosarcoidosis.

Histiocytosis X

The most frequent changes on plain skull films are the solitary calvarial lesions of eosinophilic granuloma. These appear as irregular areas of rarefaction without surrounding sclerosis and beveled margins on tangential views (Fig. 5-34). These lesions occur in the frontal bones more commonly than any other part of the body and may be multiple. Sellar erosive changes may also be seen.

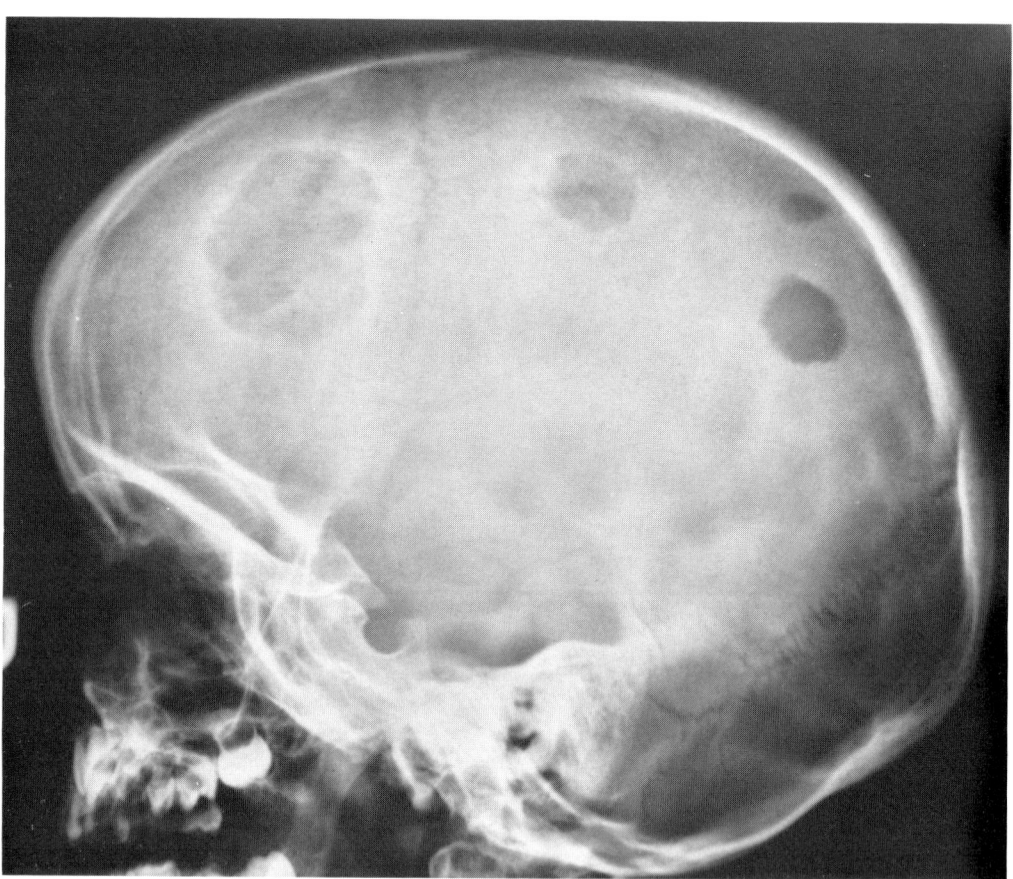

Fig. 5-34. Skull film—histiocytosis X. Lateral skull film shows multiple irregular areas of rarefaction.

CT will usually be abnormal in those patients with clinical involvement of the pituitary or hypothalamus. This usually reveals an enhancing suprasellar mass, occasionally with distortion of the third ventricle (Fig. 5-35).

In the typical case, metrizamide cisternography and angiography are not indicated.

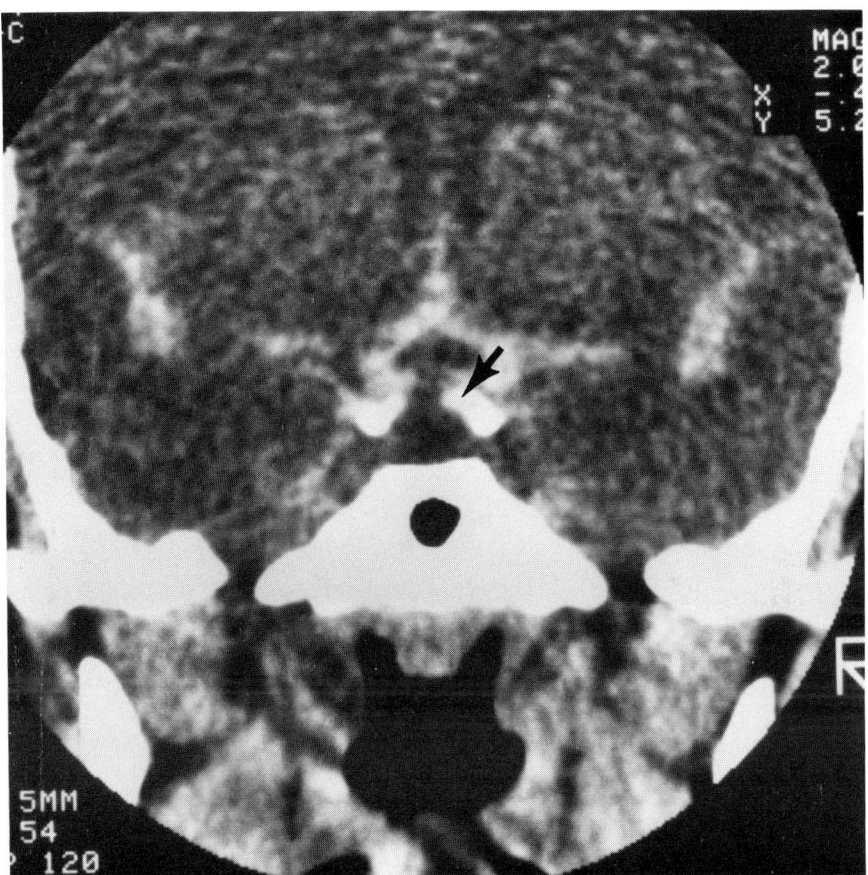

Fig. 5-35. CT—metrizamide cisternogram—histiocytosis X. Coronal section through sella demonstrates metrizamide outlining optic chiasm and enlarged pituitary stalk and gland (arrow).

"Empty sella" syndrome

Radiologically, ESS presents a diverse picture. There is often enlargement of the sella turcica with erosion of the lamina dura. The dorsum sella retains its normal curvature, and there is approximation of the anterior and posterior clinoids. All degrees of sellar deformity can occur, including posterior displacement, demineralization of the dorsum sella, and erosion of the entire sella turcica. On the basis of skull x-ray examinations (or tomography) alone, the sellar enlargement associated with the ESS is indistinguishable from that resulting from a pituitary tumor.

The typical appearance of an empty sella on the coronal view of a high-resolution CT scan is that of a low-density area within the confines of the sella turcica. The density is consistent with that of CSF (Fig. 5-36). The undisplaced pituitary stalk is visualized entering the sella, a finding referred to as the infundibular sign of an empty sella. This sign is helpful in distinguishing ESS from intrasellar cystic lesions presenting with low density on the CT scan. In cases in which the plain CT scan does not verify the diagnosis, metrizamide cisternography is indicated. This technique has completely replaced pneumoencephalography. The presence of a significant quantity of metrizamide in the empty sella confirms the diagnosis (see Fig. 16-4).

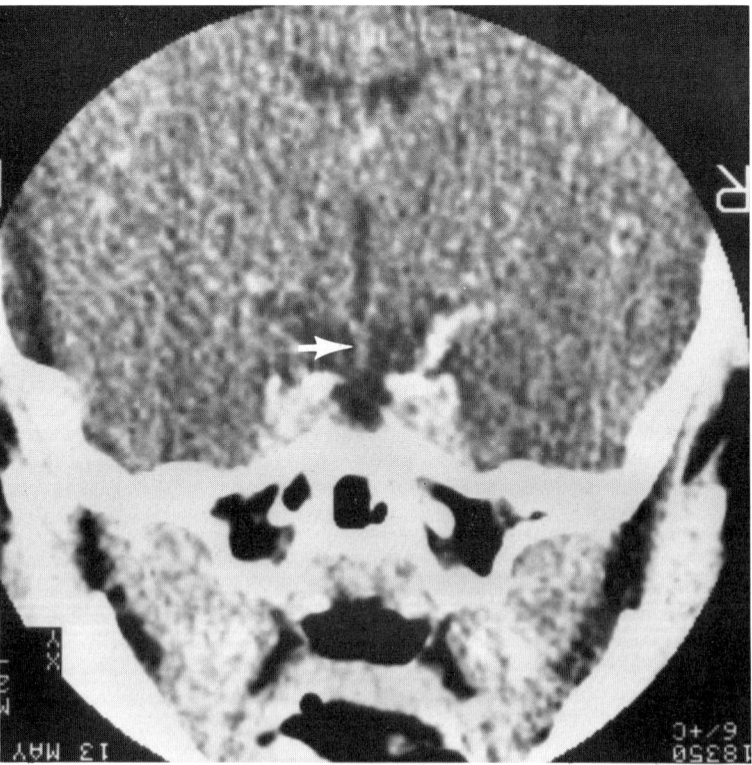

Fig. 5-36. CT—empty sella. Enhanced coronal scan reveals area of CSF density within sella turcica. Note undisplaced pituitary stalk entering sella (arrow).

Metrizamide cisternography has proven to be a valuable diagnostic procedure in patients with CSF leaks (rhinorrhea). The exact site of the leak may be demonstrated, or if not the leak site, the entry of the metrizamide into a paranasal sinus (which serves to identify the intracranial fossa the leak is coming from)—information that is valuable in planning surgical treatment designed to close the leak (Fig. 5-37).

CSF rhinorrhea has been reported in patients with the ESS, and in these cases, metrizamide cisternography will usually confirm this entity as the cause of the CSF leak by demonstrating metrizamide in the sphenoid sinus. CSF rhinorrhea has also been reported in patients with large prolactinomas treated with bromocriptine, presumably because reduction in the size of the tumor exposes an area of erosion into the dura and bony sella floor allowing egress of CSF.[2,7,20,38] Metrizamide cisternography would be expected to be of value in this situation by demonstrating metrizamide in the sphenoid sinus.

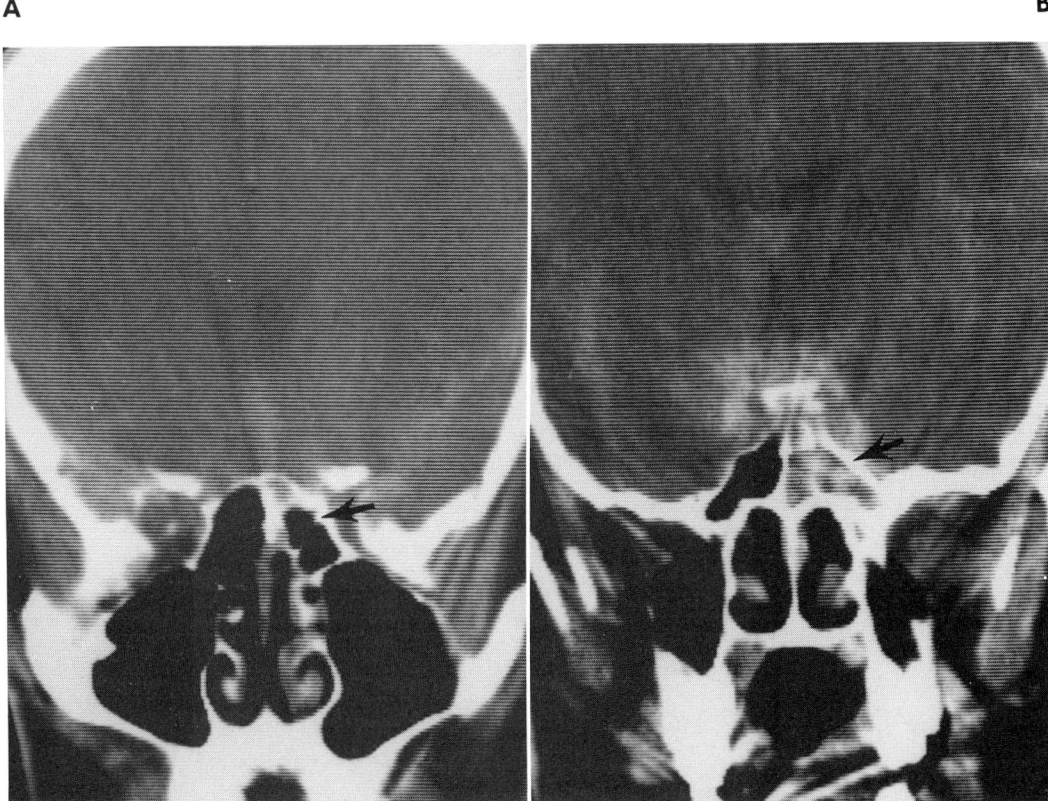

Fig. 5-37. CT-metrizamide cisternogram—CSF rhinorrhea. **A,** CT before intrathecal administration in patient with CSF rhinorrhea. Arrow points to aerated sphenoid sinus. **B,** Sphenoid sinus fills with metrizamide (arrow) and thus demonstrates site of leak.

REFERENCES

1. Baker HL Jr: The angiographic delineation of sellar and parasellar masses. *Radiology* 104:67, 1972.
2. Baskin DS, Wilson CB: CSF rhinorrhea after bromocriptine for prolactinoma, letter. *N Engl J Med* 306:178, 1982.
3. Boggan JE, Tyrrell JB, Wilson CB: Transsphenoidal microsurgical management of Cushing's disease: Report of 100 cases. *J Neurosurg* 59:195, 1983.
4. Brooks BS, El Gammal T, Hungerford GD, et al: Radiologic evaluation of neurosarcoidosis: Role of computed tomography. *AJNR* 3:513, 1982.
5. Byrd SE, Bentson JR, Winter J, et al: Giant intracranial aneurysms simulating brain neoplasms on computed tomography. *J Comput Assist Tomogr* 2:303, 1978.
6. Close HG: The incidence of adenoma of the pituitary body in some types of new growth. *Lancet* 1:732, 1934.
7. Cole IE, Keene M: Cerebrospinal fluid rhinorrhoea in pituitary tumors. *J R Soc Med* 73:244, 1980.
8. Costello RT: Subclinical adenoma of the pituitary gland. *Am J Pathol* 12:205, 1936.
9. Davis PC, Hoffman JC Jr, Tindall GT, et al: Prolactin-secreting pituitary microadenomas: Inaccuracy of high-resolution CT imaging. *AJNR* 5:721, 1984.
10. Di Chiro G, Nelson KB: The volume of the sella turcica. *AJR Rad Ther Nucl Med* 87:989, 1962.
11. Doppman JL, Oldfield E, Krudy AG, et al: Petrosal sinus sampling for Cushing syndrome: Anatomical and technical considerations. *Radiology* 150:99, 1984.
12. Faria MA Jr, Tindall GT: Transsphenoidal microsurgery for prolactin-secreting pituitary adenomas: Results in 100 women with the amenorrhea-galactorrhea syndrome. *J Neurosurg* 56:33, 1982.
13. George AE: Radiologic diagnosis of pituitary tumors. *Semin Reproductive Endocrinol* 2(1):47, 1984.
14. Goodman SS, Margulies ME: Boeck's sarcoid simulating a brain tumor. *Arch Neurol Psychiatry* 81:419, 1959.
15. Hamberger CA, Hammer G, Norlen G, et al: Transantrosphenoidal hypophysectomy. *Arch Otolaryngol* 74:2, 1961.
16. Hardy J: Transphenoidal microsurgery of the normal and pathological pituitary. *Clin Neurosurg* 16:185, 1969.
17. Kaufman B: Magnetic resonance imaging of the pituitary gland. *Radiol Clin North Am* 22:795, 1984.
18. Kovacs K, Ryan N, Horvath E, et al: Pituitary adenomas in old age. *J Gerontol* 35:16, 1980.
19. Kricheff II, Schotland, DL: Tumor stain in a pituitary adenoma. *Radiology* 82:11, 1964.
20. Landolt AM: Cerebrospinal fluid rhinorrhea: A complication of therapy for invasive prolactinomas. *Neurosurgery* 11:395, 1982.
21. Lawrence WP, El Gammal T, Pool WH Jr, et al: Radiological manifestations of neurosarcoidosis: Report of three cases and review of literature. *Clin Radiol* 25:343, 1974.
22. Leeds NE, Naidich TP: Computerized tomography in the diagnosis of sellar and parasellar lesions. *Semin Roentgenol* 12:121, 1977.
23. McCormick WF, Halmi NS: Absence of chromophobe adenomas from a large series of pituitary tumors. *Arch Pathol* 92:231, 1971.
24. Miller JH, Peña AM, Segall HD: Radiological investigation of sellar region masses in children. *Radiology* 134:81, 1980.
25. Modic MT, Weinstein MA, Chilcote WA, et al: Digital subtraction angiography of the intracranial vascular system: Comparative study in 55 patients. *AJR* 138:299, 1982.
26. Ovitt TW, Christenson PC, Fisher HD III, et al: Intravenous angiography using digital video subtraction: X-ray imaging system. *AJR* 135:1141, 1980.
27. Parent AD, Bebin J, Smith RR: Incidental pituitary adenomas. *J Neurosurg* 54:228, 1981.
28. Rand RW, Hanafee WN: Cavernous sinus venography and stereotaxic cryohypophysectomy. *J Neurosurg* 26: 521, 1967.
29. Robertson WD, Newton TH: Radiologic assessment of pituitary microadenomas. *AJR* 131:389, 1978.
30. Rohatgi PK, Archutowska-Kempka M: Combined calvarial and CNS sarcoidosis: Report of two cases. *Arch Neurol* 38:261, 1981.
31. Seldinger SI: Catheter replacement of the needle in percutaneous arteriography: A new technique. *Acta Radiol* 39:368, 1953.
32. Shiu PC, Hanafee WN, Wilson GH, et al: Cavernous sinus venography. *AJR* 104:57, 1968.

33. Susman W: Pituitary adenoma. *Br Med J* 2:1215, 1933.
34. Swartz JD, Russell KB, Basile BA, et al: High-resolution computed tomographic appearance of the intrasellar contents in women of childbearing age. *Radiology* 147:115, 1983.
35. Syvertsen A, Haughton VM, Williams AL, et al: The computed tomographic appearance of the normal pituitary gland and pituitary microadenomas. *Radiology* 133:385, 1979.
36. Taveras and Wood: *Diagnostic Neuroradiology*, ed 2. Baltimore, Williams & Wilkins, vols 1 and 2.
37. Theron J, Chevalier D, Delvert M, et al: Diagnosis of small and micro pituitary adenomas by intercavernous sinus venography: A preliminary report. *Neuroradiology* 18:23, 1979.
38. Wilson JD, Newcombe RLG, Long FL: Cerebrospinal fluid rhinorrhoea during treatment of pituitary tumours with bromocriptine. *Acta Endocrinol* 103:457, 1983.

CHAPTER 6

Acromegaly

Physiology of growth hormone
Pathophysiology
Etiology of acromegaly and gigantism
Clinical features
    Acral and facial enlargement
    Headache
    Skin changes
    Peripheral nerve entrapments
    Arthralgias
    Myopathy
    Other findings
Associated medical conditions and metabolic disturbances
Prognosis
Diagnostic evaluation
    Endocrine testing
    Neuroradiologic studies
        Skull film
        CT scan
Treatment
    Criteria of cure
    Surgery
    Irradiation
        Conventional electromagnetic irradiation
        Heavy particle irradiation
    Pharmacotherapy
Therapeutic decision making
    "Virgin" acromegaly
    Persistent or recurrent acromegaly
        Following previous radiation therapy
        Following previous surgery
    Preoperative surgical therapy
Summary

Acromegaly is a disorder resulting from the excess secretion of growth hormone (GH). Although there are potentially a variety of sources of the GH, GH-secreting pituitary adenomas account for the vast majority of cases. The presence of a pathologic excess of GH results in the gross enlargement of the extremities, face, and various soft tissues of the body, resulting in a characteristic appearance. When the condition is present in childhood, before closure of the epiphyses of the long bones, there is a more proportional increase in the size of all body parts, referred to as gigantism.

Because acromegaly causes such a gross distortion of the normal appearance and limits the normal life expectancy of the patient, treatment is usually indicated. Once the diagnosis is established by the typical clinical manifestations with endocrine and neuroradiologic substantiation, the treatment options include surgery, medical therapy with dopamine agonists, and radiation therapy.

In 1886 Marie[70] described two patients with the condition he called acromegaly, deriving the name from the Greek akron (extremity) and megas (large). His detailed description of the manifestations of the disease, including the gigantic hands and feet, enlarged head, prognathous mandible, macroglossia, headaches, joint pain, and thickened skin, clearly identified the classic features of the disease. Marie did not attribute the disease to any anatomic or physiologic cause. Minkowski[61,80] in 1887 noted that an enlargement of the pituitary gland was observed in all carefully examined cases of acromegaly, but many regarded this as being a manifestation of the disease rather than a cause.

By 1909 Cushing[20,21] regarded acromegaly as a disease of pituitary hypersecretion. Finally, Cushing and Davidoff[21] in 1927 reported that the pituitary gland in acromegaly was usually enlarged by a "hyperplastic" or "adenomatous process" composed of acidophilic cells and that these cells were responsible for the hormone that caused acromegaly and gigantism in man.

PHYSIOLOGY OF GROWTH HORMONE

Normally, GH secretion by somatotrophs in the adenohypophysis is under hypothalamic control. This is a dual control mediated by somatostatin (growth hormone–inhibiting factor [GIF]) suppressing and somatocrinin (growth hormone–releasing factor [GRF]) stimulating GH secretion.[115] The belief that GRF predominates over GIF is supported by the observation that hypothalamic lesions that effect GH result in diminished or absent GH secretion. The normal secretion of GH is pulsatile with a circadian rhythm as measured by frequent sampling techniques. Periods of secretory surges or bursts occur spontaneously and result from neural inputs that arise in the hypothalamus and are believed to be mediated by GRF. The largest secretory surge commonly occurs during the first 2 hours of night sleep, sometimes in association with slow wave sleep. Other factors such as stress, exercise, hypoglycemia, and hyperglycemia influence GH release.

A variety of pharmacologic agents stimulate the release of GH in normal subjects.[72] These include certain amino acids (arginine, leucine), peptides (vasopressin, glucagon), and monoamines (levodopa, bromocriptine). Some of these substances such as levodopa and insulin are used to measure pituitary GH reserve. The mechanism and site of action of these agents has not been fully clarified. It is believed likely that the biogenic amines act on the hypothalamus to affect release of GRF.

Salmon and Daughaday[95] postulated that GH did not directly stimulate cell growth when they demonstrated in vitro that GH added to serum from a rat with pituitary function stimulated cartilaginous growth while GH alone or GH added to serum from a hypophysectomized rat did not.[95] They suggested that a "sulfation factor" was present in normal rat serum and later termed this factor somatomedin.[25] Somatomedins, which have been shown to be a family of polypeptides with both growth and anabolic effects on most tissues, are produced in the liver and are regulated by many factors including GH.[86,87] Levels of circulating somatomedins are elevated by GH, prolactin, and chorionic somatomammotropin and are depressed by steroids, estrogen, insulin deficiency, uremia, liver failure, chronic disease, and starvation.

PATHOPHYSIOLOGY

In acromegaly, the response to the administration of some of the agents mentioned above is the opposite, or paradoxical, from that which occurs in the normal subject. For instance, in most acromegalic patients there is a paradoxical inhibition of GH after the administration of dopamine agonists such as apomorphine and bromocriptine. Also the response of GH to glucose administration is altered and forms the basis for an important diagnostic test in these patients. Under normal circumstances, the oral administration of glucose results in a suppression of GH to less than 5 ng/ml and in many cases to undetectable levels. However, in acromegalic patients, the administration of glucose usually fails to suppress the levels of GH and at times causes an elevation. In normal subjects, the administration of thyrotropin-releasing hormone (TRH) has no effect on GH secretion, whereas in the majority of acromegalic patients, its administration causes an elevation in GH secretion.[4]

ETIOLOGY OF ACROMEGALY AND GIGANTISM

Acromegaly and gigantism could result either from elevated serum GH levels, an increased responsiveness of peripheral tissues to GH or excessively active GH. A case for the latter possibility is made by the recent documentation of acromegaly in five patients with apparently normal circulating immunoreactive GH levels.[6] The bioactivity of the GH was documented in vitro by a growth-promoting assay. The frequency of this apparently rare condition is unknown. There are several pituitary and extrapituitary causes of elevated serum GH levels, and these are listed as follows*:

---

*From Melmed S, Braunstein GD, Horvath E, et al: Pathophysiology of acromegaly. *Endocr Rev* 4:271, 1983.

Pituitary
    Densely granulated GH cell adenoma
    Sparsely granulated GH cell adenoma
    Mixed GH cell and prolactin cell adenoma
        Densely granulated GH and densely granulated prolactin cells
        Sparsely granulated GH and sparsely granulated PRL cells
        Sparsely granulated GH and densely granulated prolactin cells
        Densely granulated GH and sparsely granulated prolactin cells
    Acidophil stem cell adenoma
    Mammosomatotroph cell adenoma
    Plurihormonal adenoma
    GH cell carcinoma
    GH cell hyperplasia
Extrapituitary
    Eutopic GH cell adenoma
        Sphenoid sinus
        Parapharyngeal
    Ectopic GH-producing tumors
        Lung
        Ovary
        Breast
    Excess GH-releasing factor secretion
        Eutopic
            Hypothalamic hamartoma or choristoma
        Ectopic
            Pancreatic islet cell tumors
            Bronchial and intestinal carcinoid tumors

The pituitary hypersecretion of GH may be associated with densely or sparsely granulated GH cell adenomas, mixed GH cell–prolactin cell adenomas, acidophil stem cell adenomas, mammosomatotroph cell adenomas, or plurihormonal adenomas. Densely and sparsely granulated GH cell adenomas, both of which are probably variants of the same neoplasm, are the most frequent tumor types accounting for acromegaly and occur with approximately the same frequency. Separation of the two types is justified on clinical and pathologic grounds. Sparsely granulated GH cell adenomas are less differentiated than the densely granulated form and often exhibit a more rapid growth rate, present earlier to surgery, and often are invasive, causing sellar erosion and extrasellar extension.[79] Although the densely granulated adenomas are acidophilic by light microscopy, the sparsely granulated tumors are chromophobic.

Mixed GH cell–prolactin cell adenomas are composed of two distinct cell types, somatotrophs and lactotrophs. Patients harboring these tumors have elevated GH levels with clinical acromegaly or gigantism and may have blood prolactin levels that are moderately to markedly elevated or in some cases within the normal range.

Acidophil stem cell adenomas are believed to arise from a cell that is the common precursor of both GH and prolactin cells. They consist of one cell type producing both GH and prolactin. Patients with this tumor type usually have moderately elevated prolactin levels. Elevated GH levels and acromegalic features may occur, but in the majority of cases, serum GH levels are within the normal range. These tumors also may show rapid growth, often invading the sphenoid bone and cavernous sinus.[79]

Mammosomatotroph cell adenomas are more slowly growing benign tumors believed to be a mature variant of acidophil stem cell adenomas.[56] Patients who harbor this tumor and who have acromegaly have elevated serum GH levels and normal or slightly elevated serum prolactin levels.

Plurihormonal adenomas are rare tumors that have only recently been recognized.[14,44] These tumors produce two or more adenohypophysial hormones, usually GH and prolactin plus a glycoprotein hormone, and may be associated with clinical acromegaly.

GH cell carcinomas are exceptionally rare tumors that may cause acromegaly with only a few cases reported in the literature.[52,58,75,98] Pituitary carcinoma should only be diagnosed when distant metastases are present. The role of GH cell hyperplasia as a cause of acromegaly is unknown. This is a difficult diagnosis to make, since GH cells are unevenly distributed in the normal pituitary and predominate in the lateral wings. GH cell hyperplasia may occur with extrapituitary sources of GRF from bronchial carcinomas, islet cell tumors,[107] and lung or intestinal carcinoid tumors.[13,22,100,101,114]

Extrasellar GH-producing adenomas in the sphenoid sinus or parapharyngeal region have been a cause of acromegaly.[15,90] Interestingly, these ectopic sites are along the path of migration of the cells of Rathke's pouch from the pharynx to the sella turcica during embryogenesis.[76,78] Ectopic GH secretion has been reported with breast cancer,[51] normal and metastatic ovarian tissue,[51] and bronchial carcinoma.[37,102]

The great majority of cases are caused by pituitary adenomas.

As with prolactinomas and adrenocorticotropic hormone (ACTH)-producing pituitary adenomas, there is pathologic and clinical evidence that GH-secreting pituitary tumors may be caused by either a primary pituitary abnormality, by defective hypothalamic control, or by a combination of factors. Evidence that acromegaly is a primary pituitary disease includes the following:

1. The pituitary tissue surrounding a GH-secreting adenoma does not contain GH cell hyperplasia but is normal, suggesting that the gland is not under the influence of abnormal hypothalamic stimulation.[24,59] This finding is more in keeping with the notion that an adenoma arises from a locally transformed cell within the pituitary gland.[79]
2. The presence of mixed GH cell–prolactin cell adenomas suggests that the cells making up these neoplasms are derived either from a common stem cell, from two separately transformed cells, or from fusion of two separate cells. Excessive secretion of a hypothalamic factor such as GRF is unlikely to produce a neoplastic transformation of prolactin-secreting cells.[79]
3. In several large surgical series, the basal GH levels have returned to

normal following the selective removal of GH-secreting tumors,* and the GH responses to provocative stimuli, likewise, have been normalized following selective adenomectomy.[29] This evidence, however, must be viewed with caution, since basal GH levels and response to provocative tests do not return to normal in all patients following surgery.[63,99] Because the development of acromegaly is an insidious process, long-term follow-up of operated patients is needed to confirm these impressions.[79,91]

Evidence that acromegaly may result from a defect in hypothalamic control of GH secretion includes the following:

1. The rare finding of a normal pituitary gland in the presence of acromegaly strongly indicates a hypothalamic cause of the disease.[3,30] On the other hand, acromegaly in these patients could be a result of hypersensitivity of peripheral tissues to GH, ectopic sources of GRF or GH, or a small GH-secreting pituitary adenoma that may have been overlooked at surgery.

2. Hypothalamic hamartomas and choristomas associated with GH cell adenomas have been described.[5,92] These tumors may produce GRF, which could cause GH cell hyperplasia and subsequently an adenoma.

3. Serum from acromegalic patients has been shown to have GRF activity in vitro by bioassay.[38,39,103]

4. Although basal GH levels frequently return to normal following surgical removal of a GH-secreting adenoma, the postoperative responses of GH to provocative testing often remain abnormal.[32] This suggests an ongoing hypothalamic defect. Paradoxical GH stimulation by glucose in acromegalic patients is also seen in other hypothalamic disorders such as porphyria.[85]

5. There is evidence that GH secretion by pituitary adenomas is not purely autonomous but that some physiologic hypothalamic control is retained in some cases. For instance, retention of a pulsatile secretion of GH in acromegaly can occur as in the normal situation,[60] and normal GH responses to certain pharmacologic and physiologic stimuli have been noted in some acromegalic patients.[18,19] Although there is abnormal GH suppression by levodopa[12,68,71] and TRH administration,[36,47] some patients with acromegaly exhibit a normal suppression of GH secretion to beta adrenergic stimulation and alpha adrenergic blockage.[19]

6. Cell cultures of human GH adenoma cells have been shown to respond to an ectopic GRF by increased GH secretion,[113] suggestive of GRF receptors on GH adenoma cells. The presence of such receptors may be indicative of a hypothalamic role in acromegaly. Thorner et al[17,107] described a patient with acromegaly resulting from an ectopic source of

---

*See references 1, 3, 9, 40, 45, 58, and 111.

GRF in a pancreatic islet cell tumor that produced pituitary somatotroph hyperplasia. The paradoxical stimulation of GH by glucose and TRH and suppression by dopamine were reversed after removal of the tumor. This suggests that the paradoxical response of GH seen in acromegaly could result from elevated GRF levels in some patients.

Thus there is evidence that some GH cell adenomas are autonomous tumors, whereas others seem to be responsive to hypothalamic influences. Although retention of some hypothalamic control does not prove a hypothalamic cause for the disease, the data are conflicting, and no clear-cut theory of pathogenesis can be made at this time.

CLINICAL FEATURES

The principal clinical features of acromegaly are as follows:

Acral enlargement
Facial enlargement
Headache
Skin changes
   Hyperpigmentation
   Coarseness
   Oiliness
   Increased pore size
   Hyperhidrosis
Peripheral nerve entrapments
Arthralgias
Proximal muscle weakness (myopathy)
Menstrual disturbances
Galactorrhea
Decreased libido
Fatigue
Visual field defects

The onset of acromegaly is usually in the third to the fifth decade. In the rare cases in which the hypersecretion of GH occurs before puberty and epiphysial closure, the clinical syndrome that results is gigantism. Before epiphysial bone fusion, long bone growth is stimulated by the excessive GH and proportionate growth results. Associated hypogonadism delays epiphysial closure and causes a prolonged growth period that contributes to the ultimate size. If the disease begins after epiphysial closure, proliferation of only certain bony structures and soft tissues occurs. The disease progresses slowly in most cases with gradual changes in facial and acral features. Previous photos of the patient taken over a period of years are helpful in documenting and charting the course of the disease.

Two older terms occasionally heard in a clinical discussion of this disorder are *fugitive acromegaly* and *burned-out acromegaly*. *Fugitive acromegaly* is a term coined by Cushing that describes patients with the disease in whom the degree of overgrowth is slight and the period of progression of the disease is short. *Burned-out acromegaly* refers to those cases in whom obvious overgrowth

210 *Disorders of the pituitary*

ceases after a period of years. Explanations for the "burned-out" condition include cessation of GH hypersecretion because of tumor infarction and limitation of growth of acral parts despite the continued presence of excessive GH in the plasma. A brief discussion of some of the clinical features follows.

Acral and facial enlargement

The alterations in bones and soft tissues are especially marked in the hands, feet, skull, and mandible (Plate 1). The hands are described as "spadelike" and

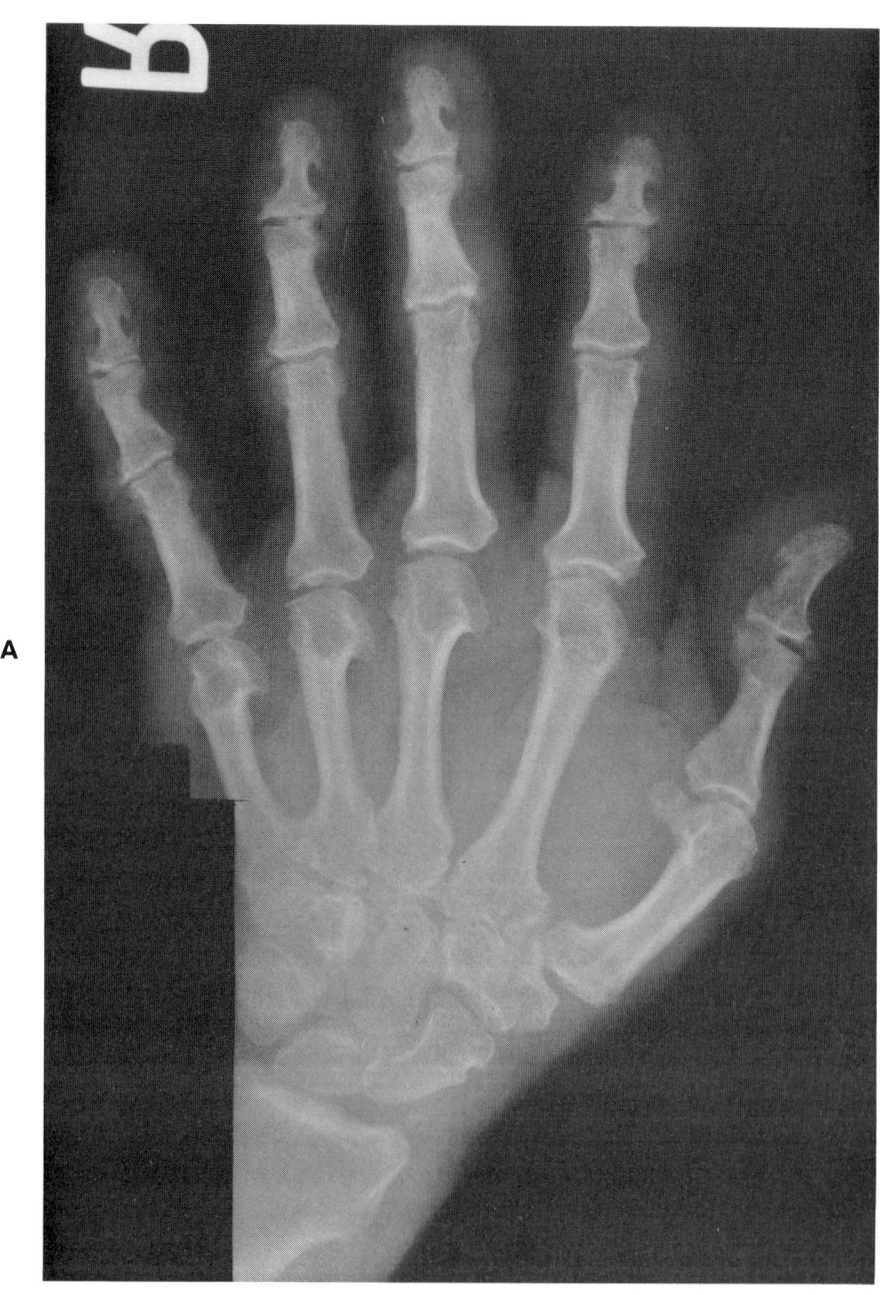

Fig. 6-1. Hand (**A**) and foot (**B**) x-ray film showing tufting.

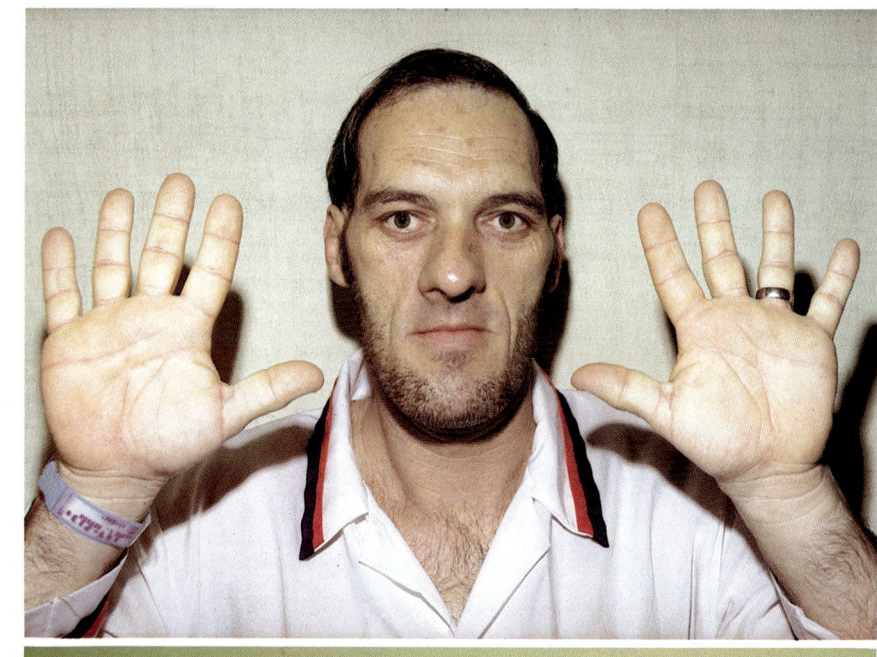

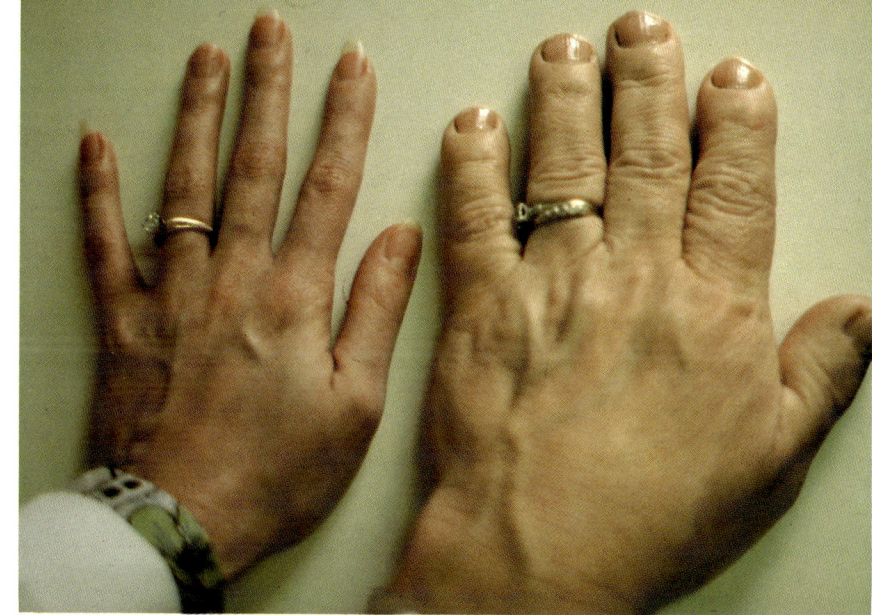

Plate 1. Adult patient with acromegaly. **A,** Typical appearance of adult patient with acromegaly. Prominence of malar, frontal, and mandibular regions and widening of digits are to be noted. Patient had 8 mm growth hormone–secreting microadenoma removed by transsphenoidal surgery. **B,** Normal subject's hand *(left)* compared with hand *(right)* of patient with well-advanced acromegaly showing "spadelike" appearance of hand with marked thickening of digits.

are characterized by a marked degree of thickening (as opposed to lengthening) of the digits. Tufting of the distal phalanges of the hands and feet is apparent on x-ray examination (Fig. 6-1). The increase in length and thickness of the mandible produces the characteristic "lantern jaw" appearance with resultant prognathism and overbite of the facial soft tissues. Overgrowth of the frontal, malar, and nasal bones account for the gross change in an individual's appearance and usually provide the clinician with an unmistakable but late guide to the diagnosis. Overgrowth of cartilage occurs in joints, nose, ears, and larynx. The latter contributes to the deep voice characteristic of acromegaly.

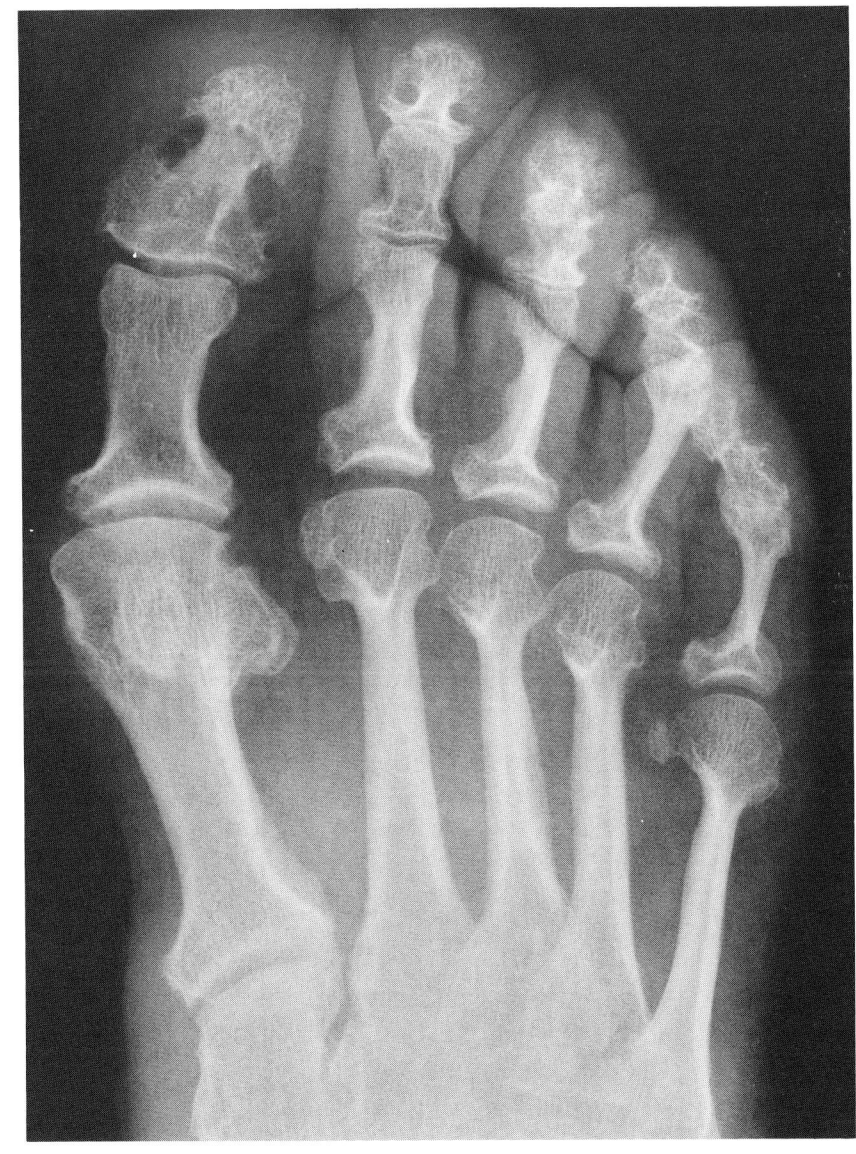

Fig. 6-1, cont'd. For legend see opposite page.

Visceromegaly results from the same tissue overgrowth and may affect the kidneys, lungs, liver, spleen, stomach, intestines, and salivary glands.

Headache

These are estimated to occur in 50% to 75% of all patients.[27,61] The headache pattern varies, the location and types of pain have no particular distinguishing features, and the mechanism for the headache is not always clear. In those patients with large tumors, stretching or distortion of the diaphragm sella (innervated by the first division of the trigeminal nerve) probably accounts for the pain and discomfort. However, this mechanism does not explain headache in patients in whom the tumor is small and completely confined to the sella.[88]

Skin changes

The majority of patients with acromegaly complain of hyperhidrosis and an oiliness of the skin associated with an unpleasant odor. The skin is coarse, and the normal skin pores and markings are accentuated. Body hair is sometimes increased in amount and excessively coarse in texture. The hyperhidrosis and oiliness occur especially in the early, more active phase of the disease.

Peripheral nerve entrapments

Numbness and tingling of one or more extremities, so-called acroparesthesias, are early symptoms of acromegaly, the most common of which is the carpal tunnel syndrome. This syndrome is characterized by numbness and tingling in the thumb and index and middle fingers and, occasionally, weakness in the thenar musculature, all of which result from compression of the median nerve beneath the transverse carpal ligament at the wrist. The syndrome is frequently bilateral, and usually the symptoms are worse at night. Although the carpal tunnel syndrome is not unique to acromegaly, acromegalic patients are more prone to develop this compression neuropathy. Possible contributing factors to its development include compression of the median nerve by overgrowth of bone and soft tissue in the carpal tunnel, involvement of the median nerve by endoneural and perineural changes that occur characteristically in acromegaly, and altered fluid balance in the carpal tunnel. Other peripheral nerve manifestations include the relatively infrequent occurrence of a peripheral neuropathy characterized by paresthesias in the hands and feet, absent deep tendon reflexes in the lower extremities, and muscle weakness and atrophy thought by some to be related to altered glucose metabolism.

Arthralgias

Articular symptoms ranging from mild joint pains to severe degrees of arthritis are common in acromegaly. Bony overgrowth leads to distortion of the articular plate and altered joint mechanics. Articular cartilage proliferation initially widens the joint space, and as the disease progresses, cartilage may become eroded with resultant disabling arthritis. Fibrous thickening of the joint capsule and related ligaments may contribute to the discomfort.

Myopathy

Acromegalic patients frequently complain of muscle weakness and fatigability. Mastaglia et al[74] studied the clinical, biochemical, electromyographic, and pathologic aspects of neuromuscular function in 11 acromegalic patients and found that the proximal muscles are commonly the site of a patchy myopathic process. Electromyography (EMG) showed significant reduction of motor unit action potentials even in cases without clinical symptoms or demonstrable weakness. An elevated creatine phosphokinase (CPK) in five of their 11 patients supported the EMG evidence of a myopathy and implies an abnormal permeability of muscle fiber membranes.

The pathophysiology of this patchy myopathy is not well understood. Copious amounts of glycogen in muscle have been observed,[74] but this is not an unexpected finding, since GH is known to promote glycogen deposition in skeletal muscle.[23] However, this does not appear to explain the muscle fiber dysfunction entirely. The severity of the myopathic process in acromegalic patients as judged by EMG does not correlate with the duration of the disease or with GH levels.[74]

Other findings

Many female patients with acromegaly complain of menstrual disturbances, whereas male acromegalic patients often have decreased libido and impotence. In 26 male patients studied by Jadresic et al,[49] no correlation between GH level or sellar size and decreased libido or impotence existed. Reduced follicle-stimulating hormone (FSH) and luteinizing hormone (LH) levels or elevated prolactin values may be responsible for these findings.[82]

Galactorrhea may be a symptom in acromegaly resulting either from prolactin production by a GH-secreting adenoma, lactogenic activity of GH, or interference with release of prolactin-inhibiting factor. Interestingly, the presence of two separate pituitary adenomas, one secreting prolactin and the other GH was documented in one case.[108]

ASSOCIATED MEDICAL CONDITIONS AND METABOLIC DISTURBANCES

The principal conditions associated with acromegaly include hypertension, abnormalities in carbohydrate metabolism, organomegaly, arteriosclerotic cardiovascular disease, and degenerative arthritis.

The association of cardiomegaly and congestive heart failure with acromegaly was described by Huckard[46] in 1895 and by Fournier[31] in 1896. Although it is a common finding in acromegaly, its pathogenesis is incompletely understood.[16] The list of proposed etiologic factors include hypertension, coronary artery disease, valvular heart disease, compensatory hypertrophy following increased work load induced by generalized splanchnomegaly and somatomegaly, and direct humoral effects of GH.[65] Some investigators have suggested that a specific heart muscle disease in acromegalic patients, "acromegalic cardiomyopathy," exists in many cases.[2,50,84,94] Although disproportionate cardiomegaly (cardiac enlargement greater than enlargement of other visceral organs) has been said to be a uniform finding in acromegaly, the autopsy study of 27 patients performed by Lie and Grossman[65] found that this was not always present. Although cardiomegaly occurred in 81% of their patients, disproportionate cardiomegaly (in comparison with hepatomegaly, splenomegaly and renomegaly) was not a uniform finding, occurring in one fourth to one third of all their cases. The cardiomegaly appeared to be related to the duration of acromegaly and was present in both hypertensive and normotensive patients. The study of Lie and Grossman did not support the common belief that premature atherosclerosis and diabetes were causally related to cardiomegaly and cardiac failure in acromegaly.[65] For instance, 33% of their patients had cardiomegaly without hypertension, atherosclerosis, or severe valvular disease, a finding which may support the notion of an acromegalic cardiomyopathy.[65]

Martins et al[73] and Savage et al[97] have shown that echocardiography is a sensitive tool for detecting cardiac abnormalities in acromegalic patients, often before they are otherwise apparent. Both of the studies included a subgroup of patients with no history of hypertension or other demonstrable cardiac disease in whom there was echocardiographic left ventricular wall thickening. Although it is generally believed that this cardiomyopathy is related to prolonged acromegaly or very high GH concentrations,[73] no actual causal relationship has been established, and successful therapy of the acromegaly has not clearly been shown to reverse the condition.[97]

Hepatomegaly often occurs, and a reversible increase in the size of the kidneys may result in significant changes in renal function.

An impaired glucose tolerance curve is present in about half the cases of acromegaly, but clinical diabetes mellitus only occurs in approximately 10% of patients. It is possible that some acromegalic patients with frank diabetes are those who have a hereditary predisposition to the disease. Diabetic retinopathy is unusual. Following successful therapy of the acromegaly, glucose tolerance usually improves coincident with the fall in GH levels.

PROGNOSIS

Acromegaly is associated with a reduced life expectancy. Of 194 cases reviewed by Wright et al,[118] 26% of the deaths occurred before the age of 50 years and 64% by the age of 60 years. The number of deaths was almost twice that expected from the general age-matched population. There were an increased number of deaths resulting from cardiovascular and respiratory disease in male patients and cerebrovascular and respiratory disease in female patients.[118] An earlier study of 100 acromegalic patients by Evans et al[28] reported 50% of deaths before the age of 50 years and 89% by the age of 60 years. The prospective study of 57 patients by McGuffin et al[77] produced a notable lack of correlation between hypertension, cardiac disease, and the GH concentration in acromegaly. It is believed that effective treatment of the disease may favorably influence overall mortality.

DIAGNOSTIC EVALUATION

The diagnosis should present no difficulty in those cases with fairly advanced clinical features. The appearance is quite typical and straightforward.[48] In the early stages of the disease however, one must be more dependent on neuroradiologic and endocrine studies to establish the diagnosis.

The only other entity that may superficially resemble acromegaly is the rare condition of pachydermoperiostitis. In this unusual condition, hypertrophic osteoarthropathy is combined with certain acromegalic features, including thickening of the skin of the hands, forearms, and legs and accentuation of facial folds.[81] Pachydermoperiostitis may occur in disorders of the lungs, most commonly bronchogenic carcinoma, but also with other intrathoracic malignancies, lung abscesses, bronchiectasis, empyema, cyanotic cardiac malformations, biliary cirrhosis, and other disorders. A familial form of pachydermoperiostitis (Touraine-Salente-Golé syndrome) is unrelated to malignancy, and neither of the forms of this disease are associated with elevated GH levels.[81]

Endocrine testing

An endocrinologic evaluation is important in establishing and confirming the diagnosis, determining the functional capacity of the normal pituitary, and evaluating the effectiveness of therapy. Endocrine studies are discussed in detail in Chapter 4. The baseline studies determine the status of pituitary endocrine function, and the special studies (GH determination, both baseline and during a glucose tolerance test, and determination of somatomedin-C levels) document the diagnosis of acromegaly. The TRH test has potential value in assessing the effectiveness of treatment and should be performed before and following therapeutic procedures, especially surgery.

A specific radioimmunoassay is available for one of the somatomedins, somatomedin-C, and is used in the diagnosis of acromegaly and in assessing clinical disease activity. Somatomedin-C levels may actually be a more accurate indicator of activity of acromegaly than levels of GH, since the acute fluctuations that occur in GH levels do not result in similar, rapid changes in somatomedin-C. Rieu et al[93] measured serum somatomedin levels in 92 acromegalic patients and found significant correlations between somatomedin and GH levels and the clinical activity of the disease. Their results indicated that measurements of serum somatomedins can be helpful in the diagnosis and assessment of the activity of the disease. Similar findings have been noted by others.[14,110] Although in untreated acromegaly somatomedin-C blood levels accurately reflect GH activity, there have been variances that do not appear to relate to any of the factors just mentioned.[104] More information related to physiology of GH can be found in Chapter 2.

216 *Disorders of the pituitary*

Neuroradiologic studies

Neuroradiologic evaluation in patients suspected of harboring a GH-producing adenoma consists of a lateral coned-down skull film centered on the sella turcica and sphenoid sinus and a high-resolution coronal computed tomographic (CT) scan (see Chapter 5).

Skull film. The skull film serves to determine the overall size of the sella, the presence and degree of surrounding bone erosion, height of the maxilla (Fig. 6-2), and the configuration of the sphenoid sinus—an important aspect of the examination if transsphenoidal surgery is selected as the treatment option.

CT scan. The definitive radiologic study is a high resolution *coronal* CT scan using 1.5 mm slices through the entire sella turcica (see Chapter 5). This important study usually confirms the presence and determines the size and configuration of the tumor and the degree of suprasellar or lateral extension. *Axial* 1.5 mm slices through the suprasellar region, sella turcica, and sphenoid sinus may provide further information concerning the configuration of the sphenoid

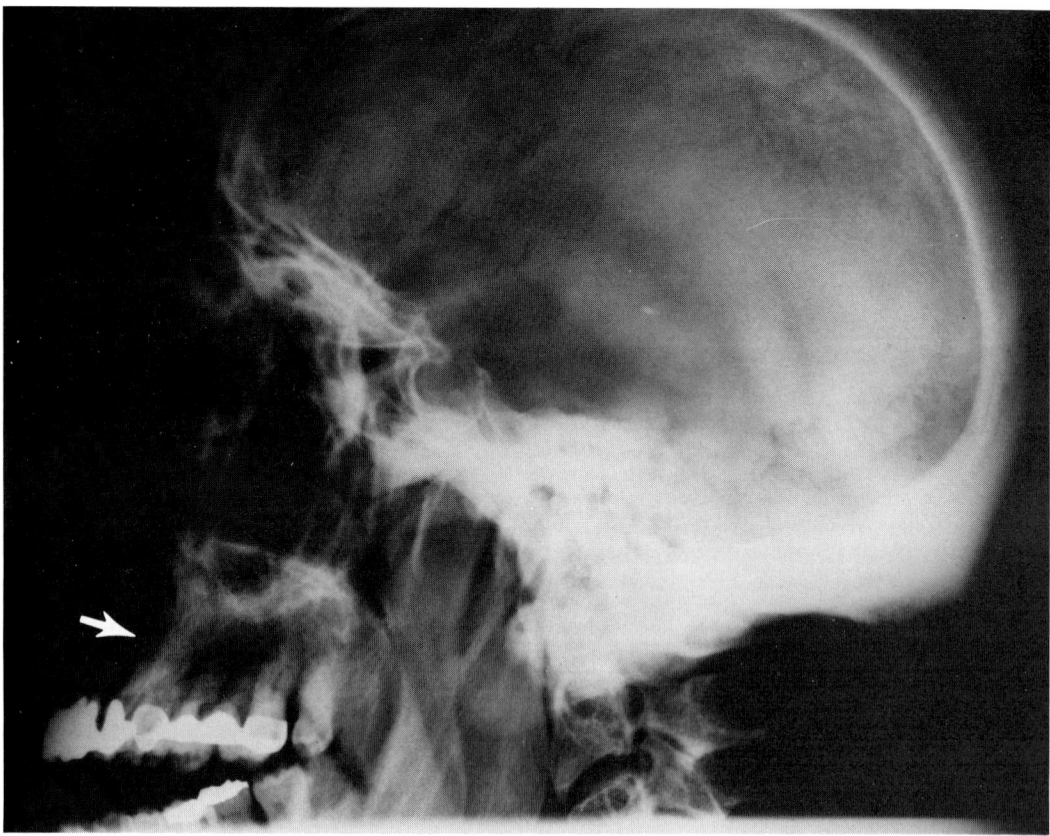

Fig. 6-2. Lateral skull film in patient with advanced acromegaly showing increased height of maxilla.

and may demonstrate erosion of the clivus or extension into the anterior, middle, or posterior cranial fossae.

Other neurodiagnostic studies such as cerebral angiography, pneumoencephalography, and polytomography are no longer recommended in the routine neuroradiologic evaluation of patients with acromegaly.

TREATMENT

In addition to the disfigurement it causes, acromegaly impairs a subject's normal health and life expectancy, and thus, most clinicians agree that definitive treatment should be started as early as possible.

Criteria of cure

Ideally, successful therapy will result in clinical improvement, reduction in basal GH levels to less than 5 ng/ml, suppression of GH levels following an oral glucose load, normalization of somatomedin-C levels, and a normal GH response to TRH administration. From a practical standpoint, most clinicians accept clinical improvement, GH levels less than 5 ng/ml, and normal glucose suppression of GH as evidence of cure.

Many treated patients report some regression in ring and shoe size, and some exhibit improvement in facial features (Fig. 6-3). Such physical changes, if present, occur more rapidly following surgical than medical or radiation therapy,

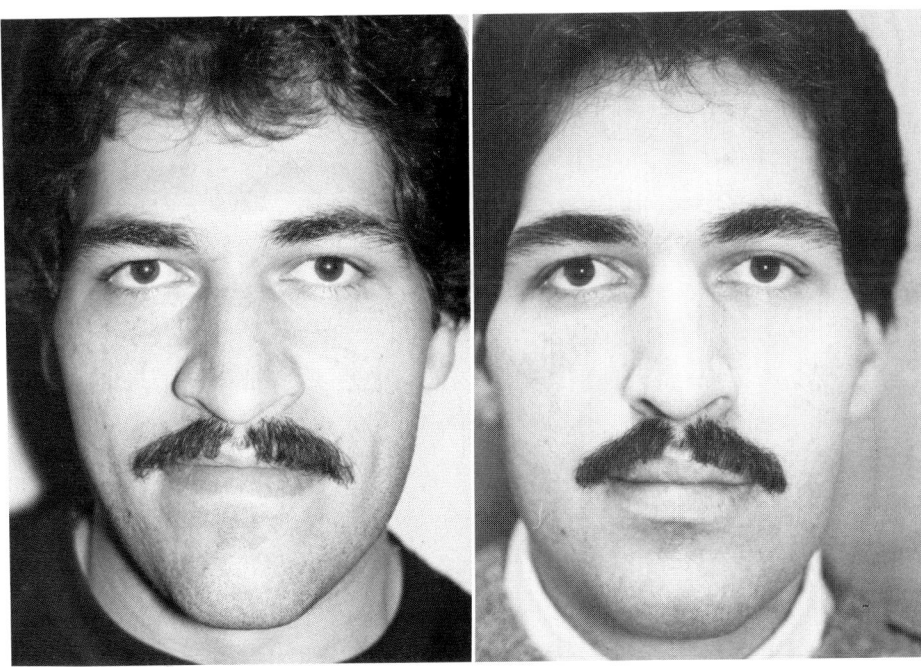

Fig. 6-3. Improvement in facial features 8 months after surgical treatment for acromegaly. **A,** Preoperative. **B,** Eight months postoperative.

probably because of the more rapid normalization of GH levels. The benefits usually occur when the disease is in a relatively early stage and are not nearly as impressive as the significant changes that occur in patients with Cushing's disease when a cure is obtained (compare Fig. 6-3 with Plate 2).

Surgery, irradiation, and pharmacotherapy are all effective therapies to treat this problem.

Surgery

We believe that surgery is the most practical option for treatment and, furthermore, that transsphenoidal surgery is currently the best surgical approach for removing pituitary tumors causing acromegaly. In experienced hands, this operation not only offers the best chance for cure of the disease but is an acceptable procedure in terms of morbidity and mortality. These latter issues, along with the technical aspects of the operation, are discussed in Chapter 12. Thus, in addressing cure rates obtainable with surgery, only series treated by the modern transsphenoidal surgical procedure will be reported. The majority of neurosurgeons experienced in the treatment of pituitary tumors currently use the transsphenoidal approach.

As shown in Table 6-1, several neurosurgeons have reported cure rates ranging from 44% to 90%. Not all have used the same criteria for cure. For instance, both Laws et al[63] and Wilson's group[9,43] use GH levels <10 ng/ml as criteria for cure, whereas most investigators use a value of <5 ng/ml. Obviously, the level arbitrarily chosen (<10 versus <5) has a significant bearing on reported cure rates. These cure rates refer mainly to immediate cures, and unfortunately not many authors have addressed the issue of long-term cure (i.e., >10 years) of acromegaly by transsphenoidal surgery (see opposite page).

The surgical results are influenced by several factors. Two important determinants, apart from the skill and experience of the surgeon, are the size and invasiveness of the tumor. For instance, Laws et al[63] obtained a cure in 87.5% of 18 patients with microadenomas, as opposed to a 68% cure rate in 39 cases with adenomas that filled the sella but remained confined by the dura, some of which had suprasellar extension.

Although not all authors agree, previous radiation or surgery appears to adversely influence the results of transsphenoidal surgery. Although Wilson's group[9,43] reported that remission was achieved in 74% of patients in whom previous therapy (irradiation, cryosurgery, and/or craniotomy) had been given, it is our belief that the true figure for cure in these patients will be considerably lower when they are followed for 5 to 10 years or longer. Any experienced surgeon appreciates the great difficulties encountered in trying to cure with transsphenoidal surgery a patient who has recurrent and/or persistent disease following a previous transsphenoidal operation. In our opinion, "cures" in this group are few and far between, and some therapy other than surgery should be seriously considered in these cases.

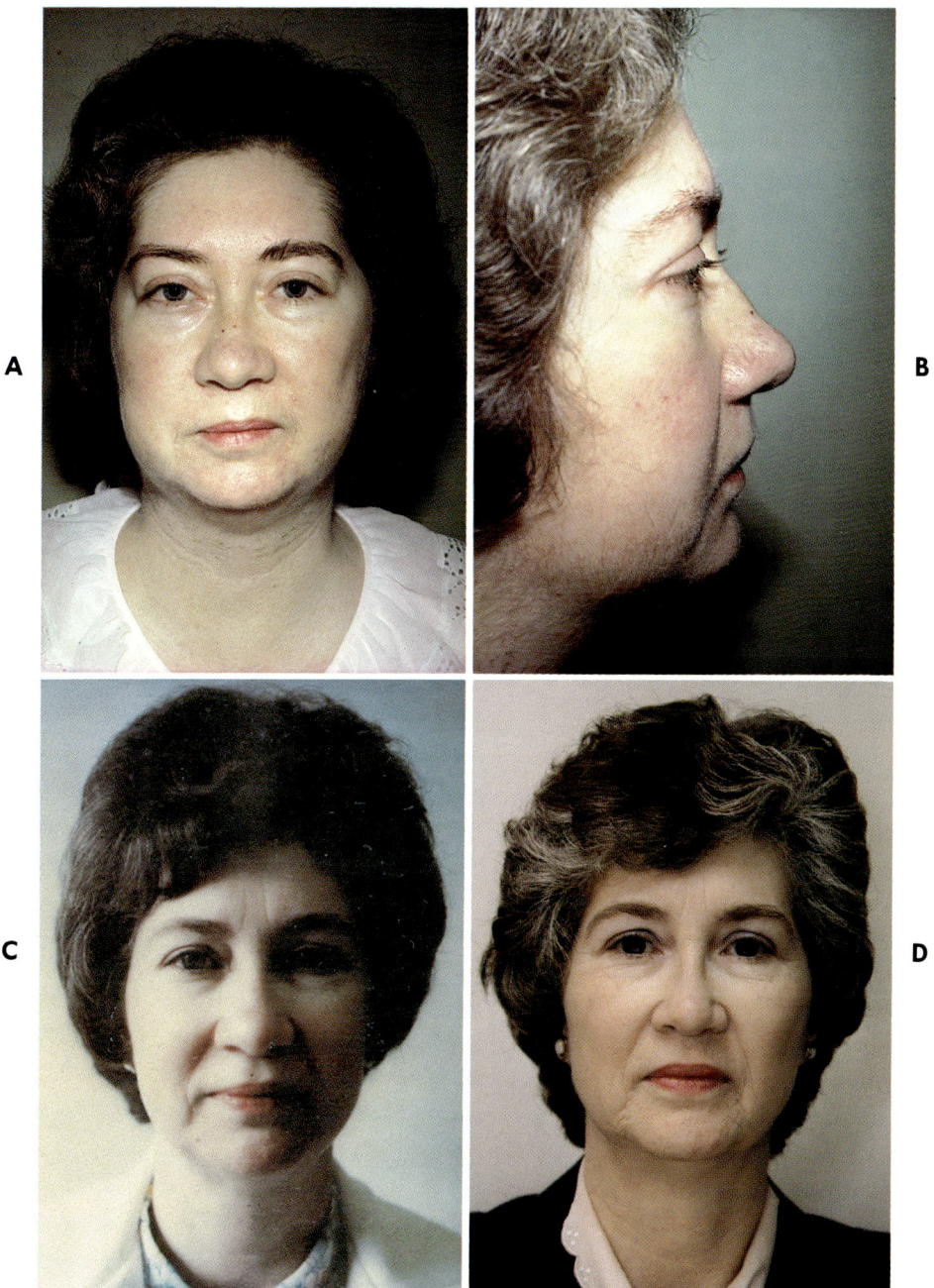

Plate 2. Adult patient with Cushing's syndrome. **A** and **B,** Typical appearance of patient with Cushing's syndrome. **C,** Same patient 1¼ years after transsphenoidal removal of 6 mm ACTH-secreting pituitary microadenoma. Both clinical response and endocrine testing indicated cure. **D,** Same patient 7 years following surgery. Curative status maintained.

Table 6-1
Results of transsphenoidal surgery in acromegaly

Series	Number of cases	Number cured	Percentage	Surgically related hypopituitarism	Incidence of postoperative CSF rhinorrhea (%)	Surgical mortality (%)	Level of GH used as criteria for cure (ng/ml)
Arafah, 1980[3]	25	17	68	12	0	0	<5
Balagura, 1981[7]	132	—	58	*	*	*	<5
Bøhmer, 1974[11]	23	16	70	17	0	0	<6
Emory series, 1985	64	45	70	8	0	0	<5
Faglia, 1978[29]	18	12	67	17§	†	†	<10
Garcia-Uria, 1978[33]	41	31	78	10	10	0	<10
Giovanelli, 1976[35]	27	12	44	*	11	0	<10
Giovanelli, Fahlbusch, et al, (1980)[34]	57	47	82	7	2	0	<5**
Hardy, 1979[41]	120	94	78	11	0.8	0.8	<5
Laws, 1979[63]	80	53	66	16	1.3	0	<10
Leavens, 1977[64]	16	12	75	‖	12.5	0	<5
Lüdecke, 1976[69]	80	70	87.5	*	*	0	<5
Quabbe,¶ 1982[89]	152	83 (GH <5) 121 (<10)	55 80	17	2.6	—	<5
Teasdale, 1982[105]	28	19	68	25‡	0	0	<10
Tucker, 1980[109]	32	24	75	13	3	0	<5
Williams, 1975[117]	59	39	66	*	1.7	0	<5
Wilson et al, 1982[9]	137	106	77	2	5	0	<10

*Incidence not clear from report.
†Not mentioned in report.
‡Seven patients, or 25%, were "hypoadrenal" postoperatively, and 4, or 14%, were "hypothyroid." It is not clear whether some of these patients were both "hypoadrenal" and "hypothyroid."
§One pituitary-target organ axis only was impaired in three patients.
‖All but two of the 16 patients required cortisone and thyroid replacement after surgery.
¶Cooperative Study involving 12 German Clinics.
**Or <10 but suppressed with glucose load.

These impressions regarding the effect of previous treatment do not apply to patients treated medically, for there is not information available that provides data as to the effect of medical treatment for acromegaly on the cure rate that is achieved with subsequent transsphenoidal surgery.

Although transsphenoidal surgery provides an impressive cure rate as evidenced by immediate reductions in GH, the important question to be answered is how effective this treatment modality is over a long period of time (i.e., >10 years). In our opinion, it is reasonable to assume that if a patient remains free of the disease following surgery for a period of 10 years, the prospects for tumor recurrence after this interval of time are very low.

Relatively few series have addressed the issue of long-term results in acromegaly following transsphenoidal surgery. The principal reason for the relative dearth of long-term studies is the fact that a number of neurosurgeons, even those with considerable experience, have not used the operation long enough to have a large series treated longer than 10 years. In a relatively small series, Knappe et al[55] maintained normalization of GH in nine of 10 patients 10 years following transsphenoidal surgery.

Irradiation

There are two general types of radiation therapy that have been used to treat acromegaly, conventional electromagnetic and heavy particle irradiation. A description of these types of irradiation and results in the treatment of this condition are found in Chapter 13.

Conventional electromagnetic irradiation. As an example of what can be achieved, Eastman et al[26] reported results indicating that conventional radiation therapy is an effective mode of therapy for pituitary tumors causing acromegaly and, furthermore, there is the obvious implication that it would be an appropriate therapeutic option to use as primary therapy for these patients. Against this argument is the fact that radiation requires a relatively long period of time before the effects are seen, and more importantly, there are the serious delayed risks of radiation in patients who are expected to survive long periods after administration of the therapy. Thus, although the immediate and short-term risks of transsphenoidal surgery are greater than with conventional radiation therapy, the potential long-range consequences of radiation, in our opinion, outweigh any therapeutic advantages of this mode of treatment when used as primary therapy. It would seem preferable to reserve radiation as a primary therapy in those acromegalic patients with surgically incurable tumors or when surgery cannot be performed because of poor health.

Heavy particle irradiation. The experiences of both Kjellberg et al[54] and Lawrence, Linfoot et al[61,62,67] indicate that good control of acromegaly can be achieved by *heavy particle therapy* with an acceptable incidence of side effects. As a primary form of therapy for acromegaly, however, this treatment modality is not used as much today as it was 10 to 12 years ago. Its relative decline is related to increasing use of transsphenoidal surgery and to increasing concerns over the long-term effects of high doses of irradiation.

Pharmacotherapy

Over the years, a number of pharmacologic agents have been used for the treatment of acromegaly. These have included estrogen, chlorpromazine, antiserotonin drugs, and dopamine agonists. The most effective and practical pharmacologic agents currently in use are the long-acting dopamine agonists such as bromocriptine or lergotrile. Clinical studies have shown that bromocriptine has a beneficial effect on the disease as evidenced by symptomatic improvement and reduction in elevated GH levels. Bromocriptine was effective in lowering serum GH levels in up to 75% of patients, but in only 20% were the levels reduced to normal in the series reported by Besser et al.[10] Shrinkage in size of the tumor has been reported in isolated cases.[83,112] However, it may turn out that the tumors that exhibit shrinkage are those that secrete both GH and prolactin.[57] Hyperprolactinemia was present in two patients with acromegaly in whom there was radiologic evidence of shrinkage in the series of Wass et al.[112] One relatively recent study showed no significant beneficial effects of bromocriptine in 18 patients.[66] However, this study has been criticized by Thorner et al[106] for several reasons, the main one being that an inadequate dose of bromocriptine was used. Progressive enlargement of the sella despite treatment that restored serum GH levels to normal has also been reported.[96]

The amount of bromocriptine required for therapeutic responses in acromegaly is usually much higher than that which is effective in hyperprolactinemic states, and dosages from 15 to 50 mg/day are commonly needed. As with patients harboring prolactinomas, continuous treatment with bromocriptine is required as withdrawal of the drug is associated with a prompt return of elevated serum GH levels. This finding emphasizes the major shortcoming of bromocriptine therapy for acromegaly, namely *that the drug is not tumoricidal*. Bromocriptine may serve a tumoristatic role in some cases, but it does not effect tumor kill. Although bromocriptine is therapeutically beneficial, it is our opinion that it should not be used as primary therapy for pituitary tumors causing acromegaly in otherwise healthy subjects. The drug is not tumoricidal and effects only a partial reduction of GH in the majority of cases. Its high cost, side effects, and the probable necessity for lifelong continuation of the drug are also distractors.

Nevertheless, it is our opinion that bromocriptine may have an important role in acromegaly under certain special clinical situations. These include (1) patients who are not candidates for other forms of therapy—This would include patients who are not surgical candidates either for reasons of poor health or advanced age; (2) those who fail to achieve a cure by transsphenoidal surgery and who are to be treated with radiation—In these cases, bromocriptine may provide symptomatic relief from the disease until the radiation therapy becomes clinically apparent in 2 to 4 years; and (3) those who receive the drug as a preoperative adjunct to surgery—In these cases, daily administration of bromocriptine for 6 to 8 weeks before surgery might cause shrinkage of the tumor, theoretically making total excision easier and more certain. However, this issue requires considerably more study before determining its clinical usefulness. In all these above situations, it appears that a clinical trial of the drug is necessary to predict which patients will respond.

THERAPEUTIC DECISION MAKING

The availability of more than one effective treatment modality in acromegaly stresses the need for appropriate and thoughtful therapeutic decision making on the part of the physician.

"Virgin" acromegaly

The "virgin" acromegalic patient has never received definitive therapy for the disease. If the patient is healthy and the diagnosis is confirmed and the CT appearance does not indicate a surgically inaccessible or invasive tumor, the best therapeutic option currently available is transsphenoidal surgery performed by an experienced surgeon. A realistic cure rate in this group of patients is on the order of 70% to 75%.

In "virgin" acromegalic patients who are in poor or unstable health or who do not wish to undergo a surgical procedure, primary treatment with conventional or heavy particle irradiation therapy is appropriate. The expense and long distance involved in obtaining heavy particle therapy makes this form of treatment available to only a minority of patients. Thus from a practical standpoint, supervoltage conventional radiotherapy is a reasonable and appropriate form of treatment for this group. Bromocriptine can be administered during the initial years after delivery of therapy for symptomatic relief until the effects of radiation become manifest if the patient is a bromocriptine responder.

Persistent or recurrent acromegaly following previous surgical and/or radiation therapy

Following previous radiation therpy. In patients who do not achieve a cure following conventional x-ray therapy, transsphenoidal microsurgery should be considered as the therapeutic option of choice. Although the previous radiotherapy can potentially leave some scarring in the sella that may affect the cure rate, it is our opinion that transsphenoidal surgery is the best therapeutic option in this group.

Following previous surgery. Experience has shown that transsphenoidal surgery in patients who have undergone previous surgery is not likely to result in a cure. For this reason, the appropriate treatment in persistent or recurrent acromegaly following surgery is radiation, possibly in conjunction with bromocriptine.

Preoperative surgical therapy

In recent years, there has been interest in shrinking pituitary adenomas with bromocriptine before transsphenoidal surgery in the hope that this change would facilitate surgery and thus enhance the cure rate. This therapeutic approach has been aimed more at prolactinomas than GH-producing tumors.[8] Even in prolactinomas where dramatic preoperative reductions in tumor size during bromocriptine therapy have been achieved, there is no clear evidence that the tumor is easier to remove or that the cure rate is enhanced. In fact, there is the possibility that long-term preoperative treatment might reduce the chances of obtaining a cure. Weiss[116] believes that preoperative bromocriptine treatment of acromegalics may improve surgical cure rates, but in our opinion, more study and documentation is necessary before recommending bromocriptine as preoperative therapy.

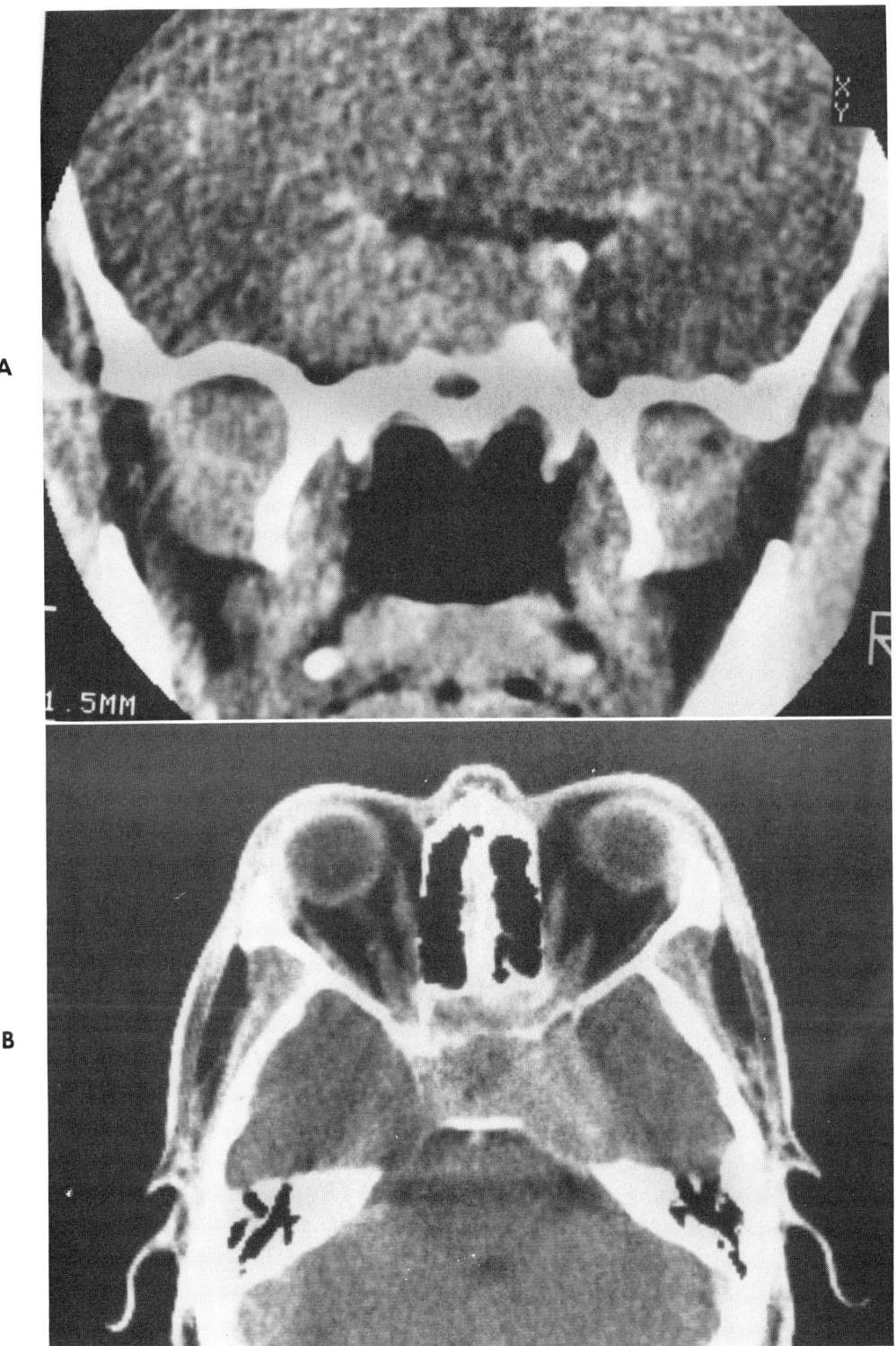

Fig. 6-4. CT scans of 39-year-old woman with acromegaly. Preoperative coronal (**A**) and axial (**B**) views show large sellar mass with extension into region of cavernous sinus and medial portion of middle cranial fossa.

Continued.

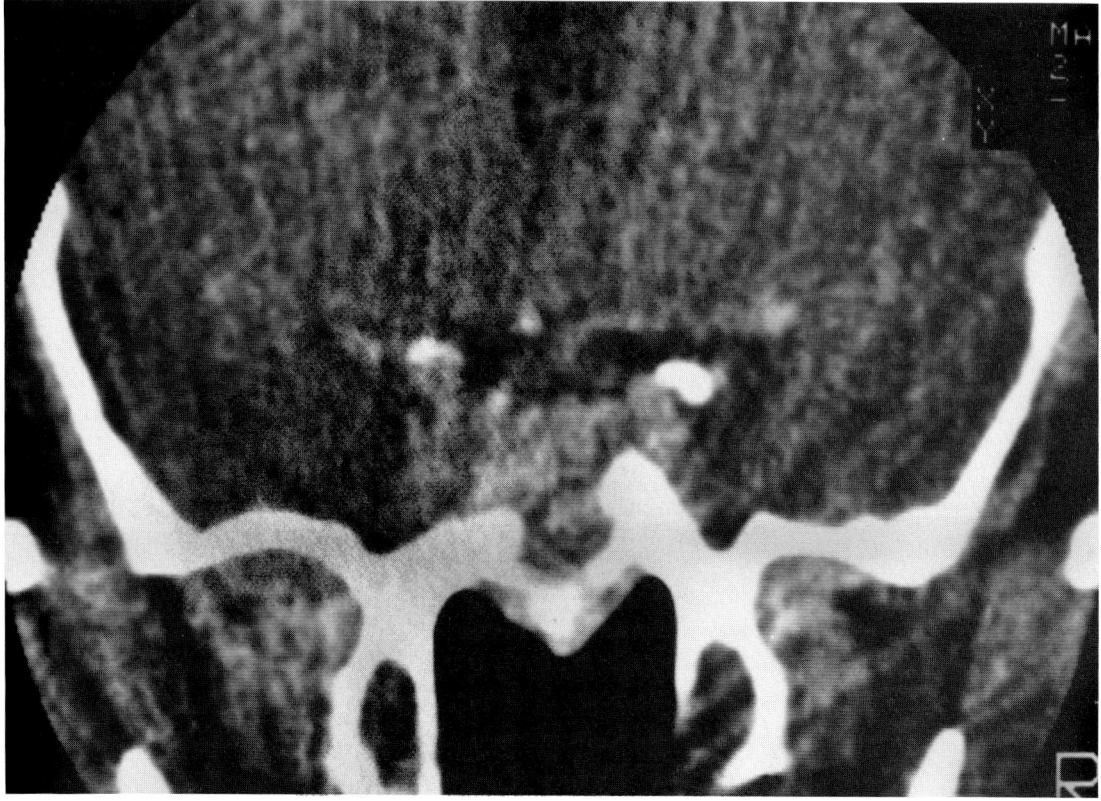

Fig. 6-4, cont'd. Postoperative coronal scan (**C**) shows residual tumor, but mass is much smaller than on preoperative scans.

Case study

The following case summary illustrates some of the problems that may be encountered in the management of these cases:

> A 39-year-old woman was noted by her physician to have the physical stigmata of acromegaly. A serum GH level was found to be 68.5 ng/ml. During the glucose suppressibility test, the level rose to 74.5 ng/ml. A CT of the sella showed a large sellar mass extending laterally to the left with erosion of the sellar floor and soft tissue within the sphenoid sinus (Fig. 6-4, *A* and *B*).
>
> The patient elected a surgical option despite the fact that she was advised that the appearance of the tumor on the CT scan indicated that a cure may not be achieved. She underwent transsphenoidal surgery, and a subtotal removal of a GH-secreting pituitary adenoma that had invaded the dura, cavernous sinus, bone, and sphenoid sinus was performed.
>
> The patient had no difficulties with her operative procedure, but the GH level remained elevated to 29.8 ng/ml. A postoperative CT showed residual tumor (Fig. 6-4, *C*). Options discussed with the patient at this time were radiation therapy or medical treatment with bromocriptine. She refused radiation and chose to use bromocriptine. The drug was given in a dosage of 20 mg/day in divided doses for 8 months without any change in the GH level. At that time, the patient underwent radiation therapy with some symptomatic improvement and a subsequent fall of the serum GH level to 12 ng/ml.

This case demonstrates the options available for treating acromegaly. Not all GH-secreting tumors are responsive to bromocriptine. The GH level may decline further with time following radiation. The patient continues to be followed.

SUMMARY

Acromegaly is a disease caused by excessive secretion of GH, nearly always by a pituitary adenoma. It is a disorder that produces characteristic clinical features and associated systemic changes that, when established, should present no diagnostic problems. The laboratory diagnosis is based on persistent elevations of GH, failure of oral glucose to suppress the elevated GH levels, and elevated somatomedin-C levels. Neuroradiologic studies consist of a lateral skull film and a high-resolution coronal CT scan.

There is good evidence that acromegaly shortens life primarily through adverse effects on the cardiovascular system. Thus some form of treatment is mandatory, and effective options include transsphenoidal surgery, irradiation, and pharmacotherapy. In the healthy "virgin" acromegalic patient, it is our opinion that transsphenoidal surgery is the treatment of choice; but in patients with recurrent or persistent disease, radiation in conjunction with bromocriptine is probably the best course to recommend.

REFERENCES

1. Allen JP, Cook DM, Greer MA, et al: Evidence that acromegaly is not a hypothalamic disease. *Trans Assoc Am Physicians* 86:272, 1973.
2. Aloia JF, Field RA: The heart and the endocrine system: Part 1. Effect of the pituitary on the heart and great vessels, in Conn HL, Horwitz O (eds): *Cardiac and Vascular Disease*. Philadelphia, Lea & Febiger, 1971, vol 2.
3. Arafah BM, Brodkey JS, Kaufman B, et al: Transsphenoidal microsurgery in the treatment of acromegaly and gigantism. *J Clin Endocrinol Metab* 50:578, 1980.
4. Arosio M, Giovanelli MA, Riva E, et al: Clinical use of pre- and postsurgical evaluation of abnormal GH responses in acromegaly. *J Neurosurg* 59:402, 1983.
5. Asa SL, Bilbao JM, Kovacs K, et al: Hypothalamic neuronal hamartoma associated with pituitary growth hormone cell adenoma and acromegaly. *Acta Neuropathol* 52:231, 1980.
6. Ashcraft MW, Hartzband PI, Van Herle AJ, et al: A unique growth factor in patients with acromegaloidism. *J Clin Endocrinol Metab* 57:272, 1983.
7. Balagura S, Derome P, Guiot G: Acromegaly: Analysis of 132 cases treated surgically. *Neurosurgery* 8:413, 1981.
8. Barrow DL, Tindall GT, Kovacs K, et al: Clinical and pathological effects of bromocriptine on prolactin secreting and other pituitary tumors. *J Neurosurg* 60:1, 1984.
9. Baskin DS, Boggan JE, Wilson CB: Transsphenoidal microsurgical removal of growth hormone–secreting pituitary adenomas. *J Neurosurg* 56:634, 1982.
10. Besser GM, Wass JAH, Thorner MO: Bromocriptine in the medical management of acromegaly. *Adv Biochem Psychopharmacol* 23:191, 1980.
11. Bøhmer T, Berdal P, Haugen HN: Transsphenoidal subtotal hypophysectomy in the treatment of acromegaly. *Acta Endocrinol* 77:477, 1974.
12. Boyd AE, Lebovitz HE, Pfeiffer JB: Stimulation of human-growth-hormone secretion by L-dopa. *N Engl J Med* 283:1425, 1970.
13. Buse J, Buse MG, Roberts WJ Jr: Eosinophilic adenoma of the pituitary and carcinoid tumor of the recto-sigmoid area. *J Clin Endocrinol Metab* 21:735, 1961.
14. Clemmons DR, Van Wyk JJ, Ridgway EC, et al: Evaluation of acromegaly by radioimmunoassay of somatomedin-C. *N Engl J Med* 301:1138, 1979.
15. Corenblum B, LeBlanc FE, Watanabe M: Acromegaly with an adenomatous pharyngeal pituitary. *JAMA* 243:1456, 1980.
16. Courville C, Mason VR: The heart in acromegaly. *Arch Intern Med* 61:704, 1938.
17. Cronin MJ, Rogol AD, Dabney LG, et al: Selective growth hormone and cyclic AMP stimulating activity is present in a human pancreatic islet cell tumor. *J Clin Endocrinol Metab* 55:381, 1982.
18. Cryer PE, Daughaday WH: Regulation of growth hormone secretion in acromegaly. *J Clin Endocrinol Metab* 29:386, 1969.
19. Cryer PE, Daughaday WH: Adrenergic modulation of growth hormone secretion in acromegaly: Suppression during phentolamine and phentolamine-isoproterenol administration. *J Clin Endocrinol Metab* 39:658, 1974.
20. Cushing H: The hypophysis cerebri: Clinical aspects of hyperpituitarism and of hypopituitarism. *JAMA* 53:249, 1909.
21. Cushing H, Davidoff LM: The pathological findings in four autopsied cases of acromegaly with a discussion of their significance. Monograph no. 22, The Rockefeller Institute for Medical Research (New York), Baltimore, Waverly Press, 1927.
22. Dabek JT: Bronchial carcinoid tumour with acromegaly in two patients. *J Clin Endocrinol Metab* 38:329, 1974.
23. Daughaday WH: The adenohypophysis, in Williams RH (ed): *Textbook of Endocrinology*, ed 5. Philadelphia, WB Saunders Co, 1974.
24. Daughaday WH: Pathophysiology of acromegaly, in Givens JR (ed): *Hormone-Secreting Pituitary Tumors*. Chicago, Year Book Medical Publishers Inc, 1982.
25. Daughaday WH, Hall K, Raben MS, et al: Somatomedin: Proposed designation for sulfation factor. *Nature* 235:107, 1972.
26. Eastman RC, Gorden P, Roth J: Conventional supervoltage irradiation is an effective treatment for acromegaly. *J Clin Endocrinol Metab* 48:931, 1979.
27. Eskildsen PC, Svendsen PA, Vang L, et al: Long-term treatment of acromegaly with bromocriptine. *Acta Endocrinol* 87:687, 1978.
28. Evans HM, Briggs, JH, Dixon JS: The physiology and chemistry of growth hormone, in Harris GW, Donovan BT (eds): *The Pituitary Gland*. Berkeley, Calif., University of California Press, 1966, vol 1.
29. Faglia G, Paracchi A, Ferrari C, et al: Evaluation of the results of trans-sphenoidal surgery in acromegaly by assessment of the growth-

hormone response to thyrotrophin-releasing hormone. *Clin Endocrinol* 8:373, 1978.
30. Feingold KR, Goldfine ID, Weinstein PR: Acromegaly with normal growth hormone levels and pituitary histology: Case report. *J Neurosurg* 50:503, 1979.
31. Fournier JBC: Acromegalie et troubles cardiovasculaires. Thesis. Paris, 1896, 1938.
32. Frohman LA: Diseases of the anterior pituitary, in Felig P, Baxter J, Brondus AE, et al (eds): *Endocrinology and Metabolism.* New York, McGraw-Hill Inc, 1981.
33. García-Uría J, del Pozo JM, Bravo G: Functional treatment of acromegaly by transsphenoidal mirosurgery. *J Neurosurg* 49:36, 1978.
34. Giovanelli MA, Fahlbusch R, Gaini SM, et al: Surgical treatment of growth hormone–secreting microadenomas, in Faglia G, Giovanelli MA, MacLeod RM (eds): *Pituitary Microadenomas.* Proceedings of the Serono Symposia, London. Academic Press Inc, 1980, vol 29.
35. Giovanelli MA, Motti EDF, Paracchi A, et al: Treatment of acromegaly by transsphenoidal microsurgery. *J Neurosurg* 44:677, 1976.
36. Gomez-Pan A, Tunbridge WMG, Duns A, et al: Hypothalamic hormone interaction in acromegaly. *Clin Endocrinol* 4:455, 1975.
37. Greenberg PB, Beck C, Martin TJ, et al: Synthesis and release of human growth hormone from lung carcinoma in cell culture. *Lancet* 1:350, 1972.
38. Hagen TC, Lawrence AM, Kacherian RE, et al: A dialyzable heat stable factor in acromegalic plasma associated with increased *in vitro* growth hormone release. *Proc Soc Exp Biol Med* 141:536, 1972.
39. Hagen TC, Lawrence AM, Kirsteins L: *In vitro* release of monkey pituitary growth hormone by acromegalic plasma. *J Clin Endocrinol Metab* 33:448, 1971.
40. Hardy J: Transsphenoidal microsurgical treatment of pituitary tumors, in Linfoot JA (ed): *Recent Advances in the Diagnosis and Treatment of Pituitary Tumors.* New York, Raven Press, 1979.
41. Hardy J, Somma M: Acromegaly: Surgical treatment by transsphenoidal microsurgical removal of the pituitary adenoma, in Tindall GT, Collins WF (eds): *Clinical Management of Pituitary Disorders.* New York, Raven Press, 1979.
42. Heitz PU: Multihormonal pituitary adenomas. *Horm Res* 10:1, 1979.
43. Hoi Sang U, Wilson CB, Tyrrell JB: Transsphenoidal microhypophysectomy in acromegaly. *J Neurosurg* 47:840, 1977.
44. Horvath E, Kovacs K, Scheithauer BW, et al: Pituitary adenomas producing growth hormone, prolactin, and one or more glycoprotein hormones: A histologic, immunohistochemical, and ultrastructural study of four surgically removed tumors. *Ultrastruct Pathol* 5:171, 1983.
45. Hoyte KM, Martin JB: Recovery from paradoxical growth hormone responses in acromegaly after transsphenoidal selective adenomectomy. *J Clin Endocrinol Metab* 41:656, 1975.
46. Huchard H: Anatomic pathologigue, lesions et troubles cardiovasculaires de l'acromegalie. *J Practiciens* 9:249, 1895.
47. Irie M, Tsushima T: Increase of serum growth hormone concentration following thyrotropin-releasing hormone injection in patients with acromegaly or gigantism. *J Clin Endocrinol Metab* 35:97, 1972.
48. Jackson IMD: Growth-hormone–secreting pituitary adenomas, in Post KD, Jackson IMD, Reichlin S (eds): *The Pituitary Adenoma.* New York, Plenum Medical Book Co, 1980.
49. Jadresic A, Banks LM, Child DF, et al: The acromegaly syndrome: Relation between clinical features, growth hormone values and radiological characteristics of the pituitary tumours. *Q J Med* 51:189, 1982.
50. Jonas EA, Aloia JF, Lane FJ: Evidence of subclinical heart muscle dysfunction in acromegaly. *Chest* 67:190, 1975.
51. Kaganowicz A, Farkouh NH, Frantz AG, et al: Ectopic human growth hormone in ovaries and breast cancer. *J Clin Endocrinol Metab* 48:5, 1979.
52. Kernohan JW, Sayre GP: Tumors of the pituitary gland and infundibulum, in *Atlas of Tumor Pathology.* Section X, Fascicle 36. Washington, D.C., Armed Forces Institute of Pathology, 1956.
53. Kinnman J: The prognosis in acromegaly treated by transanthro-sphenoidal operation. *Acta Otolaryngol* 82:420, 1976.
54. Kjellberg RN, Kliman B: Proton radiosurgery for functioning pituitary adenoma, in Tindall GT, Collins WF (eds): *Clinical Management of Pituitary Disorders.* New York, Raven Press, 1979.
55. Knappe G, Rohde W, Mennig H, et al: Ten years' follow-up of transsphenoidal pituitary surgery in acromegaly. *Endokrinologie* 79:423, 1982.
56. Kovacs K, Horvath E, Ezrin C: Pituitary adenomas. *Pathol Annu* 12:341, 1977.
57. Lamberts SWJ, Verleun T, Oosterom R: The interrelationship between the effects of soma-

tostatin and human pancreatic growth hormone–releasing factor on growth hormone release by cultured pituitary tumor cells from patients with acromegaly. *J Clin Endocrinol Metab* 58:250, 1984.
58. Landolt AM: Ultrastructure of human sella tumors: Correlations of clinical findings and morphology. *Acta Neurochir* 22(suppl):1, 1975.
59. Landolt AM: Pituitary adenomas: Clinico-morphologic correlations. *J Histochem Cytochem* 27:1395, 1979.
60. Lawrence AM, Goldfine ID, Kirsteins L: Growth hormone dynamics in acromegaly. *J Clin Endocrinol Metab* 31:239, 1970.
61. Lawrence JH, Tobias CA, Linfoot JA, et al: Successful treatment of acromegaly: Metabolic and clinical studies in 145 patients. *J Clin Endocrinol Metab* 31:180, 1970.
62. Lawrence JH, Tobias CA, Linfoot JA, et al: Heavy-particle therapy in acromegaly and Cushing's disease. *JAMA* 235:2307, 1976.
63. Laws ER Jr, Piepgras DG, Randall RV, et al: Neurosurgical management of acromegaly: Results in 82 patients treated between 1972 and 1977. *J Neurosurg* 50:454, 1979.
64. Leavens ME, Samaan NA, Jesse RH, et al: Clinical and endocrinological evaluation of 16 acromegalic patients treated by transsphenoidal surgery. *J Neurosurg* 47:853, 1977.
65. Lie JT, Grossman SJ: Pathology of the heart in acromegaly: Anatomic findings in 27 autopsied patients. *Am Heart J* 100:41, 1980.
66. Lindholm J, Riishede J, Vestergaard S, et al: No effect of bromocriptine in acromegaly: A controlled trial. *N Engl J Med* 304:1450, 1981.
67. Linfoot JA: Heavy ion therapy: Alpha particle therapy of pituitary tumors, in Linfoot JA (ed): *Recent Advances in the Diagnosis and Treatment of Pituitary Tumors*. New York, Raven Press, 1979.
68. Liuzzi A, Chiodini PG, Botalla L, et al: Inhibitory effect of L-dopa on GH release in acromegalic patients. *J Clin Endocrinol Metab* 35:941, 1972.
69. Lüdecke D, Kautzky R, Saeger W, et al: Selective removal of hypersecreting pituitary adenomas? An analysis of endocrine function, operative and microscopical findings in 101 cases. *Acta Neurochir* 35:27, 1976.
70. Marie P: Sur deux cas d'acromegalie: Hypertropie singuliere non congential des extremites supericures, infericures et cephalique. *Rev Med Paris* 6:297, 1886.
71. Martin JB: Pathophysiology of growth hormone regulation, in Tolis G, Labrie F, Martin JB, et al (eds): *Clinical Neuroendocrinology: A Pathophysiological Approach*. New York, Raven Press, 1979.
72. Martin JB: Management of hypersecretory pituitary adenomas. *Clin Neurosurg* 27:99, 1980.
73. Martins JB, Kerber RE, Sherman BM, et al: Cardiac size and function in acromegaly. *Circulation* 56:863, 1977.
74. Mastaglia FL, Barwick DD, Hall R: Myopathy in acromegaly. *Lancet* 2:907, 1970.
75. McCarty KS Jr, Bredesen DE, Vogel FS: Neoplasms of the anterior pituitary. *Neurosurgery* 3:96, 1978.
76. McGrath P: Volume and histology of the human pharyngeal hypophysis. *Aust NZ J Surg* 37:16, 1967.
77. McGuffin WL Jr, Sherman BM, Roth J, et al: Acromegaly and cardiovascular disorders: A prospective study. *An Intern Med* 81:11, 1974.
78. Melchionna RH, Moore RA: The pharyngeal pituitary gland. *Am J Pathol* 14:763, 1938.
79. Melmed S, Braunstein GD, Horvath E, et al: Pathophysiology of acromegaly. *Endocr Rev* 4:271, 1983.
80. Minkowski O: Uber einem Fall von adromegalie. *Klin Wochenschr* 24:371, 1887.
81. Nelson DH: Diseases of the anterior lobe of the pituitary gland, in Wintrobe MM, Thorn GW, Adams RD, et al (eds): *Harrison's Principles of Internal Medicine*, ed 7. New York, McGraw-Hill Book Co, 1974.
82. Nelson JC, Kollar DJ, Lewis JE: Growth hormone secretion in pituitary disease. *Arch Intern Med* 133:459, 1974.
83. Oppizzi G, Liuzzi A, Chiodini P, et al: Dopaminergic treatment of acromegaly: Different effects on hormone secretion and tumor size. *J Clin Endocrinol Metab* 58:988, 1984.
84. Pepine CJ, Aloia J: Heart muscle disease in acromegaly. *Am J Med* 48:530, 1970.
85. Perlroth MG, Tschudy DP, Waxman A, et al: Abnormalities of growth hormone regulation in acute intermittent porphyria. *Metabolism* 16:87, 1967.
86. Phillips LS, Vassilopoulou-Sellin R: Somatomedins: (First of two parts). *N Engl J Med* 302:371, 1980.
87. Phillips LS, Vassilopoulou-Sellin R: Somatomedins: (Second of two parts). *N Engl J Med* 302:438, 1980.
88. Pickett JBE, Layzer RB, Levin SR, et al: Neuromuscular complications of acromegaly. *Neurology* 25:638, 1975.
89. Quabbe HJ: Treatment of acromegaly by transsphenoidal operation, 90-yttrium implantation and bromocriptine: Results in 230 patients. *Clin Endocrinol* 16:107, 1982.

90. Rasmussen P, Lindholm J: Ectopic pituitary adenomas. *Clin Endocrinol* 11:69, 1979.
91. Reichlin S: Etiology of pituitary adenomas, in Post KD, Jackson IMD, Reichlin S (eds): *The Pituitary Adenoma*. New York, Plenum Medical Book Co, 1980.
92. Rhodes RH, Dusseau JJ, Boyd AS Jr, et al: Intrasellar neural-adenohyophyseal choristoma: A morphological and immunocytochemical study. *J Neuropathol Exp Neurol* 41:267, 1982.
93. Rieu M, Girard F, Bricaire H, et al: The importance of insulin-like growth factor (somatomedin) measurements in the diagnosis and surveillance of acromegaly. *J Clin Endocrinol Metab* 55:147, 1982.
94. Robinowitz D, Sper SP, Bladsoe T: The pituitary gland, in Harvey AM (ed): *The Principles and Practice of Medicine*, ed 18, New York, Appleton-Century-Crofts, 1972.
95. Salmon WD Jr, Daughaday WH: A hormonally controlled serum factor which stimulates sulfate incorporation by cartilage in vitro. *J Lab Clin Med* 49:825, 1957.
96. Salti IS: Bromocriptine fails to stop growth of eosinophilic adenomas in acromegaly, letter. *N Engl J Med* 301:386, 1979.
97. Savage DD, Henry WL, Eastman RC, et al: Echocardiographic assessment of cardiac anatomy and function in acromegalic patients. *Am J Med* 67:823, 1979.
98. Scheithauer BW: Surgical pathology of the pituitary and sellar region, in Laws ER Jr, Randall RV, Kern EB, et al (eds): *Management of Pituitary Adenomas and Related Lesions with Emphasis on Transsphenoidal Microsurgery*. New York, Appleton-Centruy-Crofts, 1982.
99. Schuster LD, Bantle JP, Oppenheimer JH, et al: Acromegaly: Reassessment of the long-term therapeutic effectiveness of transsphenoidal pituitary surgery. *Ann Intern Med* 95:172, 1981.
100. Sonksen PH, Ayres AB, Braimbridge M, et al: Acromegaly caused by pulmonary carcinoid tumours. *Clin Endocrinol* 5:503, 1976.
101. Southern AL: Functioning metastatic bronchial carcinoid with elevated levels of serum and cerebrospinal fluid serotonin and pituitary adenoma. *J Clin Endocrinol Metab* 20:298, 1960.
102. Sparagana M, Phillips G, Hoffman C, et al: Ectopic growth hormone syndrome associated with lung cancer. *Metabolism* 20:730, 1971.
103. Stachura ME, Frohman LA, Dharivial APS: Effect of purified hypothalamic extract acromegalic plasma on growth hormone synthesis and secretion in vitro. *Endocrinology* 88:81A, 1971.
104. Stonesifer LD, Jordan RM, Kihler PO: Somatomedin C in treated acromegaly: Poor correlation with growth hormone and clinical response. *J Clin Endocrinol Metab* 53:931, 1981.
105. Teasdale GM, Hay ID, Beasttall GH, et al: Cryosurgery or microsurgery in the management of acromegaly. *JAMA* 247:1289, 1982.
106. Thorner MO, Besser GM, Wass JAH, et al: Bromocriptine in acromegaly, letter. *N Engl J Med* 305:1092, 1981.
107. Thorner MO, Perryman RL, Cronin MJ, et al: Somatotroph hyperplasia: Successful treatment of acromegaly by removal of a pancreatic islet tumor secreting a growth hormone–releasing factor. *J Clin Invest* 70:965, 1982.
108. Tolis G, Bertrand G, Carpenter S, et al: Acromegaly and galactorrhea-amenorrhea with two pituitary adenomas secreting growth hormone or prolactin: A case report. *Ann Intern Med* 89:345, 1978.
109. Tucker H, Grubb SR, Wigand JP, et al: The treatment of acromegaly by transsphenoidal surgery. *Arch Intern Med* 140:795, 1980.
110. Van Wyk JJ, Underwood LE: Relation between growth hormone and somatomedin. *Annu Rev Med* 26:427, 1975.
111. Wanski ZJ, Robinson AG, Jannetta PJ: Selective total removal of a growth-hormone–secreting adenoma: Evidence that acromegaly is a primary pituitary disease. *Metabolism* 28:624, 1979.
112. Wass JAH, Thorner MO, Charlesworth M, et al: Reduction of pituitary-tumour size in patients with prolactinomas and acromegaly treated with bromocriptine with or without radiotherapy. *Lancet* 2:66, 1979.
113. Webb CB, Thominet JL, Frohman LA: Ectopic growth hormone–releasing factor stimulates growth hormone release from somatotroph adenomas in vitro. *J Clin Endocrinol Metab* 56:417, 1983.
114. Weiss L, Ingram M: Adenomatoid bronchial tumors: A consideration of the carcinoid tumors and the salivary tumors of the bronchial tree. *Cancer* 14:161, 1961.
115. Weiss MH: Medical and surgical management of functional pituitary tumors. *Clin Neurosurg* 28:374, 1981.
116. Weiss MH: Personal communication, 1983.
117. Williams RA, Jacobs HS, Kurtz AB, et al: The treatment of acromegaly with special reference to trans-sphenoidal hypophysectomy. *Q J Med* 44:79, 1975.
118. Wright AD, Hill DM, Lowy C, et al: Mortality in acromegaly. *Q J Med* 39:1, 1970.

CHAPTER 7

Cushing's syndrome and Nelson's syndrome

Physiology of ACTH and cortisol secretion
Cushing's syndrome
  History
  Pathophysiology
  Clinical features
  Prognosis
  Diagnostic evaluation
    Endocrine tests
    Neuroradiologic evaluation
      Skull films
      CT scan
      Selective venous catheterization and sampling for ACTH
  Treatment
    Criteria of cure
    Transsphenoidal surgery
    Irradiation
    Pharmacotherapy
      Adrenal toxins
      Serotonin antagonists
      Dopamine agonists
    Therapeutic decision making
Nelson's syndrome
  Clinical features
  Diagnostic evaluation
  Treatment
    Surgery
    Irradiation
    Pharmacotherapy
  Therapeutic decision making
Summary

Cushing's syndrome, which results from hypercortisolism, is a disorder characterized by distinctive clinical features and associated systemic changes that, when well established, present few diagnostic problems. Noniatrogenic Cushing's syndrome may be the result of an adrenal tumor, an ectopic source (tumor) of adrenocorticotropic hormone (ACTH) production, or a pituitary source of excessive ACTH, usually from a pituitary adenoma. When the disorder is caused by a pituitary source, it is referred to as Cushing's disease and this source accounts for approximately 70% of the cases of Cushing's syndrome.

Nelson's syndrome is a clinical condition characterized by hyperpigmentation associated with an enlarging ACTH-secreting pituitary tumor following bilateral adrenalectomy for hypercortisolism. Current opinion holds that the pituitary tumor associated with Nelson's syndrome was present and responsible for the Cushing's disease before the adrenalectomy. Because the use of adrenalectomy for hypercortisolism has declined in recent years, one can expect a parallel decrease in the incidence of Nelson's syndrome. Because of the close relationship between Cushing's and Nelson's syndromes, they are both described and discussed in this chapter.

PHYSIOLOGY OF ACTH AND CORTISOL SECRETION

The regulation of pituitary ACTH secretion is dependent on corticotropin-releasing hormone (CRH, CRF). This substance is produced in neurons of the medial basal hypothalamus.[4] Recently, CRH has been isolated from sheep hypothalamic extracts, characterized as a 41-amino acid polypeptide,[74,80] and synthesized.[67] Rat CRH, which is identical in structure to human CRH, has also been isolated, characterized, and synthesized.[66,71] When CRH is released into the portal circulation, it stimulates corticotrophs in the adenohypophysis to release ACTH, which in turn activates the adrenal cortex to increase the synthesis and release of cortisol. Cortisol acts at both the hypothalamic and pituitary levels to regulate feedback inhibition of ACTH secretion. ACTH secretion is also altered by other substances (e.g., norepinephrine, vasopressin, progesterones, prostaglandins) that exert direct effects at the level of the pituitary, although the physiologic importance of these substances is uncertain. A more detailed discussion of the physiologic regulation of ACTH and cortisol secretion is presented in Chapter 2.

CUSHING'S SYNDROME
History

In an outstanding article published in 1932, Cushing detailed the case histories of several patients with a "polyglandular disorder" characterized by a number of distinctive features including, among others, a peculiar adiposity of the face, neck and trunk with sparing of the extremities, hypertrichosis of the face and trunk in women and preadolescent boys, purple stria, and hypertension.[11] His report was based on 12 patients, most of whom had been reported as separate case reports by other authors. In those patients in whom autopsies were done, a pituitary adenoma was found in six and a normal pituitary gland in two cases. The tumor was a basophilic adenoma in three, an undifferentiated adenoma in two, and an adenomatous-like lesion in one case. The adrenals showed cortical hyperplasia in two cases, a small adenoma in one case (which also had an undifferentiated adenoma of the pituitary), and no abnormality in four cases. Cushing concluded that this "obscure polyglandular syndrome," which was later to bear his name, was related to a pituitary rather than an adrenal source. He used the term *pituitary basophilism* to categorize this clinical condition. Particularly germane and prophetic were his concluding remarks,

> The fact, that the peculiar polyglandular syndrome . . . may accompany a basophil adenoma in the absence of any apparent alteration in the adrenal cortex other than a possible secondary hyperplasia, will give pathologists reason in the future more carefully to scrutinize the anterior-pituitary for lesions of similar composition.[11]

Although he believed that most cases of this disorder arose from basophilic adenomas of the pituitary gland, studies by others suggested that only a minority of cases had pituitary tumors, thus casting doubt on Cushing's conclusions. The doubt arose in large measure because there were no associated abnormalities seen on skull x-ray films and other neurodiagnostic studies (pneumoencephalograms and/or cerebral angiograms). This lack of radiologic abnormality led many in the years subsequent to Cushing's observations to the conclusion that no pituitary tumor was present. (However, currently, it is well known that the majority of pituitary adenomas causing Cushing's disease are too small to produce abnormalities on routine skull films and pneumoencephalograms.) Furthermore, for some years following Cushing's publication, it was considered that the basophilic changes in the pituitary were in fact a result of excessive cortisol secretion.

The pituitary again became the focus of interest in the etiology of Cushing's disease when it was shown that these patients have elevated plasma ACTH levels and a high "set point" for feedback inhibition of ACTH-cortisol secretion and that about 15% of cases develop pituitary ACTH-secreting tumors following adrenalectomy (i.e., Nelson's syndrome.)[45,46] As knowledge accumulated, the three basic causes of hypercortisolism—adrenal tumors, pituitary adenomas, and ectopic sources of ACTH—and their relative frequencies were identified. With this information has come the confirmation of Cushing's theory regarding small pituitary adenomas as a cause for many if not the majority of cases of the "polyglandular syndrome" that we now justifiably term Cushing's syndrome. In current practice, Cushing's syndrome is referred to as Cushing's disease when caused by a pituitary source, either a tumor or hyperplasia. Hardy[18-26] contributed significantly to the elucidation of pituitary microadenomas as a cause for Cushing's disease with his early transsphenoidal surgical observations. His microsurgical approach not only afforded an effective means for treating the disorder but also permitted unequivocal documentation of ACTH-secreting microadenomas as a cause of Cushing's disease.

Pathophysiology

The pathophysiologic derangement responsible for spontaneously occurring Cushing's syndrome is excessive cortisol secretion by the adrenal cortex. Iatrogenic Cushing's syndrome results from excessive administration of exogenous corticosteroids.

The causes of the spontaneously occurring syndrome include a pituitary tumor or hyperplasia, an adrenal tumor, or an ectopic ACTH-producing nonpituitary tumor.[54] Increased ACTH secretion by a pituitary adenoma or hyperplasia accounts for approximately 60% to 70% of all cases of Cushing's syndrome (Cushing's disease). Primary hypersecretion of cortisol from an adrenal adenoma or carcinoma and elaboration of excessive ACTH from ectopic nonpituitary tumors account for the remaining cases of Cushing's syndrome. As would be expected, the incidence of the various causes varies among different reports. In a series of 108 patients reported by Orth and Liddle,[61] the incidence was pituitary, 60%; adrenal, 25%; and ectopic, 15%. It is our impression that the incidence of a pituitary cause is higher and ectopic sources lower than the figures cited by Orth and Liddle.

There is considerable interest and controversy among endocrinologists and neurosurgeons regarding the possible etiologic factors of the adenomas responsible for Cushing's disease. The basic issue is whether the pathologic changes in the pituitary (i.e., tumor and/or hyperplasia) that account for the excessive ACTH secretion arise de novo or whether they occur as a result of dysfunction of either the hypothalamus or higher cerebral centers. A number of observations have been cited to support the concept of a neural cause of Cushing's disease. As an example, Heinbecker[24] noted histologic abnormalities (i.e., atrophy) in the hypothalamus of patients dying with Cushing's syndrome. Castor et al,[7] however, reported that thalamic and hypothalamic lesions can be produced during either ACTH or cortisone therapy, indicating that these lesions may be a result rather than a cause of hypercortisolism. Additional observations that suggest a hypothalamic and/or central nervous system (CNS) origin include (1) the discovery of basophilic adenomas in patients without clinical or laboratory evidence of an endocrinopathy;[24,32,76] (2) the fact that pituitary adenomas associated with Cushing's disease are not entirely autonomous and that a variety of agents,[44] including thyrotropin-releasing hormone (TRH),[37,40,62] luteinizing hormone-releasing hormone (LHRH),[62] vasopressin,[35,40] cyproheptadine,[36,37] bromocriptine,[43] and glucocorticoids,[45] exert an effect on ACTH secretion by the tumor; and (3) the occurrence of sleep abnormalities in some patients with active and inactive Cushing's disease that may reflect altered CNS mechanisms.[38] For instance, electroencephalogram (EEG) studies performed on sleeping patients with Cushing's disease have demonstrated a significant reduction in the portion of time spent in slow wave sleep.[38,39] These responses are believed to be mediated via higher CNS centers. Furthermore, treatment with the serotonin antagonist, cyproheptadine, has been reported to reverse the EEG abnormalities, reduce the levels of ACTH and cortisol, initiate return of dexamethasone suppressibility, and produce medical remission in some patients with Cushing's disease and Nelson's syndrome.[36] Also persistence of a cortisol-ACTH feedback abnormality following removal of a pituitary adenoma has been corrected by cyproheptadine.[44] The site of action of cyproheptadine is unknown but is presumed to be at some level of the CNS. Although abnormalities of the hypothalamus and other areas of the CNS may exist, Martin[54] stresses that this information does not prove that Cushing's disease is a result of a hypothalamic CNS lesion.

In support of the de novo origin of pituitary pathologic findings in Cushing's disease is the fact that most patients with proven microadenomas do not develop recurrent pituitary microadenomas or hyperplasia after transsphenoidal surgery. Furthermore, the majority of patients remain cured of their disease over relatively long follow-up periods. If a hypothalamic or other CNS mechanism were responsible for the neoplastic or hyperplastic change, it would be expected that there would be a high incidence of recurrent Cushing's disease following successful surgical treatment. Also the rare report of Cushing's disease caused by an ectopic pituitary adenoma supports the notion that the disorder does not arise at the hypothalamic/CNS level.[2,29] It is possible that multiple etiologic factors exist for the development of Cushing's disease.

Lamberts et al[42] hypothesized that Cushing's disease may be caused by two types of ACTH-secreting pituitary tumors. Based on studies in 15 patients, they divided the cases into two histologically different groups based on the presence or absence of neural tissue in the adenoma. In nine adenomas, no neural tissue was present (group-1), but in the tissue removed from the other six patients, argyrophilic nerve fibers were identified in the adenoma (group-2). These investigators also found distinct clinical and endocrinologic differences between these two groups. A normal cortisol secretion rate following surgery was achieved in all but one group-1 patients but in only one of the six patients in group-2. Hyperprolactinemia was present in three of the six patients of group-2, whereas all patients of group-1 had normal prolactin levels. Bromocriptine preoperatively suppressed ACTH secretion in all group-2 patients but had no effect in four of nine group-1 patients who were tested. Lamberts et al[42] believe the group-2 tumors originate from the intermediate lobe and may be preceded by a hypothalamic-dependent hyperplastic lesion and that the group-1 cases arise in the anterior lobe. Their results imply that most ACTH-secreting pituitary adenomas are located in the anterior pituitary gland and are readily managed by transsphenoidal surgery; whereas those originating from the intermediate lobe may be associated with multiple microadenomas and/or hyperplastic cell nests, and transsphenoidal surgery can be expected to be less successful. Furthermore, this latter entity might be recognized clinically by the suppression of plasma ACTH levels following administration of bromocriptine.

Clinical features

Cushing's syndrome occurs in all races and ages and both sexes but has been reported with greatest frequency in women between the ages of 20 and 60 years. The principal clinical findings of Cushing's syndrome include the following*:

>Obesity
>Hirsutism
>Hypertension
>Amenorrhea
>Oligomenorrhea
>Impotence (men)
>Plethoric appearance
>Purple striae
>Mental symptoms—emotional lability, depression, psychosis
>Poor wound healing or severe infections
>Weakness
>Muscle wasting
>Acne, skin pigmentation, or rash
>Back pain resulting from vertebral compression fractures
>Purpura or easy bruisability
>Ankle edema
>Headache
>Neurologic symptoms or signs
>Virilism
>Exophthalmos

Various associated medical conditions and metabolic disturbances are as follows:

>Impaired glucose tolerance
>Hypertension, left ventricular hypertrophy
>Edema
>Hypokalemia
>Osteoporosis
>Protein loss/muscle wasting
>Maldistribution of adipose tissue
>Erythrocytosis, lymphopenia, eosinopenia

As with acromegaly, recognition of the clinical features in patients in whom the disease is well developed is usually relatively easy; whereas in the early stages, establishing a clinical diagnosis is often difficult. In the latter cases, the neuroradiologic and particularly the endocrine studies are essential in establishing the diagnosis.

The weight gain results from the accumulation of adipose tissue—particularly in the facial, nuchal, truncal, and girdle areas—producing an appearance referred to as centripetal obesity. The face, instead of being round or "moon-faced," as popularly described, has a wide, rectangular appearance caused by extension of

---

*Adapted from Plotz CM, Knowlton AI, Ragan C: *Am J Med* 13:598, 1952.

prominent cheek fat pads over the mandible, with obliteration of the normal angle between the mandible and the horizontal plane of the chin (Plate 2, *A*). Another characteristic finding caused by an abnormal accumulation of adipose tissue are the supraclavicular fat pads that appear as convexities in the region adjacent to the base of the neck. Some clinicians consider the supraclavicular fat pads to be present more consistently and to be more valuable diagnostically in Cushing's syndrome than the dorsal nuchal fat pad prominence ("buffalo hump") that is inconsistently present.

The numerous abnormal skin and subcutaneous tissue changes seen in Cushing's syndrome are a result of protein wasting. The tissues do not have the strength and healing potential found in normal subjects. Consequently, surgeons find that the tissues of patients with Cushing's syndrome tear easily, hold sutures poorly, heal slowly, and are more susceptible to infections than are normal subjects. The relative ease with which these individuals bruise results from poor tensile strength of the skin and subcutaneous tissues including increased capillary fragility. The weakened skin and subcutaneous tissues are stretched by the accumulation of adipose tissue, producing the stretched streaks and capillaries known as purple striae.

The loss of bone matrix leads to generalized osteoporosis, which in turn sets the stage for compression fractures of the vertebra and occasional pathological fractures of the extremities. The occurrence of a compression fracture of a vertebral body is usually associated with severe back pain, some loss of height, and occasional kyphosis if anterior wedging from a fracture of the vertebra occurs. Hypercalciuria, which occurs with urinary calcium values of 150 to 300 mg/day, is probably caused by the mobilization of calcium from bone.[46] Renal stones occur in about 20% of patients with long-standing Cushing's syndrome. Approximately 90% of patients will have some degree of impaired glucose metabolism. However, in most patients, the impairment is usually manifested by an abnormality of the glucose tolerance test rather than by clinically apparent diabetes mellitus.

The majority of patients (approximately 85%) with Cushing's syndrome have hypertension and associated left ventricular hypertrophy. Although excessive mineralocorticoid production has been implicated in the pathogenesis of the hypertension associated with Cushing's syndrome,[9,10,53,69] evidence obtained by some investigators has indicated that an abnormality of the renin-angiotensin system resulting from glucocorticoid excess is responsible.[12,33,34] The latter conclusion is primarily based on measurements of plasma renin activity, plasma renin concentration, and plasma renin substrate in both dexamethasone-treated rats[33] and patients with Cushing's syndrome.[34] Krakoff et al believe the elevated plasma renin substrate levels found in their patients may have contributed to increased angiotensin formation and that glucocorticoid-induced hypertension may be initiated by alterations in vascular responsiveness to pressor agents.[34] Also the drug saralasin, which is a competitive antagonist of angiotensin II, produces a hypotensive response in hypertensive patients with Cushing's disease.[12]

A wide range of psychopathologic findings may be encountered in patients with Cushing's syndrome.[65] Many patients are emotionally labile, easily irritated, and a few are psychotic. In the past, one of the frequent causes of death was suicide. Studies by Regestein et al[65] indicate that excessive steroids arouse dormant, previously unexpressed mental disturbances rather than cause a specific psychologic abnormality.[65] The fact that the psychopathologic condition may fluctuate with steroid levels was illustrated by one of their patients whose endogenous depression was relieved following surgical removal of an adrenal adenocarcinoma, only to recur with increased steroid output by subsequent metastases. Serum potassium depletion associated with steroid excess has been implicated as a mediator in some steroid psychoses.[60,65] Although steroids appear to nonspecifically exacerbate a variety of dormant, mental disturbances, there is a tendency for patients with Cushing's syndrome to develop either agitation or endogenous depression.[63,65]

Prognosis

Cushing's syndrome is a devastating illness with only rare spontaneous remissions. Plotz et al[63] evaluated 114 autopsied cases—seven from their series and 107 from the literature—and found that the major causes of death were infection, complications of cardiovascular disease, and neoplasms. They determined that 50% of patients were dead within an average of 5 years from the onset of symptoms. Also suicide was found to be a relatively frequent cause of death. A high incidence of both arteriosclerosis and osteoporosis was noted in their study. Fortunately, advances in therapeutic measures and the availability of more effective antibiotics have improved the prognosis for these patients. With the exception of those with adrenal carcinoma and the ectopic ACTH syndrome, most patients are benefited and many are cured by current therapy.[14]

Diagnostic evaluation

Endocrine tests. There are two important phases in the endocrine evaluation of patients with Cushing's syndrome: establishing the diagnosis of hypercortisolism and identifying the cause of the disease. Although establishing the diagnosis of hypercortisolism is not usually difficult, finding the *source* of the disease (i.e., ectopic, pituitary, or adrenal) is more difficult. (The endocrine evaluation of Cushing's syndrome/disease is discussed in detail in Chapter 4.)

These investigations are extremely important, and the results usually form the sole basis for therapeutic decision making.[45] For instance, suppression by high-dose dexamethasone (but not with low-dose) in a patient with classic features, even in the presence of a negative high-resolution computed tomographic (CT) scan, is considered an adequate indication to proceed with transsphenoidal exploration of the pituitary gland.

Neuroradiologic evaluation. Neuroradiologic assessment in patients with Cushing's disease consists of a lateral skull film centered on the sella turcica and sphenoid sinus; a high-resolution coronal CT scan; and on occasions, selective venous sampling for ACTH levels.

Skull films. The skull x-ray examination usually is not valuable from a diagnostic standpoint, since most of the pituitary adenomas causing Cushing's disease are not large enough to produce bony abnormalities that can be detected on routine plain films. In a study by MacErlean et al,[51] plain skull films from 86 patients with pituitary-dependent Cushing's syndrome included only nine that could be unequivocally called abnormal. Tyrrell et al[78] found that none of their 20 patients with Cushing's disease had generalized enlargement of the sella turcica that could be determined on plain skull x-ray films. However, polytomography showed sellar changes consistent with a pituitary microadenoma in 12 of the 20 patients. The experience with radiographic studies of Salassa et al[68] in 32 patients with Cushing's disease was somewhat similar. All their patients had negative skull x-ray examinations, but 12 had either positive or highly suggestive changes on polytomography. However, for reasons discussed in Chapter 5, polytomography is no longer recommended in the routine neuroradiologic evaluation of patients with suspected pituitary adenomas. Skull x-ray films provide the surgeon with valuable information regarding the configuration of the sphenoid sinus and thus should be routinely obtained once the decision to perform surgery has been made. Carotid angiography and pneumoencephalography are no longer indicated in the routine neuroradiologic evaluation of patients with Cushing's disease.

CT scan. A high-resolution coronal CT scan should be a routine study in the evaluation of all patients with Cushing's disease. However, because of the small size of many of these tumors, a significant number of patients, perhaps as many as 50%, will have either a negative or an equivocal CT scan. For instance, Boggan et al[3] found that 73% of 100 histologically confirmed tumors were below the size of 10 mm, with an average size of 5 mm.[3] This finding emphasizes the important point that in the management of these cases, the major determinant in deciding whether or not the patient has pituitary Cushing's disease is the endocrinologic rather than the radiologic data. If positive, the CT is valuable in confirming the diagnosis of a microadenoma and, more importantly, in determining the location of the tumor within the pituitary gland. However, the decision for a definitive treatment program, which in turn necessitates that the source of the disorder be identified, is usually based on the results of the endocrine studies.

Selective venous catheterization and sampling for ACTH. Sampling provides valuable information regarding location of ACTH-producing tumors in special cases.[8,15,31] It helps the physician locate extrapituitary lesions but is also useful in confirming a pituitary source of excessive ACTH; some investigators believe that the test will lateralize the side of the pituitary microadenoma.[52]

Treatment

Because of the poor prognosis of untreated Cushing's disease,[63] it is recommended that some type of definitive therapy be instituted in all patients after the appropriate studies have confirmed the diagnosis and identified the source of the disorder.

Criteria of cure. Before discussing effective therapeutic options available for Cushing's disease, it is important to discuss what constitutes the criteria of

Table 7-1

Results of transsphenoidal surgery in Cushing's disease

Series	Number of patients	Number cured	Percentage	Surgically related hypopituitarism (%)	Incidence of CSF leak and/or meningitis (%)	Surgical mortality (%)	Diabetes insipidus
Boggan et al, 1983[3]	100	78	78	14†	2	1	*
Emory series, 1985	25	19	76	12‡	0	0	4
Guthrie et al, 1981[16]	12	9	75	0	0	0	0
Hardy, 1982[22]	75	63	84	*	*	2.6	6
Kageyama, Kuwayama, 1985[41]	98	81	83	*	*	*	*
Salassa, et al 1978[68]	18	16	89	*	*	†	0
Lüdecke, 1976[49]	15	14	93	93‡	*	*	*

*Incidence either not mentioned or not clear in report.
†Authors state that during past 4½ years "250 patients with pituitary adenomas have been operated . . . with mortality of 1.1%. Complications have been rare and permanent diabetes insipidus has not occurred in any of the patients with microadenomas."
‡Panhypopituitarism in those patients who had total hypophysectomy.

cure in this disorder. We would concur with Boggan et al,[3] who define "endocrinological remission" as the resolution of symptoms and signs of hypercortisolism, the return of plasma ACTH and cortisol levels to normal, and the return of normal cortisol suppression after the administration of low-dose dexamethasone. To this list, we would add a return of the normal circadian rhythm of ACTH secretion.

The therapeutic options available for primary therapy of pituitary Cushing's disease are transsphenoidal surgery, irradiation, and pharmacotherapy.

Transsphenoidal surgery. The results of several large current series would indicate that this form of therapy, when used by an experienced surgeon, yields cure rates that are superior to any other form of treatment. Analysis of several series summarized in Table 7-1 illustrates that immediate cure rates ranging from 75% to 93% can be obtained.

In those patients in whom transsphenoidal surgery results in a cure, significant regression of the features of the disease can be expected over a period of a year or so (Plate 2, *B* and *C*). In cases that obtain a cure, virtually all the stigmata of the disorder will regress.

Surgical experience has shown that the majority of tumors causing Cushing's disease are very small, and even an experienced surgeon occasionally will encounter difficulty finding the tumor in the normal pituitary gland. In adult cases in which this situation occurs and in which laboratory tests indicate that the patient has a pituitary source of hypercortisolism, it is our opinion that one should proceed with a *complete hypophysectomy,* provided this option was agreed on by the patient before the surgery. Subsequent pathologic examination of the entire gland will frequently reveal the presence of a very small microadenoma, often no larger than 2 mm in greatest diameter. In Boggan et al[3] series of 100 cases, total hypophysectomy was performed in 12 cases because no abnormal tissue could be identified during the transsphenoidal operation.

However, in children and young adults in whom *no tumor* is found at surgery, it is our opinion that total *hypophysectomy should not be performed.* In these cases, postoperative irradiation is probably the best option to employ. As will be discussed later, Cushing's disease in children appears to be more responsive to x-ray treatment than it is in adults.

Bilateral adrenalectomy as a primary treatment modality for pituitary-dependent Cushing's disease is not, in our opinion, an appropriate option for two important reasons. First, although the procedure relieves the hypercortisolism, it leaves a large number of ACTH-producing adenomas untreated; thus one can expect a certain incidence of patients to develop Nelson's syndrome (see below). The pituitary adenoma associated with the latter is frequently aggressive, invasive, and commonly incurable. Secondly, bilateral adrenalectomy is technically a more difficult operation to perform and is more difficult for the patient than a transsphenoidal operation. Although not recommended as a primary treatment procedure, adrenalectomy may have a place in the treatment of certain patients with persistent or recurrent Cushing's disease.

Irradiation. The types of irradiation therapy and the results in Cushing's disease are covered in some detail in Chapter 13. In general, the results of conventional electromagnetic irradiation as primary therapy for Cushing's disease differ in adults and children, with a better cure rate being reported in children. Approximately 15% of adults will be cured by conventional irradiation and an additional 30% will be improved.[61] The average time to clinical or biochemical remission varies from a few months to a year. Jennings, Liddle, and Orth[27] treated 15 children (age range 7½ years to 18½ years) with conventional irradiation in doses ranging from 3500 to 4950 rads. Twelve of the patients were cured within 18 months of receiving therapy. There were no complications of therapy and no progressive pituitary enlargement or hyperpigmentation. The reason for the difference in responsiveness to irradiation between the two age groups is unclear.

Kjellberg[30] reports that approximately 65% of patients treated with proton beam irradiation underwent remission with restoration of normal clinical and laboratory findings, and another 20% were improved such that no further treatment was considered desirable. Thirteen percent of the group required replacement endocrine therapy, and an additional 13% developed impaired pituitary reserve. Using alpha particle irradiation (5000 to 15,000 rads), Linfoot[47,48] "treated successfully" 40 of 42 (95%) patients between 1972 and 1978. He concludes that the results of this therapy are comparable to that reported for transsphenoidal surgery.

In our opinion, the reported results of conventional irradiation in *adult* Cushing's disease are such that this form of treatment cannot reasonably be recommended as primary therapy, especially since other effective therapeutic options are available. The results in a small series of children, on the other hand, indicate that conventional irradiation may be a reasonable option for primary treatment in this age group. However, Styne et al[75] reported a series of 15 children and adolescents with Cushing's disease treated by transsphenoidal adenomectomy, in which all but one had correction of their hypercortisolism. In their series, no microadenoma was found in one patient, and one required a second operation because of incomplete removal of the tumor at the initial operation. These authors believe the low morbidity and failure rates combined with the preservation of pituitary function and rapid amelioration of signs make surgery the preferred initial treatment, even in children.

The results of heavy particle therapy appear to be superior to conventional therapy in adult Cushing's disease. However, we hesitate to recommend this form of therapy because of the relative inaccessibility of this treatment method to the average patient, the potential danger of the large amount of irradiation delivered to a small focused area, and the relative superiority of transsphenoidal surgery.

Pharmacotherapy. Many drugs have been used in Cushing's disease with variable results. As shown in Table 7-2, these drugs can be divided into adrenal toxins, serotonin antagonists, and dopamine agonists.

Table 7-2
Pharmacologic agents used in Cushing's disease

Drug category	Drug name
Adrenal toxins	Mitotane (o, ṕ DDD)
	Aminoglutethimide
	Metyrapone
Serotonin antagonists	Cyproheptadine
	Metergoline
Dopamine agonists	Bromocriptine

Adrenal toxins. Although these agents have been effective in some cases, the frequency of side effects is relatively high and temporary adrenal insufficiency is common. o, ṕ DDD, or mitotane, is an adrenal toxin that was first used for treating adrenal carcinoma and in 1961 recommended by Southern et al[73] for the treatment of Cushing's disease. Temple et al[77] reported four patients in whom the therapeutic objective of reducing cortisol secretion without producing aldosterone deficiency was achieved after several months of treatment with mitotane.

In a fifth patient in their series in whom bilateral adrenalectomy was to be performed, treatment was administered for 1 month before surgery to provide information about the morphologic changes induced by the drug. Electron microscopy in this case revealed degenerative changes in the mitochondria of the zona fasciculata with sparing of the zona glomerulosa. The authors observed no prohibitive toxic side effects. Luton et al[50] treated 62 patients with mitotane, 16 of whom also received cobalt irradiation of the pituitary. Following an initial treatment period averaging 8 months, a remission was achieved in 38 of the 46 patients given the drug alone and in all patients who received the drug combined with irradiation. However, 60% of their patients became either mitotane resistant or suffered a relapse. Only 17% remained controlled for more than 2 years after a single 8-month period of medication. In their series, side effects (e.g., nausea, anorexia, vomiting, and hypersialorrhea) were reported in about one third of cases. However, these complications did not make it necessary to interrupt therapy for more than a few days in any case.

Another adrenal toxin, metyrapone, was used successfully by Jeffcoate et al[26] in the long-term management of 13 patients with Cushing's disease. The drug is an inhibitor of adrenocortical steroid C-11 beta hydroxylation. Jeffcoate et al recommended the use of metyrapone to control the clinical manifestations of Cushing's disease as an adjunct to definitive treatment, either pituitary irradiation or transsphenoidal surgery. In their opinion, subsequent surgery is greatly simplified and less hazardous in patients on an effective dosage of metyrapone.

Aminoglutethimide, which was developed as an anticonvulsant in the 1950s, was withdrawn from clinical use after reports that it caused adrenal insufficiency.[25] The drug was subsequently shown to suppress synthesis of all adrenal steroid hormones by inhibiting the first step in their metabolic pathway, the enzymatic conversion of cholesterol to pregnenolone.[5] It was suggested that aminoglutethimide might be used to achieve a "medical adrenalectomy" in patients with metastatic breast cancer.[17] The results have shown that oral aminoglutethimide is at least as effective as surgical adrenalectomy in producing responses in patients with metastatic breast cancer.[72] Thus the drug is effective in inhibiting adrenal steroid function. Most of the clinical experience with the drug, which has been in metastatic breast cancer rather than in patients with Cushing's syndrome, indicates that there is a relatively low incidence of side effects and that most of them are "moderate in nature."[72]

Serotonin antagonists. Since experimental evidence suggests a role for serotonin in the regulation of ACTH release, Krieger et al[36] administered cyproheptadine, an antiserotonergic agent, to three patients with Cushing's disease for a period of 3 to 6 months. Symptomatic improvement occurred, and urinary corticosteroid excretion and cortisol secretory rates returned to normal. The usual dosage of cyproheptadine is 24 mg/day; and when effective, normal dexamethasone suppressibility and stress responsiveness appear within 6 months, and resumption of menses occurs in some patients.[1,35,37] The drug is also effective in some cases of Nelson's syndrome, but as with Cushing's disease, cessation of therapy is accompanied by the prompt return of the clinical features of the disease. Other investigators have had either little or no success with cyproheptadine.[70,79]

Dopamine agonists. Bromocriptine has been reported to be effective in the therapy of some patients, but the data remain contradictory.

In commenting on the medical treatment of Cushing's disease, Martin[54] believes that the drugs discussed above may be useful in preparation of a patient for surgery or in combination with radiation therapy but is of the opinion that the present evidence does not indicate that they will have a major function as primary therapy for the disorder. We agree fully with Martin's assessment of the role of medical treatment for Cushing's disease.

To summarize, the most effective therapeutic option currently available for Cushing's disease is transsphenoidal surgery performed by an experienced pituitary surgeon. Immediate cure rates on the order of 75% can be achieved. In adult patients in whom transsphenoidal exploration fails to reveal a tumor, total hypophysectomy is an appropriate procedure, whereas in children and young adults, this should not be done. Rather, in this latter group, postoperative pituitary irradiation is recommended, and it would be appropriate to use pharmacotherapy while awaiting the therapeutic effects of irradiation.

Therapeutic decision making. When endocrine tests clearly indicate that the pituitary is the source of Cushing's syndrome in patients who have not received definitive treatment, most physicians would recommend transsphenoidal surgery. In persistent and/or recurrent Cushing's disease following definitive treatment more than one therapeutic option may be reasonable. This diagnosis is made by documenting return of hypercortisolism and recurrence of the clinical findings associated with the disease. The results of a dexamethasone suppression test and metyrapone test are similar to those found before initial treatment. Following successful transsphenoidal microsurgery, it has been our experience as well as that of most surgeons, that patients may require a year or even longer to reestablish a normal endogenous secretory pattern of cortisol and, consequently, will require steroid replacement during this period of time. Thus whenever a patient *does not require* maintenance cortisone in the relatively early postoperative period, the physician should be suspicious that the disease may not be cured.

The ideal therapy for proven recurrent or persistent Cushing's disease is not a totally settled issue. First, thorough endocrine testing should be repeated to reestablish the diagnosis. It is our opinion that reoperation (i.e., transsphenoidal surgery) with total hypophysectomy is indicated in those adult patients in whom only adenomectomy with sparing of the normal pituitary gland was performed at the original operation. If a total hypophysectomy fails to cure the disease, conventional irradiation to the sellar region is recommended. If a total hypophysectomy was performed at the original operation, then conventional irradiation without consideration of reoperation is a reasonable option to pursue. Another option in these cases may be to perform a complete adrenalectomy rather than use pituitary irradiation. In the report by Prinz et al,[64] adrenalectomy provided remission in all 11 patients who had failed other therapies (including one patient who had had transsphenoidal surgery) for pituitary-dependent Cushing's disease.[64] Others may prefer to use pituitary irradiation along with adrenalectomy. Since the effects of irradiation require a considerable period (2 to 4 years) to become manifest, medical treatment with either cyproheptadine or metyrapone can be initiated to reduce the clinical manifestations of the disease while awaiting the therapeutic effects of irradiation.

NELSON'S SYNDROME

Nelson's syndrome was first described by Nelson et al[58,59] in 1958. In their original report, they presented a patient in whom bilateral adrenalectomy successfully relieved hypercortisolism but who 2 years postoperatively developed increasing cutaneous pigmentation.[58] The pigmentation involved the extensor surfaces of the limbs, as well as scars and striae, particularly over exposed areas of the body. The patient had failing vision because of an invasive pituitary tumor that was ultimately shown to be a chromophobe adenoma. A craniotomy with partial resection of the tumor was performed, followed by a course of irradiation. At the time of their report, the patient was alive and vision had improved, but there had been an increase in the degree of cutaneous pigmentation.

Clinical features

The time course of development of the syndrome ranges from 1 to 16 years following adrenalectomy, and the pituitary adenomas are estimated to be locally invasive 10% to 25% of the time.[55] However, the relatively poor results of treatment, especially surgery, would imply that a much higher percentage of these tumors are invasive and thus probably incurable.

Apart from the cutaneous pigmentation and the previous history of Cushing's disease treated by adrenalectomy, there are no distinctive clinical features of Nelson's syndrome. As with any pituitary tumor, mass effects such as headaches and visual disturbances can result from involvement of adjacent anatomic structures. In addition to visual impairment, there may be oculomotor or other cranial nerve palsies caused by lateral or posterior extension of the tumor. In the series of 19 cases of Nelson's syndrome reported by Wilson et al,[82,83] three patients initially had diplopia and an additional two patients had loss of vision. Cavernous sinus involvement in two patients accounted for trigeminal neuralgia.

It has been suggested that pituitary irradiation before adrenalectomy *prevents* the development of Nelson's syndrome,[61] although at least two cases have been reported in which it failed to do so.[56] For a further and more thorough discussion of this issue, the reader is referred to Chapter 13.

The plasma ACTH concentration in Nelson's syndrome is elevated. The hyperpigmentation of the syndrome, however, is a result of increased plasma beta melanocyte–stimulating hormone (β-MSH).[13]

Diagnostic evaluation

The diagnosis of Nelson's syndrome is made on the basis of the following criteria:
1. Previous history of hypercortisolism (Cushing's disease/syndrome) treated "successfully" by bilateral adrenalectomy
2. Progressive cutaneous pigmentation
3. Elevated plasma ACTH levels
4. CT and clinical evidence of a pituitary adenoma

Treatment

The treatment options for the pituitary tumors causing Nelson's syndrome as with Cushing's disease are surgery, irradiation, and pharmacotherapy. However, in general, the results of treatment of these patients are relatively dismal, and long-term cures are uncommon. The best that can be achieved in most of the patients is symptomatic relief and control of the disease for variable periods of time.

Surgery. In the absence of significant lateral extension of the tumor, transsphenoidal surgery can be considered as an appropriate option. The results of a relatively large series (19 cases) reported by Wilson et al[82,83] typify the results that can be obtained within a center where a large volume of modern transsphenoidal surgery is performed. At the time of surgery, the surgeon reported a gross total removal in 14 of the 19 cases. However, using return of plasma ACTH levels to normal as the sole criteria of success, only four patients were cured by operation; one of these four died later (? cause), and another exhibited panhypopituitarism. Of their 19 patients, four were dead as a result of their tumors at the time of the report. Similarly, only three of nine patients operated on by Müller et al[57] showed normal ACTH levels postoperatively. A moderately optimistic report on the effects of transsphenoidal surgery for Nelson's syndrome was recently published by Wislawski et al.[84] These authors achieved clinical remission in eight of ten patients for periods ranging from 6 months to 10 years. However, as noted previously, others have not achieved this degree of success with surgery in this disorder.

Thus the cure rate with surgery in Nelson's syndrome is not comparable to the surgical results in other endocrinopathies associated with pituitary tumors (e.g., Cushing's disease, acromegaly). In fact, these rather bleak figures might raise the question of whether surgery has a role in this disorder. If surgery is chosen as the treatment option, it should, in our opinion, be followed with a full course of irradiation, since experience has shown that this combination of therapies (surgery followed by irradiation) can provide reasonable control of the disease for variable but usually relatively long periods of time.[57,81]

Irradiation. Radiation therapy is a reasonable option for treatment of this condition either following surgery or as primary therapy. The results of this form of treatment are discussed in more detail in Chapter 13. Suffice it to say, however, that it is probably the most effective way to obtain long-term control (not cure) of the disease and, in our opinion, should be considered in all cases of Nelson's syndrome either as adjunctive or primary treatment.

Satisfactory results have also been reported with radioactive yttrium implantation.[6] Although this form of therapy would seem to have a very limited applicability, given the current interest in brachytherapy (i.e., stereotaxic insertion of radioactive "seeds") of brain tumors in general, it may be that a variation of this form of therapy could be considered in cases that progress despite surgery and conventional radiation.

Pharmacotherapy. Cyproheptadine has been reported to have some effectiveness in the therapy of Nelson's syndrome.[1,28] Patients with elevated ACTH levels have been reported to have a significant suppression of these levels along with a decrease in skin pigmentation. Patients have been demonstrated, at 6 to 12 months after initiating therapy, to have normal suppressibility of ACTH by dexamethasone along with a restoration of normal cortisol circadian rhythm.[1] Aronin and Krieger[1] reported a patient who maintained clinical and laboratory remission for 18 months after withdrawal of cyproheptadine. However, patients generally undergo an exacerbation of the disease process when therapy is discontinued.

We believe that medical therapy in Nelson's syndrome is comparable to the situation in Cushing's disease. It should be considered adjunctive in the majority of cases, particularly in patients receiving radiation therapy. The drug may help in patients with progressive disease in whom both surgery and irradiation have been used. It may be used as a primary therapy in patients who for one reason or another are not candidates for surgery (i.e., poor medical condition) and who do not wish to have irradiation. Although these drugs may be useful in preparing a patient for surgery alone or in combination with radiation therapy, the evidence does not indicate that they will have a major function in the primary therapy for this disorder.[54]

Therapeutic decision making

Therapeutic decision making in well-documented cases of Nelson's syndrome relies almost entirely on a review of a high-resolution coronal CT scan. In patients who harbor a small- or moderate-sized tumor on CT scan that does not appear to involve the cavernous sinus and who have not had previous pituitary surgery, transsphenoidal surgery is an appropriate option. In some patients in this group, a cure may be obtainable. We also believe that surgery is a reasonable option in patients who have had previous pituitary irradiation and who still fit the CT criteria of a small- or moderate-sized, noninvasive tumor. Although we incline toward surgery in previously untreated cases, we cannot argue too strongly against pituitary irradiation as a primary treatment option, especially in view of the relatively poor surgical results reported in the literature.

In patients in whom the CT scan indicates a large tumor or a smaller lesion with obvious cavernous sinus invasion, primary treatment should be pituitary irradiation in conjunction with pharmacotherapy (e.g., cyproheptadine). In the larger tumors, transsphenoidal surgery may be considered as a debulking procedure to enhance the effectiveness of irradiation. In these cases, the major therapeutic tool is irradiation, with both surgery and pharmacotherapy considered only as adjunctive treatment.

In patients with large and/or invasive tumors who have had a full course of pituitary irradiation, the effective therapeutic options are limited. In these cases, one can consider interstitial irradiation (brachytherapy) as the primary therapeutic modality. The radioactive seeds can either be inserted stereotactically via the transnasal route or can be placed into the residual tumor bed following partial debulking of the tumor by transsphenoidal surgery. Obviously, brachytherapy performed either stereotactically or placed at open operation requires that the surgical team be thoroughly experienced and skilled in the use of this procedure and in the safe handling of radioactive isotopes.

SUMMARY

Cushing's syndrome is a devastating condition characterized by distinctive clinical features and associated systemic changes.

The pathophysiologic derangement responsible for spontaneously occurring Cushing's syndrome is excessive cortisol secretion by the adrenal cortex. The causes of the syndrome include a pituitary tumor or hyperplasia; an adrenal tumor; or an ectopic, nonpituitary ACTH-producing tumor. Increased ACTH secretion by a pituitary adenoma or hyperplasia accounts for approximately 60% to 70% of all cases of Cushing's syndrome (Cushing's disease). Iatrogenic Cushing's syndrome results from excessive administration of exogenous corticosteroids.

Cushing's syndrome is a serious medical problem, and it is estimated that approximately 50% of patients with no definitive therapy are dead within an average of 5 years from the onset of symptoms.

Because of the poor prognosis of untreated Cushing's disease, it is appropriate that some type of definitive therapy be instituted in all patients after studies have confirmed the diagnosis and identified the source of the disorder.

The diagnosis of Cushing's disease is made by documentation of elevated plasma ACTH levels and excess cortisol production, as well as abnormal cortisol secretory dynamics. In the majority of cases, plasma ACTH and cortisol levels suppress after high doses of dexamethasone. This latter result is usually the important decision maker in terms of identifying the pituitary as the source of the disease. Because of the small size of most of the pituitary adenomas causing Cushing's disease, radiologic studies, including high-resolution CT scans, are frequently nondiagnostic.

Of all the treatment options (medical therapy, irradiation, and transsphenoidal surgery) available for Cushing's disease, transsphenoidal surgery offers the best chance for cure of the disease. Immediate cure rates in patients who are found to have adenomas range from 75% to 93% in the hands of experienced pituitary surgeons. For recurrent or persistent Cushing's disease, reoperation (i.e., transsphenoidal) with total hypophysectomy is indicated in those adult patients that only adenomectomy with sparing of the gland was performed at the original operation. If a total hypophysectomy was performed at the original operation, then conventional irradiation without consideration of reoperation is a reasonable option to pursue.

Nelson's syndrome was first described in 1958 as a clinical condition characterized by hyperpigmentation associated with an enlarging ACTH-secreting pituitary adenoma following adrenalectomy.

The treatment options for the pituitary tumors causing Nelson's syndrome are surgery, irradiation, and pharmacotherapy. In general, the results of treatment of these patients are relatively poor, and long-term cures are uncommon. The best that can be achieved in most of the patients is symptomatic relief and control of the disease for variable periods of time. Fortunately, the incidence of Nelson's syndrome can be expected to decline significantly in the future because of the decreasing use of bilateral adrenalectomy for hypercortisolism.

REFERENCES

1. Aronin N, Krieger DT: Sustained remission of Nelson's syndrome after stopping cyproheptadine treatment. *N Engl J Med* 302:453, 1980.
2. Bergenstal DM, Hertz R, Lipsett MB, et al: Chemotherapy of adrenocortical cancer with o, ṕ DDD. *Ann Intern Med* 53:672, 1960.
3. Boggan JE, Tyrrell JB, Wilson CB: Transsphenoidal microsurgical management of Cushing's disease: Report of 100 cases. *J Neurosurg* 59:195, 1983.
4. Carey RM, Varma SK, Drake CR Jr, et al: Ectopic secretion of corticotropin-releasing factor as a cause of Cushing's syndrome: A clinical, morphologic, and biochemical study. *N Engl J Med* 311:13, 1984.
5. Cash R, Brough AJ, Cohen MNP, et al: Aminoglutethimide (Elipten-Ciba) as an inhibitor of adrenal steroidogenesis: Mechanism of action and therapeutic trial. *J Clin Endocrinol* 27:1239, 1967.
6. Cassar J, Doyle FH, Lewis PD, et al: Treatment of Nelson's syndrome by pituitary implantation of yttrium-90 or gold-198. *Br Med J* 2:269, 1976.
7. Castor CW, Baker BL, Ingle DJ, et al: Effect of treatment with ACTH or cortisone on anatomy of the brain. *Proc Soc Exp Biol Metab* 76:353, 1951.
8. Corrigan DF, Schaaf M, Whaley RA, et al: Selective venous sampling to differentiate ectopic ACTH secretion from pituitary Cushing's syndrome. *N Engl J Med* 296:861, 1977.
9. Cost WS: Mineralocorticoid excess syndrome presumably due to excessive secretions of corticosterone. *Lancet* 1:362, 1963.
10. Crane MG, Harris JJ: Desoxycorticosterone secretion rates in hyperadrenocorticism. *J Clin Endocrinol Metab* 26:1135, 1966.
11. Cushing H: The basophil adenomas of the pituitary body and their clinical manifestations (pituitary basophilism). *Bull Johns Hopkins Hosp* 50:137, 1932.
12. Dalakos TG, Elias AN, Anderson GH Jr, et al: Evidence for an angiotensinogenic mechanism of the hypertension of Cushing's syndrome. *J Clin Endocrinol Metab* 46:114, 1978.
13. Daughaday WH: The adenohypophysis, in Williams RH (ed): *Textbook of Endocrinology*, ed 5. Philadelphia, WB Saunders Co, 1974.
14. Feldman JM: Cushing's disease: A hypothalamic flush? *N Engl J Med* 293:930, 1975.
15. Findling JW, Aron DC, Tyrrell JB, et al: Selective venous sampling for ACTH in Cushing's syndrome: Differentiation between Cushing's disease and the ectopic ACTH syndrome. *Ann Intern Med* 94:647, 1981.
16. Guthrie FW Jr, Ciric I, Hayashida S, et al: Pituitary Cushing's syndrome and Nelson's syndrome: Diagnostic criteria, surgical therapy, and results. *Surg Neurol* 16:316, 1981.
17. Hall T, Barlow J, Griffiths C, et al: Treatment of metastatic breast cancer with aminoglutethimide, abstract. *Clin Res* 17:402, 1969.
18. Hardy J: Transphenoidal microsurgery of the normal and pathological pituitary. *Clin Neurosurg* 16:185, 1969.
19. Hardy J: Transsphenoidal hypophysectomy. *J Neurosurg* 34:582, 1971.
20. Hardy J: Transsphenoidal surgery of hypersecreting pituitary tumors, in Kohler PO, Ross GT (eds): *Diagnosis and Treatment of Pituitary Tumors*. Amsterdam, Excerpta Medica, 1973.

21. Hardy J: Transsphenoidal microsurgical removal of microadenoma, in Krayenbuhl H, Maspes PE, Sweet WH (eds): *Progress in Neurological Surgery*. Basel, Switzerland, S Karger, 1975.
22. Hardy J: Cushing's disease: 50 years later. Presidential Address, Proceedings of the Seventeenth Canadian Congress of Neurological Sciences. *Can J Neurol Sci* 9:375, 1982.
23. Hardy J: Microsurgery of the hypophysis: Subnasal transsphenoidal approach with television magnification and televised radiofluoroscopic control, in Rand RW (ed): *Microneurosurgery*, ed 3, St. Louis, The CV Mosby Co, 1984.
24. Heinbecker P: The pathogenesis of Cushing's syndrome. *Medicine* 23:225, 1944.
25. Hughes SWM, Burley DM: Aminoglutethimide: A 'side effect' turned to therapeutic advantage. *Postgrad Med J* 46:409, 1970.
26. Jeffcoate WJ, Rees LH, Tomlin S, et al: Metyrapone in long-term management of Cushing's disease. *Br Med J* 2:215, 1977.
27. Jennings AS, Liddle GW, Orth DN; Results of treating childhood Cushing's disease with pituitary irradiation. *N Engl J Med* 297:957, 1977.
28. Jialal I, Pillay NL: Cyproheptadine therapy in Cushing's disease and Nelson's syndrome. *S Afr Med J* 57:305, 1980.
29. Kammer H, George R: Cushing's disease in a patient with an ectopic pituitary adenoma. *JAMA* 246:2722, 1981.
30. Kjellberg RN, Kliman B: Proton radiosurgery for functioning pituitary adenoma, in Tindall GT, Collins WF (eds): *Clinical Management of Pituitary Disorders*. New York, Raven Press, 1979.
31. Kley HK, Stolze T, Krüskemper HL: Jugular-vein sampling of ACTH. *N Engl J Med* 297:731, 1977.
32. Kovacs K, Horvath E, Bayley TA, et al: Silent corticotroph cell adenoma with lysosomal accumulation and crinophagy: A distinct clinicopathologic entity. *Am J Med* 64:492, 1978.
33. Krakoff LR: Measurement of plasma renin substrate by radioimmunoassay of angiotensin: I. Concentration in syndromes associated with steroid excess. *J Clin Endocrinol Metab* 37:110, 1973.
34. Krakoff L, Nicolis G, Amsel B: Pathogenesis of hypertension in Cushing's syndrome. *Am J Med* 58:216, 1975.
35. Krieger DT: Medical treatment of Cushing's disease, in Tolis G (ed): *Clinical Neuroendocrinology: A Pathophysiological Approach*. New York, Raven Press, 1979.
36. Krieger DT, Amorosa L, Linick F: Cyproheptadineinduced remission of Cushing's disease. *N Engl J Med* 293:893, 1975.
37. Krieger DT, Condon EM: Cyproheptadine treatment of Nelson's syndrome: Restoration of plasma ACTH circadian periodicity and reversal of response to TRF. *J Clin Endocrinol Metab* 46:349, 1978.
38. Krieger DT, Glick SM: Growth hormone and cortisol responsiveness in Cushing's syndrome: Relation to a possible central nervous system etiology. *Am J Med* 52:25, 1972.
39. Krieger DT, Glick SM: Sleep EEG stages and plasma growth hormone concentration in states of endogenous and exogenous hypercortisolemia or ACTH elevation. *J Clin Endocrinol Metab* 39:986, 1974.
40. Krieger DT, Luria M: Plasma ACTH and cortisol responses to TRF, vasopressin or hypoglylcemia in Cushing's disease and Nelson's syndrome. *J Clin Endocrinol Metab* 44:361, 1977.
41. Kuwayama A, Kageyama N: Current management of Cushing's disease, parts 1 and 2. in Tindall GT (ed): *Contemporary Neurosurgery*, Baltimore, Williams & Wilkins, 1985, vol 7.
42. Lamberts SWJ, de Lange SA, Stefanko SZ: Adrenocorticotropin-secreting pituitary adenomas originate from the anterior or the intermediate lobe in Cushing's disease: Differences in the regulation of hormone secretion. *J Clin Endocrinol Metab* 54:286, 1982.
43. Lamberts SWJ, Klijn JGM, de Quijada M, et al: The mechanism of the suppressive action of bromocriptine on adrenocorticotropin secretion in patients with Cushing's disease and Nelson's syndrome. *J Clin Endocrinol Metab* 51:307, 1980.
44. Lankford HV, Tucker HSG, Blackard WG: A cyproheptadine-reversible defect in ACTH control persisting after removal of the pituitary tumor in Cushing's disease. *N Engl J Med* 305:1244, 1981.
45. Liddle GW: Tests of pituitary-adrenal suppressibility in the diagnosis of Cushing's syndrome. *J Clin Endocrinol Metab* 20:1539, 1960.
46. Liddle GW, Melmon KL: The adrenals, in Williams RH (ed): *Textbook of Endocrinology*, ed 5. Philadelphia, WB Saunders Co, 1974.
47. Linfoot JA: Heavy ion therapy: Alpha particle therapy of pituitary tumors, in Linfoot JA (ed): *Recent Advances in the Diagnosis and Treatment of Pituitary Tumors*. New York, Raven Press, 1979.
48. Linfoot JA: Alpha particles versus conventional radiotherapy to the pituitary region: A comparison of risk-benefit. *Clin Neurosurg* 27:83, 1980.

49. Lüdecke D, Kautzky R, Saeger W, et al: Selective removal of hypersecreting adenomas. *Acta Neurochir* 35:27, 1976.
50. Luton JP, Mahoudeau JA, Bouchard P, et al: Treatment of Cushing's disease by o, ṕ DDD: Survey of 62 cases. *N Engl J Med* 300:459, 1979.
51. MacErlean DP, Doyle FH: The pituitary fossa in Cushing's syndrome: A retrospective analysis of 93 patients. *Br J Radiol* 49:820, 1976.
52. Manni A, Latshaw RF, Page R, et al: Simultaneous bilateral venous sampling for adrenocorticotropin in pituitary-dependent Cushing's disease: Evidence for lateralization of pituitary venous drainage. *J Clin Endocrinol Metab* 57:1070, 1983.
53. Marquezy RA, Bricaire H, Laudat MH, et al: Adéno-carcinome de la surrénale avec syndrome a'hyperandrogénie et syndrome d'hyperminéralocorticism: Elimination urinaire du composé S et de la tétrahydro S, de la desoxycorticostérone et de la tétrahydrodesoxycorticostérone. *Ann Endocrinol* 26:247, 1965.
54. Martin JB: Management of hypersecretory pituitary adenomas. *Clin Neurosurg* 27:99, 1980.
55. Molitch ME: ACTH-secreting adenomas, in Post KD, Jackson IMD, Reichlin S (eds): *The Pituitary Adenoma*. New York, Plenum Medical Book Co, 1980.
56. Moore TJ, Dluhy RG, Williams GH, et al: Nelson's syndrome: Frequency, prognosis, and effect of prior pituitary irradiation. *Ann Intern Med* 85:731, 1976.
57. Müller OA, Baur X, Fahlbusch R, et al: Diagnosis and treatment of ACTH-producing pituitary tumors, in Fahlbusch R, von Werder K (eds): *Treatment of Pituitary Adenomas*. Stuttgart, Georg Thieme, 1978.
58. Nelson DH, Meakin JW, Dealy JB, et al: ACTH-producing tumor of the pituitary gland. *N Engl J Med* 259:161, 1958.
59. Nelson DH, Meakin JW, Thorn GW: ACTH-producing pituitary tumors following adrenalectomy for Cushing's syndrome. *Ann Intern Med* 52:560, 1960.
60. Op de Coul AAW: The effect of ACTH and corticosteroids on the brain. *Psychiatr Neurol Neurochir* 69:385, 1966.
61. Orth DN, Liddle GW: Results of treatment in 108 patients with Cushing's syndrome. *N Engl J Med* 285:243, 1971.
62. Pieters GFFM, Smals AGH, Benraard TJ, et al: Plasma cortisol response to thyrotropin-releasing hormone and luteinizing hormone–releasing hormone in Cushing's disease. *J Clin Endocrinol Metab* 48:874, 1979.
63. Plotz CM, Knowlton AI, Ragan C: The natural history of Cushing's syndrome. *Am J Med* 13:597, 1952.
64. Prinz RA, Brooks MH, Lawrence AM, et al: The continued importance of adrenalectomy in the treatment of Cushing's disease. *Arch Surg* 114:481, 1979.
65. Regestein QR, Rose LI, Williams GH: Psychopathology in Cushing's syndrome. *Arch Intern Med* 130:114, 1972.
66. Rivier J, Spiess J, Vale W: Characterization of rat hypothalamic corticotropin-releasing factor. *Proc Natl Acad Sci USA* 80:4851, 1983.
67. Rivier J, et al: in Blaha, Malor (ed): *Seventeenth European Peptide Symposium,* Prague, Czechoslovakia, Aug 29-Sept 3, 1982. Berlin, Walter de Gruyter & Co. (In press.)
68. Salassa RM, Laws ER Jr, Carpenter PC, et al: Transsphenoidal removal of pituitary microadenoma in Cushing's disease. *Mayo Clin Proc* 53:24, 1978.
69. Schambelan M, Slaton PE Jr, Biglieri EG: Mineralocorticoid production in hyperadrenocorticism: Role in pathogenesis of hypokalemic alkalosis. *Am J Med* 51:299, 1971.
70. Scott R, Espiner EA, Donald RA: Cyproheptadine for Cushing's disease. *N Engl J Med* 296:57, 1977.
71. Shibahara S, Morimoto Y, Furutani Y, et al: Isolation and sequence analysis of the human corticotropin-releasing factor precursor gene. *EMBO J* 2:775, 1983.
72. Smith IE, Fitzharris BM, McKinna JA, et al: Aminoglutethimide in treatment of metastatic breast carcinoma. *Lancet* 2:646, 1978.
73. Southren AL, Weisenfeld S, Laufer A, et al: Effect of o, ṕ DDD in a patient with Cushing's syndrome. *J Clin Endocrinol Metab* 21:201, 1961.
74. Spiess J, Rivier J, Rivier C, et al: Primary structure of corticotropin-releasing factor from ovine hypothalamus. *Proc Natl Acad Sci USA* 78:6517, 1981.
75. Styne DM, Grumbach MM, Kaplan SL, et al: Treatment of Cushing's disease in childhood and adolescence by transsphenoidal microadenomectomy. *N Engl J Med* 310:889, 1984.
76. Susman W: Adenomata of the pituitary, with special reference to pituitary basophilism of Cushing. *Br J Surg* 22:539, 1934-35.
77. Temple TE Jr, Jones DJ Jr, Liddle GW, et al: Treatment of Cushing's disease: Correction of hypercortisolism by o, ṕ DDD without induction of aldosterone deficiency. *N Engl J Med* 281:801, 1969.

78. Tyrrell B, Brooks RM, Fitzgerald PA, et al: Cushing's disease: Selective trans-sphenoidal resection of pituitary microadenomas. *N Engl J Med* 298:753, 1978.
79. Tyrrell JB, Brooks RM, Forsham PH: More on cyproheptadine. N Engl J Med 295:1137, 1976.
80. Vale W, Spiess J, Rivier C, et al: Characterization of a 41-residue ovine hypothalamic peptide that stimulates secretion of corticotropin and β-endorphin. *Science* 213:1394, 1981.
81. Wilson CB, Dempsey LC: Transsphenoidal microsurgical removal of 250 pituitary adenomas. *J Neurosurg* 48:13, 1978.
82. Wilson CB, Tyrrell JB, Fitzgerald PA, et al: Neurosurgical aspects of Cushing's disease and Nelson's syndrome, in Tindall GT, Collins WF (eds): *Clinical Management of Pituitary Disorders*. New York, Raven Press, 1979.
83. Wilson CB, Tyrrell JB, Fitzgerald PA, et al: Cushing's disease and Nelson's syndrome. *Clin Neurosurg* 27:19, 1980.
84. Wislawski J, Kasperlik-Zaluska AA, Jeske W, et al: Results of neurosurgical treatment by a transsphenoidal approach in 10 patients with Nelson's syndrome. *J Neurosurg* 62:68, 1985.

CHAPTER 8

Prolactinoma

Physiology of prolactin
Pathophysiology
Potential medical problems associated with hyperprolactinemia
Clinical features
Diagnostic evaluation
   Endocrinologic studies
   Neuroradiologic evaluation
Treatment
   Criteria for cure
   Surgery
   Pharmacotherapy
   Irradiation
Therapeutic decision making
   Microadenomas
   Recurrent prolactinoma following surgery
   Recurrent hyperprolactinemia following treatment
   Macroprolactinoma
   Preoperative use of bromocriptine
   Pseudoprolactinoma
Summary

Prolactin-secreting tumors (prolactinomas) are the most commonly encountered hyperfunctional pituitary tumor and account for approximately 25% of all pituitary tumors. The tumors are associated with hyperprolactinemia, which in turn causes galactorrhea (about 30%) and impairment of the menstrual cycle in women and impotency, galactorrhea (rarely), and hypogonadism in men.

In 1954 Forbes et al[22] demonstrated a relationship between pituitary tumors and the symptoms—amenorrhea and galactorrhea. In their original report, 8 of 15 patients had an enlargement of the sella turcica, and in 3 of the latter, a pituitary tumor was found. The authors suggested that lactation in these patients was the result of an excess production of prolactin by the tumor. Although prolactin was discovered in 1928 in extracts of the bovine pituitary, definite identification and measurement in human blood was not achieved until 1970. A sensitive bioassay reported in 1970 demonstrated that prolactin was present in human blood as a substance distinct from growth hormone.[27] In 1971 Friesen, Fournier, and Desjardins[34] isolated small quantities of prolactin from pituitary extracts, developed a radioimmunoassay for the human hormone, and measured it in plasma. Once a reliable assay became available, it soon became apparent that a significant number of patients with proven pituitary tumors had significant elevations of serum prolactin.

An interesting, and at the time unexplained, observation was made by Ehni and Eckles[18] in 1959 in a group of 17 women undergoing pituitary stalk section as palliative therapy for metastatic breast cancer. The intent of the surgery was to produce a functional hypophysectomy by interruption of the stalk and portal system. Postoperatively, four of the patients developed lactation. The authors speculated that "lactogenic hormone" elaborated by the surviving adenohypophysis produces and maintains lactation in the human breast following interruption of the stalk. Since then, it has been determined that interruption of the delivery of prolactin inhibiting factor (PIF) by stalk section allows the surviving adenohypophysis to secrete an unrestrained release of prolactin, thus accounting for lactation in stalk-sectioned women.

PHYSIOLOGY OF PROLACTIN

Prolactin is a polypeptide trophic hormone secreted by the erythrosinophilic subtype of acidophilic cells in the adenohypophysis.[28] Its release into the systemic circulation is under the dual control of hypothalamic neurohormones that act as releasing and inhibiting factors.[38] The dominant modulator is PIF, which is necessary to prevent an unrestrained release of prolactin by the adenohypophysis. Thus lesions such as pituitary stalk section or certain hypothalamic lesions that interfere with the normal production or delivery of PIF to the anterior lobe increase serum prolactin.[57,63] The prolactin inhibitory mechanism is dopaminergic in nature,[15] and there is some evidence to suggest that PIF is dopamine.[43] A prolactin-releasing factor (PRF), possibly regulated by serotonin, has been identified in hypothalamic extracts but has not been characterized. Thyrotropin-releasing hormone (TRH) is a potent stimulator of prolactin release from the pituitary but is not believed to be the physiologic PRF. This issue is also discussed in Chapter 2. These physiologic features serve as a basis for understanding both normal and abnormal responses of prolactin secretion to various pharmacologic agents and explain some changes in prolactin secretion associated with pituitary tumors.

The only established function of prolactin is in the initiation and maintenance of lactation provided the glandular breast tissue has been appropriately primed by the interaction of several other hormones including estrogen, progestins, corticosteroids, GH, and insulin.[15] Prolactin is also necessary in small amounts for progesterone production by granulosa cells. Although other functions of prolactin are not clear, the only clear clinical impairment resulting from elevated levels in women is suppression or interference with the menstrual cycle resulting in amenorrhea and infertility.

Several possible mechanisms may be responsible for the inhibitory effect of elevated serum prolactin levels on the normal functioning of the menstrual cycle.[26] First, prolactin could act at the hypothalamic level to interfere with either the tonic or the cyclic release of gonadotropin releasing hormone (luteinizing hormone–releasing hormone, [LHRH]). Secondly, elevated prolactin concentrations could act at the pituitary level to desensitize the gland to the action of LHRH, leading to impaired pituitary gonadotropin secretion. A third possibility is that elevated levels of serum prolactin act at the ovarian level to interfere with steroid production. The latter mechanism has received more support than the other two mechanisms mentioned above.[8,47]

Although the function of prolactin in men is unclear, the hormone is believed to be necessary for normal sperm production. Hyperprolactinemia inhibits 5-alpha-reductase, an enzyme that converts testosterone to the biologically active dihydrotestosterone, a hormone that needs to be in high concentrations within the testicular tubules for spermatogenesis to occur.[9] In men, impotence has been ascribed to elevated levels of prolactin, although this relationship is not established definitely.

Spontaneous galactorrhea occurs in about 35% of women with hyperprolactinemia,[24] and only rarely in men.[20]

PATHOPHYSIOLOGY

As shown in the following list and as indicated by many reports in the literature,* there are numerous causes for hyperprolactinemia:

    Pituitary tumors
      Prolactinomas
      Other ("stalk phenomenon")
    Destructive lesions of hypothalamus
    Parasellar tumors, aneurysms, and cysts—("stalk phenomenon")—(e.g., meningiomas, craniopharyngiomas, Rathke's pouch cysts
    Pharmacologic
      Monoamine depleting drugs (reserpine, methyldopa)
      Dopaminergic blocking drugs (haloperidol, chlorpromazine, pimozide)
      Histamine$_2$ blockers (cimetidine)
      Opiates (morphine, methadone)
    Oral contraceptives
    "Empty sella" syndrome
    Hypothyroidism, primary
    Idiopathic galactorrhea with amenorrhea (Argonz/del Castillo syndrome)
    Postpartum (Chiari-Frommel syndrome†)
    Repetitive and excessive breast stimulation
    Polycystic ovary syndrome
    "Idiopathic"
    Miscellaneous—(renal failure, chest wall lesions, trauma)

---

*See references 2, 11, 23-26, 29, 35, 36, 44, 48, 57, 58, and 63.
†Persistent galactorrhea and amenorrhea beginning after childbirth.

In practice, the three most commonly identifiable etiologic factors are ingestion of certain drugs, particularly phenothiazines; primary hypothyroidism; and pituitary tumors.[21,35,44] When the level of prolactin is modestly elevated (25 to 100 ng/ml), it is not possible to differentiate between these 3 conditions on the basis of prolactin levels alone. However, when the level is >150 ng/ml, the hyperprolactinemia with few exceptions is caused by a prolactin-secreting pituitary adenoma.

Elevated serum prolactin levels in patients with pituitary tumors occur as a result of one of two mechanisms.[36] The first results from the fact that certain tumors autonomously secrete excessive quantities of prolactin. The second mechanism is caused by mechanical impairment of the hypothalamus and/or stalk in such a manner as to diminish the secretion and delivery of PIF, thus resulting in unrestrained overproduction of prolactin by the normal adenohypophysis.

Pituitary tumors that autonomously secrete prolactin, termed prolactinomas, account for about 70% of chromophobe adenomas.[23,35] Currently, prolactinomas are the most frequently diagnosed functional pituitary tumors and represent approximately 25% of all pituitary tumors.[48,49,51] Hardy has shown that these tumors are usually located in the lateral wings of the pituitary gland,[31] which corresponds to the distribution of the majority of lactotrophs in the gland.

In patients with pituitary tumors, it is difficult to identify the underlying mechanism for elevated prolactin levels whenever the values are only moderately elevated (i.e., <100 ng/ml). Elevations of this magnitude in patients with pituitary tumors can result from compression of the stalk and/or hypothalamus as well as autonomous secretion by the tumor. Thus any structural lesion (e.g., craniopharyngioma, aneurysm, nonfunctional pituitary adenoma) exerting even minimal pressure on the pituitary stalk and/or inferior hypothalamus can cause modest elevations of prolactin. On the other hand, as mentioned above, when the fasting level exceeds 150 ng/ml, one can reasonably assume that the mechanism for the hyperprolactinemia is autonomous secretion by a prolactin-secreting pituitary adenoma.

There has been an apparent increase in the number of pituitary adenomas, especially microprolactinomas, in women of childbearing age, whereas the incidence in men and older women appears to have remained stable. Whether this increase is prompted by exposure to certain etiologic factors is controversial. The administration of estrogen to laboratory animals has been associated with an increased incidence of pituitary adenomas, but currently, no clear relationship has been identified between oral contraceptives and prolactinomas despite widespread use of these drugs.

POTENTIAL MEDICAL PROBLEMS ASSOCIATED WITH HYPERPROLACTINEMIA

Since the publication of a study showing that hyperprolactinemic women may exhibit decreased bone density, there has been concern that these patients may be at future risk for osteopenia and secondary fractures. Klibanski et al[37] measured bone densities in 14 women aged 20 to 40 years with moderate elevations of serum prolactin (22 to 99 ng/ml) and found that all patients had a significant reduction in bone density when compared with age-matched normal controls. The patients also had reduced estradiol levels, which accompanied the hyperprolactinemic state and probably accounted for the reduced bone density. Others have shown that the majority of hyperprolactinemic women have estradiol levels in the early follicular or postmenopausal range. Fearful that long-standing hyperprolactinemia may lead to unfavorable bony changes, Klibanski et al recommended that medical treatment (i.e., bromocriptine) may be indicated in patients with sustained hyperprolactinemia. Based on the findings of this single study and the rationale regarding therapy, many endocrinologists concerned with the possibility of patients developing future osteoporosis currently recommend that treatment of the hyperprolactinemic state is probably indicated.

Schlechte et al[54] did not find a correlation between hypoestrogenemia and reduced bone density. These authors believe other factors are responsible for the demineralization. In their study the reduction of bone mineral content was specifically related to hyperprolactinemia and was not seen in amenorrheic patients with normal prolactin levels. Interestingly, 38 women with prolactin-secreting pituitary tumors studied 2 to 5 years after transsphenoidal surgery had significantly diminished bone mineral content whether they were cured or had persistent amenorrhea and hyperprolactinemia.[54]

In our opinion, sustained hyperprolactinemia, particularly the modest elevations reported by Klibanski et al,[37] does not constitute a serious health hazard. There is no proof that these women actually exhibit a higher incidence of symptomatic osteoporosis. Thus it does not seem appropriate to treat all women with hyperprolactinemia because of the threat of this potential complication.

CLINICAL FEATURES

As with other hyperfunctional pituitary adenomas, prolactinomas may be evidenced by symptoms of endocrinopathy (resulting from hyperprolactinemia), mass effects, or both. Mass effects of prolactinomas are identical to those produced by nonfunctional tumors and are discussed in Chapter 4. The clinical findings incurred by hyperprolactinemia differ between sexes. In women, the principal findings consist of galactorrhea and reproductive dysfunction including amenorrhea or oligomenorrhea and infertility.

Galactorrhea consists of a white milky discharge. It may occur spontaneously or may require mild nipple stimulation. Galactorrhea occurs in approximately 30% of women of childbearing age who have proven prolactinomas.[25] It is not known why only some patients develop galactorrhea, but its occurrence does not appear to be related to serum prolactin levels. Amenorrhea or oligomenorrhea is a more consistent clinical finding and occurs in approximately 95% of women with hyperprolactinemia caused by a prolactinoma.[19]

Prolactinomas tend to be larger in men than in women at the time they come to medical attention. The reason for this difference in size at the time of presentation is unknown, but may be related to the fact that prolactinomas in women are detected earlier because of the more apparent symptoms resulting from the endocrinopathy. It has been suggested that the tumors in men may be more aggressive than those occurring in women,[30] again possibly a result of the earlier detection in women. Since the tumors are usually larger in men, the clinical picture is often dominated by hypopituitarism and symptoms resulting from mass effects. Men with prolactinomas may also present with decreased libido, impotency, and oligospermia. As expected, the incidence of galactorrhea in men is much lower than in women.[9,20] Carter et al[9] reported this finding in three of 22 men with prolactinomas. The mechanism of the impotency is not clear, but it does not appear to be a result of hypopituitarism or reduced levels of testosterone, although the latter is not an infrequent finding in these patients. However, restoration of lowered testosterone levels does not necessarily cure the impotency. It has been suggested that the impotency may result from a direct effect of prolactin on the central nervous system.[9,30]

DIAGNOSTIC EVALUATION

The endocrinopathy associated with prolactinomas is caused by the resultant hyperprolactinemia and is symptomatically identical to that produced by any other cause of elevated serum prolactin levels. Thus in the diagnostic workup of patients with hyperprolactinemia resuting from a suspected pituitary tumor, it is essential to obtain a detailed history and to perform appropriate tests to identify the cause of the elevated serum prolactin levels.

Because hyperprolactinemia can result from a wide variety of causes, including impingement of the pituitary stalk by any mass, it is occasionally difficult to make a positive diagnosis of a prolactinoma, particularly in cases of small microadenomas with serum levels of prolactin below 150 ng/ml.

The term *pseudoprolactinoma* is applied to any intrasellar or parasellar lesion other than a prolactin-secreting pituitary adenoma that causes elevation of serum prolactin by interfering with the delivery of PIF through pituitary stalk compression. The pseudoprolactinoma may be a nonfunctional pituitary adenoma, craniopharyngioma, tuberculum sella meningioma, aneurysm, or any one of several other lesions. Although serum prolactin levels are elevated, they rarely exceed 150 ng/ml. With prolactin levels of this magnitude, it is impossible to distinguish clinically between a lesion producing hyperprolactinemia by stalk compression and a true prolactinoma associated with a relatively low output of prolactin. Differentiation can be achieved only by surgical biopsy followed by immunohistologic evaluation of the tumor cells for prolactin granules. The clinical importance of the pseudoprolactinoma is seen when bromocriptine therapy is chosen for treatment in a patient with a pituitary tumor in whom the levels of serum prolactin are relatively low (i.e., <150 mg/ml) (see case summary on p. 277). There is no clinical way to determine if the tumor in this situation is a prolactinoma; thus failure of the patient to respond to bromocriptine by tumor shrinkage may be caused by the fact that the lesion is a pseudoprolactinoma.

Only *one* definite criteria indicates that the patient has a prolactinoma, the consistent elevation of serum prolactin levels above 150 ng/ml. The clinical syndrome alone is not adequate to make the diagnosis of prolactinoma because hyperprolactinemia from any cause may result in amenorrhea, galactorrhea, and infertility in women and impotence in men.

Although a few endocrinologists might argue that levels of prolactin above 150 ng/ml might be seen in patients with conditions other than tumors (and that the level for the positive diagnosis of a prolactinoma should be 200 or even 300 ng/ml), for practical purposes, when the level is greater than 150 ng/ml, one can reasonably assume that the patient has a prolactinoma. Very high serum prolactin levels (i.e., >1000 ng/ml) are believed to indicate tumor extension into the cavernous sinus.

Endocrinologic studies

The recommended endocrinologic studies are discussed in Chapter 4. In addition to the routine baseline endocrine tests, it is our recommendation that fasting serum prolactin values be obtained on at least two occasions. As with other pituitary tumors, the endocrine evaluation serves to establish and confirm the diagnosis of a prolactinoma, determine the functional capacity of the remaining pituitary gland, and evaluate therapy. Baseline endocrine studies are especially important in patients who undergo surgery, since comparison with postsurgical endocrine values will determine both the effectiveness of the procedure and, importantly, whether the surgery caused impairment in pituitary endocrine function.

Neuroradiologic evaluation

Neuroradiologic evaluation in patients with suspected prolactinomas consists of a lateral skull x-ray and a high-resolution coronal computed tomographic (CT) scan. The CT scan, which is the definitive radiologic procedure, will establish the diagnosis in most cases (except in some cases of very small microadenomas) and will determine the size and configuration of the adenoma and the degree of suprasellar or lateral extension. The use and limitations of CT are discussed in Chapter 5.

Any mass lesion in the vicinity of the stalk may be associated with a modest elevation in serum prolactin (usually <150 ng/ml) because of the stalk phenomenon. Therefore in patients with suspected prolactinomas in whom serum prolactin values are <150 ng/ml and in whom there is concern that the sellar or parasellar mass could conceivably be an aneurysm, it would be wise to obtain angiographic studies. Currently, a digital intravenous angiogram (DIVA) is an appropriate study for this purpose, since it provides adequate vascular imaging of the intracranial circulation to enable one to exclude the diagnosis of an aneurysm.

TREATMENT

Many factors enter into the therapeutic decision-making process in patients with prolactinomas, and when these are considered, it is easy to understand why treatment of this entity is a source of much controversy. Factors to consider include the availability of more than one effective therapeutic option; the variability in the natural history of prolactinomas, particularly microprolactinomas; and the issue of whether the hyperprolactinemic state constitutes a genuine health hazard.

Although one can assume that large prolactin-secreting macroadenomas started as microadenomas, we are not able to predict with accuracy which tumors will progress. The variability in the natural history of these lesions was addressed in a study by Weiss et al.[65] These investigators prospectively followed 27 women with symptomatic microprolactinomas who elected to have no treatment for 6 years. In only three of the 27 patients was there significant growth of the tumor during this period. Progressive growth in these three patients was not signaled by a significant increase in prolactin levels but rather by radiologic studies, principally the CT scan. These three patients subsequently underwent transsphenoidal surgery with normalization of their prolactin levels. Six patients experienced a progressive fall in prolactin levels, and the remaining 18 patients had no change in their radiologic studies, physical findings, or endocrine status. Although serial prolactin determinations were not helpful in predicting progressive growth of tumors, all six patients who exhibited a decline in their hyperprolactinemia had initial serum prolactin levels below 150 ng/ml. The results of this study in a relatively small number of cases would indicate that the short-term risk of progressive enlargement of a microprolactinoma is approximately 10%. Certainly, therapeutic decisions must be individualized for each patient after considering their health, tumor size, prolactin level, desire for pregnancy, and psychologic state.

Criteria for cure

The criteria for cure in patients with prolactinomas include total removal or complete destruction of the tumor mass, normalization of prolactin levels, relief of symptoms, and no evidence of recurrence over a follow-up period of at least 5 years. We do not believe that restoration of pituitary endocrine function, particularly restoration of impaired prolactin reserve as measured by stimulation tests (e.g., TRH, chlorpromazine tests [see Chapter 4]), should be included among the criteria for cure because these tests may remain abnormal in patients in whom all the other criteria for cure are met. Also there is no information available to indicate whether or not those patients who continue to have impaired prolactin reserve following treatment are those who are most likely to develop recurrence of disease.

Although normalization of prolactin levels is considered one of the criteria for cure, it is necessary to qualify this statement. As will be discussed later, it is possible to normalize prolactin levels with pharmacotherapy and yet not achieve eradication of the tumor. On the other hand, it is not uncommon to perform a "gross total removal" of a small- or moderate-sized tumor and yet not achieve normal serum prolactin values postoperatively. In these latter cases, it is possible that all tumor was removed and that the persistent hyperprolactinemia reflects stalk damage either from the tumor or surgery or both. If the elevated prolactin levels continue to fall gradually or remain unchanged on subsequent follow-up evaluation, it is likely that stalk damage was the causative factor for the persistent postoperative hyperprolactinemia. However, if subsequent prolactin levels begin to increase, it indicates that regrowth of residual tumor was responsible for the failure to normalize the prolactin in the immediate postoperative period. The problem of post-treatment hyperprolactinemia is discussed on pp. 263 and 264.

There are three effective therapeutic options for prolactinomas: transsphenoidal surgery, pharmacotherapy, and irradiation. Another option that a patient may choose, particularly in the case of a microprolactinoma, is *no therapy* with periodic follow-up and assessment of tumor size, clinical symptoms, and serum prolactin levels. This negative option for treatment is not unreasonable because, as discussed earlier, a study of the relatively short-term natural history of the microprolactinoma indicates that a significant number of cases may show no substantial growth over a period of several years.

Surgery

Transsphenoidal surgery is a safe and effective means of therapy in many patients with prolactinomas.* In our opinion, the major factors that influence the results of transsphenoidal surgery are the preoperative level of serum prolactin, the tumor size, and the direction of extrasellar extension if the tumor extends outside the confines of the sella turcica.

The direction of extrasellar tumor extension influences not only the surgical results but also the surgical approach. Tumors that invade the dura of the cavernous sinus are not surgically resectable by most criteria and, in our opinion, are incurable by any operative approach. Many tumors that extend into the anterior, middle, or posterior cranial fossae are better dealt with by craniotomy than transsphenoidal surgery.

Many authors have categorized their surgical results in terms of the preoperative serum prolactin levels. Good results can be achieved with transsphenoidal surgery, especially in patients in whom the preoperative serum prolactin levels are <200 ng/ml, as shown in Table 8-1. In patients with pretreatment prolactin levels <200 ng/ml, the immediate normalization of serum prolactin and symptomatic relief is in the neighborhood of 80%. Unfortunately, the results in patients with prolactinomas in whom the levels of serum prolactin are >200 ng/ml, and especially when the levels are >1000 ng/ml, are relatively poor. This is probably caused by the fact that many of the latter tumors are invasive (i.e., into the walls of the cavernous sinus) and thus defy any attempt at total surgical extirpation. As shown in Table 8-1 in the series of Hardy[32] and Bertrand et al,[7]

---

*See references 4, 7, 10, 16, 17, 19, 31-33, 39, 49, 51, 52, and 66.

Table 8-1
Results of transsphenoidal surgery in prolactinomas

Series	Total number of cases	Preoperative prolactin levels (ng/ml)	Number of cases	Number cured	Surgically related hypopituitarism	Number of complications	Year report published	Mortality
Bertrand et al, 1983[7]	90	<200	50	41 (82%)	3 (3.3%)	2† (2.2%)	1983	0
		>200, >500	18	9 (50%)				
		>500, <1000	11	4 (36%)				
		>1000	9	2 (22%)				
Emory Series, 1985	211	<200	130	104 (80%)	15 (7%)	5 (2.4%)	1985	0
		>200, <500	44	17 (39%)				
		>500, <1000	14	3 (21%)				
		>1000	23	0 (0%)				
Hardy, 1983[32]	266	<250	188	147 (78%)	44* (14.7%)	7* (2.3%)	1983	1
		>250, <500	33	16 (48%)				
		>500, >1000	28	6 (21%)				
		>1000	17	1 (6%)				

*Based on 300 cases (women) in his series; complete preoperative and postoperative prolactin levels in 266 of these 300 cases.
†Only two complications—one CSF rhinorrhea and one diplopia—appeared serious; also reported 30 instances of diabetes insipidus, all transient and six nasal septal perforations, all asymptomatic.

and our own, levels of preoperative prolactin <200 ng/ml are associated with immediate cure rates of 80% (78% to 82%). However, the rate drops to 39% to 50% with preoperative prolactin values between 200 (and in Hardy's series, 250 ng) and 500 ng/ml. Cure rates ranging from 21% to 36% are obtained in patients whose preoperative serum prolactin values range from 500 to 1000 ng/ml. Serum prolactin values above 1000 ng/ml are associated with a very low cure rate. There were no cures in this group in the Emory series, and Hardy reports only one cure in 17 (6%) cases. Bertrand et al cured two of nine for an incidence of 22%.

There are many other series reporting the results of transsphenoidal surgery. These series usually divide the patients into two groups with the point of division being a preoperative serum prolactin level of 200 ng/ml. The only reason for not citing these other series in Table 8-1 is that further subdivision above a preoperative serum prolactin level >200 ng/ml was not made. In these series (which include reports by Landolt;[39] Post et al;[52] Dominique, Richmond, and Wilson;[17] Aubourg et al;[4] Werder et al;[66] among others), the "immediate" cure rates in those cases whose preoperative serum prolactin was <200 ng/ml ranged from 75% to 88%.

Thus one can surmise from the results shown in Table 8-1 that the results of surgery, particularly when preoperative values are greater than 500 ng/ml, are poor. We would conclude that for these patients surgery is probably not the best option and pharmacotherapy on a daily basis may be the most appropriate therapeutic option.

The surgical cure rate is also related to size of the tumor, which in turn bears some relationship to preoperative serum prolactin levels. In the first 100 women with verified prolactinomas treated at our institution, 81% of 72 patients with preoperative serum prolactin levels <200 ng/ml had microadenomas, and 86% of 28 patients with levels >200 ng/ml had tumors >10 mm in diameter.[19] Thus in our experience, the preoperative serum prolactin level is related to the size of the tumor, and both of these factors have a distinct bearing on the results of surgery. In the Chang et al[10] series of patients undergoing transsphenoidal surgery, cure (as expressed by return of menses) was obtained in 16 of 17 patients (94%) with tumors less than 10 mm in diameter (microadenoma) but in only two of seven patients (29%) with macroadenomas (>10 mm).

Most of the surgical reports of prolactinomas have been limited to the results in women, and only a few authors have addressed the issue in men. As already mentioned, most men with prolactinomas seek medical attention with larger tumors (related to the later clinical presentation in male patients), and as would be expected, the cure rates in general are not as favorable as they are in women. For instance, Serri et al[56] reported the results of transsphenoidal surgery in 15 men with prolactinomas in whom prolactin levels ranged from 85 to 6240 ng/ml. Postoperatively, normal prolactin levels were obtained in only four of the 15 patients (27%). In nine of their patients with postoperative hyperprolactinemia, the values were in excess of 200 ng/ml.

A recent report by Serri et al[55] reviewing Hardy's series emphasizes the necessity for long-term follow-up in assessing the true cure rate in patients undergoing transsphenoidal surgery for prolactinomas. In evaluating prognosis for these patients after transsphenoidal surgery, they found that 12 of 24 patients with microprolactinomas and four of five patients with macroprolactinomas had recurrence of hyperprolactinemia 6.2 ± 1.5 years after surgery.[55] Although clinical and biologic features before surgery could not predict the long-term outcome, the immediate postoperative level of prolactin was significantly lower in patients in whom normal prolactinemia was maintained than in those who relapsed. It should be stressed that in their study there was no radiologic evidence of tumor recurrence in any patient and no relationship between the occurrence of pregnancy after surgery and the recurrence of hyperprolactinemia. The explanation for the recurrent hyperprolactinemia is unknown. Recurrent tumors too small to be detected and a primary hypothalamic defect that induced hyperplasia of normal pituitary lactotrophs were possible mechanisms suggested by the authors, but at the present time, there are no hard facts to explain the recurrent hyperprolactinemia.

Pharmacotherapy

In the past, a variety of hormonal therapies were used in patients with amenorrhea and galactorrhea, most without affecting the underlying disorder. More recently dopamine agonists such as levodopa and ergot alkaloids have undergone therapeutic trials with more encouraging results. Most noteworthy,

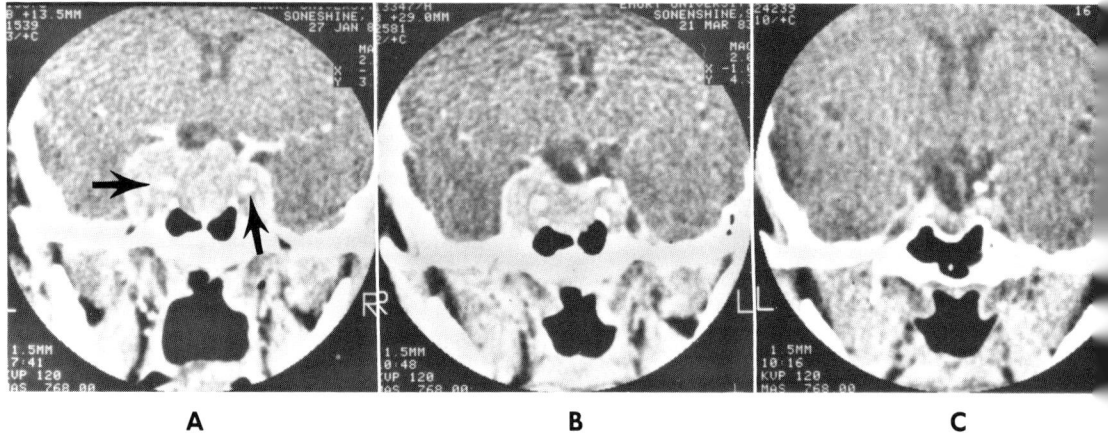

Fig. 8-1. Serial CT scans illustrating response of invasive prolactinoma to bromocriptine. Patient is 21-year-old man who was seen with complaints of headaches and bitemporal hemianopsia associated with serum prolactin value of 3200 ng/ml. **A,** Contrast-enhanced coronal CT before treatment showing invasive tumor. Carotid arteries (arrows) can be visualized within the tumor. **B,** Scan performed 3 months after initiation of bromocriptine treatment shows significant reduction of tumor. Patient had complete resolution of his visual field defect. **C,** Striking reduction in tumor 15 months after starting therapy. Serum prolactin value was reduced to 256 ng/ml. Patient's visual fields remain normal, and he is presently being followed on bromocriptine.

bromocriptine is a potent inhibitor of the synthesis and release of prolactin by the pituitary gland and has beneficial therapeutic effects in the majority of cases of prolactinomas.* Bromocriptine administered orally on a daily basis usually results in a significant reduction or normalization of elevated serum prolactin levels, provides symptomatic relief including cessation of galactorrhea and resumption of menses, and may initiate a return of fertility. The pathologic changes underlying these favorable clinical changes include a reduction in cytoplasmic volume resulting from a reduction of ribosomes, rough endoplasmic reticulum, and Golgi complexes.[5,53,61] There is, however, no evidence of lysosomal accumulation, necrosis, vascular or endothelial cell damage, platelet aggregation, or thrombosis. An example of a striking result of bromocriptine therapy of a prolactinoma is shown in Fig. 8-1. Available data would indicate that these favorable regressive changes persist in the majority of patients for several years as long as the drug is taken on a regular daily basis.

However, as indicated by the pathologic changes referred to previously, bromocriptine is *not tumoricidal*. Consequently, when the drug is withdrawn, one can expect the tumor to reexpand, the symptoms to recur, and the hyperprolactinemia to return in the majority of patients with prolactinomas (Fig. 8-2).

There do not appear to be many serious side effects of the drug. The initial

---

*See references 3, 8, 12, 14, 45, 46, 50, 58-60, and 64.

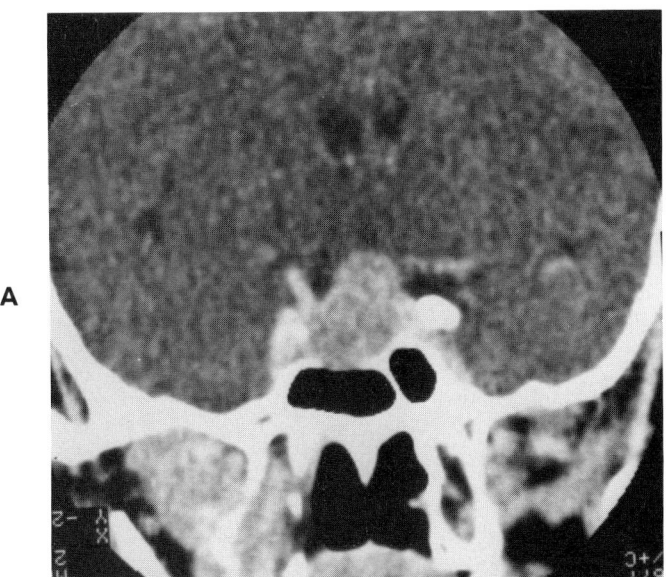

Fig. 8-2. Serial CT scans demonstrating return of tumor size to pretreatment dimensions following discontinuation of bromocriptine. Patient is 34-year-old man who came to medical attention with headaches, hypopituitarism, and a serum prolactin level of 3150 ng/ml. **A,** Contrast-enhanced coronal CT scan before treatment shows a large pituitary tumor with suprasellar extension. *Continued.*

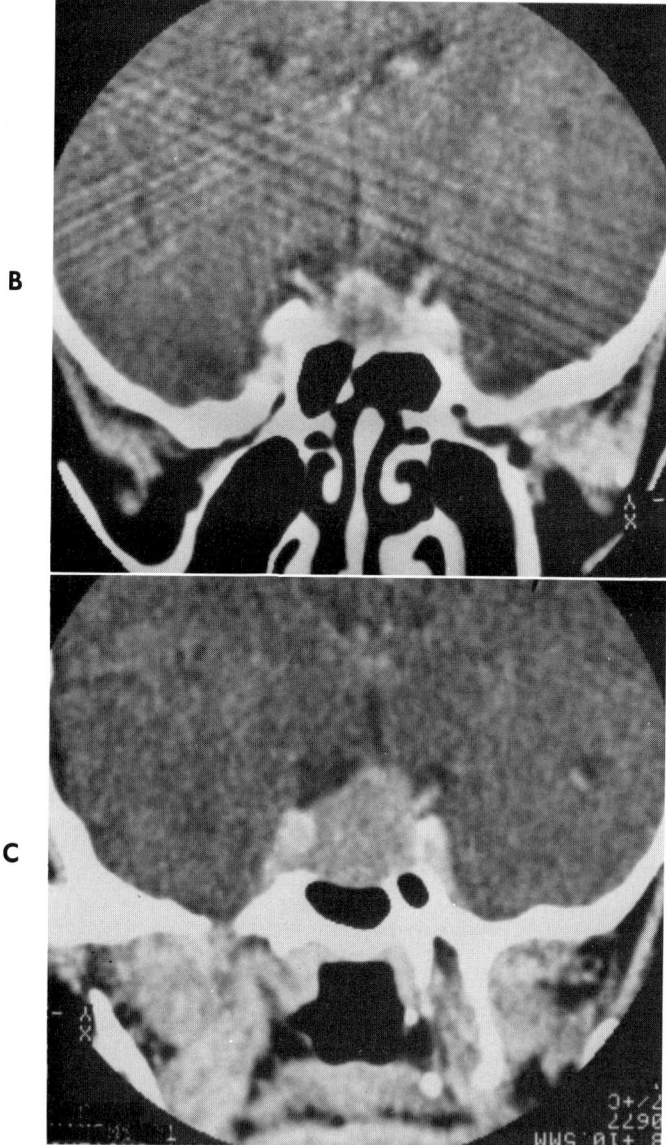

Fig. 8-2, cont'd. B, Scan performed 3 weeks after initiation of bromocriptine therapy shows a significant reduction in tumor size. Six weeks after beginning of therapy, patient developed a rash, and his endocrinologist discontinued bromocriptine. **C,** Scan performed 10 days after discontinuation of bromocriptine reveals return of adenoma to its pretreatment size.

syncopal symptoms that may occur soon clear, and the gastrointestinal discomforts can usually be controlled by taking the drug with food. In patients who take the medication in an effort to restore fertility, evidence would indicate that the drug has no adverse effects on the fetus. The collective world experience, documented by Sandoz, of 1410 pregnancies in 1335 women who conceived while taking bromocriptine has failed to demonstrate any increased incidence of fetal abnormalities or multiple births.[62]

There is some theoretical concern over the long-term (i.e., several years) effects of a potent dopamine agonist drug such as bromocriptine on the brain. Whether this therapy will permanently inhibit the normal endogenous production of dopamine in important brain centers such as the substantia nigra is unknown at present. Should this occur, it is conceivable that permanent neurologic sequelae (i.e., Parkinsonism) could result.

Also data are currently available that suggest the prolonged and regular use of bromocriptine in patients with microprolactinomas may result in lower cure rates in patients who, for whatever reason(s), later choose to have transsphenoidal surgery. Landolt compared the surgical results in patients with microprolactinomas treated for at least 1 year with bromocriptine with the results in patients who had received no bromocriptine.[41] The success rate in the bromocriptine-treated patients was 44% compared with 78% in those who had not received bromocriptine. He attributed the reduced cure rate in the bromocriptine-treated patients to fibrosis induced by the drug, which in turn prevented the surgeon from obtaining a complete removal of tumor. In a subsequent study, Landolt and Osterwalder[42] showed that there was a significant increase in perivascular fibrous tissue in the treated group as compared to those patients who did not receive bromocriptine. They postulated that the shrinkage of tumor cells induced by bromocriptine caused enlargement of the extracellular and perivascular spaces, which filled by the deposition of collagen, thus producing a more dense consistency of the adenoma. These studies have generated much interest and raise more issues and questions than answers. The possibility that bromocriptine may adversely affect later surgical cure rates has great impact among endocrinologists and neurosurgeons and obviously requires more study in larger patient populations before all the facts of this issue are available for analysis.

Cerebrospinal fluid (CSF) rhinorrhea during bromocriptine therapy of large prolactinomas has been reported.[6,13,40,67] This relatively rare complication is believed to develop as a result of shrinkage of a responsive tumor, thus exposing a defect in the dura and sella floor.

Another relative disadvantage of bromocriptine is that it is moderately expensive; however, the same criticism can be applied to other treatment modalities.

Irradiation

Although this mode of therapy has some effectiveness, it is generally not recommended as primary treatment in the majority of patients with prolactinomas. In fact, there are relatively few data available on the use of irradiation as primary therapy in prolactinomas. This subject is discussed in Chapter 13.

Among the patients with prolactinomas reported by Antunes et al[1] were six patients treated by irradiation alone. These authors tended to use radiotherapy in patients with high-grade tumors and high prolactin concentrations. Although a reduction in prolactin levels was obtained, normalization of serum prolactin was not achieved in any of the six patients.

Irradiation is an effective and reasonable option in patients with recurrent or persistent disease following other forms of therapy, especially transsphenoidal surgery.

THERAPEUTIC DECISION MAKING

As with other hyperfunctional pituitary tumors the availability of more than one effective treatment modality creates a need for the physician to make appropriate decisions regarding therapy in these patients. The following clinical presentations represent the majority of patients requiring treatment.

Microadenomas

The majority of microadenomas will be seen in young women who have impairment of the reproductive cycle with or without galactorrhea. Occasionally, men with impotence and hypogonadism will be found to have a microprolactinoma. However, most men who have this symptom complex on the basis of prolactin-secreting adenomas will have macroadenomas rather than microadenomas.

Young women with amenorrhea either with or without galactorrhea. In these cases, decision making is influenced by the patient's desire for pregnancy. If the patient does not desire pregnancy, we believe that the best two options are careful and periodic follow-up with no therapy or transsphenoidal surgery. We do not endorse the use of bromocriptine in treating these cases, primarily because it may jeopardize the chances for a surgical cure if the patient later decides to have surgery, which many patients later choose when pregnancy is desired.[41,42]

As indicated in the study by Weiss et al,[65] the majority of microprolactinomas do not seem to follow a steady growth curve. In fact, one can expect that in a significant percentage of patients with microprolactinomas, serial CT scans at 6 or 12 month intervals may show *no* increase in size of the tumor, thus providing a good rationale for follow-up observation in young women with this lesion who do not desire pregnancy.

Transsphenoidal surgery is also a good option in these patients, since the best chance for a cure is in the small tumor with values of serum prolactin <200 ng/ml. This choice is often made by young women regardless of whether or not pregnancy is desired after becoming fully informed of the risks and benefits of all therapies and the likely natural history of the lesion. Although immediate cure rates of approximately 80% have been reported in these cases, it is important to realize that many of these women may symptomatically "recur" as indicated in the report by Serri et al.[55] It should be stressed, however, that in their report there was recurrent hyperprolactinemia but no actual evidence of tumor regrowth. Obviously, the implications of this study have a great impact on patients contemplating surgery as a therapeutic option, and it is important that these results be verified in a larger series of cases and by other investigators.

Women with microprolactinomas desiring pregnancy. Currently, it is our opinion that transsphenoidal surgery is the most appropriate option in this group. As already indicated, surgery will restore normal menses in approximately 80% of the patients. The advantage of surgery over pharmacotherapy is that it eradicates the tumor and eliminates the possibility of having to manage any complication related to the tumor that may arise during pregnancy. For instance, if bromocriptine is chosen as primary therapy in these patients, it will normalize serum prolactin and restore menses, allowing the woman to achieve pregnancy despite the fact that the tumor is still present. After the patient becomes pregnant, bromocriptine is discontinued. In these cases, there is always the possibility that the tumor will enlarge significantly during pregnancy and become symptomatic by producing mass effects. Should this happen, the physician must make a decision as to how to deal with the lesion (i.e., surgery versus pharmacotherapy) during the pregnancy, a situation that is avoided if surgery was chosen as the initial therapeutic option. Experience indicates, however, that there is relatively little chance that during pregnancy a microprolactinoma will enlarge to the point of causing significant mass effects.

The following case illustrates some of the points just discussed:

Prolactin microadenoma with negative CT—recurrent hyperprolactinemia after a period of "cure"

A 25-year-old woman was referred with a 5-year history of amenorrhea and a 3-month history of galactorrhea. On examination, the patient was slightly overweight, and a milky discharge could be expressed from either nipple. The examination was otherwise negative.

The serum prolactin was 80 ng/ml, and a coronal CT scan (Fig. 8-3) of the pituitary was negative. The patient was taking no medications and did not have hypothyroidism. It was believed likely that the patient had a microadenoma that was too small to be detected by the CT scan.

The options (i.e., no therapy but close follow-up, pharmacotherapy, and transsphenoidal surgery) were discussed, and the patient chose surgery. The patient desired fertility and did not want to use a medical option.

Transsphenoidal surgery was performed, and a 7 mm microadenoma was excised with preservation of the remaining gland. Postoperatively, the patient did well. Serum prolactin 6 days following surgery was 16 ng/ml. The patient's galactorrhea cleared, and she resumed normal menstrual periods. Sixteen months after surgery, she delivered a normal baby girl. Following delivery, she had galactorrhea, which has been persistent, and 9 months later her menstrual periods became irregular. Three years after surgery, a serum prolactin was 70 ng/ml, and a CT scan was normal. She continues to be followed in the clinic.

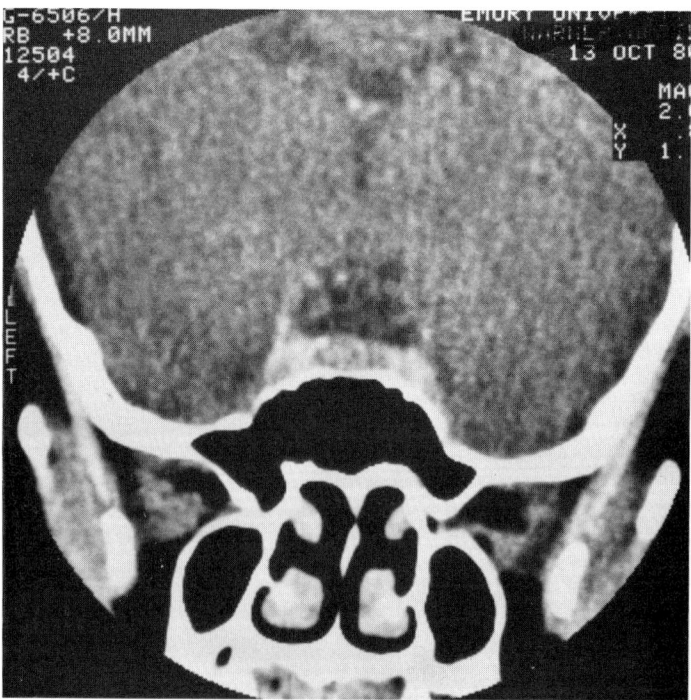

Fig. 8-3. Negative CT scan in patient with microprolactinoma. Contrasted coronal CT showing a gland of normal dimensions without focal abnormalities.

This case emphasizes two important points. First, the patient had a definite microprolactinoma despite the negative high-resolution CT scan. The diagnosis was made by the presence of hyperprolactinemia in the absence of another cause, not the CT scan. Secondly, despite a "cure" characterized by normalization of serum prolactin and achievement of pregnancy, the patient 4 years later has had a recurrence of hyperprolactinemia. Tests so far have failed to reveal recurrent tumor. This case is similar to those discussed in the report by Serri et al.[55]

Recurrent prolactinoma following surgery

The diagnosis of recurrent tumor (or a regrowth of tumor missed at the initial operation) is established by CT scanning and progressive rises in serially determined serum prolactin levels. In these patients, it is highly *unlikely* that further surgery, even when performed by an experienced surgeon, will result in a cure. Although pharmacotherapy and radiation are both effective and appropriate options in these patients, it is our practice to use only pharmacotherapy as treatment and, if it is effective as measured by significant reduction in serum prolactin levels and favorable changes on the CT scan, to continue to use it for as long as it remains effective. Radiation is reserved for those patients who do not achieve a good therapeutic result with bromocriptine or in those in whom the drug later fails to control tumor growth.

Recurrent hyperprolactinemia following treatment (recurrence of tumor not verified)

Bromocriptine is probably the treatment of choice in patients who have initial success with surgical therapy but who later develop hyperprolactinemia as illustrated in the 25-year-old woman presented above. The clinician may also choose to follow the patient and periodically check for the possibility of tumor recurrence and not initiate any therapy as long as no tumor is obvious.

Macroprolactinoma

In general, therapeutic decisions need to be individualized in these patients because some tumors will obviously be invasive and others, although associated with high values of prolactin, will show CT characteristics that would suggest that total excision may be possible. We have arbitrarily listed three categories of patients basing the division primarily on the level of serum prolactin. The reader should realize that this method of grouping is relatively arbitrary and that factors (e.g., appearance on the CT scan) other than the level of serum prolactin enter into the therapeutic decision-making process in these patients.

Subgroup 1—serum prolactin levels between 200 and 500 ng/ml. In many of these cases, tumors are of moderate size, and invasiveness is not apparent. If the CT scan shows that the extrasellar extension is directly suprasellar, the tumor measures less than 2.5 cm in its greatest diameter, and there is no obvious invasion of the cavernous sinus, it is our opinion that transsphenoidal surgery is a reasonable therapeutic option. In the hands of an experienced pituitary surgeon, the cure rate in this group is approximately 50%. If surgery fails to cure the patient and the surgeon either leaves behind obvious tumor or the 3-month postoperative CT scan confirms the presence of residual tumor, the recommended treatment is the same as that cited earlier (i.e., recurrent prolactinomas following previous surgery).

Subgroup 2—serum prolactin levels between 500 and 1000 ng/ml. Many of these tumors are large and invasive; in fact, extremely high levels of serum prolactin usually indicate that the tumor has already involved the cavernous sinus. An example of such a case is shown in Fig. 8-1. Although cavernous sinus invasion cannot always be determined by CT, such involvement is confirmed if a contrasted coronal CT scan shows the internal carotid artery surrounded by tumor. Therapeutic decisions in this group should all be individualized and will rely considerably on CT findings. Despite the high prolactin levels, some tumors may appear on CT to be noninvasive, and in these cases, it is appropriate to recommend surgery. In cases such as that illustrated in Fig. 8-1, it is impossible to achieve a surgical cure, and thus options other than surgery should be chosen. In general, the most appropriate therapeutic option in this group is the regular use of bromocriptine.

The following example illustrates a case in which medical management was selected:

Large prolactinoma with serum prolactin level greater than 500 ng/ml

The patient is a 32-year-old policeman who was seen with complaints of slight visual impairment described as "blind spots," primarily in his right eye. Neuroophthalmologic examination showed a bitemporal superior quadrantanopsia with acuity 20/40 OD; 20/30 OS. A CT scan (Fig. 8-4, *A*) showed a large pituitary tumor with suprasellar extension. The serum prolactin was 540 ng/ml.

The options (surgery versus pharmacotherapy) were discussed with the patient. He was told that the literature indicated that the chances for a surgical cure (with prolactin levels above 500 ng/ml [see Table 8-1]) were on the order of 25%. The patient chose bromocriptine, and therapy was begun with low dosages gradually building up to a total daily dosage of 7.5 mg/day.

The patient noted almost immediate subjective improvement in his vision. Eight weeks after starting therapy, the serum prolactin level was 35 ng/ml, and the neuroophthalmologic examination was normal. A CT scan (Fig. 8-4, *B*) showed significant reduction in size of the tumor. The patient continues therapy and will be followed periodically in the clinic.

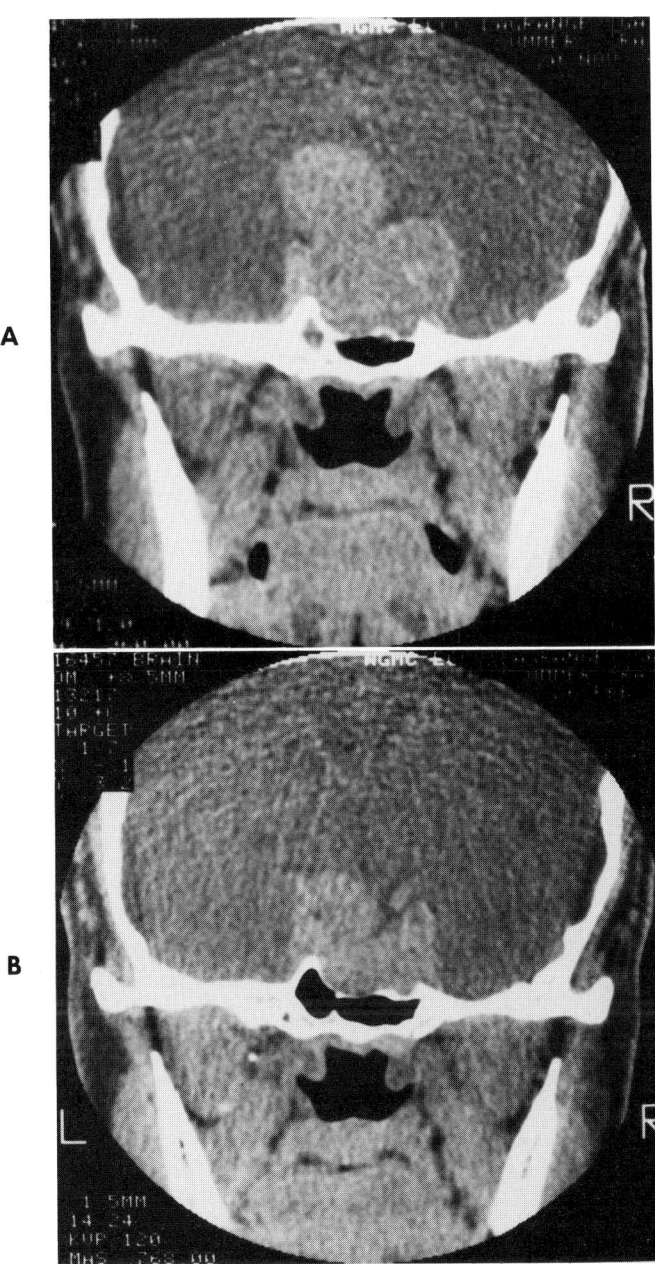

Fig. 8-4. CT scan of macroprolactinoma treated with bromocriptine. **A,** Pretreatment contrast-enhanced coronal scan shows large pituitary adenoma with significant suprasellar extension. **B,** Scan performed 6 weeks after initiation of bromocriptine shows significant reduction in size of tumor.

Subgroup 3—serum prolactin levels greater than 1000 ng/ml. Serum prolactin levels of this magnitude indicate invasiveness. The chances of surgical cure are so low in this group that we cannot recommend surgery as an appropriate treatment. Pharmacotherapy is the best option, and when and if this choice fails to control the tumor, irradiation should be employed.

Preoperative use of bromocriptine

Also to be considered in macroprolactinomas is the possibility that preoperative treatment with bromocriptine will cause enough reduction in tumor size that subsequent management by surgery will provide a better chance of achieving a cure. We have had some experience with this method of therapy and *are not convinced* that this approach enhances therapeutic success.[5,61]

The following case illustrates an example of this therapeutic approach:

> A 23-year-old woman sought medical help because of headaches, amenorrhea, and galactorrhea. She had a serum prolactin level of 9800 ng/ml, and a CT scan (Fig. 8-5, *A*) showed a large pituitary adenoma with marked suprasellar extension. Bromocriptine therapy was initiated (2.5 mg t.i.d.), followed by a reduction in the prolactin level to 310 ng/ml. A CT performed 3 weeks after starting bromocriptine showed a dramatic reduction in the size of the tumor (Fig. 8-5, *B*). After 6 weeks of therapy, the patient underwent transsphenoidal removal of all visible tumor with continuation of bromocriptine up to the morning of surgery. Postoperatively, the patient had improvement in her headache but continued to have amenorrhea and galactorrhea. The postoperative serum prolactin climbed to 3000 ng/ml, and a CT scan showed residual tumor (Fig. 8-5, *C*). Bromocriptine therapy was reinstituted. After 2 years of postoperative bromocriptine therapy, her serum prolactin is 22 ng/ml, the amenorrhea and galactorrhea have ceased, and the CT shows no evidence of residual tumor (Fig. 8-5, *D*). She is presently being maintained on bromocriptine and is followed in the clinic.

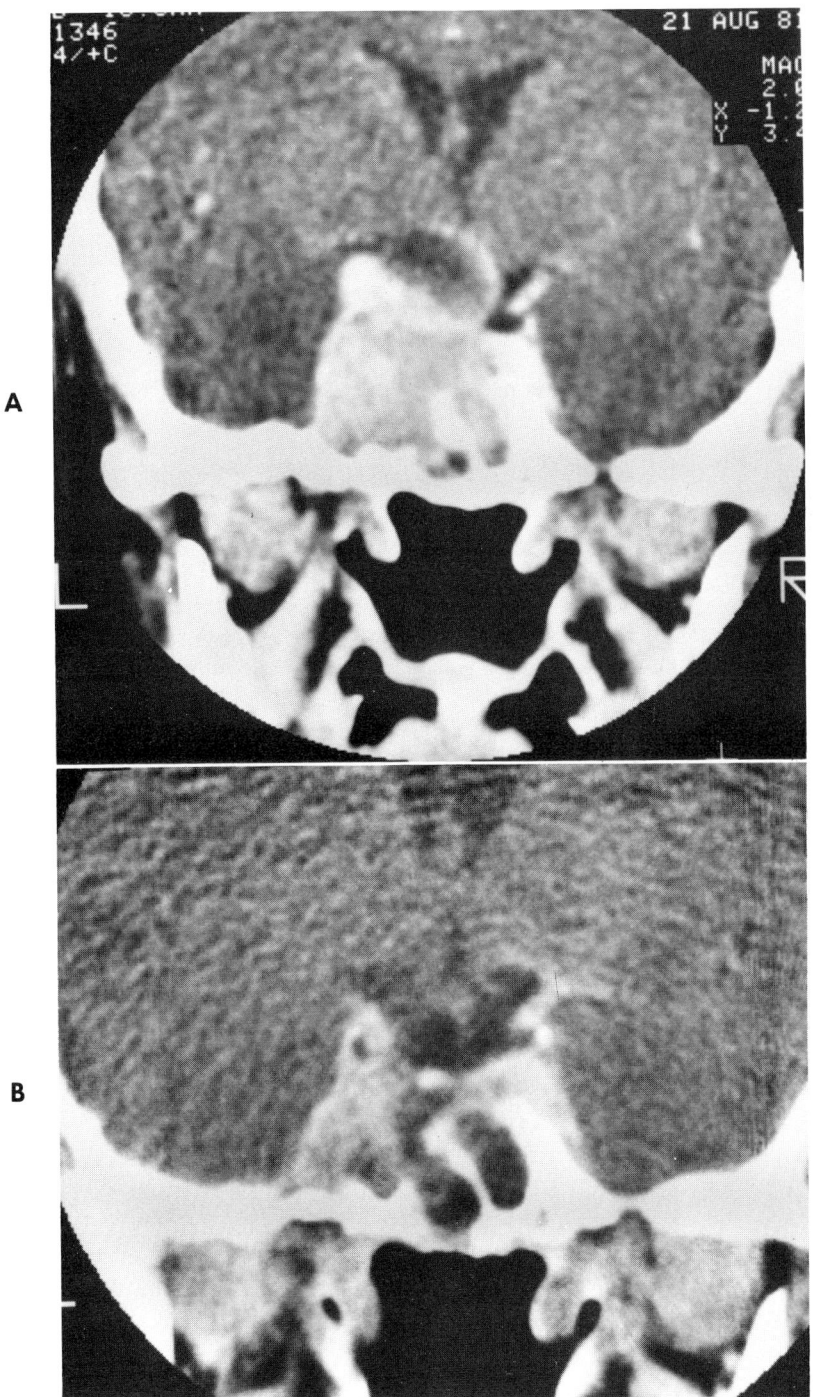

Fig. 8-5. CT in patient treated preoperatively with bromocriptine. **A,** Contrasted coronal CT shows large pituitary adenoma with significant suprasellar extension. **B,** Scan performed after 3 weeks of bromocriptine therapy shows a dramatic reduction in tumor size.
Continued.

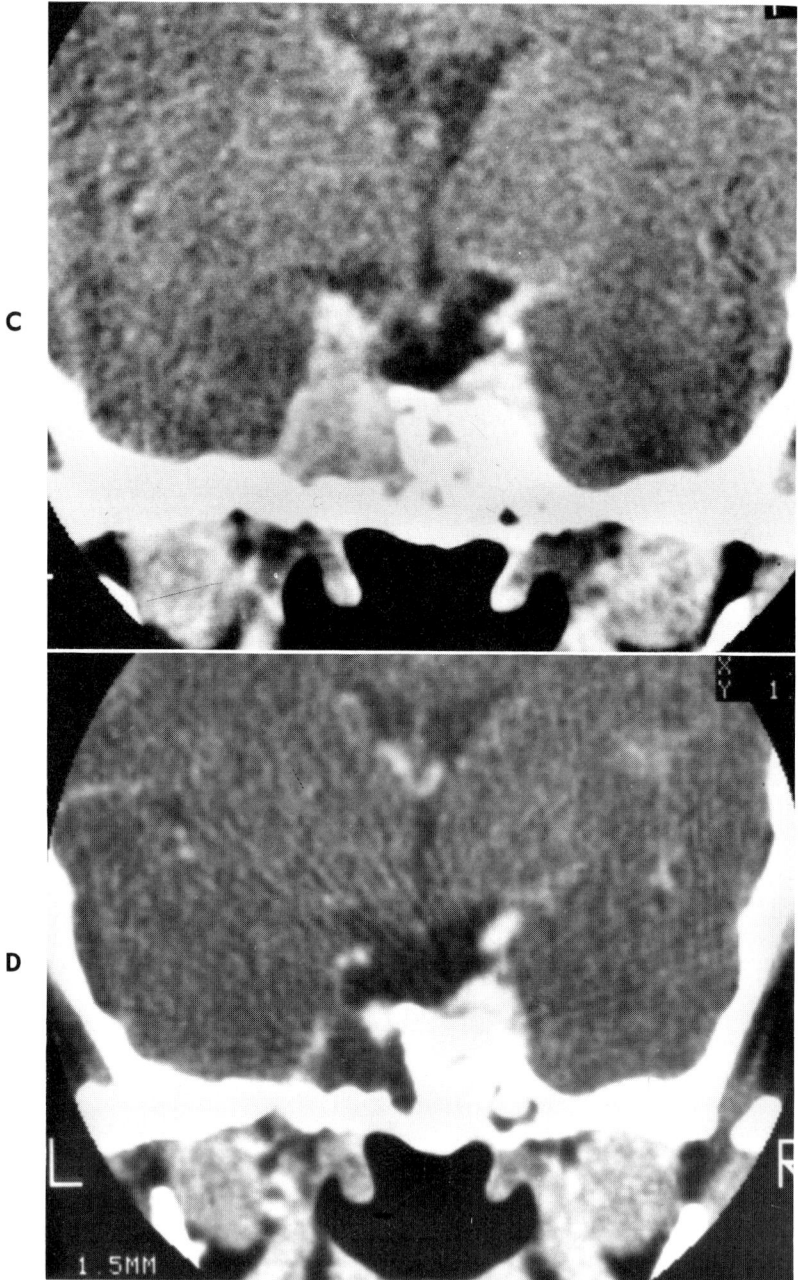

Fig. 8-5, cont'd. C, Postoperative CT indicates residual enhancing tumor. **D,** Following postoperative bromocriptine therapy, there is no demonstrable tumor on CT.

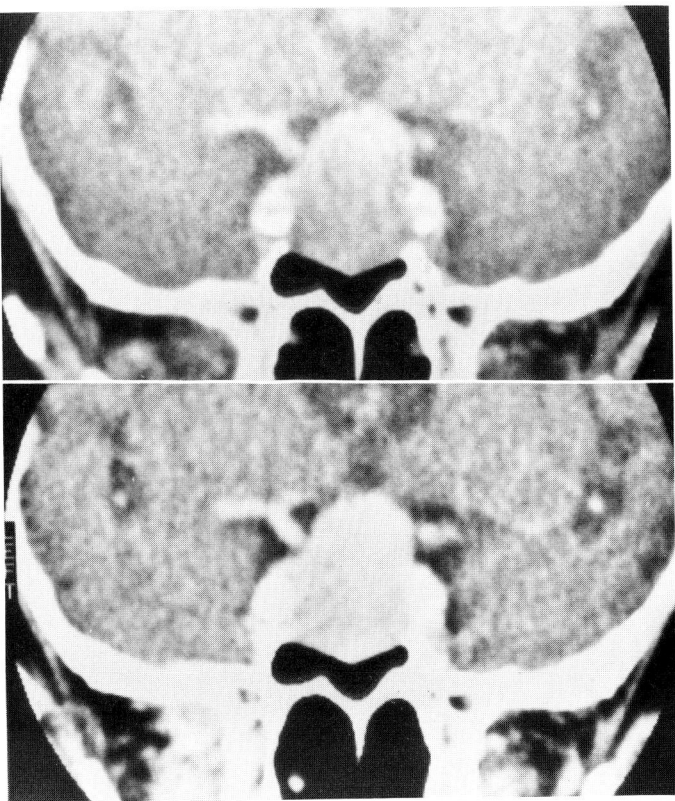

Fig. 8-6. CT of "pseudoprolactinoma" treated with bromocriptine and surgery. *Top,* Contrast-enhanced coronal CT showing large pituitary adenoma. *Bottom,* CT performed 6 weeks after institution of bromocriptine therapy (but before surgery) shows no change in size of tumor.

"Pseudoprolactinoma"

It is important to exercise caution in assuming that all hyperprolactinemia is a result of prolactinomas, as the following case illustrates:

> A 42-year-old man came to medical attention because of headaches and visual loss. Neuroophthalmologic examination revealed a bitemporal hemianopsia and visual acuity of 20/40 OU. He had a serum prolactin level of 113 ng/ml, and a CT scan that showed a large pituitary adenoma (Fig. 8-6, *A*). After discussing the options for treatment, it was decided to treat the patient with bromocriptine (2.5 mg t.i.d.) before surgery in an attempt to shrink the mass and make total excision more feasible. After 6 weeks of treatment with bromocriptine, a CT revealed no change in the size of the tumor from the pretreatment scan (Fig. 8-6, *B*), although the prolactin level dropped to 43 ng/ml. The patient underwent transsphenoidal surgery with a gross total removal of the tumor. Pathologic examination of the tumor indicated that it was a null cell adenoma without any prolactin granules identified by immunocytochemistry. Postoperatively, the patient experienced relief of his headaches, the visual fields returned to normal, and the serum prolactin dropped to 2 ng/ml. Three years after surgery, he has no evidence of recurrence of tumor on CT and maintains a normal serum prolactin level.

This case is an example of a "pseudoprolactinoma" with the hyperprolactinemia resulting from pituitary stalk impingement rather than autonomous secretion of prolactin by the tumor. When treating a presumed prolactinoma with bromocriptine, careful follow-up is necessary to be certain the drug is having the desired therapeutic effect.

SUMMARY

The diagnosis of prolactinomas is established by the level of serum prolactin and high-resolution coronal CT scanning. Hyperprolactinemia, which is associated with demineralization of bone, is a potential complication, but whether this observation translates into a genuine health hazard is as yet unproven. The therapy of prolactinomas is a controversial issue. The three effective options include surgery, pharmacotherapy, and irradiation. There are no simple, general statements to be made that will encompass therapeutic recommendations for all patients except to state that therapeutic decisions depend on many factors and many of the decisions are made on an individualized basis.

REFERENCES

1. Antunes JL, Housepian EM, Frantz AG, et al: Prolactin-secreting pituitary tumors. *Ann Neurol* 2:148, 1977.
2. Argonz J, del Castillo EB: A syndrome characterized by estrogenic insufficiency, galactorrhea and decreased urinary gonadotropin. *J Clin Endocrinol Metab* 13:79, 1953.
3. Aronoff SL, Daughaday WH, Laws ER Jr: Bromocriptine treatment of prolactinomas, letter. *N Engl J Med* 300:1391, 1979.
4. Aubourg PR, Derome PJ, Peillon F, et al: Endocrine outcome after transsphenoidal adenomectomy for prolactinoma: prolactin levels and tumor size as predicting factors. *Surg Neurol* 14:141, 1980.
5. Barrow DL, Tindall GT, Kovacs K, et al: Clinical and pathological effects of bromocriptine on prolactin-secreting and other pituitary tumors. *J Neurosurg* 60:1, 1984.
6. Baskin DS, Wilson CB: CSF rhinorrhea after bromocriptine for prolactinoma, letter. *N Engl J Med* 306:178, 1982.
7. Bertrand G, Tolis G, Montes J: Immediate and long-term results of transsphenoidal microsurgical resection of prolactinomas in 92 patients, in Tolis G, et al (eds): *Prolactin and Prolactinomas.* New York, Raven Press, 1983.
8. Besser GM, Thorner MO: Bromocriptine in the treatment of the hyperprolactinaemia-hypogonadism syndromes. *Postgrad Med J* 52(suppl 1):64, 1976.
9. Carter JN, Tyson JE, Tolis G, et al: Prolactin-secreting tumors and hypogonadism in 22 men. *N Engl J Med* 299:847, 1978.
10. Chang RJ, Keye WR Jr, Young JR, et al: Detection, evaluation, and treatment of pituitary microadenomas in patients with galactorrhea and amenorrhea. *Am J Obstet Gynecol* 128:356, 1977.
11. Chiari J: Bericht uber die in den Jahren 1848 bis inclusive 1951 an der gynakologishen Abteilung in Wien beobachteten Frauenkrankheiten im engern Sinne des Wortes, in Chiari J, Braun C, Spath J: *Klinik der Geburtshilfe und Gynakologie*. Stuttgart, Ferdinand Enke Verlag, 1855.
12. Chiodini P, Liuzzi A, Cozzi R, et al: Size reduction of macroprolactinomas by bromocriptine or lisuride treatment. *J Clin Endocrinol Metab* 53:737, 1981.
13. Cole IE, Keene M: Cerebrospinal fluid rhinorrhoea in pituitary tumors. *J R Soc Med* 73:244, 1980.
14. Corenblum B, Webster BR, Mortimer CB, et al: Possible anti-tumour effect of 2-bromo-ergocryptine (CB-154, Sandoz) in two patients with large prolactin-secreting pituitary adenomas, (abstract). *Clin Res* 23:614A, 1975.
15. Daughaday WH: The adenohypophysis, In Williams RH (ed): *Textbook of Endocrinology,* ed 5. Philadelphia, WB Saunders Co, 1974.
16. Derome PJ, Peillon R, Bard RH, et al: Adénomes à prolactine: fesultats du traitement chirurgical. 120 cas féminins, 30 cas masculins. *Nouv Presse Méd* 8:577, 1979.
17. Dominque JN, Richmond IL, Wilson CB: Results of surgery in 114 patients with prolactin-secreting pituitary adenomas. *Am J Obstet Gynecol* 137:102, 1980.

18. Ehni G, Eckles NE: Interruption of the pituitary stalk in the patient with mammary cancer. *J Neurosurg* 16:628, 1959.
19. Faria MA Jr, Tindall GT: Transsphenoidal microsurgery for prolactin-secreting pituitary adenomas. *J Neurosurg* 56:33, 1982.
20. Finn JE, Mount LA: Galactorrhea in males with tumors in the region of the pituitary gland. *J Neurosurg* 35:723, 1971.
21. Fluckiger E: Drugs and the control of prolactin secretion, in Boynes AR, Griffiths K (eds): *Prolactin and Carcinogenesis. Proceedings of the Fourth Tenovus Workshop*. Cardiff, Wales, Alpha Omega Alpha Publishing, 1972.
22. Forbes AP, Henneman PH, Griswold GC, et al: Syndrome characterized by galactorrhea, amenorrhea and low urinary FSH: Comparison with acromegaly and normal lactation. *J Clin Endocrinol Metab* 14:265, 1954.
23. Franks S, Jacobs HS, Nabarro JDN: Studies of prolactin secretion in pituitary disease. *J Endocrinol* 67:55, 1975.
24. Franks S, Murray MAF, Jequier AM, et al: Incidence and significance of hyperprolactinaemia in women with amenorrhoea. *Clin Endocrinol* 4:597, 1975.
25. Franks S, Nabarro JDN, Jacobs HS: Prevalence and presentation of hyperprolactinaemia in patients with "functionless" pituitary tumours. *Lancet* 1:778, 1977.
26. Frantz AG: Prolactin. *N Engl J Med* 298:201, 1978.
27. Frantz AG, Kleinberg DL: Prolactin: Evidence that it is separate from growth hormone in human blood. *Science* 170:745, 1970.
28. Friesen HG, Fournier P, Desjardins P: Pituitary prolactin in pregnancy and normal and abnormal lactation. *Clin Obstet Gynecol* 16:25, 1973.
29. Frommel R: Über puerperale atrophie des uterus. *Ztschr Geburtsh Gynakol* 7:340, 1882.
30. Goodman RH, Molitch ME, Post KD, et al: Prolactin-secreting adenomas in the male, in Post KD, Jackson IMD, Reichlin S (eds): *The Pituitary Adenoma*. New York, Plenum Medical Book Co, 1980.
31. Hardy J: Transsphenoidal surgery of hypersecreting pituitary tumors, in Kohler PO, Ross GT (eds): *Diagnosis and Treatment of Pituitary Tumors*. International Congress Series 303, Amsterdam, Excerpta Medica, 1973.
32. Hardy J: Transsphenoidal microsurgery of prolactinomas: Report on 355 cases, in Tolis G, et al (eds): *Prolactin and Prolactinomas*. New York, Raven Press, 1983.
33. Hardy J, Beauregard H, Robert F: Prolactin-secreting pituitary adenomas: Transsphenoidal microsurgical treatment. *Clin Neurosurg* 27:38, 1980.
34. Hwang P, Guyda H, Friesen H: A radioimmunoassay for human prolactin. *Proc Natl Acad Sci USA* 68:1902, 1971.
35. Jacobs HS: Prolactin and amenorrhea. *N Engl J Med* 295:954, 1976.
36. Kleinberg DL, Noel GL, Frantz AG: Galactorrhea: A study of 235 cases, including 48 with pituitary tumors. *N Engl J Med* 296:589, 1977.
37. Klibanski A, Neer RM, Beitins IZ, et al: Decreased bone density in hyperprolactinemic women. *N Engl J Med* 303:1511, 1980.
38. Kolodny HD, Sherman L: Laboratory aids in the diagnosis of pituitary tumors. *Ann Clin Lab Sci* 4:67, 1974.
39. Landolt AM: Surgical treatment of pituitary prolactinomas: Postoperative prolactin and fertility in seventy patients. *Fertil Steril* 35:620, 1981.
40. Landolt AM: Cerebrospinal fluid rhinorrhea: A complication of therapy for invasive prolactinomas. *Neurosurgery* 11:395, 1982.
41. Landolt AM, Keller PJ, Froesch ER, et al: Bromocriptine: Does it jeopardise the result of later surgery for prolactinomas? *Lancet* 2:657, 1982.
42. Landolt AM, Osterwalder V: Perivascular fibrosis in prolactinomas: Is it increased by bromocriptine? *J Clin Endocrinol Metab* 58:1179, 1984.
43. MacLeod RM: Regulation of prolactin secretion, in Martini L, Ganong WF (eds): *Frontiers in Neuroendocrinology*. New York, Raven Press, 1976, vol 4.
44. Martin JB: Management of hypersecreting pituitary adenomas. *Clin Neurosurg* 27:99, 1980.
45. McGregor AM, Scanlon MF, Hall R, et al: Effects of bromocriptine on pituitary tumour size. *Br Med J* 2:700, 1979.
46. McGregor AM, Scanlon MF, Hall K, et al: Reduction in size of a pituitary tumor by bromocriptine therapy. *N Engl J Med* 300:291, 1979.
47. McNatty KP, Sawers RS, McNeilly AS: A possible role for prolactin in control of steroid secretion by the human graafian follicle. *Nature* 250:653, 1974.
48. Nasr H, Mozaffarian G, Pensky J, et al: Prolactin-secreting pituitary tumors in women. *J Clin Endocrinol Metab* 35:505, 1972.
49. Nielson KD, Clark K: Transsphenoidal microsurgery for selective removal of functional pituitary microadenomas. *Tex Med* 72:61, 1976.
50. Parkes D: Drug therapy—Bromocriptine. *N Engl J Med* 301:873, 1979.
51. Pearson OH, Brodkey JS, Kaufman B: Endocrine evaluation and indications for surgery of functional pituitary adenomas. *Clin Neurosurg* 21:26, 1974.

52. Post KD, Biller BJ, Adelman LS, et al: Selective transsphenoidal adenomectomy in women with galactorrhea-amenorrhea. *JAMA* 242:158, 1979.
53. Rengachary SS, Tomita T, Jefferies BF, et al: Structural changes in human pituitary tumor after bromocriptine therapy. *Neurosurgery* 10:242, 1982.
54. Schlechte JA, Sherman B, Martin R: Bone density in amenorrheic women with and without hyperprolactinemia. *J Clin Endocrinol Metab* 56:1120, 1983.
55. Serri O, Rasio E, Beauregard H, et al: Recurrence of hyperprolactinemia after selective transsphenoidal adenomectomy in women with prolactinoma. *N Engl J Med* 309:280, 1983.
56. Serri O, Somma M, Rasio E, et al: Prolactin-secreting pituitary adenomas in males: Transsphenoidal microsurgical treatment. *Can Med Assoc J* 122:1007, 1980.
57. Sherman L, Kolodny HD: The effects of drugs on human hypophysiotrophic functions, in Stoll BA (ed): *Mammary Cancer and Neuroendocrine Therapy*. London, Butterworth & Co, 1974.
58. Thorner MO, Evans WS, MacLeod RM, et al: Hyperprolactinemia: Current concepts of management, including medical therapy with bromocriptine, in Goldstein M, et al (eds): *Ergot Compounds and Brain Function: Neuroendocrine and Neuropsychiatric Aspects*. New York, Raven Press, 1980, vol 23.
59. Thorner MO, Martin WH, Rogol AD, et al: Rapid regression of pituitary prolactinomas during bromocriptine treatment. *J Clin Endocrinol Metab* 51:438, 1980.
60. Thorner MO, Perryman RL, Rogol AD, et al: Rapid changes of prolactinoma volume after withdrawal and reinstitution of bromocriptine. *J Clin Endocrinol Metab* 153:480, 1981.
61. Tindall GT, Kovacs K, Horvath E, et al: Human prolactin-producing adenomas and bromocriptine: A histological, immunocytochemical, ultrastructural, and morphometric study. *J Clin Endocrinol Metab* 55:1178, 1982.
62. Turkalj I, Braun P, Krupp P: Surveillance of bromocriptine in pregnancy. *JAMA* 247:1589, 1982.
63. Turkington RW, Underwood LE, Van Wyk JJ: Elevated serum prolactin levels after pituitary-stalk section in man. *N Engl J Med* 285:707, 1971.
64. Wass JAH, Moult PJA, Thorner MO, et al: Reduction of pituitary-tumour size in patients with prolactinomas and acromegaly treated with bromocriptine with or without radiotherapy. *Lancet* 2:66, 1979.
65. Weiss MH, Teal J, Gott P, et al: Natural history of microprolactinomas: Six-year follow-up. *Neurosurgery* 12:180, 1983.
66. Werder KV, Fahlbusch R, Landgraf R, et al: Treatment of patients with prolactinomas. *J Endocrinol Invest* 1:47, 1978.
67. Wilson JD, Newcombe RLG, Long FL: Cerebrospinal fluid rhinorrhoea during treatment of pituitary tumours with bromocriptine. *Acta Endocrinol* 103:457, 1983.

CHAPTER 9

Nonfunctional pituitary adenomas

Classification
Clinical features
Diagnostic evaluation
   Endocrinologic studies
Neuroradiologic evaluation
Treatment
   Surgical management
   Irradiation
Therapeutic decision making
   Invasive nonfunctional pituitary adenoma causing visual loss
   Nonfunctional pituitary adenoma associated with pituitary apoplexy
   Nonfunctional pituitary adenoma causing obstructive hydrocephalus
Summary

The nonfunctional pituitary adenoma is defined as a pituitary tumor that does not cause a clinically apparent endocrinopathy. Nonfunctional tumors come to medical attention either because of mass effects, usually visual impairment, or because of discovery during the course of other clinical investigations. For instance, during the evaluation of a patient with chronic headaches, "sinus" problems, or head trauma, an enlargement of the sella turcica may be found on routine skull films or a pituitary adenoma discovered on the computed tomographic (CT) scan. Patients with hyperfunctional tumors, on the other hand, seek medical attention usually because of the endocrinopathy (i.e., acromegaly, Cushing's disease) caused by the hypersecretion of a normal hormone produced by the tumor although sometimes mass effects may accompany the endocrinopathy.

    In the past, the nonfunctional pituitary adenoma, which was usually referred to as a "chromophobe adenoma," constituted a majority of clinically recognized pituitary tumors. As better understanding and more knowledge of pituitary tumors associated with Cushing's disease, acromegaly, and the amenorrhea-galactorrhea syndrome and particularly since circulating pituitary hormones could be measured, it became apparent that hyperfunctional tumors constituted a higher percentage of pituitary tumors than was formerly realized. The continued refinement of endocrinologic testing, especially the availability of serum prolactin determinations, has resulted in a further proportionate decrease in the incidence of the nonfunctional pituitary adenoma from a previous frequency of almost 90% to approximately 25% in most series. The major emphasis in this chapter will be on surgical and radiation treatment. The classification, clinical features, and diagnostic evaluation have been considered elsewhere in this book.

CLASSIFICATION

Horvath and Kovacs* have proposed a useful morphologic classification of pituitary tumors that is based on immunocytology and electron microscopy and correlates structure with clinical history, biochemical findings, and secretory activity. This classification with slight modification is listed on p. 72 of Chapter 3. Although some of the tumors cited in this table as morphologically functional may in fact be found in patients who show no clinical evidence of endocrinopathy, the majority of pituitary adenomas in the nonfunctional group are found in the null cell adenoma category. The null cell adenomas exhibit distinct morphologic features and are not associated with clinical and biochemical evidence of increased hormone production. The distinctive morphologic features of the null cell adenoma are discussed in detail in Chapter 3.

CLINICAL FEATURES

The clinical findings associated with nonfunctional pituitary tumors are related to mass effect (see Table 4-1) rather than overproduction of hormones. Mass effects result from compression of adjacent anatomic structures, primarily the optic chiasm and the normal pituitary gland. The most common objective manifestations resulting from mass effect are visual findings including *impairment of visual fields* and *loss of acuity*.

DIAGNOSTIC EVALUATION
Endocrinologic studies

In the endocrine investigation of patients with nonfunctional tumors, it is usually unnecessary to perform special testing procedures (e.g., growth hormone suppression with glucose, dexamethasone suppression of glucocorticoids) that are important in patients with hyperfunctional tumors. Nonfunctional tumors can cause elevation of serum prolactin most likely from interference with prolactin inhibiting factor (PIF) conduction (stalk phenomenon) from the hypothalamus and may be misdiagnosed as a prolactin-secreting tumor. The serum prolactin levels in this situation are rarely above 100 ng/ml. The endocrine protocol shown in Table 9-1 is recommended for the investigation of patients with a provisional diagnosis of nonfunctional pituitary adenomas.

---

*Horvath E, Kovacs K: Ultrastructural classification of pituitary adenomas. *Can J Neurol Sci* 3:9, 1976.

Table 9-1
Evaluation of pituitary hormone reserve

	Screening	Further study
Adrenal	AM cortisol, cosyntropin stimulation	ITT, metyrapone, corticotropin-releasing factor (CRF)
Thyroid	T_4 (total or free)	Thyrotropin-releasing hormone (TRH) stimulation
Gonadal	LH, FSH, testosterone (men), estradiol (women)	Gonadotropin-releasing hormone (GnRH) stimulation clomiphene
Prolactin	Baseline prolactin	Not recommended
Growth hormone	Not recommended in adults	ITT, arginine, glucagon, growth hormone-releasing factor (GHRF)
ADH	Urine volume, serum electrolytes	Water deprivation test, hypertonic saline infusion

In patients who undergo surgery, endocrine testing should be repeated approximately 7 days following surgery to determine whether or not the surgery resulted in any further endocrine deficiency (see Chapter 4 for specific tests). By repeating these tests, the surgeon can monitor the effect of the surgery on the remaining normal pituitary gland and obtain information that indicates whether the patient will require replacement therapy postoperatively. Transsphenoidal surgery in small- and moderate-sized tumors is associated with approximately a 7% incidence of damaging one or more pituitary–target organ axes. And, as would be anticipated, the incidence of damage is higher in large tumors. Thus one can anticipate that some type of endocrine replacement therapy may be required in a small number of patients following surgery.

NEURORADIOLOGIC EVALUATION

The neuroradiologic evaluation of patients with nonfunctional tumors includes a lateral skull x-ray, high-resolution coronal view CT scan, and angiographic visualization of the major arteries in the vicinity of the sella turcica (see Chapter 5).

284 *Disorders of the pituitary*

There are no distinctive radiologic abnormalities associated with nonfunctional tumors that will enable one to differentiate them from hyperfunctional pituitary tumors. As with other sellar and parasellar lesions, a good quality CT scan will define the size and extent of a nonfunctional adenoma and, in some cases, determine whether the lesion is invasive (Fig. 9-1), information that is invaluable in making therapeutic decisions.

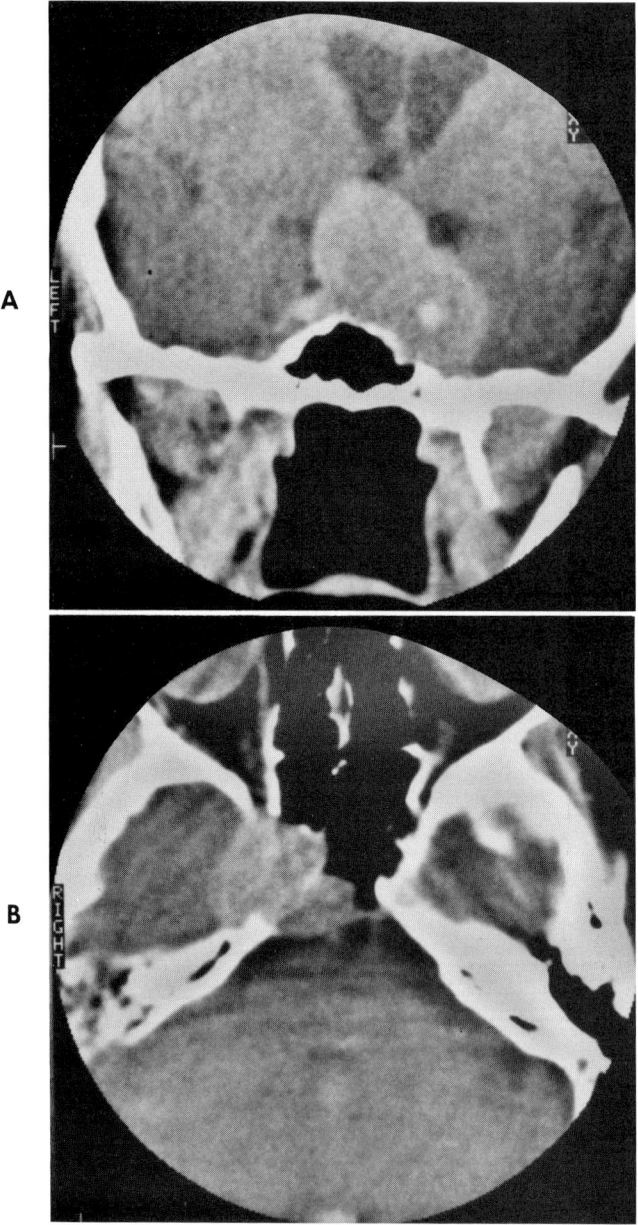

Fig. 9-1. For legend see opposite page.

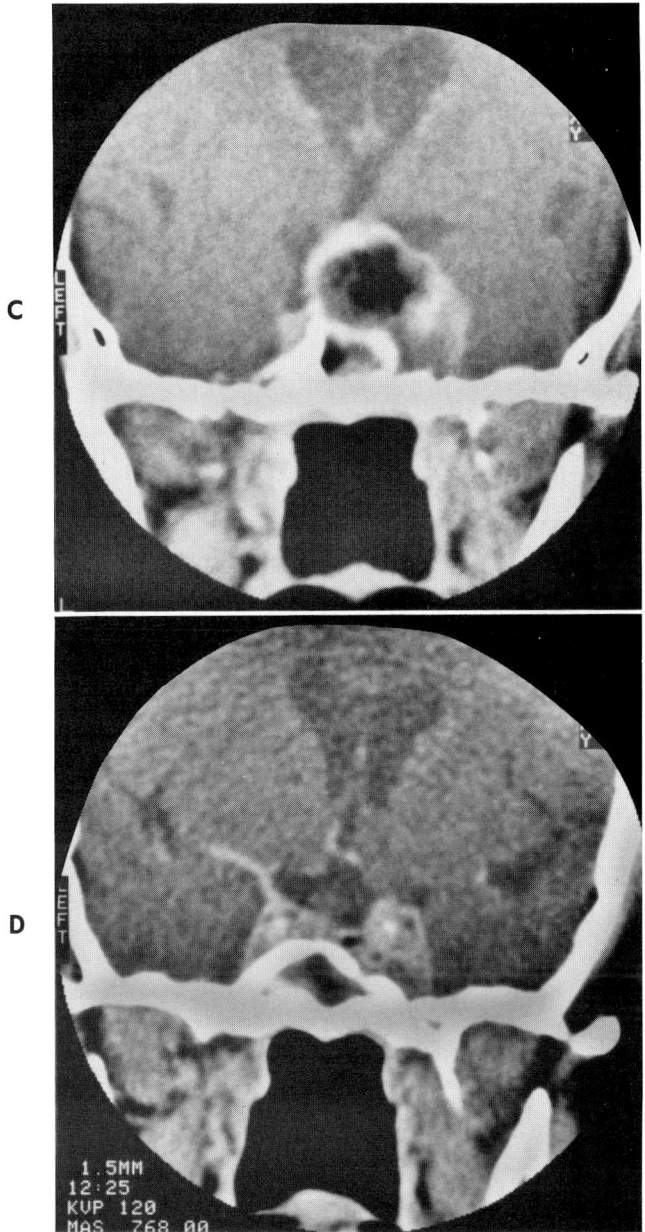

Fig. 9-1. Invasive nonfunctional pituitary adenoma. **A,** Coronal CT scan showing suprasellar and lateral extension of large tumor. Internal carotid is seen surrounded by tumor on enhanced view indicating cavernous sinus invasion by tumor. **B,** Axial view, CT scan, showing erosion of medial petrous region by lesion, again emphasizing invasiveness of tumor. **C,** Three-month postoperative coronal CT scan showing subtotal resection with little change in position in superior portion of tumor. **D,** Twelve-month postoperative coronal CT scan showing that suprasellar portion of tumor has collapsed into sella.

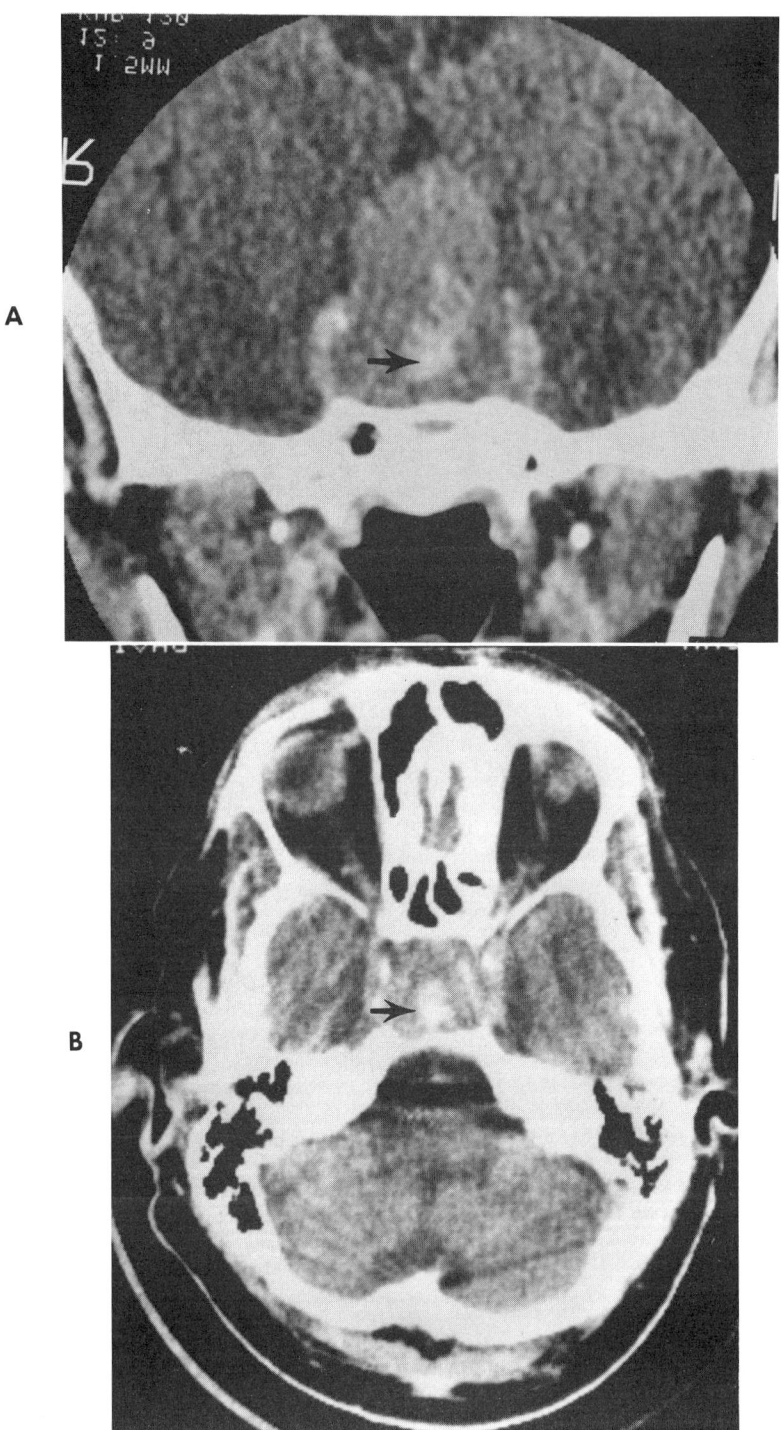

Fig. 9-2. Pituitary apoplexy. Coronal (**A**) and axial (**B**) CT scan; unenhanced views show area of increased density (arrowheads) consistent with hemorrhage within adenoma.

In patients with pituitary apoplexy, a CT scan without contrast enhancement may reveal the hemorrhage as a high-density or a mottled mixed-density lesion within the adenoma (Fig. 9-2).

Traditionally, angiography has been accomplished by arterial injections of contrast media usually via the transfemoral approach. As discussed in Chapter 5, the digital intravenous angiography (DIVA) technique, which is a relatively safe and effective method for demonstrating the major parasellar arteries, currently is recommended in these cases. Although the quality and resolution with DIVA is not comparable to that obtained with traditional angiography, it nevertheless provides adequate vascular imaging (see Fig. 5-8) to exclude the presence of an intracranial aneurysm, especially a large lesion, masquerading as a pituitary adenoma. In the rare patient with pituitary apoplexy in whom the clinical findings could also be consistent with a subarachnoid hemorrhage, conventional angiography may be indicated to exclude the presence of an intracranial aneurysm. The reason for recommending conventional angiography in this clinical situation is that if the patient does prove to have an aneurysmal subarachnoidal hemorrhage, the aneurysm may be relatively small and thus could easily be missed by the DIVA technique.

TREATMENT

Although patients with hyperfunctional tumors usually have a pharmacologic option for treatment, those with nonfunctional tumors do not, since there is no abnormal hormone level for a pharmacologic agent to suppress or control. Thus there are only two effective therapeutic options for patients with nonfunctional tumors—surgery and irradiation.

Surgical management

The surgeon should first determine if the tumor is resectable and, if so, select the operative approach, either transcranial or transsphenoidal, that has the best chance for achieving total excision with the least risk to the patient. In current practice, the modern transsphenoidal surgical approach, in our opinion, is the most appropriate and reasonable one for the majority of cases. The details of both transcranial and transsphenoidal operative techniques, potential complications, and postoperative care are described in Chapter 12. The presence of tumor invasiveness, especially of the cavernous sinus, is a major limiting factor in achieving complete excision of large pituitary tumors.

Patients with pituitary apoplexy usually require emergency management. Although some reports describe spontaneous recovery in patients with this entity,[3,15,22,25] many of these patients suffer acute visual deterioration, and the only hope for recovery is through rapid decompression of the mass lesion. Treatment consists of steroid therapy and surgical intervention. Although successful removal of the offending mass can be accomplished by the transcranial approach, transsphenoidal surgery is more commonly used because of its greater safety and relative speed.[6,23] Berti et al[2] and Zervas and Mendelson[31] have reported on the effective use of stereotaxic transsphenoidal needle aspiration for pituitary apoplexy.

The effectiveness of surgical treatment is evaluated by symptomatic relief and/or cure of the disease. These two criteria do not always correlate with each other. For instance, symptomatic relief can follow incomplete tumor removal and, conversely, total excision of the tumor, thus curing the disease may not provide satisfactory symptomatic relief (i.e., a patient with preoperative visual impairment may remain visually disabled following surgery).

Symptomatic relief following either partial or complete surgical excision of a pituitary tumor is synonymous with alleviation of the clinical findings caused by the mass effects of the tumor. The most commonly used objective parameters for evaluating symptomatic relief following surgery are visual fields and acuity. The results of a number of surgical series (Table 9-2), indicate that both the transcranial and the transsphenoidal operative techniques provide significant improvement in the majority of patients with preoperative impairment of vision

Table 9-2
Visual results following surgery for pituitary adenomas

		Visual results		
Series	Number of cases evaluated	Normalized or improved (%)	No change (%)	Worse (%)
Craniotomy series				
Cushing (Henderson, 1939)[13]	88	70.5	20.5	9
Bakay, 1950[1]	202	41	33	26
Tönnis et al, 1953[28]	?	62	31	7
Heimbach, 1959[12] Krayenbühl, 1958[16]	95	83	12	5
Guillaume and Caron, 1958[9]	70 (approx)	83	10	7
Fager et al, 1973[7]	197	45	?	9
Olivecrona, 1967[21]	136	42.7	43.4	14
Svien et al, 1965[27]	71	63.4	15.5	21.1
Ray and Patterson, 1971[24]	106	80	18	2
Transsphenoidal series				
Cushing (Henderson, 1939)[13]	159	72	24	4
Hamlin, 1962[11] Hirsch, 1957[14]	140	68		?
Demailly et al, 1967[5] Guiot, 1967[10]	63	82		18
Laws and Kern, 1976[17]	42	86	14	0
Ciric et al, 1983[4]	59*	90	10	0

Modified from Laws ER, Trautman JC, Hollenhorst RW: Transsphenoidal decompression of the optic nerve and chiasm: Visual results in 62 patients. *J Neurosurg* 46:717, 1977.
*Series included both functional and nonfunctional tumors that measured 20 mm or more in at least one diameter.

resulting from the compressive effects of the adenoma. An example of the dramatic improvement in visual acuity and fields in a patient operated on for a large tumor by the transsphenoidal method is shown in Fig. 9-3.

Cure, or control, of the disease following surgery is determined by the incidence of proven tumor recurrence. The data from Henderson's review of the Cushing series indicated that if there was recurrence, the symptoms appeared within 3 years in 70% and within 5 years in about 95% of cases.[13] There were no recurrences later than 8 years after operation.[13] Most of the data regarding recurrence were reported before availability of the CT scan and depended primarily on clinical findings. Thus it is likely that the incidence of recurrence was higher than actually reported. Additionally, there are other factors to consider. Postoperative irradiation appears to favorably influence the recurrence rate. Also pituitary tumors vary considerably in their growth potential, and consequently, it was not

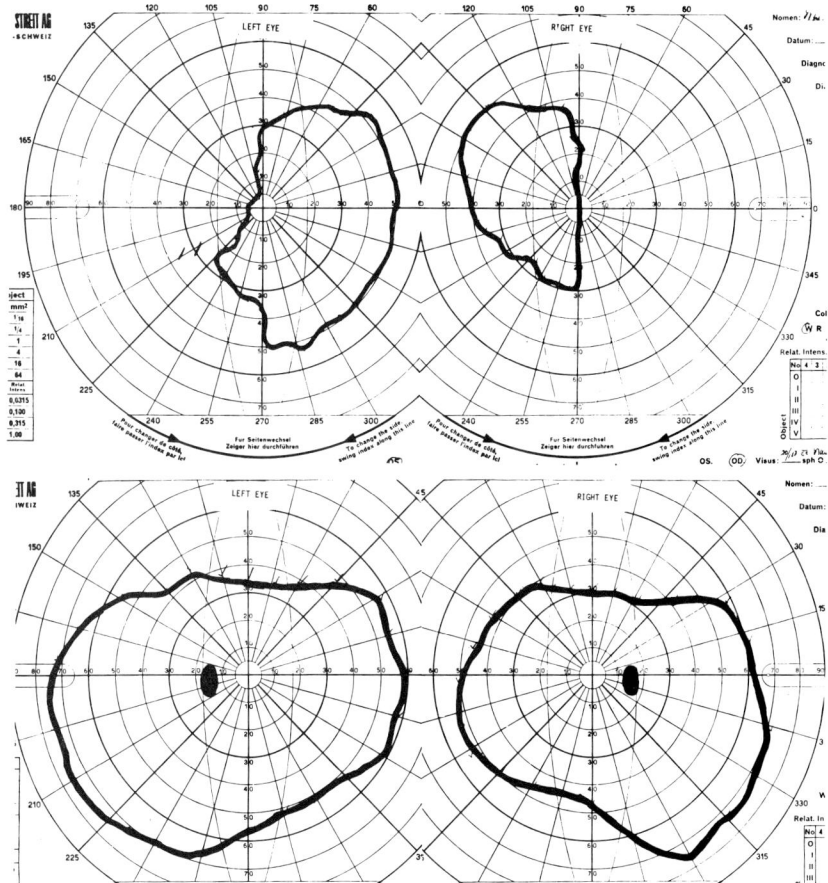

Fig. 9-3. Visual improvement following transsphenoidal removal of large nonfunctional pituitary tumor. Examination before surgery *(top)* showed bitemporal defects with acuity 20/100 OD; 20/80 OS. Visual fields 7 days after surgery *(bottom)* showed return to normal with acuity 20/25 OU.

unusual for patients to experience long-term symptomatic relief following minimal surgical removal in cases that received *no* post-operative irradiation.[8,26] As shown in Table 9-3, the incidence of recurrence following transcranial surgery varies considerably among several series and was nearly always lower in those patients who received postoperative irradiation.

Table 9-3
Recurrence rates from major published series

Authors	Number of patients	Recurrence rate (%) Without radiation	Recurrence rate (%) With radiation	Average follow-up (yr)
Cushing, 1939[13]	205	56	13	5
Bakay, 1950[1]	232	—	10-15	5
Martins et al, 1965[20]	54	—	6	—
Stern and Batzdorf, 1970[26]	64	9.4	—	5.5
Ray and Patterson, 1971[24]	146	22	8	—
MacCarty et al, 1973[19]	96	31.8	3.0	>5
Van Der Zwan[29]				6
Wirth et al, 1974[30]	157	25.8	11.7	5.3
Ciric et al, 1983[4]*	99	28	6	†

Modified from Post K: Transfrontal surgery for pituitary tumors, in Post KD, Jackson IMD, Reichlin S (eds): *The pituitary adenoma*. New York, Plenum Medical Book Company, 1980.
*Series includes both functional and nonfunctional tumors that measured 20 mm or more in at least one diameter.
†Follow-up period ranged from 6 months to 14 years.

One of several impressive series of transcranial operations for pituitary adenomas was that reported by Ray and Patterson.[24] They reported their results in 146 cases of "chromophobe adenomas" unassociated with either acromegaly or Cushing's syndrome. Their patients were treated before the availability of prolactin determinations, so it is possible that many of the nonfunctional tumors in their series, as well as others reported before 1971, were in fact prolactinomas. Significant improvement in vision occurred in 80% of the patients, and in approximately 50%, normal vision was restored. Endocrine function was measurably improved in a "substantial number of patients." The operative mortality in Ray and Patterson's series was only 1.4%, and complications consisting principally of infection, cerebrospinal fluid (CSF) leaks, and intracranial clots occurred in 12% of the cases.[24] In general, the reported operative mortality for craniotomy among many series were higher than those cited by Ray and Patterson (see Table 12-1). A review of these series indicates that the average mortality was approximately 10%.

Large series treated by transsphenoidal surgery have been reported by Henderson (Cushing series),[13] Hamlin,[11] and Hirsch.[14] These earlier series, which lacked modern sophisticated surgical instrumentation—particularly the operating microscope, were usually associated with a significantly high recurrence rate, and the latter finding was probably one of the major reasons that a number of surgeons abandoned the transsphenoidal technique (in the 1915 to 1920 era). Currently, with better instrumentation and a clearer understanding of the relationship of most of these tumors to the normal gland, an experienced surgeon has a better chance for gross total removal using the transsphenoidal as opposed to the transcranial approach. The effectiveness of transsphenoidal surgery in accomplishing a "gross total removal" in certain large adenomas is illustrated in Figs. 9-4 and 9-5.

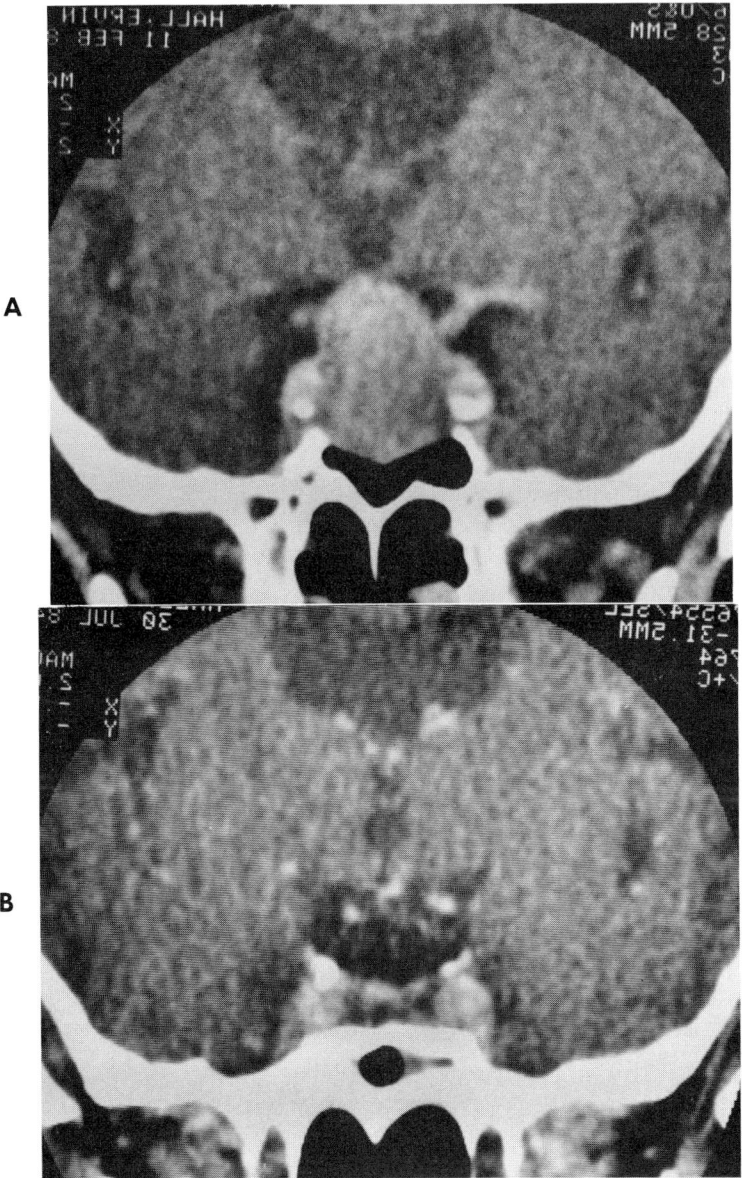

Fig. 9-4. Effectiveness of transsphenoidal surgery in removing large nonfunctional adenoma. **A,** Preoperative CT scan shows large tumor with suprasellar extension. **B,** Seventeen-month postoperative CT scan in same patient shows no evidence of tumor.

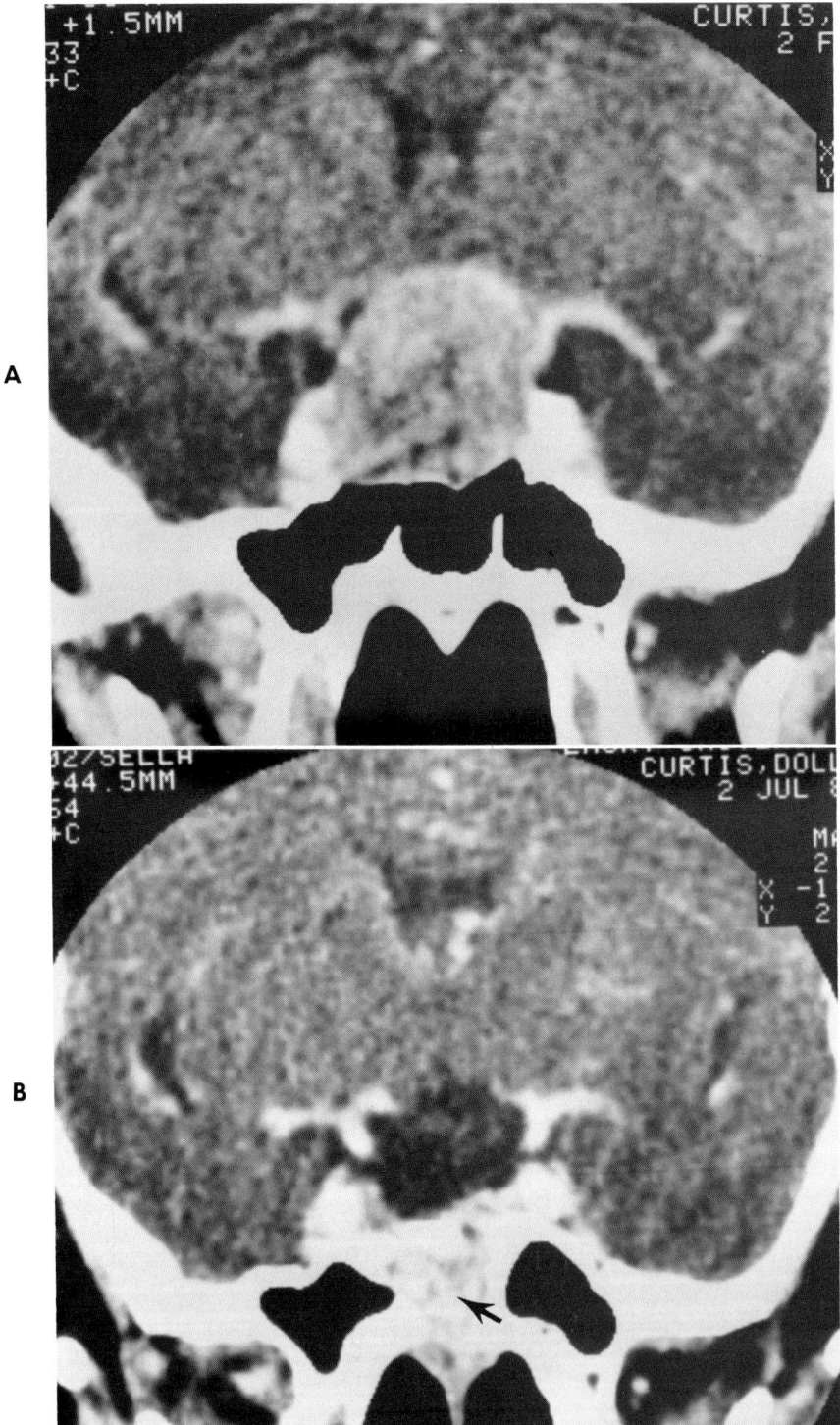

Fig. 9-5. Effectiveness of transsphenoidal surgery in removing large nonfunctional adenoma. **A,** Preoperative CT scan shows large tumor with suprasellar extension. **B,** Eighteen-month postoperative CT scan shows no residual tumor. Increased density in sphenoid sinus (arrow) is a result of scar tissue.

Furthermore, one can expect a much lower recurrence rate for transsphenoidal surgery than was obtained formerly. As an example, Ciric et al[4] reported their results using the transsphenoidal approach in 108 cases where tumors measured 20 mm or more in at least one diameter. Although their series contained both functional as well as nonfunctional tumors, their results are representative of what can be accomplished with the modern transsphenoidal operation in patients with large tumors. Using postoperative CT scan to determine completeness of tumor removal, they found no residual tumor in 57, or 62%, of 92 patients. There was an overall recurrence rate of 12.7% among 102 patients in whom a follow-up was possible. In 32 patients who did *not* receive irradiation, nine, or 28%, developed a recurrence. By way of contrast, only 4, or 6%, of 67 patients who were irradiated postoperatively experienced a recurrence.

The mortality for transsphenoidal surgery for pituitary adenomas is significantly lower than that for a craniotomy. In a recent survey of several neurosurgeons, (see Table 12-2), mortality ranged from 0 to 1.5% with an average of 0.5%. Among the fatal cases, there were usually some extenuating circumstances or contributory causes. For instance, the patients were old, in marginal health, or else had undergone previous treatments that affected the transsphenoidal operation. Complications (e.g., CSF leak, diabetes insipidus, meningitis) occurred at an average rate of 2.2%.

Thus it is clear from the figures just cited that transsphenoidal surgery performed by a neurosurgeon experienced in this operative approach carries less risk than transcranial surgery for pituitary adenomas.

Irradiation

Primary treatment of pituitary tumors by irradiation was an often-used method of therapy in the past. However, as a result of numerous advances, primarily the widespread use of the modern transsphenoidal operation, conventional irradiation as *primary and sole treatment* of pituitary adenomas other than in unusual and exceptional circumstances *has been virtually abandoned*. Heavy particle irradiation has never been used to any great extent in the treatment of nonfunctional lesions mainly because most of these lesions have been relatively large at the time of therapeutic decision making, and this is not a completely safe form of treatment for the large adenomas, especially those lesions that extend outside the confines of the sella turcica.

In previous years, particularly when craniotomy was a major method for surgical management, the majority of patients routinely received conventional irradiation to the sella region following surgery. The rationale for this method of management was related to the fact that a "gross total removal" of tumor usually was not accomplished by the transcranial approach and was supported by the finding that the recurrence rate for pituitary tumors treated by craniotomy and irradiation appeared to be significantly lower than that recorded in cases treated by craniotomy alone.

Currently, the availability of high-resolution CT scanning can, and probably should, influence the decision-making process for postoperative irradiation. If an experienced surgeon reports that "gross total removal" of tumor was accomplished by transsphenoidal surgery and the 3-month postoperative CT scan shows no definite tumor, then it is reasonable *not* to recommend irradiation to the pituitary/sella region. In these cases, follow-up visits every 3 to 6 months and a CT scan every year for at least the first 2 to 3 years postoperatively is recommended. If the CT scans for the first 2 to 3 years show no tumor, then the interval between scans can be lengthened to every 2 to 3 years. As long as no definite tumor is seen, irradiation is not recommended. If a postoperative CT scan shows persistent tumor but the patient is asymptomatic, it is reasonable, in our opinion, to withhold irradiation until a repeat scan 3 to 6 months later is obtained.

Irradiation is recommended only when documented growth is observed on serial CT scans or in patients in whom a postoperative scan is positive for recurrent tumor and who have developed new symptoms. These latter statements simply reflect our relatively conservative attitude toward the use of irradiation. Certainly, there are many experienced neurosurgeons and endocrinologists who would advise conventional irradiation in a patient who had evidence of persistent tumor on a routine 3- to 6-month postoperative CT scan regardless of whether or not the persistent tumor was causing symptoms.

The results of irradiation in nonfunctional pituitary tumors, either as primary treatment or combined with surgical therapy, indicate that among the different series (see Table 13-12), there exists a relatively wide discrepancy in recurrence rates between those patients who received postoperative pituitary irradiation as opposed to those who did not. For instance, in the Cushing series reported by Henderson,[13] there was a 5-year recurrence rate of 13% in patients operated on by craniotomy and treated with postoperative irradiation as opposed to a recurrence rate of 42.5% in those treated by surgery alone.[13] Such a marked difference, however, has not been the experience of some authors. As an example, in the large series reported by Ray and Patterson,[24] the recurrence rate was 8% in those who received postoperative irradiation as opposed to 22% in those who did not receive this adjunctive therapy. Approximately one half of the patients treated by Ray and Patterson received postoperative irradiation. However, despite these figures (8% versus 22%), these latter authors were not overly enthusiastic about the routine use of postoperative irradiation and concluded that it justifiably might be reserved until tumor recurrence becomes evident or for those cases with an invasive tumor at the first operation.

There is an extensive literature on the incidence of tumor recurrence following surgery (transcranial and transsphenoidal) either as the sole treatment or combined with irradiation. Because most of this information was gathered before the use of the modern transsphenoidal operation, the CT scan, and refined endocrinologic studies, its value is relatively limited. In many of the older series, the extent of surgery varied from a limited excision (biopsy) to a radical removal, and two important observations emerge from a review of these series. First, postoperative recurrences occurred in all patients regardless of whether irradiation was used, but in nearly every series, the rate of recurrence was lower in patients who received postoperative irradiation. Second, it was not unusual for patients to experience many years of symptomatic freedom following minimal tumor removal even in cases that received no postoperative irradiation.[8,26] This latter finding simply emphasizes a fact well known to physicians involved with pituitary disorders—pituitary adenomas can vary considerably in their growth potential.

THERAPEUTIC DECISION MAKING

Following are some examples of patients with nonfunctional tumors. These patients illustrate problems that may arise in the diagnostic/therapeutic decision-making process.

Invasive nonfunctional pituitary adenoma causing visual loss

A 51-year-old woman was referred for headaches that she had experienced for 18 months and visual loss for a period of 3 months. Examination revealed a superior bitemporal quadrantanopsia and visual acuity OD, 20/80 and OS, 20/40. Endocrine tests were normal. CT scan (see Fig. 9-1, *A*) showed a large pituitary adenoma with both suprasellar and lateral extension. The contrasted CT showed the intracavernous carotid artery surrounded by tumor, which indicated cavernous sinus invasion. The *axial* view (see Fig. 9-1, *B*) showed erosion of the medial petrous region, which further confirmed the invasiveness of the tumor.

Realizing that the tumor could not be completely removed, a transsphenoidal operation was undertaken to debulk the tumor as much as possible to relieve compression of the optic chiasm. A generous but incomplete removal resulted in resolution of the visual field defect and return of visual acuity to normal. A 3-month CT scan (see Fig. 9-1, *C*) showed that although much of the tumor had been removed, the superior portion of the lesion demonstrated relatively little change in position from its preoperative status. However, a 12-month CT (see Fig. 9-1, *D*) showed that the suprasellar portion of the tumor had largely collapsed into the sella. Postoperative irradiation was not administered. The patient was advised to have this therapy, but she refused. She is currently being followed; visual improvement has been maintained.

In this case, which represents an obvious invasive tumor and thus a lesion that cannot be totally resected, surgery was undertaken to achieve a rapid decompression of the optic nerves and chiasm and thus improve vision. It is our opinion that even if the patient had no preoperative visual impairment, we would have recommended surgery for the purpose of debulking the tumor, a procedure that is believed to enhance the effectiveness of x-ray treatment. Following debulking, a course (circa 4500 rad) of irradiation would have been recommended. Although this patient refused x-ray therapy, this recommendation would have been followed by most patients in this situation.

Nonfunctional pituitary adenoma associated with pituitary apoplexy

A 64-year-old man had a history of headaches and decreasing visual acuity for 4 months before hospitalization. Thirty-six hours before admission, his headaches became worse, and visual acuity deteriorated over a period of 1 hour. On examination, he was slightly lethargic. Visual fields could not be adequately evaluated. Visual acuity was OD 20/100; OS 20/80. An *unenhanced* CT scan (see Fig. 9-2) showed a large pituitary tumor with significant suprasellar extension. There was an area of increased density within the tumor consistent with hemorrhage.

After the usual preparations, which included obtaining blood samples for baseline pituitary–target organ axes evaluation and administering 100 mg hydrocortisone (IM), the patient was taken to surgery, and a transsphenoidal removal of the tumor was accomplished. Much of the tumor was soft, friable, and gray-white in appearance. The central portions of the tumor were purple in appearance and somewhat firmer than usual. These areas showed hemorrhagic infarction on microscopic examination.

Postoperatively, the patient's overall condition improved. He showed evidence of hypopituitarism and required thyroxine and cortisone replacement. Postoperative visual acuity was considerably improved with 20/25 OU.

Nonfunctional pituitary adenoma causing obstructive hydrocephalus

A 57-year-old man was evaluated for decreasing energy level, unsteadiness of gait, and lethargy of 3 months' duration. In the month before admission, he had developed headaches and a mild decrease in visual acuity. Mild shuffling gait, bitemporal quadrantanopsia, and slight lethargy were noted on examination. CT scan (Fig. 9-6) showed a large adenoma with significant suprasellar extension that extended into and blocked the third ventricle with resulting hydrocephalus. A biventricular-peritoneal shunt relieved the hydrocephalus, and a subsequent transsphenoidal operation accomplished a partial but generous resection of the adenoma. At the time of surgery, the tumor could be seen extending into the suprasellar area immediately anterior to a postfixed optic chiasm, which remained separated from the tumor and sella by an intact diaphragm sella. He received a full course of pituitary irradiation postoperatively. On a follow-up visit 2 years later, his condition was improved over his preoperative status.

This patient illustrates that on occasions a tumor may reach a size sufficient to block the ventricular system. In our opinion, it is necessary to perform a bilateral lateral ventricular shunt operation to relieve the hydrocephalus before any surgical attack on the tumor. For instance, the patients may deteriorate neurologically from the hydrocephalus either during or immediately following surgery for the tumor if the hydrocephalus is not shunted beforehand. In this patient, the minimal visual field defect despite the large suprasellar tumor implies a postfixed chiasm.

SUMMARY

Nonfunctional tumors constitute approximately 25% of pituitary tumors in most current series. The apparent decline in incidence in this category of pituitary tumors over the past several years is related to refinements both in endocrinologic testing and in pathologic examination techniques, both of which have shown that many pituitary tumors that in the past would have been categorized as nonfunctional indeed are functional from the standpoint of hormone secretion. The largest group of tumors formerly considered nonfunctional are the prolactinomas. Since nonfunctional tumors do not secrete hormones, which in turn can cause endo-

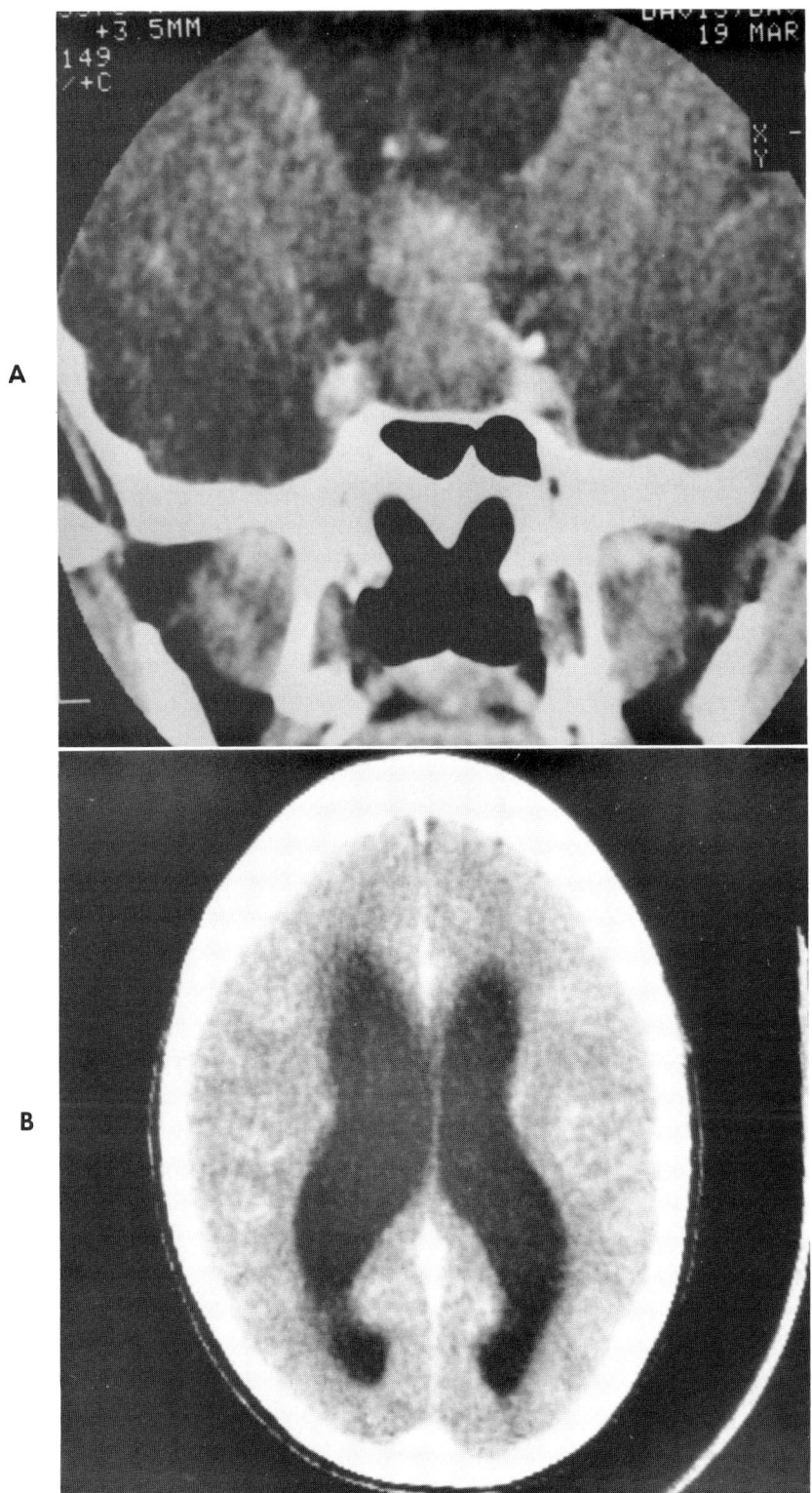

Fig. 9-6. Large pituitary tumor with significant suprasellar extension causing obstructive hydrocephalus. CT scan shows extension of tumor into third ventricle (**A**) and significant enlargement of lateral ventricles (**B**).

crinopathy, the clinical findings are those related to mass effects. Visual impairment and headache are the most common clinical manifestations. In the diagnostic evaluation of these tumors, angiographic visualization of the intracranial circulation is more important than in the hyperfunctional group because of the possibility that the nonfunctional tumor may actually be a large aneurysm. Although digital intravenous techniques usually are adequate to rule out this lesion, sometimes, especially in patients with the clinical syndrome of pituitary apoplexy, conventional (e.g., transfemoral) angiography may be necessary for more precise detail of the anatomy of the intracranial circulation.

Primary therapy for the majority of these lesions should be surgery, and currently, in most cases, the transsphenoidal approach should be used. Symptomatic relief of headaches and visual impairment can be expected in the majority of cases. Irradiation should be used as adjunctive, not primary, therapy, and we believe that a conservative attitude regarding its use is appropriate. We do not recommend *routine* postoperative irradiation in patients with large nonfunctional adenomas following transsphenoidal surgery. Rather, we believe it is appropriate to use irradiation only in cases with proven recurrent or persistent tumor that is definitely causing new clinical findings and in cases in which it appears that other therapeutic measures (i.e., repeat surgery) have little chance of success. In these cases, conventional treatment (e.g., cobalt) in a dosage of approximately 4000 to 4500 rad directed to the sellar/parasellar area in fractionated doses should be used.

REFERENCES

1. Bakay L: The results of 300 pituitary adenoma operations (Professor Herbert Olivecrona's series). *J Neurosurg* 7:240, 1950.
2. Berti G, Heisey WG, Dohn DF: Pituitary apoplexy treated by stereotactic transphenoidal aspiration. *Cleve Clin Q* 41:163, 1974.
3. Cairns H: Peripheral ocular palsies from the neuro-surgical point of view. *Trans Ophthalmol Soc UK* 58(Part 2):464, 1938.
4. Ciric I, Mikhael M, Stafford T, et al: Transsphenoidal microsurgery of pituitary macroadenomas with long-term follow-up results. *J Neurosurg* 59:395, 1983.
5. Demailly P, Guiot G, Oproiu A: Résultats visuels des exéreses d'adénomes hypophysaires par voie transphénoïdale. *Arch Ophthalmol* 27:5, 1967.
6. Ebersold MJ, Laws ER, Scheithauer BW, et al: Pituitary apoplexy treated by transsphenoidal surgery: A clinicopathological and immunocytochemical study. *J Neurosurg* 58:315, 1983.
7. Fager CA, Poppen JL, Takaoka Y: Indications for and results of surgical treatment of pituitary tumors by the intracranial approach, in Kohler PO, Ross GT (eds): *Diagnosis and Treatment of Pituitary Tumors*. Amsterdam, Excerpta Medica, 1973.
8. German WJ, Flanigan S: Pituitary adenomas: A follow-up study of the Cushing series. *Clin Neurosurg* 10:72, 1964.
9. Guillaume J, Caron JP: Remarques cliniques et chirurgicales relatives aux adénomes hypophysaires. *Neurochirurgie* 4:338, 1958.
10. Guiot G: Transsphenoidal approach in surgical treatment of pituitary adenoma: General principles and indications in nonfunctioning adenomas, in Kohler PO, Ross GT (eds): *Diagnosis and Treatment of Pituitary Tumors*. Amsterdam, Excerpta Medica, 1973.
11. Hamlin H: The case for transsphenoidal approach to hypophysial tumors. *J Neurosurg* 19:1000, 1962.
12. Heimbach SB: Follow-up studies on 105 cases of verified chromophobe and acidophile pituitary adenomata after treatment by transfrontal operation and x-ray irradiation. *Acta Neurochir* 7:101, 1959.
13. Henderson WR: The pituitary adenomata: A follow-up study of surgical results in 338 cases (Dr. Harvey Cushing's series). *Br J Surg* 26:811, 1939.
14. Hirsch O: Hypophysentumoren—Ein Grenzgebiet. *Acta Neurochir* 5:1, 1957.

15. Jefferson G: Extrasellar extensions of pituitary adenomas. *Proc Roy Soc Med* 33:433, 1940.
16. Krayenbühl H: Reflexions sur une serie de 105 cas de tumeurs de l'hypophyse: Evaluation du traitement chirurgical. *Neurochirurgie* 4:356, 1958.
17. Laws ER Jr, Kern EB: Complications of transsphenoidal surgery. *Clin Neurosurg* 23:401, 1976.
18. Laws ER, Trautmann JC, Hollenhorst RW Jr: Transsphenoidal decompression of the optic nerve and chiasm: Visual results in 62 patients. *J Neurosurg* 46:717, 1977.
19. MacCarty CS, Hanson EJ Jr, Randall RV, et al: Indications for and results of surgical treatment of pituitary tumors by the transfrontal approach, in Kohler PO, Ross GT (eds): *Diagnosis and Treatment of Pituitary Tumors*. Amsterdam, Excerpta Medica, 1973.
20. Martins AN, Kempe LG, Hayes GJ: Pituitary adenomas: Concepts based on twelve years' experience at Walter Reed General Hospital. *Acta Neurochir* 13:469, 1965.
21. Olivecrona H: The surgical treatment of intracranial tumors, in Olivecrona H, Tonnis W (eds): *Handbuch der Neurochirurgie*. Berlin, Springer-Verlag, 1967, vol 4, part 4.
22. Pelkonen R, Kuusisto A, Salmi J, et al: Pituitary function after pituitary apoplexy. *Am J Med* 65:773, 1978.
23. Post MJD, David NJ: Pituitary apoplexy: A radiographic-clinical correlation, in Smith JL (ed): *Neuro-ophthalmology 1982*. New York, Masson Publishing USA Inc, 1981.
24. Ray BS, Patterson RH Jr: Surgical experience with chromophobe adenomas of the pituitary gland. *J Neurosurg* 34:726, 1971.
25. Rovit RL, Fein JM: Pituitary apoplexy: A review and reappraisal. *J Neurosurg* 37:280, 1972.
26. Stern WE, Batzdorf U: Intracranial removal of pituitary adenomas: An evaluation of varying degrees of excision from partial to total. *J Neurosurg* 33:564, 1970.
27. Svien HJ, Love JG, Kennedy WC, et al: Status of vision following surgical treatment for pituitary chromophobe adenoma. *J Neurosurg* 22:47, 1965.
28. Tönnis W, Oberdisse K, Weber E: Bericht über 264 operierte Hypophysenadenome. *Acta Neurochir* 3:113, 1954.
29. Van Der Zwan A: Pituitary Tumors, thesis. Leiden, The Netherlands (De Kempenaer, Oegstgeest).
30. Wirth FP, Schwartz HG, Schwetschenau PR: Pituitary adenomas: Factors in treatment. *Clin Neurosurg* 21:8, 1974.
31. Zervas NT, Mendelson G: Treatment of acute haemorrhage of pituitary tumors. *Lancet* 1:604, 1975.

CHAPTER 10

Uncommon pituitary and parasellar lesions

Uncommon pituitary tumors
    Alpha subunit secreting pituitary adenoma
    TSH-secreting adenoma
    Gonadotropin (FSH- and LH-)–secreting adenoma
    Primary pituitary carcinoma
    Ectopic pituitary adenoma
    Pituitary metastases
Uncommon parasellar lesions
    Hypothalamic tumors
    Optic pathway glioma
    Germinomas and teratoid tumors
    Chordoma
    Granular cell tumor (choristoma)
    Dermoid and epidermoid cysts
    Benign cysts
    Meningiomas
Summary

Pituitary tumors commonly secrete excessive amounts of prolactin, growth hormone, or adrenocorticotropic hormone (ACTH), resulting in characteristic clinical syndromes. Occasionally, a single tumor produces both growth hormone and prolactin. On rare occasions, pituitary tumors secrete excessive quantities of thyroid-stimulating hormone (TSH), luteinizing hormone (LH), or follicle-stimulating hormone (FSH). A variety of unrelated neoplasms also occur in the parasellar region; these may alter hypophysial function. Knowledge of these pituitary and parasellar tumors and their behavior is important in establishing the differential diagnosis and determining the appropriate therapy.

UNCOMMON PITUITARY TUMORS

The glycoprotein hormones-TSH, LH, and FSH—are made up of two peptide chains with carbohydrate substituent groups attached to each chain. The carbohydrate groups include fucose, mannose, galactose, glucosamine, and galactosamine. One of the peptide chains is designated alpha and the other, beta. The amino acid sequences of the alpha chain, or subunit, appear to be identical or very similar for all three hormones. Hormonal activity in the complete molecule is conferred by the beta subunits, which have greater differences in amino acid sequences between the various hormones. When isolated, the alpha subunit lacks biologic activity, and thus its role is not clear.

Measurements of these subunits in normal human serum have documented that the alpha subunits are easily detectable, whereas the specific beta subunits are usually low or undetectable.[7,46,89,90] Elevated levels of alpha subunit have been demonstrated in patients with pituitary tumors that secrete excessive quantities of TSH, growth hormone, LH, or prolactin;[45,50,55,65] with pituitary tumors lacking clinical evidence of hypersecretion;[67] with primary hypothyroidism and primary gonadal failure;[47-49,89,90] and with a variety of malignant nonpituitary tissues.[6,69,84]

Alpha subunit secreting pituitary adenoma

Ridgeway et al[64] reported isolated hypersecretion of the alpha subunit in two men with previously diagnosed "non-functional chromophobe adenomas." Both patients had large chromophobe adenomas with suprasellar extensions and with evidence of mass effect (visual field deficit). The first patient was hypogonadal and hypothyroid, and both growth hormone and prolactin values were low. The second patient was hypogonadal and hypoadrenal. Growth hormone levels were undetectable and prolactin levels were normal. The basal serum alpha subunit concentrations in both patients were above the upper limits for normal, and after transsphenoidal surgery, the levels decreased but remained elevated.

Previous to this report, isolated alpha subunit secretion by pituitary tumors had not been recognized because of the absence of a characteristic clinical syndrome. The importance of the alpha subunit in clinical practice other than the fact that it can be elevated in association with a number of pituitary and nonpituitary tumors is that measurements of this entity may serve as a marker of treatment effectiveness, particularly in the nonfunctional pituitary tumor in which preoperative measurements of alpha subunit are elevated.

TSH-secreting adenoma

Although rare, instances of pituitary adenomas secreting elevated levels of TSH have been well documented. These lesions are associated with clinical and chemical evidence of hyperthyroidism. Clinically, the patients exhibit an increased metabolic rate, abnormal autonomic functions, tremor, heat intolerance, weight loss, and palpitations.[17] The neurologic symptoms are usually limited to tremor of the hands, exophthalmos, lid-lag, infrequent blinking, weakness of convergence, and weakness of the extremities. Mental disturbances ranging from mild emotional instability to a variety of psychotic syndromes may occur. Since the association of a pituitary adenoma and hyperthyroidism may occur by chance, definite criteria should be fulfilled to affirm the diagnosis of a TSH-secreting adenoma causing thyrotoxicosis,[5,87] and these criteria include (1) increased serum thyroxine (T_4) and/or triiodothyronine (T_3); (2) elevated or inappropriately high TSH levels, using a radioimmunoassay specific for human TSH; (3) finding of a pituitary tumor with evidence of typical thyrotrophs as defined either by morphologic fine structure or by immunohistochemistry; (4) absence of infiltrative ophthalmopathy or acropathy (hypertrophic pulmonary osteoarthropathy); (5) undetectable thyroid-stimulating immunoglobulins; and (6) disappearance of hyperthyroidism after removal of the pituitary adenoma. When all these criteria are applied, less than a dozen cases reported in the literature are unequivocal cases of TSH-thyrotoxicosis caused by a pituitary adenoma.

In most cases, the alpha subunit in the blood is elevated, and usually neither TSH nor alpha subunit levels show a rise in response to thyrotropin-releasing hormone (TRH) stimulation.[39,45,79] The pathologic features of a TSH-secreting adenoma are discussed in Chapter 3.

Benoit et al[5,33,87] reviewed 10 cases up to 1980 and added one of their own. Of the 11 surgical cases (either hypophysectomy or adenomectomy), only two patients remained euthyroid (or cured) without hypopituitarism after at least 1 year of follow-up. These two cases were treated by adenomectomy followed within a few weeks by radiation therapy. Benoit et al conclude that adenomectomy followed by irradiation appears to be the most appropriate approach to recommend in TSH-secreting pituitary adenomas. The following case from our series represents an instance of a TSH-producing adenoma that satisfied the criteria for this entity:

> The patient was a 21-year-old black man with an 18 month history of hyperthyroidism. Symptoms consisted of heat intolerance, weight loss, and occasional palpitations. He had no visual symptoms. On examination, the thyroid was soft and diffusely enlarged to approximately twice normal size. There was no exophthalmos, both eyes measuring 18 mm by exophthalmometry. He had a fine tremor of the extended extremities. Blood pressure was 118/68 mmHg, and pulse rate was 96 beats/min and regular. The skin was warm and dry. The deep tendon reflexes were bilaterally hyperactive. The heart sounds were normal. There was a systolic murmur at the apex and right second intercostal space.
>
> Laboratory results revealed a total T_4 of 16.1 mcg/dl, T_3 radioimmunoassay (RIA) 343 ng/dl, T_3 resin uptake 38.5%, and a calculated free T_4 of 4.6. Antithyroid antibodies were negative. The I^{123} thyroid uptake was elevated at 56.5% at 2 hours and 67.5% at 24 hours. TSH was greater than 50 μU/ml.

A computed tomographic (CT) scan of the pituitary (Fig. 10-1) showed a moderate-sized pituitary adenoma.

A presumptive diagnosis of TSH-secreting pituitary adenoma causing hyperthyroidism was made, and transsphenoidal surgery was recommended.

The endocrinology service felt that it would be appropriate to bring the hyperthyroidism under control before surgery, and so the patient began treatment with propylthiouracil 500 mg/day. This medication was discontinued because of nausea and abdominal cramps, and treatment was switched to methimazole, 30 mg/day. The methimazole was continued until the patient became euthyroid and was believed to be ready for surgery.

On 3/28/84 he underwent transsphenoidal surgery with removal of a discrete, 14 by 16 mm adenoma. The remaining gland, which was moderately compressed, was spared. It was felt that a complete removal of tumor was accomplished.

Dr. K. Kovacs (Toronto) kindly performed histologic examination of the excised tumor. Routine examination revealed that the tumor was a basophilic adenoma. The adenoma cells showed cytoplasmic periodic acid–Schiff (PAS) and lead hematoxylin positivity. The Grimelius technique indicated the absence of argyrophilic granules.

The immunoperoxidase technique revealed the presence of TSH, FSH, and alpha subunit in the cytoplasm of scattered adenoma cells. Immunostainings were negative for growth hormone, prolactin, ACTH, and LH.

By electron microscopy, the tumor consisted of large polar cells with long cytoplasmic processes and spherical or slightly irregular nuclei with a light chromatin substance and large, dense nucleoli. The abundant cytoplasm

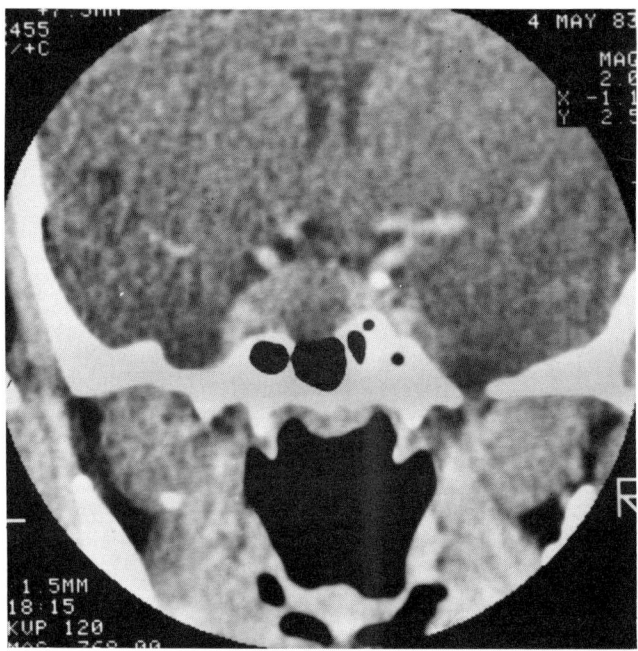

Fig. 10-1. Coronal CT scan shows moderate size adenoma. At surgery, tumor was discrete and measured 14 by 16 mm.

contained well-developed rough endoplasmic reticulum (RER) and prominent Golgi complexes. The number of secretory granules varied from cell to cell; a considerable number of cells were well granulated. The secretory granules were spherical or slightly irregular with somewhat varying electron density. The minority measured 50 to 150 nm, and the majority measured around 200 nm; numerous granules measured 150 to 350 nm.

The immunocytochemical and fine structural features of this neoplasm were consistent with the diagnosis of a *thyrotroph cell adenoma of the pituitary.*

The hospital course following surgery was unremarkable. Evaluation 20 days postoperatively revealed a normal cortisol response to insulin hypoglycemia and a normal LH, FSH, testosterone, and prolactin. The TSH level was 4 μU/ml and increased to 8 μU/ml after TRH stimulation. The T_4 was 11.0; free T_4, 1.9; and T_3 RIA, 187.

The patient continues to feel well and remains clinically and biochemically euthyroid 1 year after surgery.

Gonadotropin (FSH- and LH-)–secreting adenomas

Not surprisingly, there have been only a few well-documented reports of gonadotropin hypersecretion caused by a pituitary adenoma, and most of these have occurred in patients with primary hypogonadism.[16,27,65] Of those gonadotropin-secreting adenomas not associated with hypogonadism, most have been accompanied by FSH hypersecretion. An LH-secreting pituitary tumor without FSH hypersecretion and without hypogonadism was reported by Peterson et al.[65] Their patient was a 30-year-old, sexually potent man with an isolated LH-secreting tumor. FSH secretion was low, and the patient was azoospermic, probably a result of the decreased FSH secretion. However, the testes were normal in size, and testosterone and other testicular steroids were hypersecreted. Markedly increased serum concentration of alpha subunit peptide was present. The tumor was not completely autonomous as shown by modest (but blunted) LH and alpha subunit responses after administration of luteinizing hormone–releasing hormone (LHRH). After transsphenoidal removal of the adenoma, plasma LH and alpha subunit levels decreased but remained elevated. Irradiation to the sellar region was recommended, but the patient declined to have further treatment.

Only rarely have pituitary adenomas secreting both FSH and LH been documented.[19,80] Demura et al[19] reported a 50-year-old man who was admitted because of a left temporal hemianopsia. Previous history indicated that he had received pituitary irradiation (2000 rad) 8 years earlier and had done well until a year before admission. There was no clinical evidence of hypogonadism. Endocrine studies revealed markedly elevated plasma FSH (295 mIU/ml) and slightly elevated plasma LH (35 mIU/ml) levels. CT showed a pituitary tumor with marked suprasellar extension. The tumor was removed by craniotomy, and 2 weeks after surgery, plasma FSH and LH decreased to 19 and 22 mIU/ml, respectively. On histologic examination, the tumor consisted of 90% chromophobe and 10% eosinophilic cells. Electron microscopy revealed two sizes of secretory granules with diameters of 100 to 200 nm and 300 to 500 nm, respectively. Serum alpha subunit levels were not mentioned in the report.

As with TSH-secreting adenomas, patients with gonadotropin hypersecretion resulting from a pituitary adenoma are likely to have elevated levels of the alpha subunit indicating that excess secretion of this peptide chain may be a general phenomenon in pituitary tumors producing a glycoprotein hormone. As indicated above, in some of the reported cases of gonadotropin-secreting adenomas, there was some increase in LH and/or FSH secretion after LHRH administration.[19,80] This finding differs from that in patients with TSH-secreting adenomas in whom there is usually a lack of response to TRH administration (see p. 303).

There is no specific syndrome associated with these tumors, and because of their rarity, no meaningful results of treatment are available. Transsphenoidal surgery could be used in those cases in which it appears (from the CT scan) that the tumor might be resectable. Preoperative or postoperative serum alpha subunit measurements may serve as a marker of the effectiveness of surgery and for later follow-up of the patient in terms of recurrence.

Primary pituitary carcinoma

This entity is a distinctly rare lesion and may be impossible to diagnose by the histologic appearance alone. The presence of cellular pleomorphism, mitotic figures, and even local invasion are not conclusive evidence of malignancy, and an unequivocal diagnosis requires the demonstration of distant metastases. Scheithauer[74] has reviewed these cases and compared the gross pathologic, radiographic, and clinical features of pituitary carcinoma producing cerebrospinal metastases with those producing extracranial dissemination. In the first group (i.e., those with cerebrospinal metastases), the average age was 43 years (range 25 to 75 years), and the average duration of disease was 8 years from onset of symptoms to death. In three fourths of the cases, these tumors were endocrine inactive; the remainder of patients had acromegaly, except one with Cushing's disease. In the other group (i.e., those with extracranial dissemination), the average age was 44 years (range 7 to 75 years) with an average survival of 2½ years from onset of symptoms to death. Half of these patients had Cushing's disease, and the remainder were endocrine inactive. The most common site of blood-borne metastasis was the liver with other sites including lung, bone, myocardium, and lymph nodes.

Malignant sarcomas are quite rare but have been reported in patients previously irradiated for pituitary adenomas.[29,66]

Ectopic pituitary adenoma

Ectopic pituitary tumors have been reported to occur in various parts of the cranium including the sphenoid sinus, sphenoid wing, nasal cavity, and petrous temporal bone.[8,43,70] An ectopic pituitary adenoma probably arises from extrasellar pituitary tissue deposited along the route of fetal development.[9,22,59] Also the "ectopic tissue" could result from spread from a malignant pituitary tumor along the meninges or via the cerebrospinal fluid (CSF) or bloodstream.[56,61,62] Dislodgement of adenoma cells during surgical treatment of a pituitary adenoma could be another mechanism for the development of an ectopic neoplasm. Alternatively, ectopic adenohypophysial tissue is known to occur in the sphenoid bone or roof of the pharynx.[59] Suprasellar ectopic pituitary adenomas presumably arise from adenohypophysial cells of the pars tuberalis that normally extend above the diaphragm sella (Fig. 10-2).[8,70] Fig. 10-2 shows a CT scan and metrizamide cisternogram on a 53-year-old woman who sought medical attention because of headache and mild symptoms of diabetes insipidus. The CT revealed an enhancing suprasellar mass that was well outlined by cisternography. The sella turcica was shortened posteriorly but was not enlarged. This tumor was removed by craniotomy and proved to be an entirely suprasellar pituitary adenoma.

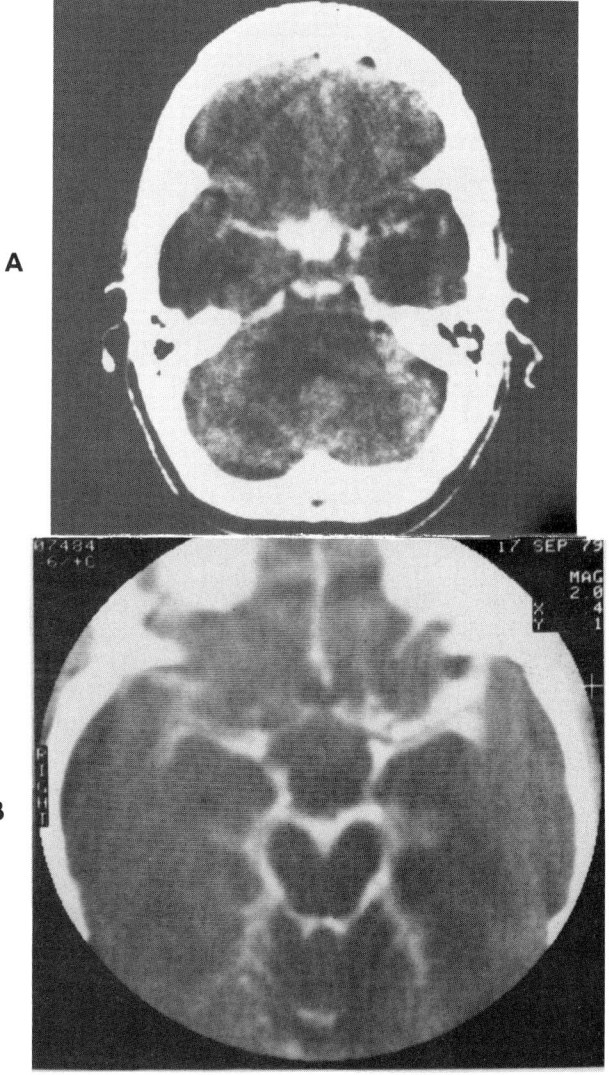

Fig. 10-2. CT and metrizamide cisternogram—ectopic suprasellar pituitary adenoma. **A,** Axial CT illustrates enhancing suprasellar mass surgically proven to be pituitary adenoma. **B,** Metrizamide CT cisternogram outlines large suprasellar mass.

Pituitary metastases

The incidence with which epithelial and hematopoietic neoplasms metastasize to the pituitary gland is largely dependent on how aggressively one searches for their presence. Autopsy series have suggested that the incidence in patients with carcinoma is below 2%,[1,51] whereas Roessman et al[68] found pituitary involvement in 26.6% of cases. Buchmann and Schwesinger[10] found pituitary metastases in 23% of patients with hematopoietic neoplasms. These patients frequently have no clinical signs of pituitary involvement, although larger suprasellar lesions may occur (Fig. 10-3).[15,44] Panhypopituitarism is rare, but diabetes insipidus occurs in 6.8% to 33% of cases.[63,74,86]

The most frequent primary tumors metastasizing to the pituitary in men are lung (62.9%), prostate (8.6%), and stomach (7.5%); whereas in women they are breast (66%), lung (13.2%), and stomach (7.5%).[86] With hematopoietic neoplasms, hypophysial involvement is more common with lymphoblastic leukemia (33.3%), non-Hodgkin's lymphoma (29%), and myeloblastic leukemia (21%) than in patients with Hodgkin's disease (5%).[10]

With both carcinomas and hematopoietic neoplasms, the posterior pituitary is more frequently affected than the anterior pituitary.[10,74,86]

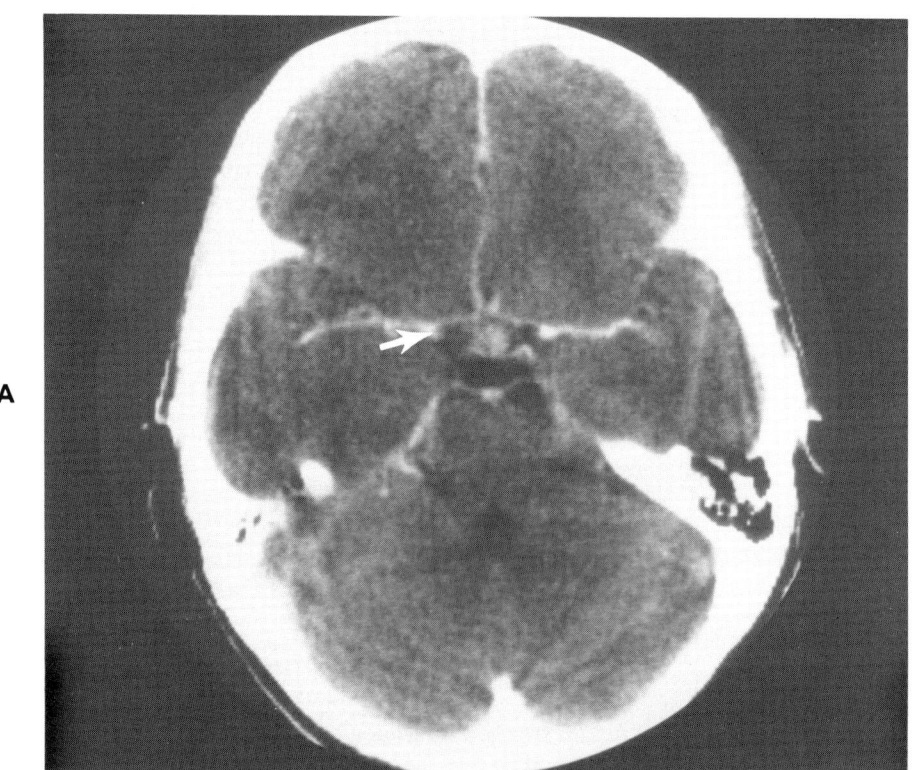

Fig. 10-3. CT and CT-metrizamide cisternogram—pituitary metastasis. **A,** Axial CT shows enhancing suprasellar mass (arrow) in patient with breast cancer.

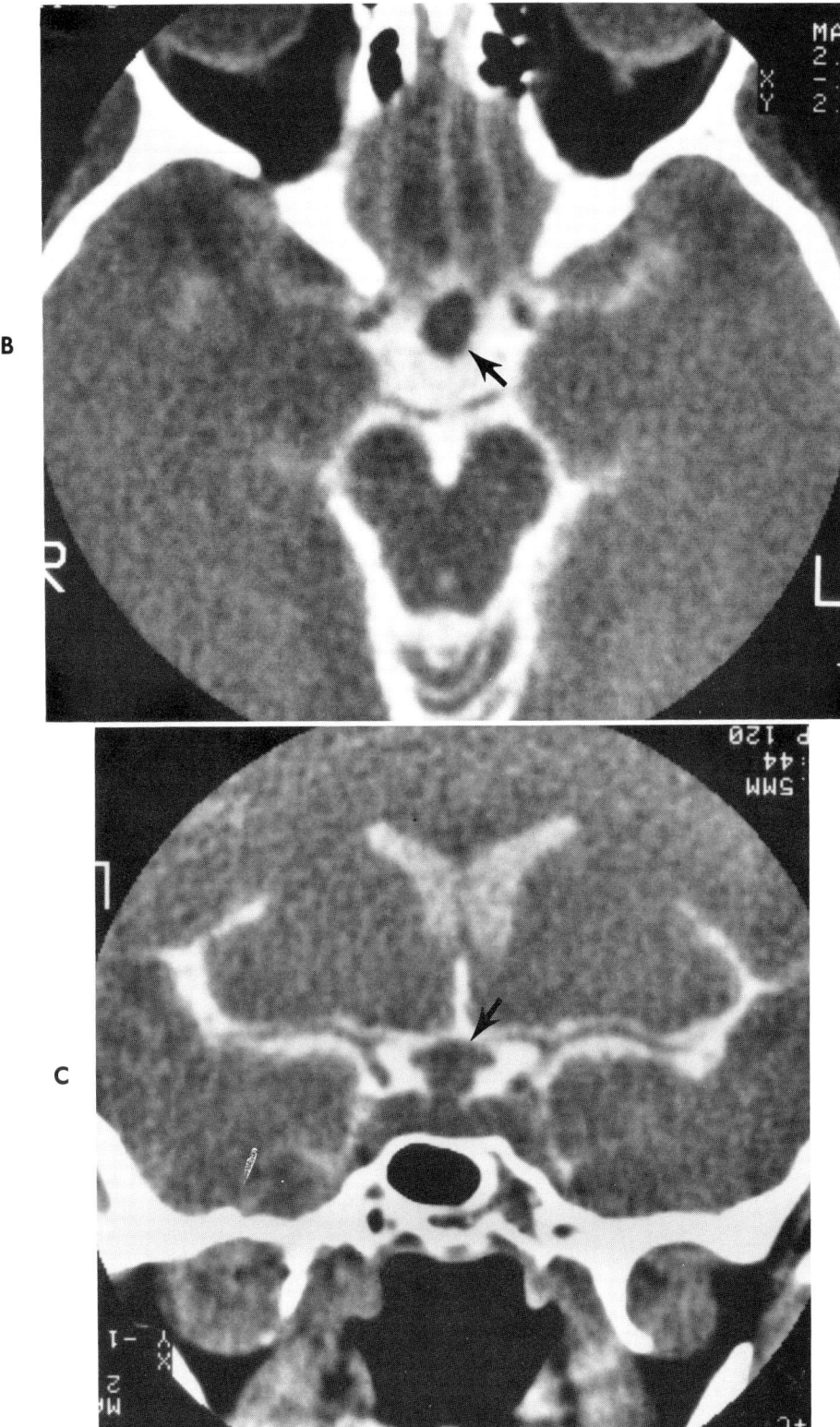

Fig. 10-3, cont'd. B, Axial CT-metrizamide cisternogram outlines suprasellar mass (arrow). **C,** Coronal view demonstrates chiasm outlined with metrizamide (arrow) below which is enlarged infundibulum.

UNCOMMON PARASELLAR LESIONS
Hypothalamic tumors

A variety of neoplasms can be found in the hypothalamus including gliomas, craniopharyngiomas, hamartomas, metastatic tumors, histiocytosis X, leukemia, ganglioneuromas, ependymomas, and medulloblastomas. The relative rarity of tumors rising in the hypothalamus is related more to the small size of this structure as compared with the rest of the brain than to any peculiar feature of this area. Although craniopharyngioma is probably the most frequently occurring tumor, this lesion does not arise within the substance of the hypothalamus and thus is an extrinsic, or extra-axial, lesion. Craniopharyngioma is discussed in Chapter 11. Likewise, the germinoma may arise in the suprasellar region and involve the hypothalamus as a result of extrinsic pressure from the suprasellar mass. The astrocytoma is the most common intrinsic tumor of the hypothalamus. All the common fibrillary astrocytic neoplasms (astrocytoma, anaplastic astrocytoma, glioblastoma multiforme) may involve the hypothalamus. A distinct type of astrocytic neoplasm, the pilocytic astrocytoma, characteristically arises in the wall of the third ventricle and the optic nerves. Clinically, there may be a long history of hypothalamic symptoms such as diabetes insipidus, obesity, bulimia, or emaciation resulting from the slow growth of these tumors. Two morphologic types of pilocytic astrocytomas have been described, the adult and juvenile pilocytic astrocytomas,[11,73] also called the spongioblastomas.[88,93] The pathologic features of these two types are described in Chapter 3.

Hamartomas are essentially non-neoplastic malformations that are characterized by an abnormal mixture of tissue indigenous to the site; grow much slower than true neoplasms; and generally, do not display a potential for malignancy. However, the separation from true neoplasm may often be difficult. The hypothalamic ganglionic hamartoma consists of redundant gray matter usually (but not always) attached to the tuber cinereum or the mammillary bodies. This lesion usually occurs in males and is classically associated with precocious puberty. The latter endocrinopathy is believed to be caused by the mechanical effects of the tumor on the hypothalamus rather than to any specific hormonal secretory effects of the hamartoma.

Optic pathway glioma

Gliomas of the optic pathways make up a relatively small portion of central nervous system neoplasms. The incidence reported by Martin and Cushing[57] and Taveras et al[85] was 0.84% and 1.7%, respectively. Approximately 75% of these lesions occur in children under the age of 12 years.[25] Neurofibromatosis is commonly associated with single (71%) or multicentric (100%) optic nerve gliomas. It is of interest that the association of neurofibromatosis is much lower in patients with chiasmal gliomas (8%).[36] The presenting signs depend on whether the tumor originates from the intraorbital or intracranial portion of the optic pathway. Progressive, painless, unilateral proptosis combined with a variable degree of visual loss is the common presenting clinical picture of the primary intraorbital gliomas.

This may be accompanied by disc swelling or optic atrophy. With chiasmal gliomas, there may be monocular or binocular visual impairment often with a hemianopsia or a homonymous field defect if there is optic tract involvement. An afferent pupillary defect (Marcus Gunn's sign) is usually present. Chiasmal gliomas may produce increased intracranial pressure and the clinical presentation of an anterior third ventricular mass.[13,52] Endocrinopathies such as precocious puberty and the diencephalic syndrome have been associated with large chiasmal gliomas in children.[18]

In adults, the differential diagnosis of optic nerve tumors is usually between a meningioma and optic glioma. Chiasmal gliomas must be distinguished from pituitary adenomas, hypothalamic gliomas, craniopharyngiomas, diaphragm sella meningiomas, aneurysms, and "ectopic pinealomas"[37] (Fig. 10-4).

Some believe the tumors of the optic nerve are quite benign with the biologic characteristics of a hamartoma,[38] whereas others regard them as having definite growth potential.[20,21,34,54,64] Radiation therapy with 4500 rad in 4 weeks is the recommended treatment for chiasmal gliomas associated with progressive visual

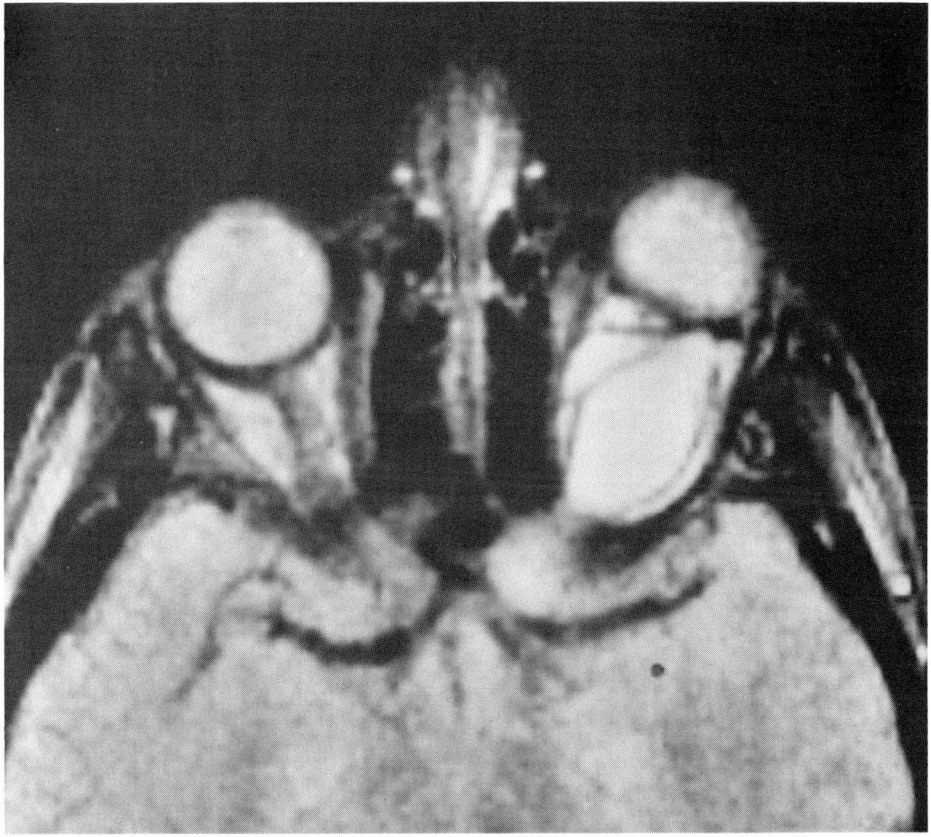

Fig. 10-4. Magnetic resonance imaging (MRI)—optic nerve glioma. Axial MRI of a biopsy verified optic nerve glioma. TE 50 ms and TR 1000 ms. Second echo demonstrates neoplasm in orbit and intracranially in optic nerve just proximal to chiasm. Ability to determine whether there is involvement of chiasm will influence therapy.

loss.[37] Likewise, there is little controversy regarding the appropriate treatment of optic nerve tumors causing disfiguring proptosis and visual loss. These are explored by a transcranial orbital approach with resection of the tumor from behind the globe to the chiasm.[35,38] Adult optic nerve tumors may require a biopsy to differentiate a glioma from a meningioma.[37] Radiation is the mainstay of therapy for chiasmal lesions, although surgery may be required to provide a diagnosis or debulking of the tumor.

Germinomas and teratoid tumors

Tumors of germ cell origin that occur in the gonads, mediastinum, and pineal region may also occur in the suprasellar or third ventricular areas, either in association with tumors of the pineal or as a solitary neoplasm (ectopic pinealoma).[40,42] A primary intrasellar position has been reported but is very rare.[28,32] Tumors of a germ cell origin in an intracranial location are a relatively common entity among the Japanese constituting 2.1% to 4.5% of all brain tumors.[83] The most common of these germ cell tumors is the germinoma, which is histologically identical to the gonadal seminoma, dysgerminoma, and mediastinal germinoma. The pathologic characteristics of these tumors are described in Chapter 3. Other teratomatous tumors that may arise in the suprasellar region include the undifferentiated embryonal cell carcinoma, the choriocarcinoma and yolk sac tumors.

The onset of symptoms is usually in the first decade of life. Although germinomas in the pineal region have a male to female ratio of 4:1 or 5:1, there appears to be no clear sex preference of the suprasellar lesions.[83] The earliest and most prominent symptom resulting from suprasellar germinomas is diabetes insipidus.[91] Another common finding is visual impairment resulting from infiltration and compression of the optic nerves, chiasm, and/or tracts. This usually produces optic atrophy and a bitemporal hemianopsia. Hypophysial dysfunction may occur with suprasellar germinomas, most commonly manifested by pituitary insufficiency and, occasionally in prepubertal patients, growth failure and dwarfism.[91] Precocious puberty is a rare endocrinologic manifestation of these neoplasms, resulting from the elaboration of HCG-secreting choriocarcinoma cells within the tumor.[91] Large tumors may produce hydrocephalus.

Suprasellar germinomas are infiltrating, nonencapsulated tumors that cannot be completely removed without producing unacceptable neurologic deficits.[91] Therefore the principles of surgical treatment include decompression of the optic apparatus and establishment of a diagnosis to differentiate the neoplasm from a craniopharyngioma or optic chiasm/hypothalamic glioma and establish the presence or absence of other types of germ cells. If the patient has hydrocephalus, a CSF shunt is placed initially and the CSF examined for the presence of tumor cells and assayed for alpha fetoprotein and HCG.

An extensive surgical procedure is not indicated for germinomas, since this is associated with an unacceptable complication rate and they are so exquisitely sensitive to radiation.[91] Since intracranial germ cell tumors are known to disseminate through the CSF pathways, the entire craniospinal axis must be irradiated. Takeuchi et al[83] recommend giving 2500 to 3000 rad to the suprasellar region, 3000 rad to the whole brain, and 2000 to 3000 rad to the spinal cord.[83] Jenkins uses a higher total dose of 5000 rad given over 5 to 6 weeks at 150 to 200 rad/day.[41]

Chordoma

A chordoma is a slowly growing, destructive and locally invasive tumor that is thought to originate from vestigial intraosseous remnants of the notocord. The anatomic sites of predilection of this tumor are the sacrococcygeal region and intracranial area. The intracranial examples comprise about 40% of all chordomas and arise on the clivus at the spheno-occipital synchondrosis.[11] Rostral growth from this area with accompanying destruction of bone may involve the sella turcica, cavernous sinuses, optic pathways, and sphenoid sinus (Fig. 10-5).

Falconer et al[24] suggested dividing chordomas into three groups. The first arises within the sella and behaves as a pituitary tumor with chiasmal compression and hypopituitarism. The second group is parasellar, characterized by ocular motor

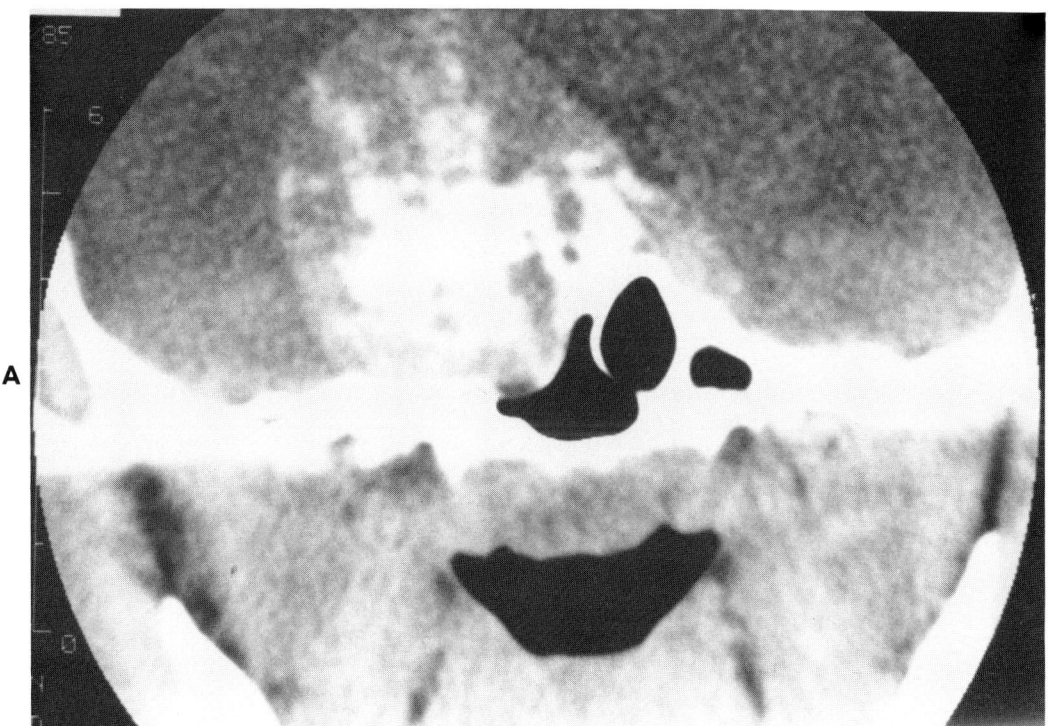

Fig. 10-5. CT and MRI—chordoma. **A,** Coronal enhanced CT scan shows large calcified and enhancing lesion eroding sella and sphenoid sinus with significant parasellar extension.
Continued.

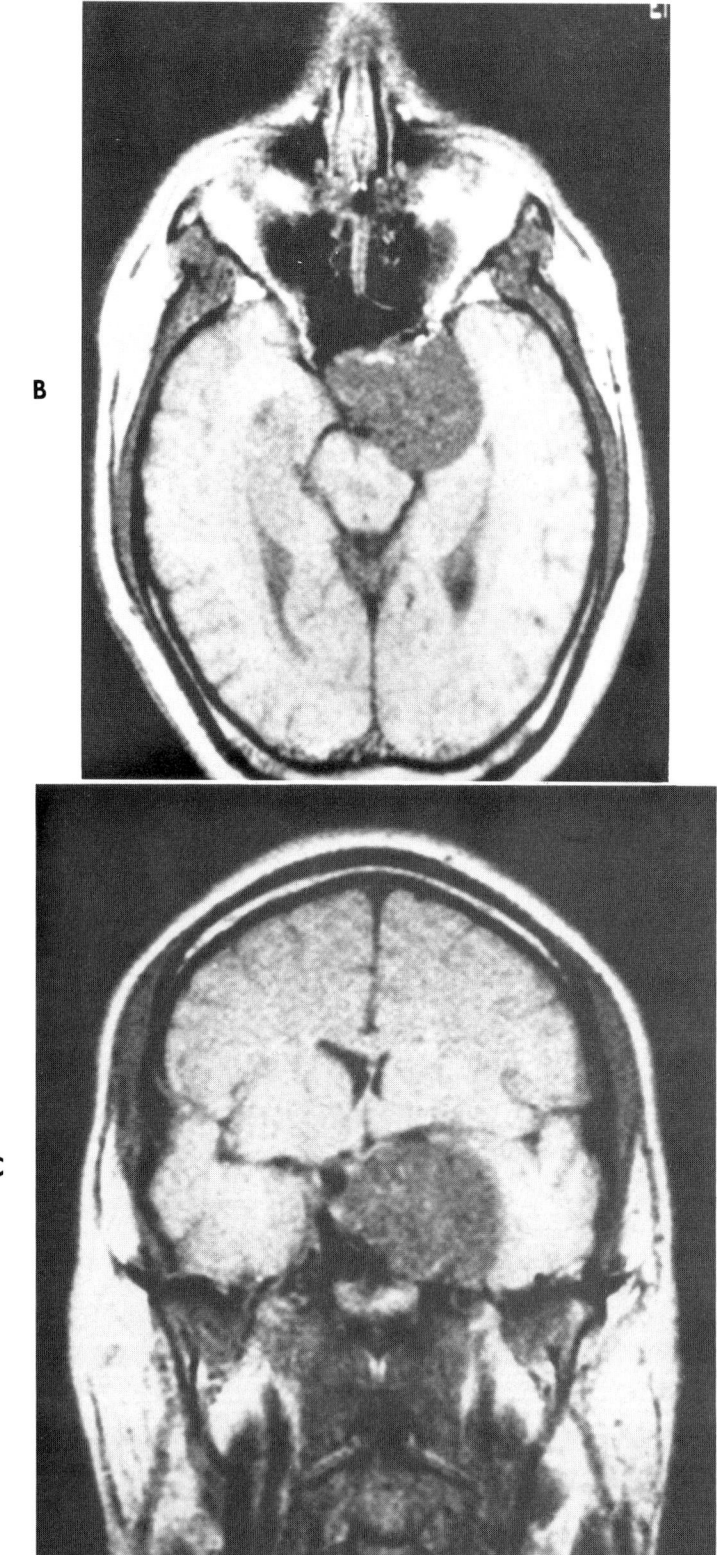

Fig. 10-5, cont'd. B, Axial MRI, TE 30 ms and TR 600 ms. First echo demonstrates area of long T1 in sellar and parasellar region on left side. Note indentation of midbrain. **C,** Coronal MRI, TE 30 ms and TR 750 ms. First echo demonstrates area of long T1 involving sella with suprasellar extension distorting third ventricle.

palsies, optic tract compression, and hypopituitarism. The third is clival and causes bilateral sixth nerve palsies and brainstem compression usually without causing hypopituitarism or chiasmal compression.

Although the cytologic features of chordomas are usually benign and mitoses are not found, the prognosis is poor because of the destructive and locally invasive characteristics of this neoplasm. As a result of their involvement of the skull base, total surgical removal is rarely, if ever, achieved. Radiation has been suggested for these tumors although the reported benefits have not been impressive.[24] The growth potential of chordomas can vary considerably from one patient to another. The gross and histologic features of this tumor are described in Chapter 3.

Granular cell tumor (choristoma)

The term *choristoma* was given by Sternberg[82] to groups of rather large round or oval cells that have a granulated cytoplasm and may be encountered incidentally on routine examination of the infundibular process.[53,73] Many authors favor a Schwann cell or perineural cell origin, but a variety of other cell types have been proposed, including pituitary cells of the intermediate lobe, glial cells (pituicytes) of the posterior lobe, or displaced basophilic rests.

Granular cell tumors of the pituitary are structurally identical to granular cell tumors found in other parts of the body, including the oral cavity, salivary glands, larynx, trachea, bronchi, gastrointestinal tract, urinary bladder, uterus, breast, and subcutaneous tissue. Neoplasms with similar morphology have been identified in the cerebral hemisphere, third ventricle, meninges of the spinal cord, and spinal and cranial nerves.

Dermoid and epidermoid cysts

Dermoid and epidermoid cysts are believed to be formed as a result of the inclusion of epithelial elements at the time of closure of the neural tube between the third and fifth fetal week.[72] Epidermoid cysts or cholesteatomas (also called ''pearly'' tumors) occur more commonly in the intracranial cavity than dermoids. The epidermoid cysts are found most frequently in the cerebellopontine angle but also occur in the suprasellar and parasellar region,[31] whereas intracranial dermoids are generally located in the posterior fossa as a midline cerebellar lesion.

These cysts present symptoms of a slowly enlarging mass. Leakage of cyst fluid from an epidermoid may produce a chemical meningitis, which may be recurrent.[11,31,75] Both dermoids and epidermoids appear as low-density masses on CT scan. These tumors are benign but will recur if incompletely removed. Malignant degeneration of both dermoids and epidermoids has been noted but is very rare.

Benign cysts

A number of different types of cysts may occur in the sellar and parasellar area. Although relatively rare, Rathke's cleft cysts, arachnoid cysts, and mucoceles are among the more common cystic lesions occurring in this region. Rathke's cleft cysts and mucoceles are each lined by epithelial cells, whereas the arachnoid cyst (see below) lacks an epithelial lining.

Rathke's cleft cysts are believed to form from remnants of Rathke's pouch caused by a persistence of the pouch between the developing anterior and intermediate lobes of the pituitary.[26,60] Some investigators have suggested that such cysts can be derived from neuroepithelium as well.[14,78] In support of this idea, Shuangshoti et al[78] emphasized that epithelial cysts of the pituitary region have a wide range of histologic features that are microscopically and histochemically indistinguishable from neuroepithelial (colloid) cysts.[78] This may explain the mode of occurrence of Rathke's cleft cysts outside the sella turcica. Incidental cysts found in 13% to 23% of routine autopsies rarely exceed 7 mm in diameter.[4,58,77,76] Although unusual, Rathke's cleft cysts may enlarge and thus compress surrounding structures such as the pituitary gland, optic nerves or chiasm, hypothalamus, or third ventricle (see Fig. 5-28).[12,71,81,92]

Fager and Carter[23] suggested that many Rathke's cleft cysts are misdiagnosed as craniopharyngiomas, a hypothesis supported by Banna's observation that 4% of 160 intracranial masses diagnosed clinically and radiologically as craniopharyngiomas were histologically proved to be Rathke's cleft cysts.[3]

Mucoceles are epithelial cysts that originate in the paranasal sinuses and are pathologically indistinguishable from Rathke's cleft cysts. This lesion may expand from a sinus with an occluded ostium and extend into the orbit or skull to compress the pituitary gland, optic nerves, or brain itself. The differentiation of a mucocele from Rathke's cleft cysts relies on the radiologic or gross observation of cyst extension from a paranasal sinus into the intracranial cavity.

Leptomeningeal or arachnoid cysts are distended areas of the subarachnoid space. They are filled with CSF and delineated on both the inner and outer aspects by a delicate arachnoid membrane sparsely populated by meningothelial cells. Enlargement is believed to occur either by an osmotic process or by a ball-valve phenomenon where CSF intermittently gains entrance to the cyst without exit.

Meningiomas

Although these tumors are not uncommon, the parasellar meningiomas that cause significant pituitary dysfunction or masquerade as pituitary tumors are relatively rare. Meningiomas that arise from the tuberculum sella and olfactory groove may occasionally cause symptoms that mimic pituitary tumors or, rarely, may cause varying degrees of hypopituitarism. Tuberculum sella meningiomas cause stretching and compression of the optic nerves and chiasm, thus producing visual field defects and loss of acuity similar to that seen with pituitary tumors. In most cases, the diagnosis can be established or suspected preoperatively on the basis of skull x-ray films and CT scan. Gregorius el al[30] reported 23 surgically treated cases of suprasellar meningiomas. There were two deaths, and vision returned to normal in 15 but remained poor in six patients.

Olfactory groove meningiomas may cause chiasmal compression when the tumor protrudes posteriorly. Symptoms such as anosmia and dementia are commonly seen with this tumor, whereas hypopituitarism occurs rarely. The diagnosis usually is readily established by CT scan.

SUMMARY

There is an intimate relationship of neural, endocrine, vascular, meningeal, and skeletal structures in the sellar region, which makes it possible for a wide variety of pathologic entities to exist in a relatively small anatomic area. Although many of the potential afflictions are rare, the physician caring for patients with pituitary disorders must be aware of these possibilities and knowledgeable in their management. Many of the unusual conditions affecting the pituitary, especially neoplasms, will cause dysfunction of surrounding anatomic structures such as the optic apparatus, hypothalamus, and pituitary stalk as a result of either mass effect or invasion. Some have characteristic presentations, whereas others are clinically indistinguishable from other parasellar lesions. In the latter case, neuroradiologic studies such as CT, metrizamide cisternography, angiography, and more recently magnetic resonance imaging (MRI) are helpful in establishing a diagnosis and planning therapy. The treatment must be individualized and will ultimately depend on the specific pathologic entity, which may require a surgical procedure for verification.

REFERENCES

1. Abrams HL, Spiro R, Goldstein N: Metastases in carcinoma: Analysis of 1000 autopsied cases. *Cancer* 3:74, 1950.
2. Allen JC, Nisselbaum J, Epstein F, et al: Alpha fetoprotein and human chorionic gonadotropin determination in cerebrospinal fluid: An aid to the diagnosis and management of intracranial germ-cell tumors. *J Neurosurg* 51:368, 1979.
3. Banna M: Craniopharyngioma: Based on 160 cases. *Br J Radiol* 49:206, 1976.
4. Bayoumi ML: Rathke's cleft and its cysts. *Edinburgh Med J* 55:745, 1948.
5. Benoit R, Pearson-Murphy BE, Robert F, et al: Hyperthyroidism due to a pituitary TSH secreting tumour with amenorrhoea-galactorrhoea. *Clin Endocrinol* 12:11, 1980.
6. Benveniste R, Linder J, Puett D, et al: Human chorionic gonadotropin α-subunit from cultured choriocarcinoma (JEG) cells: Comparison of the subunit secreted free with that prepared from secreted human chorionic gonadotropin. *Endocrinology* 105:581, 1979.
7. Binoux M, Pierce JG, Odell WD: Radioimmunological characterization of human thyrotropin and its subunits: Applications for the measurement of human TSH. *J Clin Endocrinol Metab* 38:674, 1974.
8. Bonner RA, Mukai K, Oppenheimer JH: Two unusual variants of Nelson's syndrome. *J Clin Endocrinol Metab* 49:23, 1979.
9. Borit A, Blanshard TP: Sphenoidal pituitary adenoma. *Hum Pathol* 10:93, 1979.
10. Buchmann E, Schwesinger G: Hypophyse und Hämoblastosen. *Zentralbl Neurochir* 40:35, 1979.
11. Burger PC, Vogel FS: Surgical pathology of the nervous system and its coverings. New York, John Wiley & Sons Inc, 1982.
12. Byrd SE, Winter J, Takahashi M, et al: Symptomatic Rathke's cleft cyst demonstrated on computed tomography. *J Comput Assist Tomogr* 4:411, 1980.
13. Chutorian AM, Schwartz JF, Evans RA, et al: Optic gliomas in children. *Neurology* 14:83, 1964.
14. Concha S, Hamilton BPM, Millan JC, et al: Symptomatic Rathke's cleft cyst with amyloid stroma. *J Neurol Neurosurg Psychiatry* 38:782, 1975.
15. Cox EV III: Chiasmal compression from metastatic cancer to the pituitary gland. *Surg Neurol* 11:49, 1979.
16. Cunningham GR, Huckins C: An FSH and prolactin-secreting pituitary tumor: Pituitary dynamics and testicular histology. *J Clin Endocrinol Metab* 44:248, 1977.
17. Daughaday WH: The adenohypophysis, (Chapter 2). in Williams RH (ed): *Textbook of Endocrinology,* ed 5. Philadelphia, WB Saunders Co, 1974.

18. DeSousa AL, Kalsheck JE, Mealey J Jr, et al: Diencephalic syndrome and its relation to opticochiasmatic glioma: Review of twelve cases. *Neurosurgery* 4:207, 1979.
19. Demura R, Kubo O, Demura H, et al: FSH and LH secreting pituitary adenoma. *J Clin Endocrinol Metab* 45:653, 1977.
20. Dodge HW Jr, Love JG, Craig WM, et al: Gliomas of the optic nerves. *Arch Neurol Psychiatry* 79:607, 1958.
21. Dosoretz DE, Blitzer PH, Wang CC, et al: Management of glioma of the optic nerve and/or chiasm: An analysis of 20 cases. *Cancer* 45:1467, 1980.
22. Erdheim J: Ueber einen Hypophysentumor von ungewohnlichem. *Sitz Beitr Pathol Anat* 46:233, 1909.
23. Fager CA, Carter H: Intrasellar epithelial cysts. *J Neurosurg* 24:77, 1966.
24. Falconer MA, Bailey IC, Duchew LW: Surgical treatment of chordoma and chondroma of the skull base. *J Neurosurg* 29:261, 1968.
25. Fowler FD, Matson DD: Gliomas of the optic pathways in childhood. *J Neurosurg* 14:515, 1957.
26. Frazier CH, Alpers BJ: Tumors of Rathke's cleft (hitherto called tumors of Rathke's pouch). *Arch Neurol Psychiatry* 32:973, 1934.
27. Friend JN, Judge DM, Sherman BM, et al: FSH-secreting pituitary adenomas: Stimulation and suppression studies in two patients. *J Clin Endocrinol Metab* 43:650, 1976.
28. Ghatak NR, Hirano A, Zimmerman HM: Intrasellar germinomas: A form of ectopic pinealoma. *J Neurosurg* 31:670, 1969.
29. Greenhouse AH: Pituitary sarcoma: A possible consequence of radiation. *JAMA* 190:269, 1964.
30. Gregorius FK, Hepler RS, Stern WE: Loss and recovery of vision with suprasellar meningiomas. *J Neurosurg* 42:69, 1975.
31. Guidetti B, Gagliardi FM: Epidermoid and dermoid cysts: Clinical evaluation and late surgical results. *J Neurosurg* 47:12, 1977.
32. Guiffrè R, di Lorenzo N: Evolution of a primary intrasellar germinomatous teratoma into a choriocarcinoma. *J Neurosurg* 42:602, 1975.
33. Hamilton CR Jr, Adams LC, Maloof F: Hyperthyroidism due to thyrotropin-producing pituitary chromophobe adenoma. *N Engl J Med* 283:1077, 1970.
34. Heiskanen O, Raitta C, Torsti R: The management and prognosis of gliomas of the optic pathways in children. *Acta Neurochir* 43:193, 1978.
35. Housepian EM: Intraorbital tumors, in Schmidek HH, Sweet WH (eds): *Current Techniques in Operative Neurosurgery*. New York, Grune & Stratton Inc, 1977.
36. Housepian EM: Management and results in 114 cases of optic glioma (abstract). *Neurosurgery* 1:67, 1977.
37. Housepian EM, Marquardt MD, Behrens M: Optic gliomas, in Wilkins RH, Rengachary SS (eds): *Neurosurgery*. New York, McGraw-Hill Inc, 1985.
38. Hoyt WF, Baghdassarian SA: Optic glioma of childhood: Natural history and rationale for conservative management. *Br J Ophthalmol* 53:793, 1969.
39. Jackson IMD: Thyrotropin- and gonadotropin-secreting pituitary adenomas, in Post KD, Jackson IMD, Reichlin S (eds): *The Pituitary Adenoma*. New York, Plenum Medical Book Co, 1980.
40. Jellinger K: Primary intracranial germ cell tumours. *Acta Neuropathol* 25:291, 1973.
41. Jenkin RDT, Simpson WJK, Keen CW: Pineal and suprasellar germinomas: Results of radiation treatment. *J Neurosurg* 48:99, 1978.
42. Kageyama N, Belsky R: Ectopic pinealoma in the chiasma region. *Neurology* 11:318, 1961.
43. Kammer H, George R: Cushing's disease in a patient with an ectopic pituitary adenoma. *JAMA* 246:2722, 1981.
44. Kistler M, Pribram HW: Metastatic disease of the sella turcica. *AJR* 123:13, 1975.
45. Kourides IA, Ridgway EC, Weintraub BD, et al: Thyrotropin-induced hyperthyroidism: Use of alpha and beta subunit levels to identify patients with pituitary tumors. *J Clin Endocrinol Metab* 45:534, 1977.
46. Kourides IA, Weintraub BD, Levko MA, et al: Alpha and beta subunits of human thyrotropin: Purification and development of specific radioimmunoassays. *Endocrinology* 94:1411, 1974.
47. Kourides IA, Weintraub BD, Re RN, et al: Thyroid hormone, oestrogen, and glucocorticoid effects on two different pituitary glycoprotein hormone alpha subunit pools. *Clin Endocrinol* 9:535, 1978.
48. Kourides IA, Weintraub BD, Ridgway EC, et al: Increase in the beta subunit of human TSH in hypothyroid serum after thyrotropin-releasing hormone. *J Clin Endocrinol Metab* 37:836, 1973.
49. Kourides IA, Weintraub BD, Ridgway EC, et al: Pituitary secretion of free alpha and beta subunit of human thyrotropin in patients with thyroid disorders. *J Clin Endocrinol Metab* 40:872, 1975.
50. Kourides IA, Weintraub BD, Rosen SW, et al:

Secretion of alpha subunit of glycoprotein hormones by pituitary adenomas. *J Clin Endocrinol Metab* 43:97, 1976.
51. Kovacs K: Metastatic cancer of the pituitary gland. *Oncology* 27:533, 1973.
52. Lloyd LA: Gliomas of the optic nerve and chiasm in childhood. *Trans Am Ophthalmol Soc* 71:488, 1973.
53. Luse SA, Kernohan JW: Granular-cell tumors of the stalk and posterior lobe of the pituitary gland. *Cancer* 8:616, 1955.
54. MacCarty CS, Boyd AS Jr, Childs DS Jr: Tumors of the optic nerve and optic chiasm. *J Neurosurg* 33:439, 1970.
55. MacFarlane IA, Beardwell CG, Shalet SM, et al: Glycoprotein hormone α-subunit secretion by pituitary adenomas: Influence of external irradiation. *Clin Endocrinol* 13:215, 1980.
56. Martin NA, Hales M, Wilson CB: Cerebellar metastasis from a prolactinoma during treatment with bromocriptine: Case report. *J Neurosurg* 55:615, 1981.
57. Martin P, Cushing H: Primary gliomas of the chiasm and optic nerves in their intracranial portion. *Arch Ophthalmol* 52:209, 1923.
58. McGrath P: Cysts of sellar and pharyngeal hypophyses. *Pathology* 3:123, 1971.
59. Melchionna RH, Moore RA: The pharyngeal pituitary gland. *Am J Pathol* 14:763, 1938.
60. Naiken VS, Tellem CBM, Meranze DR: Pituitary cyst of Rathke's cleft origin with hypopituitarism. *J Neurosurg* 18:703, 1961.
61. Ogilvy KM, Jakubowski J: Intracranial dissemination of pituitary adenomas. *J Neurol Neurosurg Psychiatry* 36:199, 1973.
62. Ogilvy KM, Jakubowski J, Shortland JR: Spinal subarachnoid spread of pituitary adenoma. *J Neurol Neurosurg Psychiatry* 37:1186, 1974.
63. Oi S, Ciric I, Mayer TK: Metastatic breast carcinoma in the pituitary gland. *No To Shinkei* 30:69, 1978.
64. Oxenhandler DC, Sayers MP: The dilemma of childhood optic gliomas. *J Neurosurg* 48:34, 1978.
65. Peterson RE, Kourides IA, Horwith M, et al: Luteinizing hormone-and α-subunit–secreting pituitary tumor: Positive feedback of estrogen. *J Clin Endocrinol Metab* 52:692, 1981.
66. Powell HC, Marshall LF, Ignelzi RJ: Post-irradiation pituitary sarcoma. *Acta Neuropathol* 39:165, 1977.
67. Ridgway EC, Klibanski A, Ladenson PW, et al: Pure alpha-secreting pituitary adenomas. *N Engl J Med* 304:1254, 1981.
68. Roessmann U, Kaufman B, Friede RL: Metastatic lesions in the sella turcica and pituitary gland. *Cancer* 25:478, 1970.
69. Rosen SW, Weintraub BD: Ectopic production of the isolated alpha subunit of the glycoprotein hormones: A quantitative marker in certain cases of cancer. *N Engl J Med* 290:1441, 1974.
70. Rothman LM, Sher J, Quencer RM, et al: Intracranial ectopic pituitary adenoma: Case report. *J Neurosurg* 44:96, 1976.
71. Rout D, Das L, Rao VRK, et al: Symptomatic Rathke's cleft cysts. *Surg Neurol* 19:42, 1983.
72. Rubinstein LJ: *Tumors of the Central Nervous System*. Second Series, Fascicle 6, Washington, D.C., Armed Forces Institute of Pathology, 1972.
73. Russell DS, Rubinstein LJ: *Pathology of Tumors of the Nervous System*. Baltimore, Williams & Wilkins, 1977.
74. Scheithauer BW: Surgical pathology of the pituitary and sellar region, in Laws ER, Randall RV, Kern EB et al (eds): Management of pituitary adenomas and related lesions with emphasis on transsphenoidal surgery. New York, Appleton-Century-Crofts, 1982.
75. Schwartz JF, Balentine JD: Recurrent meningitis due to an intracranial epidermoid. *Neurology* 28:124, 1978.
76. Shanklin WM: On the presence of cysts in the human pituitary. *Anat Rec* 104:379, 1949.
77. Shanklin WM: The incidence and distribution of cilia in the human pituitary with a description of micro-follicular cysts derived from Rathke's cleft. *Acta Anat* 11:361, 1951.
78. Shuangshoti S, Netsky MG, Nashold BS Jr: Epithelial cysts related to sella turcica: Proposed origin from neuroepithelium. *Arch Pathol* 90:444, 1970.
79. Smallridge RC, Wartofsky L, Dimond RC: Inappropriate secretion of thyrotropin: Discordance between the suppressive effects of corticosteroids and thyroid hormone. *J Clin Endocrinol Metab* 48:700, 1979.
80. Snyder PJ, Sterling FH: Hypersecretion of LH and FSH by a pituitary adenoma. *J Clin Endocrinol Metab* 42:544, 1976.
81. Steinberg GK, Koenig GH, Golden JB: Symptomatic Rathke's cleft cysts: Report of two cases. *J Neurosurg* 56:290, 1982.
82. Sternberg C: Ein choristom der neurohypophyse bei ausgebrecteten oedamen zbl sllg path. *Path Anat* 31:585, 1921.
83. Takeuchi J, Handa H, Nagata I: Suprasellar germinoma. *J Neurosurg* 49:41, 1978.
84. Tashjian AH Jr, Weintraub BD, Barowsky NJ, et al: Subunits of human chorionic gonadotropin: Unbalanced synthesis and secretion by clonal cell

strains derived from a bronchogenic carcinoma. *Proc Natl Acad Sci USA* 70:1419, 1973.
85. Taveras JM, Mount LA, Wood EH: The value of radiation therapy in the management of glioma of the optic nerves and chiasm. *Radiology* 66:518, 1956.
86. Teears RJ, Silverman EM: Clinicopathologic review of 88 cases of carcinoma metastatic to the pituitary gland. *Cancer* 36:216, 1975.
87. Tolis G, Bird C, Bertrand G, et al: Pituitary hyperthyroidism: case report and review of the literature. *Am J Med* 64:177, 1978.
88. Turner OA, Laird AT: Meningioma with traumatic etiology: Report of a case. *J Neurosurg* 24:96, 1966.
89. Vaitukaitis J, Robbins JB, Nieschlag E, et al: A method for producing specific antisera with small doses of immunogen. *J Clin Endocrinol Metab* 33:988, 1971.
90. Vaitukaitis JF, Ross GT, Reichert LE Jr, et al: Immunologic basis for within and between species cross-reactivity of luteinizing hormone. *Endocrinology* 91:1337, 1972.
91. Walsh JW: Suprasellar germinomas, in Wilkins RH, Rengachary SS (eds): *Neurosurgery*, New York, McGraw-Hill Inc, 1985.
92. Yoshida J, Kobayashi T, Kageyama N, et al: Symptomatic Rathke's cleft cyst: Morphological study with light and electron microscopy and tissue culture. *J Neurosurg* 47:451, 1977.
93. Zülch KJ: Some remarks on the spongioblastoma of the brain. *Acta Neurochir Suppl* 10:121, 1964.

CHAPTER 11

Craniopharyngioma

Embryogenesis
Pathology
Clinical features
   Visual pathways
   Pituitary stalk and/or gland
   Hypothalamus
   Increased ICP caused by obstructive hydrocephalus
Diagnostic evaluation
   Neuro-ophthalmologic evaluation
   Endocrinologic evaluation
   Neuroradiologic evaluation
Treatment and results
Surgical techniques
   Subfrontal and pterional approaches
   Surgical techniques
   Surgical goals
   Transsphenoidal approach
   Other approaches
   Shunting techniques
Results of surgery
   "Radical" approach
   "Conservative" approach
   Tumor-brain interface
Postoperative management
Irradiation therapy
   Primary irradiation
   Secondary irradiation
   Interstitial irradiation
   Recurrent craniopharyngioma
Summary

Craniopharyngiomas comprise approximately 2.5% of all brain tumors.[49] They appear to occur more frequently in the Japanese race and also in children with a reported incidence of 8% and 9% of all intracranial tumors, respectively.[55] These tumors exhibit a bimodal age incidence with one peak in the first decade of life and a second peak in the fifth to seventh decades.[44] Approximately 50% occur in subjects under 20 years of age. Males and females are affected equally. Craniopharyngiomas make up approximately 20% of sellar-chiasmal tumors of adults.[45,58] They are the most common nonglial tumors in children and comprise about one half of sellar-chiasmal tumors in this age group.[24,29,43]

Zenker[64] described a cystic suprasellar lesion containing both cholesterol crystals and squamous epithelium from an autopsy account in 1857. In 1932 Cushing[3] suggested the name "craniopharyngioma," since he believed it was most descriptive and indicated the origin of this tumor from the craniopharyngeal duct. Craniopharyngioma implies an origin from the pharynx rather than the primitive buccal cavity. Despite the criticism, the term *craniopharyngioma* became and remains generally accepted because of its widespread use.[14]

Lewis[36] performed the first successful transcranial resection of a craniopharyngioma in 1910. Cushing[15] was the first to operate on these tumors via the transsphenoidal route, but because of the relatively high mortality associated with this operation, he abandoned this approach in favor of the transcranial operation. Following the introduction of glucocorticosteroids to clinical medicine in the early 1950s, more aggressive surgical procedures were attempted.[23,62] In addition to the use of steroids, the introduction of the operating microscope and microtechniques has had a significant impact on the management of craniopharyngiomas.

Procedures used in the diagnostic evaluation of craniopharyngiomas include skull films, computed tomography (CT), and, in special situations, metrizamide cisternography and angiography. The management of craniopharyngiomas is a controversial issue. Therapeutic options range from radical surgery alone to irradiation with or without a surgical procedure. As this controversy is not readily resolved by the available literature, a perspective on therapeutic decision making is presented and options discussed.

EMBRYOGENESIS

The embryologic development of the pituitary gland (see Chapter 1) begins approximately on day 24 when a diverticulum (Rathke's pouch) arises from the stomodeum, the primitive buccal cavity, and grows toward the primitive brain.[34] As Rathke's pouch matures, its neck narrows and eventually is obliterated. By the fifth week, Rathke's pouch makes contact with the infundibulum, a ventral diverticulum of the diencephalon. The ectoderm of Rathke's pouch develops into the anterior lobe of the pituitary gland (adenohypophysis), and the neuroectoderm of the infundibulum evolves into the posterior lobe (neurohypophysis).

It is believed that craniopharyngiomas arise from squamous epithelial nests persisting after most of the cells of the embryonic invaginated stomodeum have differentiated into the adenohypophysis. Small clusters of these squamous epithelial cells, presumably persistent primitive cells, can be seen along the stalk and less commonly in the adenohypophysis of normal subjects. Interestingly, these squamous cell nests have been described primarily after the first decade[25] and have been noted with increasing frequency with each succeeding decade.[40] At postmortem examination, these epithelial nests are identified in one third to one fourth of adults[11,40] and 3% of newborns.[16] Thus on the basis of these observations, it could be argued that it is not necessary to postulate an embryonic origin for such cells, since they could appear later in life as a result of either cellular alteration or metaplasia from pituitary cells, which are also of ectodermal origin.[25]

The course of the stalk of Rathke's pouch is sometimes perpetuated by a canal in the sphenoid bone. The pharyngeal pituitary, which is a structure that may be found between the nasal septum and the pharyngeal tonsil, occurs along the course of the stalk of Rathke's pouch.[47]

PATHOLOGY

The gross and microscopic pathology of craniopharyngiomas is discussed fully in Chapter 3. Craniopharyngiomas are most commonly found in the suprasellar region but also appear as intrasellar masses or within the third ventricle. They vary considerably in size and may extend under the frontal or temporal lobes or rarely into the posterior fossa.

Grossly, craniopharyngiomas are often both solid and cystic and are said to have a rim of gliotic brain tissue around them. Sweet[60] believes that this rim of tissue, which he calls the "functionless glia," provides a margin of safety between the tumor and vital structures, thus allowing the surgeon the opportunity to achieve a radical removal.

As discussed in Chapter 3, Kahn[25] distinguishes between childhood and adult types of craniopharyngiomas. Whether these differing histologic patterns have clinical significance is uncertain.

CLINICAL FEATURES

Because of the usual location of craniopharyngiomas in the suprasellar region and their intimate relationship to several important anatomic structures, a great variety of clinical findings may be evident at the time of the patient's presentation. The clinical features can be divided into four major categories depending on which anatomic structures are primarily involved. These categories include (1) visual disturbances that result from involvement of the optic nerves, chiasm, or tract; (2) endocrine dysfunction resulting from compression of the pituitary gland, stalk, and/or the ventral basal hypothalamus; (3) increased intracranial pressure (ICP) from obstruction of the cerebrospinal fluid (CSF) pathways at the foramina of Monro or aqueduct of Sylvius; and (4) symptoms such as somnolence, autonomic seizures, and chronic hypernatremia that indicate intrinsic hypothalamic involvement.[52]

Psychiatric manifestations may also occur in association with craniopharyngiomas. The tumors which produce psychiatric abnormalities usually extend

Table 11-1

Clinical findings in craniopharyngiomas

	Incidence (%)	
Clinical findings	**Children**	**Adults**
Visual		
Decreased acuity	82	88-93
Visual field defects	60-80	90-95
Bitemporal hemianopia	24-52	50-60
Homonymous hemianopsia	1.5-8.3	6-28
Papilledema	27-53	12-17
Optic atrophy	55	37-43
Cranial nerve palsies	25	33
Endocrine		
Diabetes insipidus	9-13	16
Hypopituitarism	9	7
Retarded bone age	42-67	—
Adiposity	5	15
Psychiatric disturbances		
Mental deterioration	6	18-26
Korsakoff's syndrome	—	25

posteriorly toward the brainstem and hippocampus.[5,24] Adults have a higher incidence of psychiatric symptoms than children. The psychiatric manifestations are varied and include, among others, dementia, apathy, depression, memory disturbances, and hypersomnia.[3] Korsakoff's syndrome has been reported to occur in as many as 25% of adults.[25] In Banna's series[4] of 84 adults with craniopharyngiomas, mental symptoms occurred in 22 patients (26%), and in 10 of these patients, these symptoms were the initial manifestations of the lesion. In a retrospective study, Bartlett[6] found that the presence of mental symptoms suggested an ominous prognosis. Table 11-1 outlines the incidence of various clinical findings for both adults and children.[4,5,21,22,25,46,58] The duration of symptoms before diagnosis is quite variable and may have some relationship to prognosis. Bartlett[6] believes that patients coming to medical attention with symptoms of more than 2 years' duration have a longer survival after treatment than those with symptoms present for less than this period of time.

Although the duration of symptoms may be present for approximately the same amount of time, the clinical presentations differ somewhat between adults and children. For instance, very young children with craniopharyngiomas initially have signs of hydrocephalus (increasing head circumference and/or increased ICP); older children may manifest prominent endocrinopathies with failure to thrive, abnormal water metabolism, and/or short stature[44]; and teenage children and adults may primarily experience visual disturbances.[4,5,44]

The most common initial symptoms in all patients are headache and visual impairment. At the time of diagnosis, 75% to 95% of patients complain of headaches, 67% have visual disturbances and 30% to 38% suffer from vomiting.[3] In the following sections, the clinical features will be considered in detail according to the anatomic structure(s) involved.

Visual pathways

Visual symptomatology associated with craniopharyngiomas is variable, depending on the exact location and compressive effect of the tumor. In children, progressive visual loss may go unnoticed until a parent or teacher observes a change in behavior attributable to partial blindness. Visual field defects are seen in 90% to 95% of adults and 60% to 80% of children[21,54,63] and most commonly consist of a bitemporal hemianopsia. Because of the tendency to compress the posterior and superior aspects of the optic chiasm, the inferior temporal quadrants are more likely to be involved than the superior quadrants, which is just the opposite from that caused by pituitary adenomas where the greater loss of vision is in the superior temporal quadrants. Extension of tumor posteriorly with damage to the optic tracts can result in an incongruous homonymous hemianopsia. Occasionally, a junctional scotoma or combination of unilateral visual loss with a contralateral superior temporal quadrantanopsia (see Chapter 4) may be seen. This visual defect anatomically indicates the lesion is situated at the junction of the optic nerve and chiasm. Craniopharyngioma is one of the more common causes of a junctional scotoma.

Papilledema and optic atrophy are seen more commonly in children, a fact probably related to failure of children to complain about visual symptoms until the latter are well advanced. Cranial nerve palsies are seen in 25% of children and 33% of adults.[3,56] Although the parasellar cranial nerves are most commonly affected, involvement of the seventh and eighth cranial nerves has also been reported.[1,39]

Pituitary stalk and/or gland

Pituitary endocrine involvement is manifested by diabetes insipidus and/or varying degrees of hypopituitarism. As would be expected, purely intrasellar craniopharyngiomas produce a more severe degree of panhypopituitarism than primarily suprasellar lesions. The incidence of endocrine dysfunction reported among the various series bears a strong correlation with the extensiveness and sophistication of the endocrine evaluation. Approximately 70% of all patients are discovered to have some endocrine abnormality with a higher incidence of dysfunction occurring in children.[5,24,58] In most patients, pituitary-gonadal axis involvement is reflected by a gonadotropin deficiency. About 65% of patients have decreased growth hormone; 45%, decreased adrenocorticotropic hormone (ACTH); and 15%, impaired function of the pituitary-thyroid axis.[63] Growth is impaired in about 25% of children,[24,43,63] yet retarded bone age is found in as many as 62% of this group. Diabetes insipidus is slightly more common in adults, whereas panhypopituitarism is slightly more common in children.

Pituitary endocrine deficiency, particularly in the pituitary-adrenal axis, was one of the major causes of poor surgical results before the early 1950s. Thus the introduction of cortisone had a major and favorable impact in the management and ultimate outcome of these patients. In fact, total resection of craniopharyngiomas with anticipated good postoperative results became a realistic surgical goal only after the routine use of cortisone as a perioperative adjunct.

Hypothalamus

Hypothalamic involvement, usually manifested by somnolence and polyuria[21] occurs in each age group but is probably more common in children. Dysfunction tends to occur with tumors that extend superiorly and posteriorly. Disturbances of hypothalamic function such as diabetes insipidus, autonomic seizures, and chronic hypernatremia are rarely seen as presenting problems in patients with a craniopharyngioma and are more likely to be associated with infiltrative tumors (e.g., glioma) or postoperative lesions (trauma) of the hypothalamus.[42] Symptoms such as drowsiness in the absence of increased ICP and persistently subnormal temperature may result from a craniopharyngioma, but such symptoms are rare.[42] Manifestations of pituitary endocrine deficiency may also be caused by involvement of hypothalamic nuclei.

Increased ICP caused by obstructive hydrocephalus

Clinical findings that reflect obstructive hydrocephalus include headache, nausea, vomiting, and lethargy. These findings are not peculiar to craniopharyngiomas but can occur with any lesion that obstructs intracranial CSF pathways. Craniopharyngiomas usually cause hydrocephalus by blocking the third ventricle. ICP elevations with paralysis of the sixth cranial nerve and papilledema occur with craniopharyngiomas more commonly than with other parasellar lesions.

DIAGNOSTIC EVALUATION
Neuro-ophthalmologic evaluation

Because of the relatively high incidence of visual manifestations associated with craniopharyngiomas, it is important to perform a thorough neuro-ophthalmologic assessment in addition to neurologic and physical examinations in these patients. Although this may not be possible in some patients as a result of age, lack of cooperation, or a rapidly deteriorating condition, an effort should nevertheless be made to obtain this data. A neuro-ophthalmologic examination (see Chapter 4) will provide not only an indication of the extent of involvement of the visual pathways, but when obtained before treatment, will serve as yet another baseline to evaluate the effect of treatment on these relatively sensitive visual anatomic structures.

Endocrinologic evaluation

The primary goal of endocrinologic testing is to determine whether or not there is any evidence of hypothalamic and/or pituitary endocrine deficiency. From an endocrine standpoint, craniopharyngiomas are nonfunctional tumors. Thus abnormally high levels of growth hormone and ACTH do not occur. However, the level of serum prolactin may be elevated because of impingement of the tumor on the hypothalamus and/or pituitary stalk, thus impairing the delivery of prolactin-inhibiting factor (PIF).[41] When elevated by this mechanism, the level of serum prolactin rarely exceeds 150 ng/ml.

An adequate assessment of pituitary endocrine function can be obtained by determining endocrine data that measure pituitary–target organ axes. These tests are described in Chapter 4. Subnormal values in any of the axes imply a deficiency in pituitary endocrine function, which in turn indicates involvement of the hypothalamus, pituitary stalk, pituitary gland, or a combination of these structures. The evaluation of posterior lobe function is also described in Chapter 4.

Neuroradiologic evaluation

The neuroradiologic evaluation of craniopharyngiomas is outlined in Chapter 5. Valuable and recommended studies in these patients include plain skull x-ray films (Fig. 11-1) and high-resolution CT (Fig. 11-2).

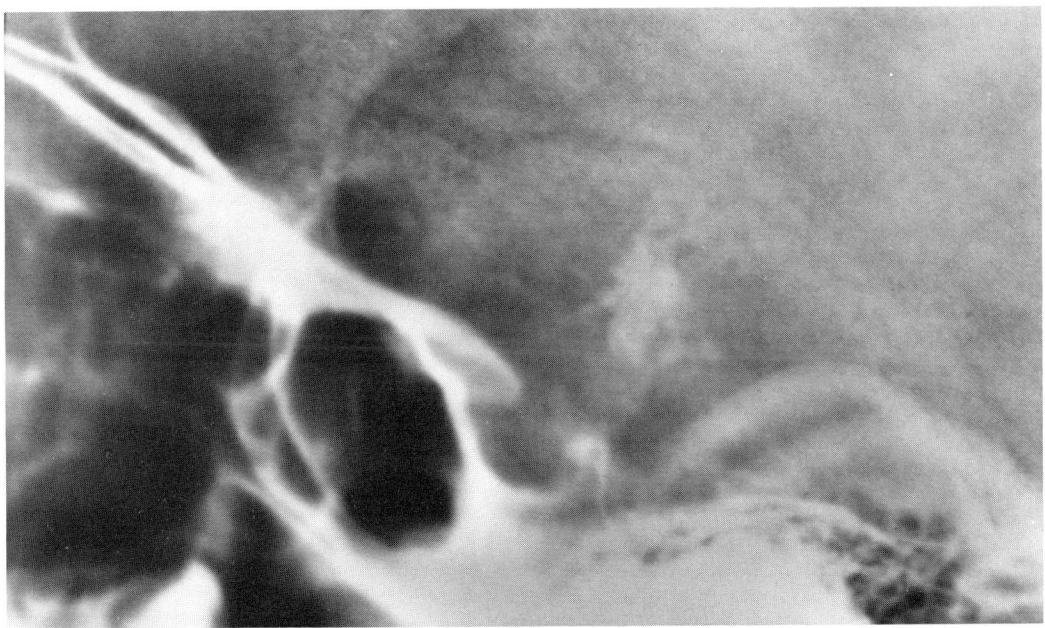

Fig. 11-1. Lateral skull x-ray film showing suprasellar calcification in craniopharyngioma. Sella is normal.

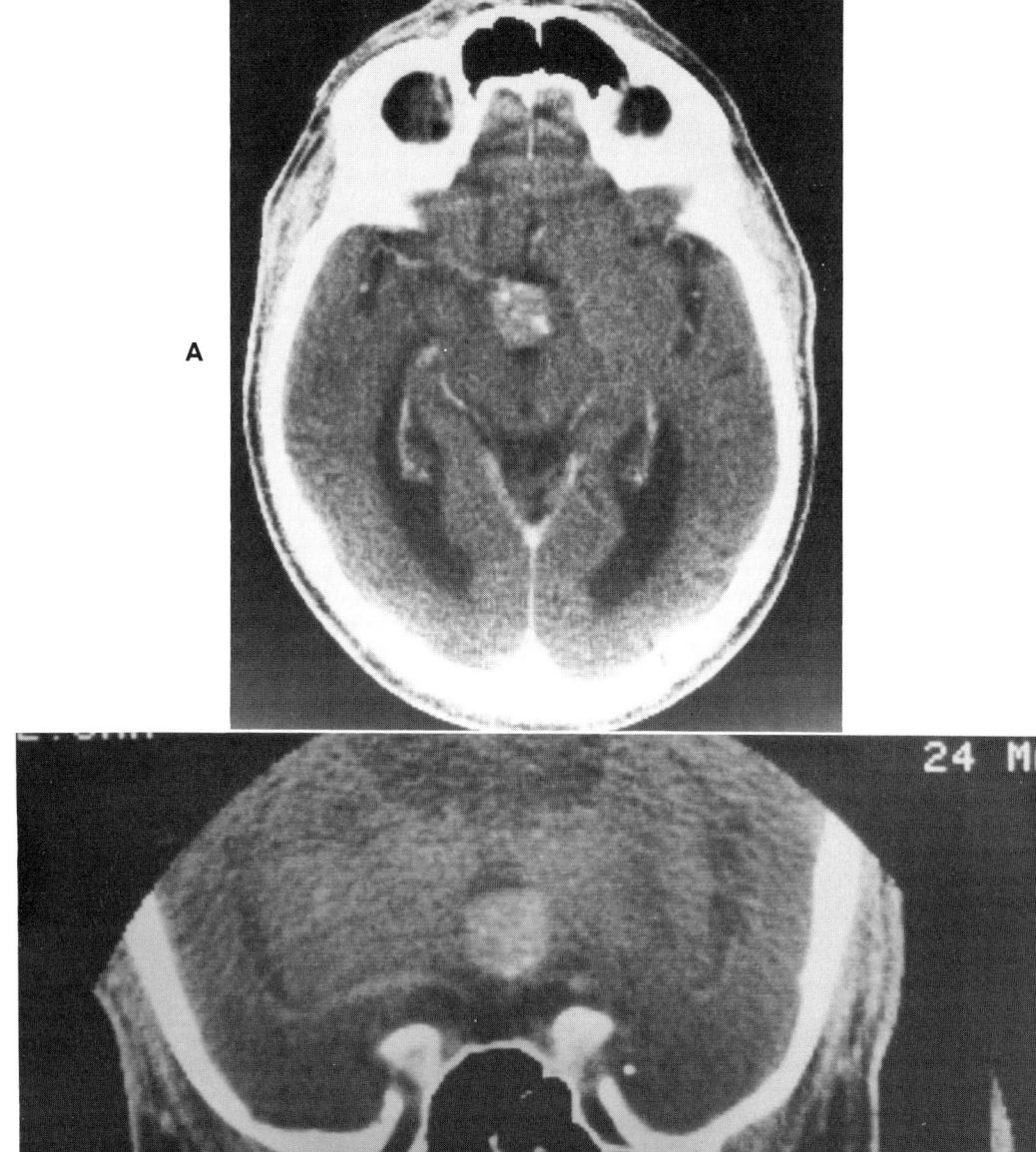

Fig. 11-2. Axial (**A**) and coronal (**B**) CT scans showing suprasellar craniopharyngioma.

Additionally, CT scans are valuable postoperatively in determining the extent of tumor removal. In patients who are doing well postoperatively, it is our opinion that a routine postoperative scan to determine whether residual tumor remains should be delayed at least 3 months after surgery to avoid artifactual changes related to the surgical procedure such as minor degrees of bleeding in the vicinity of the tumor, enhancement of the tumor capsule, and edema. Most, if not all, of these changes should have cleared by a period of 3 months, and a true assessment of any residual tumor can then be made by the scan. The CT scan is the most valuable means for long-term follow-up of patients following surgery in terms of detecting recurrent tumor and/or cysts.

In special circumstances, positive contrast cisternography and cerebral angiography will add further information. Metrizamide cisternography is reserved for those cases in which a high-resolution CT scan does not clearly define the extent and relationship of the lesion to the optic chiasm. We rarely use angiography in the diagnostic workup of patients with suspected craniopharyngiomas. This procedure is occasionally useful if there is doubt about the pathologic nature of the lesion from the plain skull films and CT or if determination of the degree of vascularity is believed to be important.

TREATMENT AND RESULTS

Comparison of the various treatment modalities available for a patient with craniopharyngioma is difficult for several reasons. First, there is considerable variability in the natural history of craniopharyngiomas. For instance, cases have been reported in which close observation over a period of many years failed to show progression of disease despite the fact that the patient had no definitive treatment.[6,54] Admittedly, the latter situation is relatively uncommon. Secondly, one must consider the relative rarity of the disease. Kjellberg[27] has presented figures indicating that if the number of patients seen clinically with a craniopharyngioma were equally divided among the practicing neurosurgeons in the United States, each neurosurgeon would see about one case every 10 years. Although the incidence is higher at certain medical institutions, these centers usually average about five cases per year.[27] Because of the relative scarcity of cases, it is difficult for any given neurosurgical center to complete a statistically sound prospective trial of the merits of different treatments. Thus evaluation of therapies is dependent on retrospective comparisons of results of different methods of treatment from different centers. Lastly, there is considerable variation among cases not only in natural history but in age of presentation, clinical findings, and size, type (i.e., predominantly solid or cystic), and location of the tumor.

Surgical results depend on numerous factors including the experience and expertise of the surgeon; the size, location, and consistency (i.e., solid versus cystic) of the tumor; whether the operating microscope was used; and the surgical approach. When comparing results of radical excision with other modalities, it is important to determine if the radical excision was the first definitive procedure or if it followed previous surgery or radiation therapy.

Notwithstanding the rare case that seems to show no progression over a period of several years, it is our opinion that some type of definitive treatment is indicated in patients with craniopharyngiomas. The only exceptions may be an elderly patient with a slow-growing tumor producing relatively little disability or a patient with an associated but unrelated serious, unstable medical condition. The only effective therapeutic options are surgery and irradiation. As a general rule, most experienced physicians consider surgery as the choice for primary therapy and irradiation as adjunctive therapy. Nevertheless, there are authoritative physicians who would take exception to this statement and consider irradiation as a primary treatment modality; however, they represent a minority viewpoint.

SURGICAL TECHNIQUES

Before 1952, which was the year that cortisone became available for clinical use, the surgical management of craniopharyngiomas, whether radical or conservative, could best be described as hazardous. As an example, in 1949 Gordy, Peet, and Kahn[17] reported a series of 51 cases with an operative mortality of 41% principally as a result of hypothalamic-pituitary trauma incident to surgical manipulation. This manipulation was believed to cause further impairment of the normal pituitary adrenocortical responses to stress. The major complications of surgical importance included disturbances of vasomotor control, temperature regulation, salt and water metabolism, and carbohydrate metabolism. The availability of adrenal substitution therapy in the form of cortisone or ACTH offered a means of preventing and controlling many of these complications, particularly in patients with preoperative impairment of the pituitary-adrenal axis.

Today, surgery is an appropriate option in patients with craniopharyngiomas. The surgeon should approach the lesion with the attitude that a gross total removal using microtechniques should be attempted. Although immediate mortality and morbidity may be higher with "radical" surgery, the long-term result is unquestionably better than in cases with only partial resection. Furthermore, the operating microscope should be used in removing the tumor, and the surgeon should be skilled in microtechniques.

Subfrontal and pterional approaches

The surgical approach for excision of a craniopharyngioma is influenced by the exact location of the lesion. The majority of these tumors are approached via either a subfrontal or pterional (frontotemporal) approach.[22,50,59,61] These exposure techniques are described in Chapter 12.

Although many neurosurgeons advocate attacking these tumors from the nondominant hemisphere, Sweet[60] recommends using the side of maximal visual impairment, which is the side where the larger mass of tumor nearly always lies. Retraction of the frontal lobe may be facilitated by the use of mannitol, furosemide, hyperventilation, and lumbar puncture drainage of CSF.

Surgical techniques

Technical principles that should be strictly followed if the goal is to achieve gross total removal ("radical" approach) include adequate exposure; gentle tissue handling; establishing tissue planes; emptying the central portion of the tumor to reduce its bulk, followed by meticulous dissection of the capsule; and slowly bringing the capsule into the operative field without undue tugging.

The most delicate part of the dissection is freeing the optic nerves, chiasm, inferior hypothalamus, and the carotid arteries from the tumor. Here, the use of the operating microscope, self-retaining retractors, bipolar coagulation, and the laser aid significantly in achieving tumor removal. The tumor will usually be visualized beneath the optic nerves and chiasm, and the initial attack is made on the part of tumor that is most accessible. Drainage of cystic portions of tumor usually improves the exposure. From this point on, the surgeon performs slow meticulous piecemeal removal of the tumor with the goal of removing as much of the lesion as possible with minimal traction on the tumor. The use of wire-loop cautery with the cautery set on the cutting mode is not safe in this situation because of the depth of the lesion and the close relationship to many important anatomic structures. Some neurosurgeons may find the ultrasonic aspirator (Cavitron) to be helpful; however, it has been our experience that because of the limited exposure and the relative depth of the lesion, the instrument is too large and cumbersome to be of much value in tumor removal.

Steady, meticulous piecemeal cauterization of the tumor with bipolar microforceps followed by removal of the cauterized tissue with either suction or microscissors is a safe and effective method of removal. Surgeons experienced with the surgical laser will find it a valuable method of tumor removal. When using the laser in this location, extreme caution must be exercised in order to protect normal structures such as the optic nerve from irreversible damage by the laser beam.

Surgical goals

Although the neurosurgeon, in our opinion, should work with the objective of achieving a gross total removal of the tumor, this goal should be tempered with realism. Tumors that extend beyond the surgeon's vision and cannot be delivered with very gentle traction usually cannot be totally removed without putting the patient at great risk from the standpoint of visual loss, hypothalamic injury, or damage to a major vessel or cranial nerve. For instance, if a piece of capsule beneath and behind the chiasm extends out of the field of vision and is firmly attached to some nonvisualized structure, the surgeon should not blindly try to pull it free if there is any significant degree of resistance. It is our opinion that in this situation, the surgeon should be content with performing as much of a partial resection as can safely be done. It has been our experience over the years that more often than not, *gross total resection* of a craniopharyngioma (at least in adults) *is not possible*. Furthermore, it appears that gross total removal in general appears more achievable in children than in adults.

The majority of craniopharyngiomas are resected via either a subfrontal or "generous" pterional approach. Alternative approaches are available depending on the tumor's location. Craniopharyngiomas may extend posterior to the chiasm in a location that cannot easily be seen from the subfrontal approach. In these cases, a subtemporal approach may give access to the lesion. Also, lesions posterior to the chiasm may still be approached subfrontally but may require opening of the lamina terminalis before the tumor mass can be resected.[42]

Transsphenoidal approach

Transsphenoidal surgery has limited applicability in these cases because of the predominantly suprasellar location of the majority of these tumors. As emphasized recently by Laws,[35] enlargement of the sella by the tumor is the critical feature allowing for successful transsphenoidal management (Figs. 11-3 and 11-4). His publication contains several important technical points regarding this

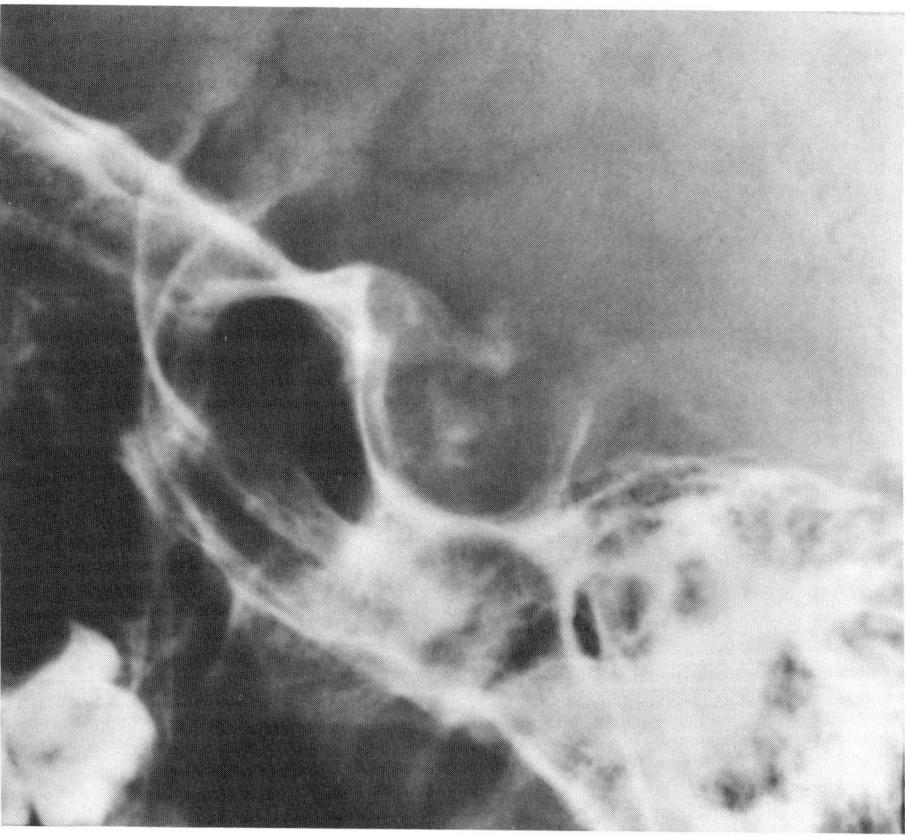

Fig. 11-3. Lateral skull x-ray film showing calcification in intrasellar craniopharyngioma. Sella is enlarged and dorsum sella is thinned.

operative approach in cases of craniopharyngiomas that have significant intrasellar extension. Hardy[20] has also addressed the issue of transsphenoidal surgery in craniopharyngiomas and believes that these lesions can be approached in this fashion even if there is a suprasellar extension, provided the sella is abnormally enlarged. Most neurosurgeons, however, believe that this approach should be reserved for tumors that are exclusively intrasellar because of the relatively poor exposure to vital suprasellar structures that is provided by transsphenoidal surgery.

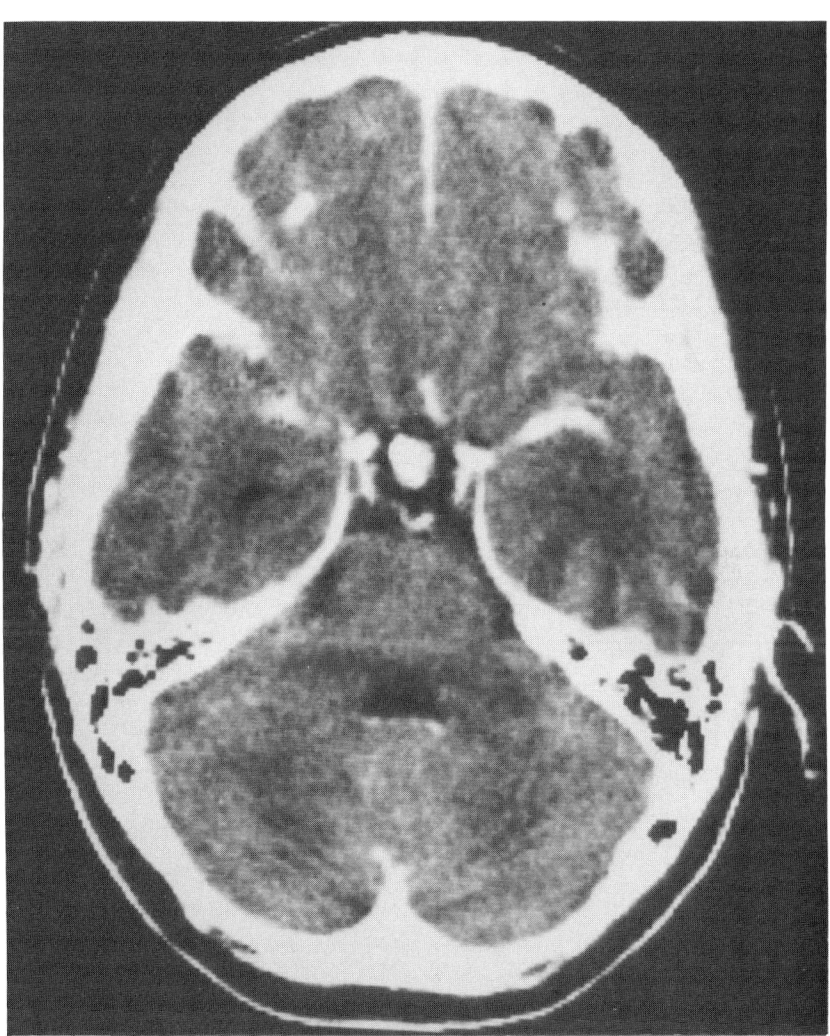

Fig. 11-4. Axial view CT scan showing intrasellar craniopharyngioma.

Other approaches

Craniopharyngiomas situated within the third ventricle can be approached via the dilated lateral ventricle or through the corpus callosum.[60] It should be pointed out, however, that both the transcallosal and transventricular approaches have the highest morbidity and mortality of all surgical approaches to this tumor in this location. For instance, all five of Northfield's patients in whom the transventricular approach was performed died.[48] The mortality is also high with this approach when only biopsies are attempted.[48] In another series in which four patients were operated via the transcallosal or transventricular approach, three died in the first postoperative week.[38] In view of the aforementioned, it is our opinion that either the transcallosal or transventricular approach should be considered only in very unusual circumstances.

Shunting techniques

Ventricular shunting is recommended in patients with significant degrees of hydrocephalus. If the hydrocephalus is caused by a tumor in the third ventricle obstructing the outlet of the lateral ventricles, bilateral lateral ventricular shunts should be placed and joined up with a "Y" or "T" connector to the valve. Shunting can be directed into the peritoneum or right auricle depending on the preference of the surgeon. Ventricular-pleural shunts have been advocated by some neurosurgeons, but there appears to be a greater number of complications with shunts placed in the pleural cavity.

If hydrocephalus is present and there is no obstructive lesion in the third ventricle, it is likely that the hydrocephalus is on an absorptive basis presumably resulting from previous leakage of tumor cyst contents into the subarachnoid space. In these cases, single lateral ventricular catheter placement (usually the right side) will be adequate for shunting.

The decision to perform a shunting procedure in patients with hydrocephalus is made on the basis of the clinical findings and the CT scan. It is imperative that the neurosurgeon ensure that the skin incision(s) used for ventricular shunt placement and the course of the tubing do not interfere with nor jeopardize the incision to be used for any subsequent definitive operation on the craniopharyngioma.

In grossly cystic craniopharyngiomas such as that illustrated in Fig. 11-5 in which complete resection is impossible, Gutin[18] has advocated placing a ventricular catheter into the cystic cavity and connecting it to a subcutaneous reservoir for aspiration as needed. A variation of this procedure was proposed by Symon,[61] who advocated placement of a Silastic catheter into the cavity.[61] The catheter is attached to a Rickham reservoir, which lies in the temporalis muscle, and is aspirated as needed.

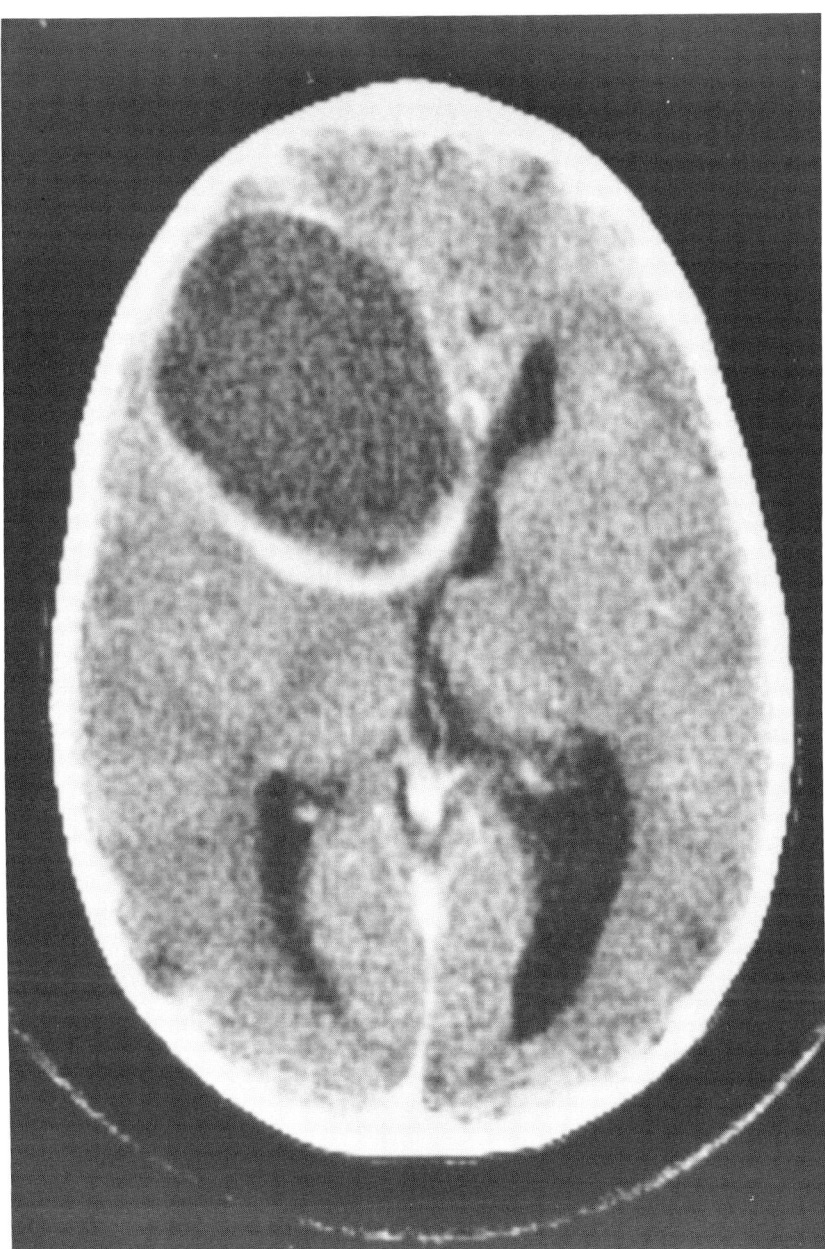

Fig. 11-5. Axial view CT scan showing huge cystic craniopharyngioma occupying virtually all of one frontal lobe.

RESULTS OF SURGERY

Over the past several years, a number of series have reported the results of surgery for craniopharyngiomas. In general, most series are relatively small and often are mixed between children and adults. As in virtually any neurosurgical procedure, series of craniopharyngiomas reported many years ago, particularly before the era of microneurosurgery, were associated with a higher mortality and morbidity than currently prevails. Also, in craniopharyngioma surgery, the significant and favorable impact that cortisone replacement made in the early 1950s has already been mentioned. Currently, many neurosurgeons advocate an aggressive, so-called radical operation, whereas others practice a more conservative approach in the surgery of these lesions.

In the "radical" procedure, the surgeon's goal is to achieve a gross total removal of the tumor; whereas in the "conservative" approach, the aim is to surgically remove enough of the lesion to provide symptomatic relief but not to attempt gross total removal. In general, surgeons who advocate the radical approach are of the opinion that a surgical plane exists between the tumor and surrounding nervous structures and that with persistent, gentle microsurgical techniques, the tumor can usually be totally excised.

"Radical" approach

Series that typify the "radical" approach include among others that of Matson[43] (and the subsequent follow-up of his series by Katz[26]), Sweet,[59,60] Symon,[61] Hoffman et al,[22] and Patterson and Danylevich.[50] The surgical approach in these series was either subfrontal or temporal, usually subfrontal. Also a comment will be made (see p. 337) on the results of the transsphenoidal approach to these lesions with a view toward total excision. Because of the many variables among reported cases, along with anecdotal reports, we found it virtually impossible to summarize all of the reported material into a single meaningful table.

Matson and Criger[43] in 1969 reported the relatively early results of radical surgery in 50 children. Of this number, 33 were alive and relatively well at the time of his report. His operative mortality was 10%. In 1975 Katz[26] re-evaluated the late results of Matson's radical removals in 34 children, 33 (66%) of whom were then living and well. A total of nine recurrences had developed in the survivors, and the mortality for reoperation in these cases was 25%. Kahn et al[25] had a 17% mortality in their adult patients, with overall favorable results in 23 of 40 (58%) long-term survivors. In 1977 Hoffman et al[22] reviewed 48 pediatric cases. A gross total tumor removal was accomplished in 17 cases, and the operative mortality was 6% (three deaths). Significantly, 34 patients were living and well at the time of their report.

Patterson and Danylevich[50] achieved total excision in nine of 11 patients in whom this was attempted. They used a subfrontal craniotomy approach and removed the tumor through the lamina terminalis and sphenoid sinus. After tumor exposure and opening of the sphenoid sinus from above, the tumor was removed by pushing pieces down and away from the chiasm and hypothalamus toward the sphenoid sinus, from which the pieces of tumor were extracted. In their report, the individual case history of each of the 11 patients is presented. Postoperative follow-up CT scans showed no tumor in seven and residual tumor in two cases. In two cases, follow-up scan results are not provided.

Sweet[59] reports 40 cases of radical removal with three deaths (7.5%). In 32 of 43 cases, the radical operation was the first craniotomy. The recurrence rate is not entirely clear from this report, although the author lists in a table that 80% of patients are "alive for stated interval," which in his table is greater than 10 years. In the text, the author states that "no patient who has lived more than 10 years has as yet had a recurrence."

Laws[35] reported his experiences with transsphenoidal surgery for craniopharyngiomas in 26 patients whose ages ranged from 13 to 66 years. Previous treatment with craniotomy significantly affected the results. In 14 of the 26 cases, the patients had no prior definitive treatment, and in this group, Laws was able to accomplish a "nearly complete removal" in all but one patient. On the other hand, in 12 patients who had a previous craniotomy, radical transsphenoidal tumor removal was achieved in only one case. He had one death and two serious complications (CSF leak).

Hardy and Vezina[19,20] and Lichter et al[37] have also discussed the surgical treatment of craniopharyngiomas via the transsphenoidal approach.

Recurrences after gross total removal have been observed in virtually all major series in which the patients have been followed for 5 or more years. Although recurrence after total removal usually occurs within 3 years after treatment,[56] Bartlett[6] reported three clinical recurrences at 15, 20, and 21 years. The recurrences may be attributed to microscopic remnants of tumor, most likely "pegs" left embedded in gliotic hypothalamic tissue. However, recurrence may result from extensions of tumor not visualized and thus not excised at the initial operation.

"Conservative" approach

The "conservatives" believe that every scrap of tumor cannot realistically be removed and that to attempt to do so involves considerable risk to the hypothalamus, optic apparatus, and neighboring major blood vessels. Often the conservative surgical approach is combined with the routine use of irradiation beginning shortly after surgery.

McKissock and Ford[46] reported a total of 100 operated cases of craniopharyngiomas of which 55 had a radical procedure and 45, conservative surgery. In the 55 with radical surgery, there was a 30% mortality. Forty-five were treated by minor surgical procedures (such as burr hole aspiration of the cyst or aspiration at craniotomy with or without shunt [Torkildsen]) followed by irradiation. On follow-up of 55 radical treatments, only 12 remained alive, well, and working at periods of 1 to over 10 years. Of 45 with conservative treatment, 33 (73%) were alive, well, and working at periods of 1 to over 10 years.

Hoff and Patterson[21] reviewed a mixed series of children and adults. Of 19 patients treated by craniotomy and radiation therapy and followed 10 or more years, 12 (63%) had evidence of recurrence and four patients with "total" removal were living and well more than 10 years after surgery. Nevertheless, the tumor recurred in 72% of patients within 5 years in those patients treated with partial removal and no postoperative irradiation. In a later publication from the same institution, Patterson and Danylevich[50] offered the opinion that the results just cited were unsatisfactory and stimulated the authors to attempt more aggressive surgery in craniopharyngiomas.

In general, and as might be expected, those series advocating a more aggressive surgical approach with a goal of achieving gross total removal have a significantly better chance of long-term cure but, in some instances, a higher immediate morbidity and mortality than series reporting a more conservative approach. Although higher for radical than for conservative surgery, the operative mortality for radical surgery in experienced hands is less than 8%.[10,22,26,56]

Tumor-brain interface

The issue of the "plane" between the tumor and surrounding brain structures, especially the hypothalamus, has been the subject of some discussion, and the issue would remain a largely academic one were it not for the fact that the existence of this plane is felt to be such by some authorities that it serves as the basis for their recommendation that a radical gross total removal be attempted in the majority of cases involving craniopharyngiomas. Landolt[33] studied biopsies of five craniopharyngiomas with electron microscopy and in three cases found extensive glial tissue on that aspect of the retrochiasmatic portion of the tumor in contact with the brain. In general, he found that the basal membranes of the epithelial tumor cells were separated from the basal membranes of the glia by a few collagen fibers. Sweet[60], who is a strong advocate of using the intervening plane to effect total tumor removal, believes that this observation of Landolt may possibly be the plane of cleavage that helps the surgeon remove neoplastic cells from the glia. On the other side of the argument, the presence of the layer of gliosis surrounding and penetrating the tumor may be a feature that precludes total removal of that portion of tumor adjacent to brain.[51,57]

Sweet[60] actually regards this "functionless glial layer" as providing a significant margin of safety between the growing epithelial cells to be excised and the vitally important thalamohypothalamic and visual structures, which should be preserved intact. Others, however, believe that "islands of tumor cells" remaining within functioning thalamus and hypothalamus following surgery account for recurrences.[28]

POSTOPERATIVE MANAGEMENT

In the postoperative management, it is important to determine whether all tumor was actually removed in those cases in which the surgeon thought that a gross total removal was accomplished. It is equally important in those cases in which a partial resection was performed to determine the amount and extent of persistent tumor. This information is best obtained with a high-resolution CT scan, and unless clinically indicated earlier, we recommend obtaining a CT scan

3 to 4 months after surgery. By this time, most if not all of the early postoperative changes related to minor bleeding and edema will have disappeared and a more accurate baseline postoperative CT scan can be obtained.

If the postoperative CT scan shows no tumor, the patient is followed at regular intervals with careful monitoring of clinical findings. In these cases, unless there is the development of new clinical findings, a CT scan can be performed at 12- to 18-month intervals.

If the 3-month postoperative CT scan shows persistent tumor but the patient is clinically stable, it is our recommendation that no further therapy for the tumor be initiated at this time. However, if the patient develops progressive clinical findings related to the lesion and/or serial CT scans show progressive enlargement of a solid as opposed to cystic tumor, a full course of conventional x-ray treatment to the tumor should be administered.

Special situations may arise, and these should be addressed. If the tumor recurs, but is largely cystic, the surgeon has the option of stereotaxic aspiration followed by the instillation of a radioactive substance. Obviously, this should be done by a surgeon familiar with either classic stereotaxic or CT-directed techniques and who is experienced with the use and handling of isotopes. This method of therapy is further discussed in Chapter 13.

IRRADIATION THERAPY

The use of irradiation as a treatment for craniopharyngioma was first described by Carpenter et al[12] in 1937. Since then there have been steady improvements and refinements in this treatment modality.

For purposes of this discussion we will divide irradiation therapy into two categories—primary, or definitive, and secondary, or adjunctive. Primary, or definitive, radiotherapy is that administered as the main treatment modality to a patient with a craniopharyngioma and includes those patients treated in this fashion either with no biopsy or in those in whom the only surgery was to establish a tissue diagnosis. Secondary, or adjunctive, radiotherapy is that delivered to patients in whom surgery was used as the primary treatment modality but in whom only a partial resection was accomplished or in whom a symptomatic recurrence has developed. There is considerably more experience with adjunctive as opposed to definitive radiotherapy.

Primary irradiation

The two major advocates of this method of treatment are Kramer and Bloom, who recommend "radical" radiotherapy following establishment of a positive tissue diagnosis by "conservative" surgery.

Kramer[30,31,32] reported his experience with radiotherapy in 43 patients over a 20-year period. Of the total, 30 patients were alive from 1 to 20 years after treatment, and 13 were dead—five because of unrelated disease; two, recurrent disease; three, from the radiation (possibly); and three, postoperative. Eighteen of the 43 cases were children, and of the 18, 16 had survived and were either in school or leading normal adult lives without major deficits. Kramer concludes that adequate irradiation can arrest the growth of craniopharyngiomas and, if applied properly, carries a minimal risk for the patient. He also believes that recurrence is common even after total surgical excision and for this reason recommends that irradiation should always form part of the management of these patients.

Bloom[7,8,9] gives survival figures following radiation of his new cases (i.e., those treated before recurrence following previous surgery). Seventy-four percent of 46 children and 60% of 66 adults are listed as surviving 10 years following irradiation treatment.

Secondary irradiation

Richmond et al[53] reported a retrospective study of 32 children treated for craniopharyngiomas using a variety of treatment modalities. Among the group, there were 13 patients treated with subtotal resection and eight patients with only biopsy or cyst aspiration who were treated with irradiation. The outcome in this group was compared with that in 12 patients having an estimated total (eight cases) or subtotal (four cases) resection but with no postoperative irradiation. The authors found that the group receiving radiation therapy after known subtotal resection did as well as the group with estimated total removal. Furthermore, the authors obtained an excellent response in the eight patients with "conservative" surgery followed by irradiation, a finding that the authors believe provides further evidence of the efficacy of adjunctive radiotherapy.

Cabezudo et al[10] conducted a retrospective study in 45 patients with craniopharyngiomas treated by three different therapeutic approaches—total excision, subtotal excision, and surgery followed by a course of irradiation. Of the patients having total excision, 30% experienced recurrence after a mean time of 2 years as opposed to 71% of those treated by subtotal excision (mean time, 2.6 years). Significantly, of patients receiving irradiation in addition to surgery, only 6% had recurrence after a mean time of 1 year. Although one could criticize the conclusions because of the relatively short follow-up intervals, their results speak in favor of the beneficial effects of adjunctive irradiation. The operative mortality for the entire series was 8.8%.

The recurrence rate of 71% after subtotal excision obtained by Cabezudo is similar to that reported by others reporting subtotal excision without adjunctive radiotherapy.[2,21,22]

Of particular interest in regard to the neurologic and psychophysiologic sequelae in patients treated by different modalities was the recent report by Cavazzuti et al.[13] They compared a group (group 1) of patients treated with radiation alone or by radiation plus conservative surgical procedures (e.g., biopsy, cyst aspiration, shunting) with a group (group 2) in whom radical tumor resection was attempted by craniotomy (subfrontal approach). They had 18 patients in group 1 and 17 in group 2. On the basis of extensive neuropsychophysiologic testing, the authors conclude that patients in group 1 showed less frontal lobe dysfunction than patients in group 2. None of group 1 patients died during the follow-up study period, whereas 11% of those treated by radical surgery died within 1 year of their surgery. Thus, in a small series, the report makes a case for treatment with radiotherapy, although the authors admit that late unfavorable outcomes (in group 1) may occur as a result of the delayed effects of radiotherapy. Therefore long-term follow-up review of these cases is indicated.

For further analysis of the results of irradiation in craniopharyngiomas and especially the complications of this form of therapy, the reader is referred to Chapter 13.

Interstitial irradiation

Another form of therapy available for treatment of certain craniopharyngiomas is interstitial, or implanted, irradiation. This is also discussed in Chapter 13.

The advantages of intracyst isotope radiotherapy are that relatively large doses of radiation can be delivered to the entire cyst capsule with, theoretically, little exposure to adjacent neural structures (provided beta emission is used).[14] The optimal candidates are those patients with large, uncontrollable cysts invading vital areas or those patients with multiple or recurrent cysts.[24]

Recurrent craniopharyngioma

The current management of proven recurrent craniopharyngiomas is not settled. Although there are advocates favoring reoperation, there are other equally experienced neurosurgeons who would not subject the patient to another major operation. The issue focuses on recurrent solid tumors, not recurrent lesions that are accompanied by significant-sized cysts. In these latter cases (i.e., cysts), repeated aspiration using a percutaneous CT-directed technique may provide palliative but effective relief for variable periods of time. In the case of recurrent solid lesions, it is our belief that after assessing the risks and benefits of reoperation, it is difficult to justify another operation. Despite the advantages of the operating microscope and the skill of some surgeons, it is less likely that a cure will be obtained on a repeat operation that carries more risk than the first procedure. If the clinical findings are progressive and threaten to disable the patient in any way, a course of irradiation is recommended.

Case study. The following case report illustrates many of the problems that may be encountered in the management of a patient with a craniopharyngioma:

> A 48-year-old female came to medical attention with a 1-year history of visual loss, headaches, loss of appetite, decreased sex drive, and constipation. On neuro-ophthalmologic examination, the patient had reduced visual acuity to 20/25 −2 OD, 20/30 OS; pallor of the optic discs; and an incongruous right homonymous hemianopsia, consistent with a lesion affecting the left optic tract and both optic nerves with greater involvement of the left. A CT scan demonstrated a large low-density suprasellar mass with an enhancing rim extending into the posterior fossa (Fig. 11-6). Laboratory studies indicated that the patient was mildly hypothyroid and hypocortisolemic.
>
> She underwent a left frontotemporal craniotomy through which the cystic component of the suprasellar mass could be seen extending from below the chiasm posteriorly around the basilar artery. The left optic nerve and tract were displaced laterally with a groove on the left optic nerve formed by

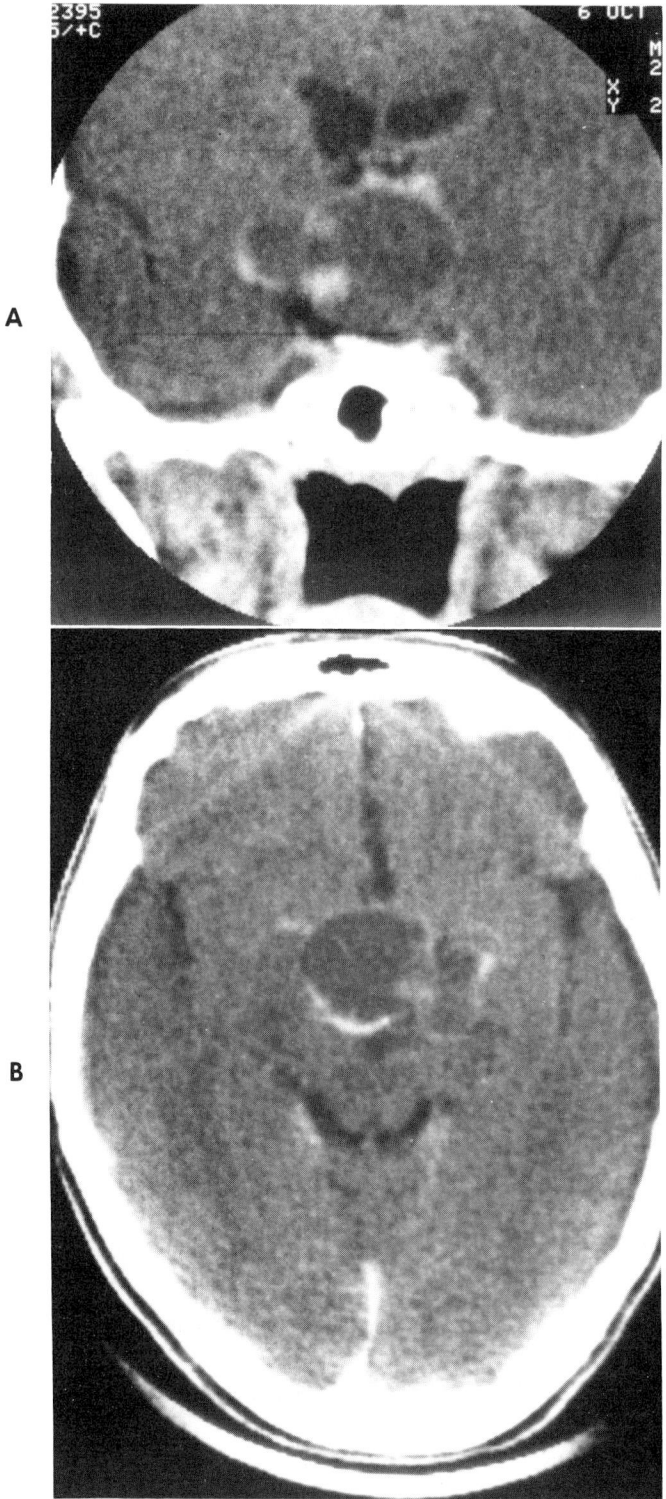

Fig. 11-6. Coronal (**A**) and axial (**B**) contrast-enhanced CT scans reveal large, cystic suprasellar mass with enhancing rim that extends into posterior fossa.

compression against the anterior cerebral artery. The tumor cyst was aspirated; but solid tumor, which proved to be a craniopharyngioma, was adherent to the undersurface of the optic chiasm, left internal carotid and anterior choroidal arteries, left third cranial nerve, hypothalamus, and basilar artery. After decompressing the cystic component of the neoplasm and removing a considerable amount of the solid tumor, it was decided that an attempt at gross total removal would not be safe. Postoperatively, the patient experienced an incomplete left third cranial nerve palsy and transient diabetes insipidus. Within 3 months of surgery, the third nerve palsy was almost entirely resolved, and the visual acuity was 20/20 -3 OD, 20/30 OS, with a subtle lower quadrantanopic defect in the right eye and no evidence of a hemianopic defect in the left eye. The patient felt much better and required no hormonal replacement therapy.

Six months after the initial operation, the patient experienced a deterioration in the visual acuity of her left eye to 20/200 associated with an enlargement of her visual field deficit. A repeat CT scan showed a recurrence of the cystic portion of the suprasellar tumor (Fig. 11-7). The patient then underwent a right frontotemporal craniotomy through which the cyst was again decompressed. The intimate relationship between the craniopharyngi-

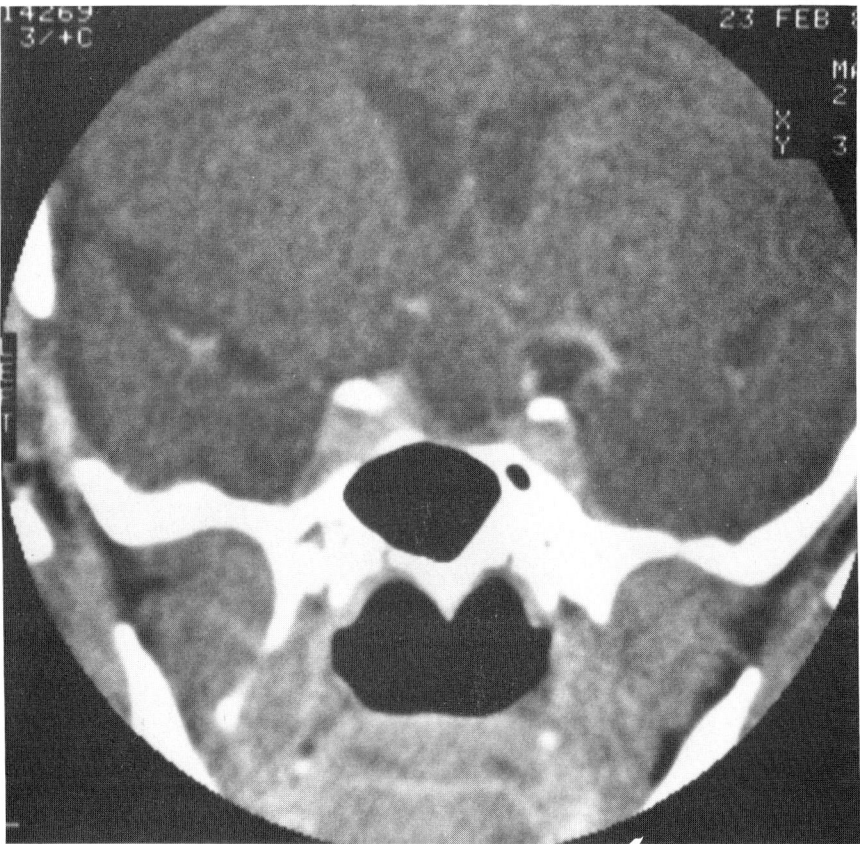

Fig. 11-7. Contrast-enhanced coronal CT scan shows recurrent suprasellar cyst.

oma and neural structures (especially the optic chiasm) precluded a total removal. In an effort to prevent the cyst from reforming, two small shunt tubes were placed into the cyst to enhance drainage into the subarachnoid space. This procedure only transiently improved her visual acuity, and radiation therapy was administered at a dosage of 180 rad/day through right and left parallel opposed portals and a single anterior portal for a total dose of 5940 rad. One month after completion of radiation therapy, the visual acuity was 20/25 +1 OD, 20/40 +1 OS with an almost complete temporal hemianopic defect in the right eye and small paracentral scotoma in the temporal half of vision of the left eye. A CT scan at this time showed a persistent tumor mass and the catheter tubes previously inserted (Fig. 11-8). The improvement in vision was believed to be in part a result of corticosteroid therapy prescribed during the period of radiation and continued in low dosages afterward. The steroids were discontinued, and the patient maintained a visual acuity of 20/30 OU with relative bitemporal field defects for 2½ years, at which time the field defects became dense and CT showed a new large suprasellar cyst distorting and blocking the third ventricle (Fig. 11-9). The patient then underwent a stereotaxic CT-directed placement of a catheter into

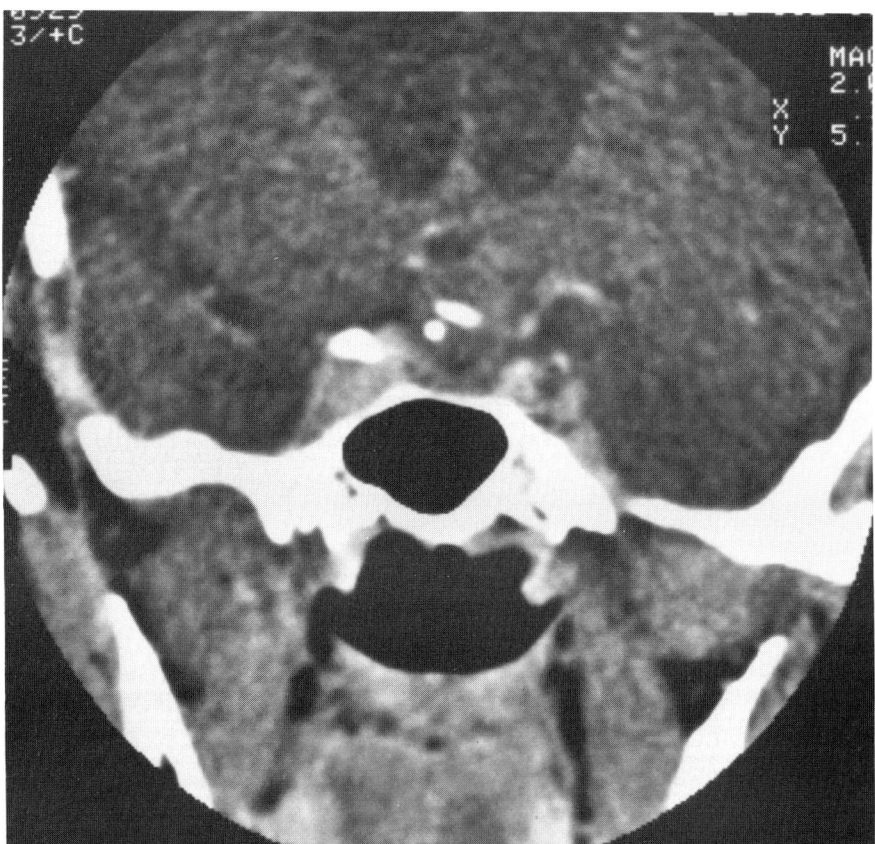

Fig. 11-8. Coronal CT demonstrates persistent cystic tumor mass with indwelling catheters.

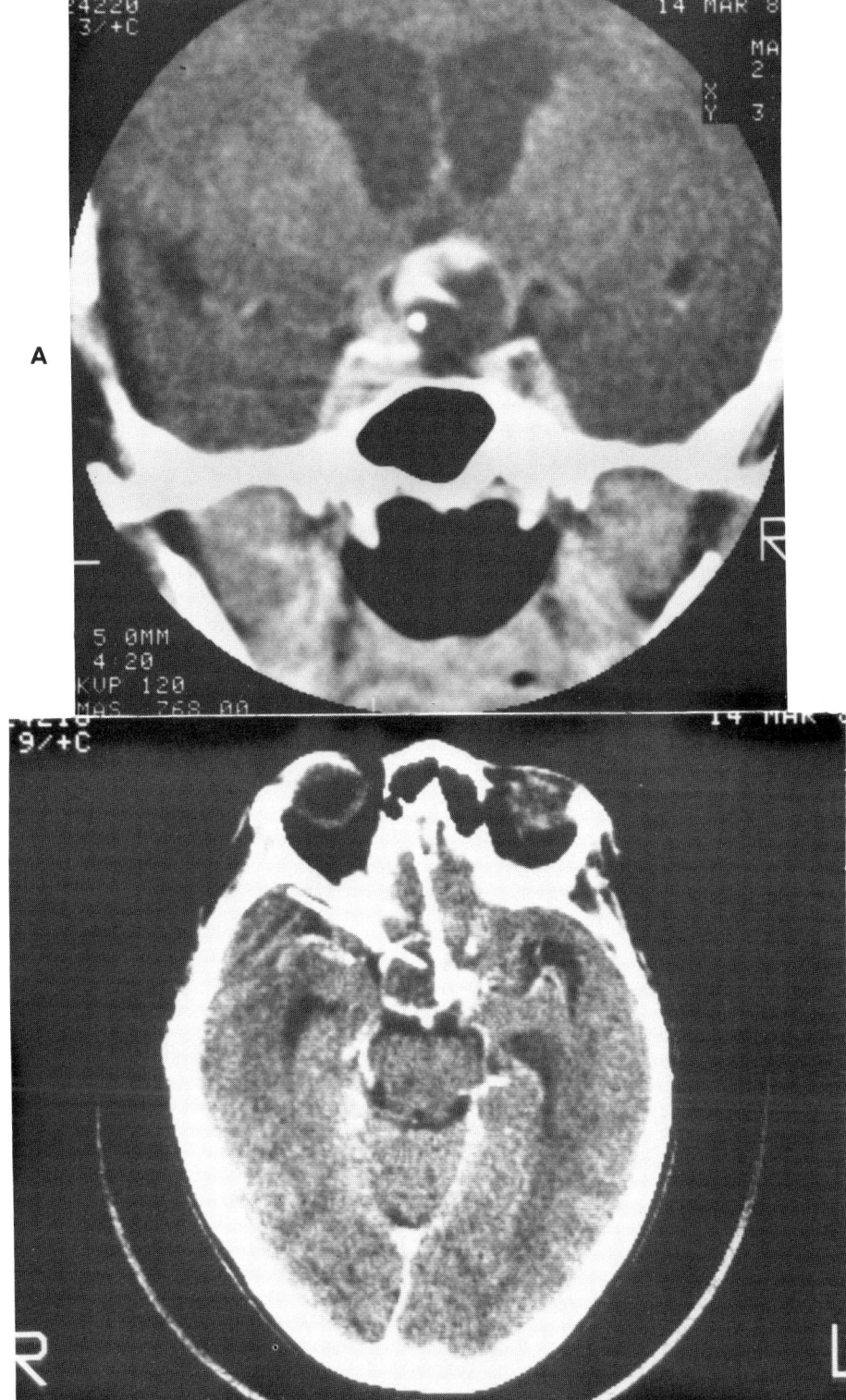

Fig. 11-9. Coronal (**A**) and axial (**B**) contrast-enhanced CT scans reveal enlarged suprasellar cystic tumor with distortion of third ventricle. Previously placed catheters are again seen entering cyst.

the cyst. The cyst was drained and the catheter attached to a reservoir placed beneath the galea. The visual field defect improved and remains stable 4 years after the initial operation. Periodic aspirations of the cyst through the reservoir and catheter have been required.

SUMMARY

In summary, surgery is an appropriate approach to overall primary treatment for adults and children unless there are extenuating or reasonable circumstances mitigating operation. The goal of surgery should be a gross total removal, but realistically, this may not always be possible. Patients with hydrocephalus should be shunted before definitive surgical treatment, and those cases with relatively rapid signs of local mass effect (i.e., visual loss) should be stabilized with steroids before surgery. If tumor removal is incomplete or the tumor recurs but in either case is *not* associated with *progressive symptomatology,* it is our recommendation that close follow-up observation be maintained. If recurrence is documented and the patient shows progressive clinical findings, conventional radiation in therapeutic effective doses should be instituted.

REFERENCES

1. Altinörs N, Senveli E, Erdogan A, et al: Craniopharyngioma of the cerebellopontine angle: Case report. *J Neurosurg* 60:842, 1984.
2. Amacher AL: Craniopharyngioma: The controversy regarding radiotherapy. *Child's Brain* 6:57, 1980.
3. Arseni C, Maretsis M: Craniopharyngioma. *Neurochirurgia* 1:25, 1972.
4. Banna M: Craniopharyngioma in adults. *Surg Neurol* 1:202, 1973.
5. Banna M, Hoare RD, Stanley P, et al: Craniopharyngioma in children. *J Pediatr* 83:781, 1973.
6. Bartlett JR: Craniopharyngiomas: An analysis of some aspects of symptomatology, radiology and histology. *Brain* 94:725, 1971.
7. Bloom HJG: Combined modality therapy for intracranial tumors. *Cancer* 35:111, 1975.
8. Bloom HJG: Recent concepts in the conservative treatment of intracranial tumours in children. *Acta Neurochir* 50:103, 1979.
9. Bloom HJG, Harmer CL: Craniopharyngioma: General aspects and treatment, in Bucalossi P, Veronesi U, Emanuelli H, et al (eds): *I Tumori Infantili*. Milan, Casa Editrice Ambrosiana, 1976.
10. Cabezudo JM, Vaquero J, Areitio E, et al: Craniopharyngiomas: A critical approach to treatment. *J Neurosurg* 55:371, 1981.
11. Carmichael HT: Squamous epithelial rests in the hypophysis cerebri. *Arch Neurol Psychiatry* 26:966, 1931.
12. Carpenter RC, Chamberlin GW, Frazier CH: The treatment of hypophyseal stalk tumors by evacuation and irradiation. *AJR* 38:162, 1937.
13. Cavazzuti V, Fischer EG, Welch K, et al: Neurological and psychophysiological sequelae following different treatments of craniopharyngioma in children. *J Neurosurg* 59:409, 1983.
14. Cobb CA, Youmans JR: Brain tumors of disordered embryogenesis in adults, in Youmans JR (ed): *Neurological Surgery,* ed 2. Philadelphia, WB Saunders Co, 1982, vol 5.
15. Cushing H: *Intracranial Tumors: Notes Upon a Series of Two Thousand Verified with Surgical-Mortality Percentages Pertaining Thereto*. Springfield, Ill., Charles C Thomas Publisher, 1932.
16. Goldberg GM, Eshbaugh DE: Squamous cell nests of the pituitary gland as related to the origin of craniopharyngiomas: A study of their presence in the newborn and infants up to age four. *Arch Pathol* 70:293, 1960.
17. Gordy PD, Peet MM, Kahn EA: The surgery of the craniopharyngiomas. *J Neurosurg* 6:503, 1949.
18. Gutin PH, Klemme WM, Lagger RL, et al: Management of the unresectable cystic craniopharyngioma by aspiration through an Ommaya reservoir drainage system. *J Neurosurg* 52:36, 1980.
19. Hardy J: Transsphenoidal hypophysectomy. *J Neurosurg* 34:582, 1971.
20. Hardy J, Vezina JL: Transsphenoidal neurosurgery of intracranial neoplasm, in Thompson RA, Green JR (eds): *Neoplasia in the Central Nervous System*. Advances in Neurology, New York, Raven Press, 1976, vol 15.

21. Hoff JT, Patterson RH: Craniopharyngiomas in children and adults. *J Neurosurg* 36:299, 1972.
22. Hoffman HJ, Hendrick EB, Humphreys RP, et al: Management of craniopharyngioma in children. *J Neurosurg* 47:218, 1977.
23. Ingraham FD, Matson DD, McLaurin RL: Cortisone and ACTH as an adjunct to the surgery of craniopharyngiomas. *N Engl J Med* 246:568, 1952.
24. Ingraham FD, Scott HW Jr: Craniopharyngiomas in children. *J Pediatr* 29:95, 1946.
25. Kahn EA, Gosch HH, Seeger JF, et al: Forty-five years' experience with the craniopharyngiomas. *Surg Neurol* 1:5, 1973.
26. Katz EL: Late results of radical excision of craniopharyngiomas in children. *J Neurosurg* 42:86, 1975.
27. Kjellberg RN: Craniopharyngiomas, in Tindall GT, Collins GT (eds): *Clinical Management of Pituitary Disorders*. New York, Raven Press, 1979.
28. Kobayashi T, Kageyama N, Yoshida J, et al: Pathological and clinical basis of the indications for treatment of craniopharyngioma. *Neurol Med Chir* 21:39, 1981.
29. Koos WT, Miller MH: *Intracranial Tumors of Infants and Children*. St. Louis, The CV Mosby Co, 1971.
30. Kramer S: Radiation therapy in the management of craniopharyngiomas, in Deeley TJ (ed): *Central Nervous System Tumors*. Kent, England, Butterworth & Co Ltd, 1974.
31. Kramer S: Craniopharyngioma: The best treatment is conservative surgery and postoperative radiation therapy, in Morley TP (ed): *Current Controversies in Neurosurgery*. Philadelphia, WB Saunders Co, 1976.
32. Kramer S, Southard M, Mansfield CM: Radiotherapy in the management of craniopharyngiomas: Further experiences and late results. *AJR* 103:44, 1968.
33. Landolt AM: Die ultrastruktur des kraniopharyngeoms. *Neurochir Psychiat* 111:313, 1972.
34. Langman J: Central nervous system, in Langman J (ed): *Medical Embryology*, ed 3. Baltimore, Williams & Wilkins Co, 1975.
35. Laws ER: Transsphenoidal microsurgery in the management of craniopharyngioma. *J Neurosurg* 52:661, 1980.
36. Lewis DD: A contribution to the subject of tumors of the hypophysis. *JAMA* 55:1002, 1910.
37. Lichter AS, Wara WM, Sheline GE, et al: The treatment of craniopharyngiomas. *Int J Radiat Oncol Biol Phys* 2:675, 1977.
38. Long DM, Chou SN: Transcallosal removal of craniopharyngiomas within the third ventricle. *J Neurosurg* 39:563, 1973.
39. Love JG, Marshall TM: Craniopharyngiomas (pituitary adamantinomas). *Surg Gynecol Obstet* 90:591, 1950.
40. Luse SA, Kernohan JW: Squamous-cell nests of the pituitary gland. *Cancer* 8:623, 1955.
41. Maira G, Di Rocca C, Anile C, et al: Hyperprolactinemia as the first symptom of craniopharyngioma. *Child's Brain* 9:205, 1982.
42. Matson DD: Craniopharyngioma, in Matson DD (ed): *Neurosurgery in Infancy and Childhood*, ed 2. Springfield, Ill., Charles C Thomas Publisher, 1969.
43. Matson DD, Crigler JF Jr: Management of craniopharyngioma in childhood. *J Neurosurg* 30:377, 1969.
44. McLone DG, Raimondi AJ, Naidich TP: Craniopharyngiomas. *Child's Brain* 9:188, 1982.
45. McKenzie KG, Sosman MC: The roentgenological diagnosis of craniopharyngeal pouch tumors. *AJR* 11:171, 1924.
46. McKissock W, Ford RK: Results of treatment of the craniopharyngiomas, abstract. *J Neurol Neurosurg Psychiatry* 29:475, 1966.
47. Melchionna RH, Moore RA: The pharyngeal pituitary gland. *Am J Pathol* 14:763, 1938.
48. Northfield DWC: Rathke-pouch tumours. *Brain* 80:293, 1957.
49. Olivecrona H: The surgical treatment of intracranial tumors, in Olivecrona H, Tonnis W (eds): *Handbuch der Neurochirurgie*. Berlin, Springer-Verlag, 1967, vol 4.
50. Patterson RH, Danylevich A: Surgical removal of craniopharyngiomas by a transcranial approach through the lamina terminalis and sphenoid sinus. *Neurosurgery* 7:111, 1980.
51. Pertuiset B: Craniopharyngiomas, in Vinken PJ, Bruyn GW (eds): *Handbook of Clinical Neurology, part III, Tumours of the Brain and Skull*. Amsterdam, NorthHolland Publishing Co, 1975, vol 18.
52. Plum F, van Uitert R: Nonendocrine diseases and disorders of the hypothalamus, in Reichlin S, Baldessarini RJ, Martin JB (eds): *The Hypothalamus*. New York, Raven Press, 1978, vol 56.
53. Richmond IL, Wara WM, Wilson CB: Role of radiation therapy in the management of craniopharyngiomas in children. *Neurosurgery* 6:513, 1980.
54. Ross-Russell RW, Pennybacker JB: Craniopharyngioma in the elderly. *J Neurol Neurosurg Psychiatry* 24:1, 1961.
55. Sano K: *Intracranial Tumors: It's Pathology and Clinic*. Tokyo, Igaku-Shoin Ltd, 1972.
56. Shapiro K, Till K, Grant DN: Craniopharyn-

giomas in childhood: A rational approach to treatment. *J Neurosurg* 50:617, 1979.
57. Shillito J Jr: The treatment of craniopharyngiomas of childhood, in Morley TP (ed): *Current Controversies in Neurosurgery*. Philadelphia, WB Saunders Co, 1976.
58. Svolos DG: Craniopharyngiomas: A study based on 108 verified cases. *Acta Chir Scand* (suppl) 403:1, 1969.
59. Sweet WH: Recurrent craniopharyngiomas: Therapeutic alternatives. *Clin Neurosurg* 27:206, 1980.
60. Sweet WH: Craniopharyngiomas, with a note on Rathke's cleft or epithelial cysts and on suprasellar cysts, in Schmidek HH, Sweet WH (eds): *Operative Neurosurgical Techniques—Indications, Methods, and Results*. New York, Grune & Stratton Inc, 1982, vol 1.
61. Symon L, Logue V, Jakubowski J: The surgical treatment of craniopharyngioma, abstract. *Neurochirurgia* 65:301, 1982.
62. Tytus JS, Seltzer HS, Kahn EA: Cortisone as an aid in the surgical treatment of craniopharyngiomas. *J Neurosurg* 12:555, 1955.
63. Waga S, Handa H: Radiation-induced meningioma: With review of the literature. *Surg Neurol* 5:215, 1976.
64. Zenker FA: Enrome crystenbilding im gehirn, vom hirnanhang ausgehend. *Arch Pathol Anat Physiol Klin Med* 11:454, 1857.

CHAPTER 12

Pituitary surgery

Anesthesia considerations
    Preoperative assessment
    Monitoring
    Positioning
Surgical approaches
Transcranial approaches
    Indications
    Frontotemporal (pterional) approach
    Subfrontal approach
    Subtemporal approach
Transsphenoidal approaches
    Indications
    Contraindications
    Sublabial transsphenoidal technique
    Hypophysectomy
    Variations
        Transnasal midline transsphenoidal approach
        Transethmoidal approach
        Transantral approach
Complications
    Operative complications—craniotomy
        Hemorrhage
        Cerebral edema, infarction, and elevated ICP
        Infection
        Damage to parasellar structures
        Operative mortality—craniotomy
    Operative complications—transsphenoidal approach
        Parasellar
        Intracranial
        Sphenoid and nasofacial
        Operative mortality—transsphenoidal approach

The evolution of various operative approaches to the pituitary comprises an interesting chapter in the history of neurosurgery. In 1889 Sir Victor Horsley performed the first operation on a pituitary tumor. Using a frontal craniotomy on a man with a mass compressing the optic chiasm, he exposed the tumor but believed that it was inoperable and did not attempt removal. By 1906 he had performed 10 operations on the pituitary with two deaths.[33] Primarily because of the high mortality and complication rate of craniotomy in the early 1900s, surgeons developed extracranial routes to the sella turcica. These approaches to the sella were transsphenoidal, thus taking advantage of the proximity of the sphenoid sinus to the sella. Historically, transsphenoidal operations were divided into superior and inferior nasal approaches. The earlier, more radical superior approaches used various incisions to turn the entire nose as a flap and gain access to the sphenoid sinus. Inferior nasal operations approached the sphenoid through incisions below the nostrils of the nose or under the upper lip.

In 1907 Schloffer[69] reported the first successful transsphenoidal operation for a pituitary tumor. His patient was a 30-year-old man with headaches and bitemporal hemianopsia from a tumor producing mass effects. In performing the operation, he reflected the nose to one side and resected the entire septum, superior and middle conchae, and ethmoid air cells (Fig. 12-1). The medial wall of the orbit was removed and the sphenoid sinus opened. The tumor was subtotally removed. Postoperatively, the patient had resolution of headaches, but the visual field deficit did not improve. A cerebrospinal fluid (CSF) leak resolved spontaneously in 2 weeks, but the patient died 2½ months after surgery because of hydrocephalus resulting from suprasellar tumor blocking the foramen of Monro.[45]

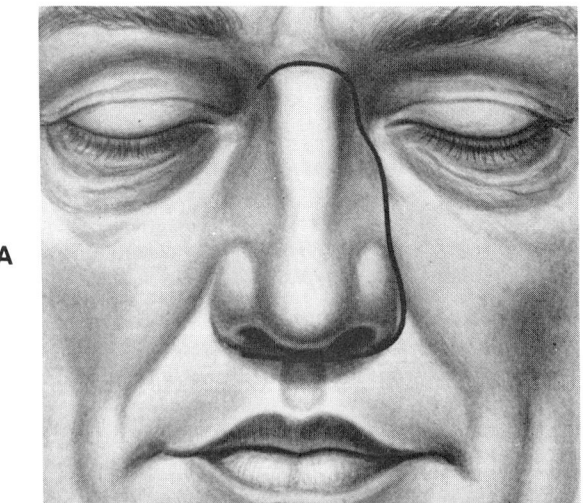

Fig. 12-1. Schloffer's first transnasal operation. **A**, Incision.

Reprinted with permission Guleke N: Die Eingriffe am Gehirnschädel, Gehirn, an der Wirbelsäule und am Rückenmark. In Allgemeine und spezielle Operationslehre, Vol. 2, 2nd ed., pp 335-343 Guleke, N., Zenker, R., eds. Berlin-Göttingen-Heidelberg: 1950, Springer.

Subsequent transnasal operations by Eiselsberg, Hochenegg, Borchardt, Loewe, and others were even more extensive than that performed by Schloffer, with opening of the frontal, ethmoid, and sphenoid sinuses after removing the septum and conchae. Not surprisingly, these early surgeons encountered many intraoperative and postoperative complications. Visualization was poor, requiring these extensive exposures. Without continuous suction, the operative field was seldom dry. Many patients developed an unpleasant nasal discharge from atrophic sinusitis. In 1911 Hirsch[30] found seven deaths within the first few postoperative days in the 22 patients in the literature. Causes of death were meningitis in one,

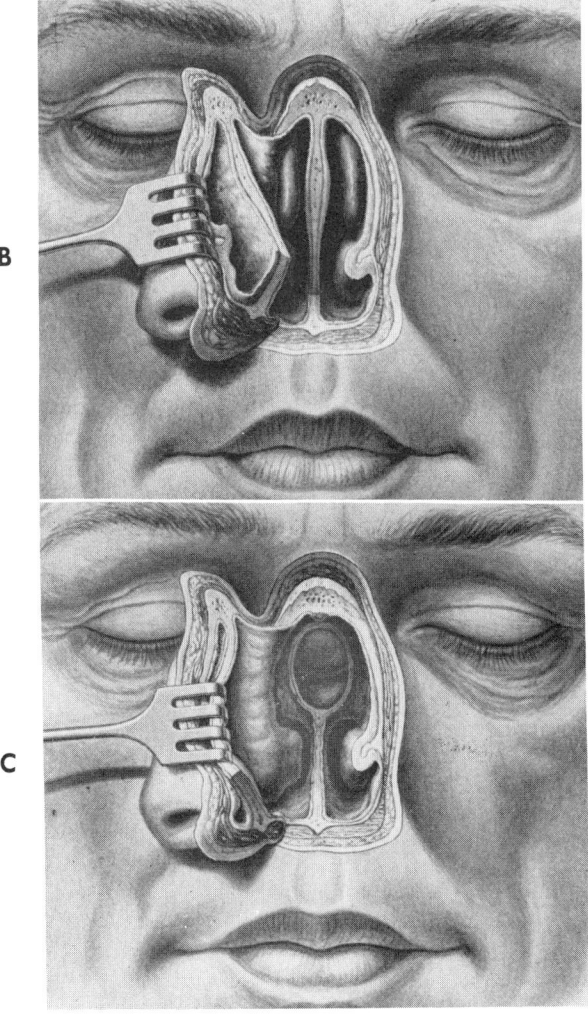

Fig. 12-1, cont'd. B, Nose has been turned exposing nasal structures. **C,** Septum has been removed and floor of sphenoid sinus and sella opened.

anemia in one, aspiration pneumonia in one, myocardial degeneration with lymphoid hyperplasia in one, and unknown in two.

Kocher's modification of the superior nasal procedure in 1909 was the first submucosal approach to the sphenoid and definitely an advance toward less mutilating operations.[42] He did not enter the nasal cavity but made incisions over the bridge of the nose to open double doorlike skin flaps. The nasal bone was cut at its base and turned downward after cutting the attachment to the septum.

The inferior nasal approaches to the sphenoid and sella are less extensive than superior nasal procedures and are still in use today. In 1910 Hirsch[29] modified his original endonasal operation and entered the sella through a transseptal approach using a nasal speculum. He based his operation on the description of a submucosal, endonasal resection of the nasal septum by Killian[41] in 1904. Later, Hirsch began adding a local radium application to remaining or recurrent tumor. He treated 413 patients with this combination between 1910 and 1956.[31] Kanavel[39,40] substituted a skin incision at the bottom of the nose under the nares and turned the nose up rather than operate through the narrow nostril. Halstead[22] used Kanavel's approach but employed a sublabial instead of intranasal incision.

Cushing[6,7] combined the advantages of the various procedures and developed a transsphenoidal operation that is essentially the same as that used today (Fig. 12-2). He made use of a sublabial incision and submucosal resection of the septum. The tissue planes were maintained by a bivalved speculum. The surgical mortality in Cushing's transsphenoidal series was 5.3%.[28] Hirsch's first combined surgical and radiotherapeutic series from 1919 to 1929 had a mortality of 4.8%.[31]

Despite these relatively impressive results in the era before the availability of antibiotics and steroids, Cushing and many other neurosurgeons abandoned the transsphenoidal procedures and again operated on pituitary neoplasms by craniotomy. A number of factors influenced this change from transsphenoidal to transcranial approaches. Perhaps the more important ones were (1) the relatively high recurrence rate of tumors related in turn to poor visualization and inability to totally resect the lesions transsphenoidally and (2) the fact that transcranial techniques were being improved and made safer. So from about 1920 until the 1960s, most neurosurgeons used the transcranial approach for pituitary tumors. However, not all neurosurgeons made the switch. Dott continued using the transsphenoidal approach and undoubtedly exerted an influence on Guiot.[18]

In the mid-1960s both Guiot and Hardy introduced innovations that rekindled interest in transsphenoidal approaches to the pituitary. Guiot's introduction of magnifying loupes,[20] intraoperative radiographs,[15,20] and image intensification,[19] and Hardy's adaptation of the operating microscope to the operation[24,25,26] plus televised fluoroscopy[27] proved that pituitary tumors, even small lesions accounting for Cushing's disease and acromegaly, could be safely and effectively treated via the transsphenoidal approach (Fig. 12-3). Contributions by Guiot and Hardy thus effected another shift, and since the late 1960s, the majority of surgeons have used transsphenoidal approaches to the pituitary.

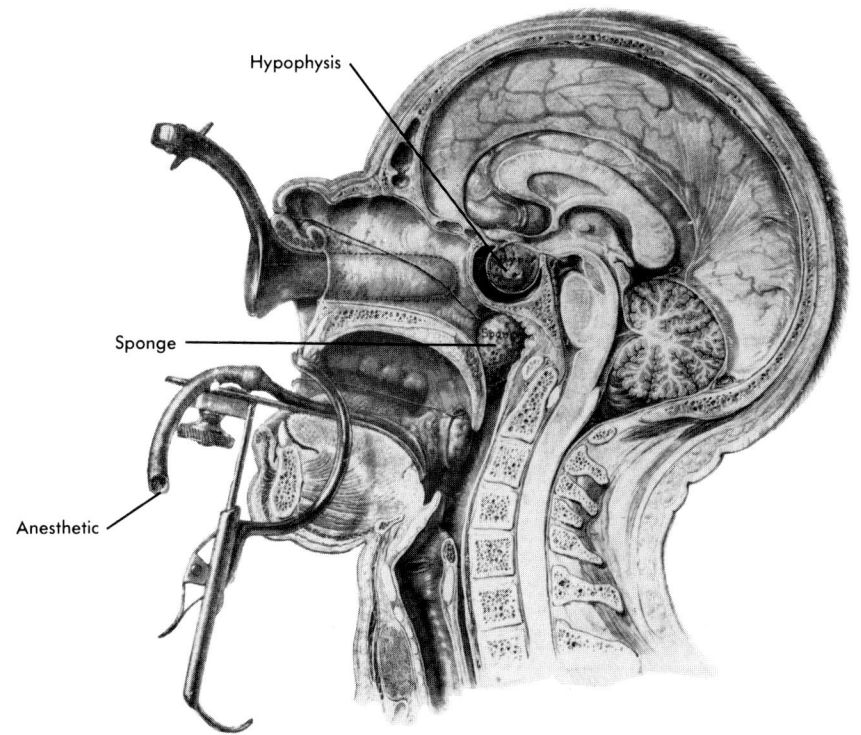

Fig. 12-2. Cushing's sublabial, transseptal pituitary operation. Self-retaining bivalved speculum is in place beneath nasal mucosa.

From Cushing H: Surgical experiences with pituitary disorders. *JAMA* 63:1515, 1914. Copyright 1914, American Medical Association.

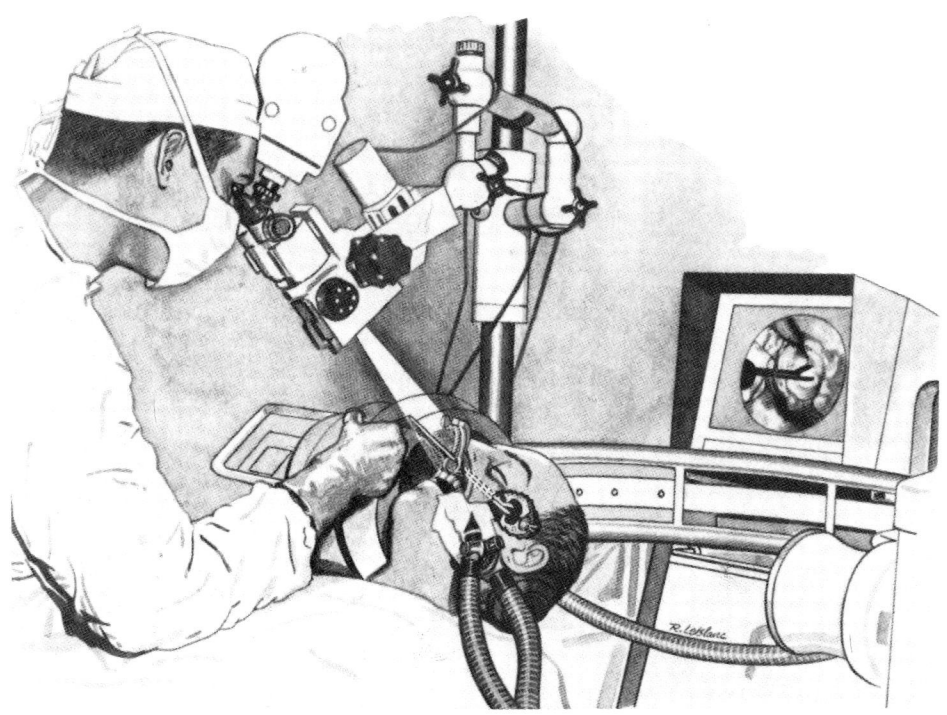

Fig. 12-3. Hardy's operative setup for transsphenoidal surgery with combined use of televised radiofluoroscopic control and operating microscope.

From Hardy J: Transsphenoidal hypophysectomy. *J Neurosurg* 34:582, 1971.

ANESTHESIA CONSIDERATIONS

Proper anesthetic management of patients undergoing pituitary surgery is an essential component of overall patient care. This management will differ somewhat depending on whether the patient is undergoing a craniotomy or transsphenoidal procedure.

Preoperative assessment

As with any other operation, preoperative evaluation of surgical patients to assess their general health and tolerance of general anesthesia is of paramount importance. The cardiovascular, respiratory, renal, hepatic, and endocrine systems should be evaluated, and a history of allergies, present medications, and prior anesthetic complications should be taken. In addition, patients with pituitary adenomas or those undergoing ablative hypophysectomies may demonstrate special or unique medical problems that could influence the method of anesthetic induction, the choice of preanesthetic medication, or choice of anesthesia itself. For instance, patients with acromegaly or gigantism frequently have associated medical conditions such as cardiomyopathy with congestive heart failure and arrhythmias or coronary artery disease with hypertension than can complicate anesthetic management.[71] Preoperative consultation with a cardiologist may be necessary to optimize the cardiac system before surgery. Acromegalic patients may have other endocrine dysfunction such as diabetes mellitus, hypothyroidism, or hyperthyroidism that require preoperative evaluation. Also the large nose, large tongue, and prognathism of the acromegalic patient may make airway management difficult.[71]

Patients with Cushing's disease also have associated conditions that may complicate anesthetic management. These patients are usually obese with thin, fragile skin that heals poorly. Special attention must be taken in positioning these patients. There is frequently hypertension and cardiac disease associated with the hypercortisolism. As with acromegalic patients, a preoperative evaluation by a cardiologist may be beneficial.

Patients with large or recurrent tumors may have varying degrees of hypopituitarism. A history of previous medication and assessment of adrenal and thyroid function is necessary. Those with hypopituitarism will already be receiving steroid replacement before surgery and will require large doses in the perioperative period because they are unable to increase their endogenous steroids during stress. In patients with normal pituitary-adrenal function, we routinely administer 100 mg hydrocortisone IM immediately before surgery, 50 mg in each liter of intravenous fluid during surgery, and 50 mg by mouth or IM every 8 hours beginning in the recovery room and continued through the second postoperative day. Thereafter the steroid dosage is tapered and subsequently discontinued or maintained at the level necessary for the patient's individual needs.

Hypophysectomy for metastatic cancer is performed on patients who usually are not in good health and who may have complicating factors such as anemia, thrombocytopenia, altered coagulation, and widespread metastases. Lung metastases may be associated with pneumonitis, pleural effusions, and decreased lung compliance—all of which complicate anesthesia. Patients with cervical spine metastases require special attention during neck movement for intubation and positioning.

Monitoring

Physiologic parameters requiring routine monitoring in patients undergoing pituitary surgery include heart rate using an esophageal stethoscope, arterial blood pressure with a cuff or direct arterial line, temperature with an esophageal temperature probe, urinary output with a Foley catheter, and electrocardiograph.

An arterial line (radial artery) for continuous blood pressure monitoring and for frequent blood sampling to check blood sugar, blood gases, and electrolytes is inserted before induction in many patients. Patients with heart disease benefit from central venous, pulmonary arterial, and capillary wedge pressure monitoring via a Swan-Ganz catheter.

On special occasions, an indwelling lumbar subarachnoid catheter or lumbar puncture needle is inserted after the patient is anesthetized. During craniotomy the removal of CSF will facilitate brain shrinkage and minimize retraction. In patients undergoing transsphenoidal surgery for pituitary tumors with suprasellar extension, the withdrawal of CSF or the infusion of sterile saline will aid in removing the tumor above the sella. In the case of an intraoperative tear of the diaphragm sella during transsphenoidal surgery, the drainage of CSF helps keep the operative field dry during closure, allows for better closure with tissue adhesive, and thus diminishes the chance of a CSF leak postoperatively.

Intracranial hypertension is unusual in patients with pituitary tumors unless suprasellar extension of the tumor obstructs the foramen of Monro and causes hydrocephalus. Under this circumstance, precautions should be taken during induction of anesthesia to prevent further increase in the intracranial pressure (ICP). These precautions include hyperventilation to a partial pressure of carbon dioxide (pco_2) of 25 to 30 mmHg before and after intubation, diuresis with mannitol (0.5 to 1 mg/kg) and furosemide (10 to 40 mg IV), and the use of intravenous lidocaine (1.5 mg/kg). These same measures should be employed during craniotomy for pituitary tumors to effect shrinkage of the brain, thus minimizing the amount of retraction needed for adequate exposure. Otherwise, induction for pituitary surgery is not significantly different from that used for general anesthesia for other operations.

356 *Disorders of the pituitary*

Positioning

The positioning of the patient for a transcranial operation will depend on the particular approach the surgeon chooses. In all cases, the head is placed in three-point fixation using a skull clamp (e.g., Mayfield). A frontotemporal (pterional) approach requires that the head be turned approximately 45 degrees to the left so that the pterion is the highest point and the patient's right shoulder is slightly elevated (Fig. 12-4). For a right subfrontal approach, the head is slightly extended and turned 10 degrees to the left with the patient supine (Fig. 12-5). The patient is placed in a lateral position for a subtemporal operation with soft padding under the axilla and with the legs flexed slightly. The long axis of the head is parallel to the floor and laterally flexed so that the vertex points slightly toward the floor (Fig. 12-6). This allows for gravity to assist in temporal lobe retraction.

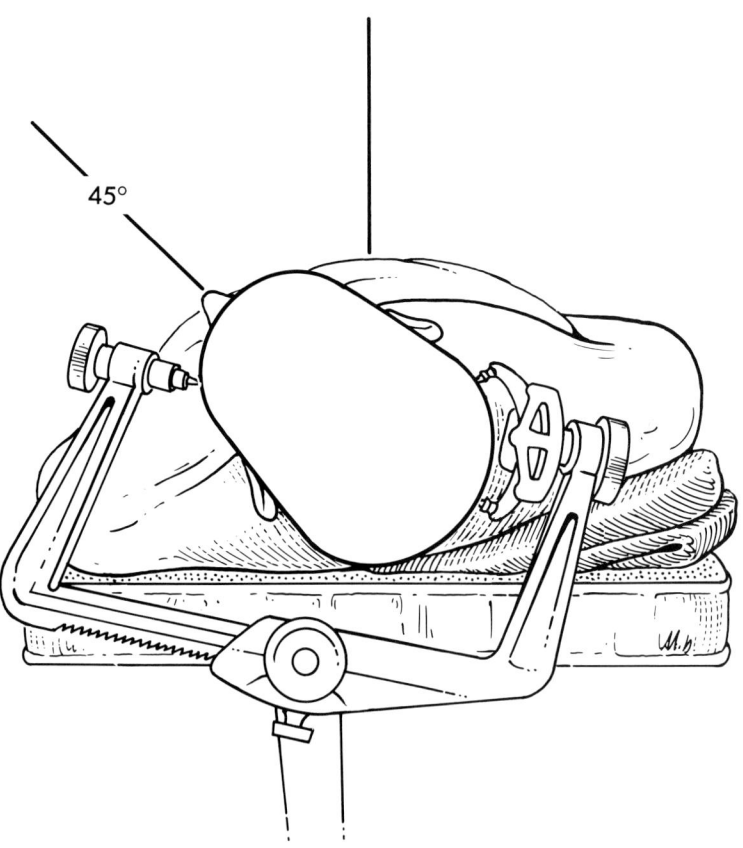

Fig. 12-4. Position of head for frontotemporal (pterional) craniotomy.

Fig. 12-5. Position of head for subfrontal approach.

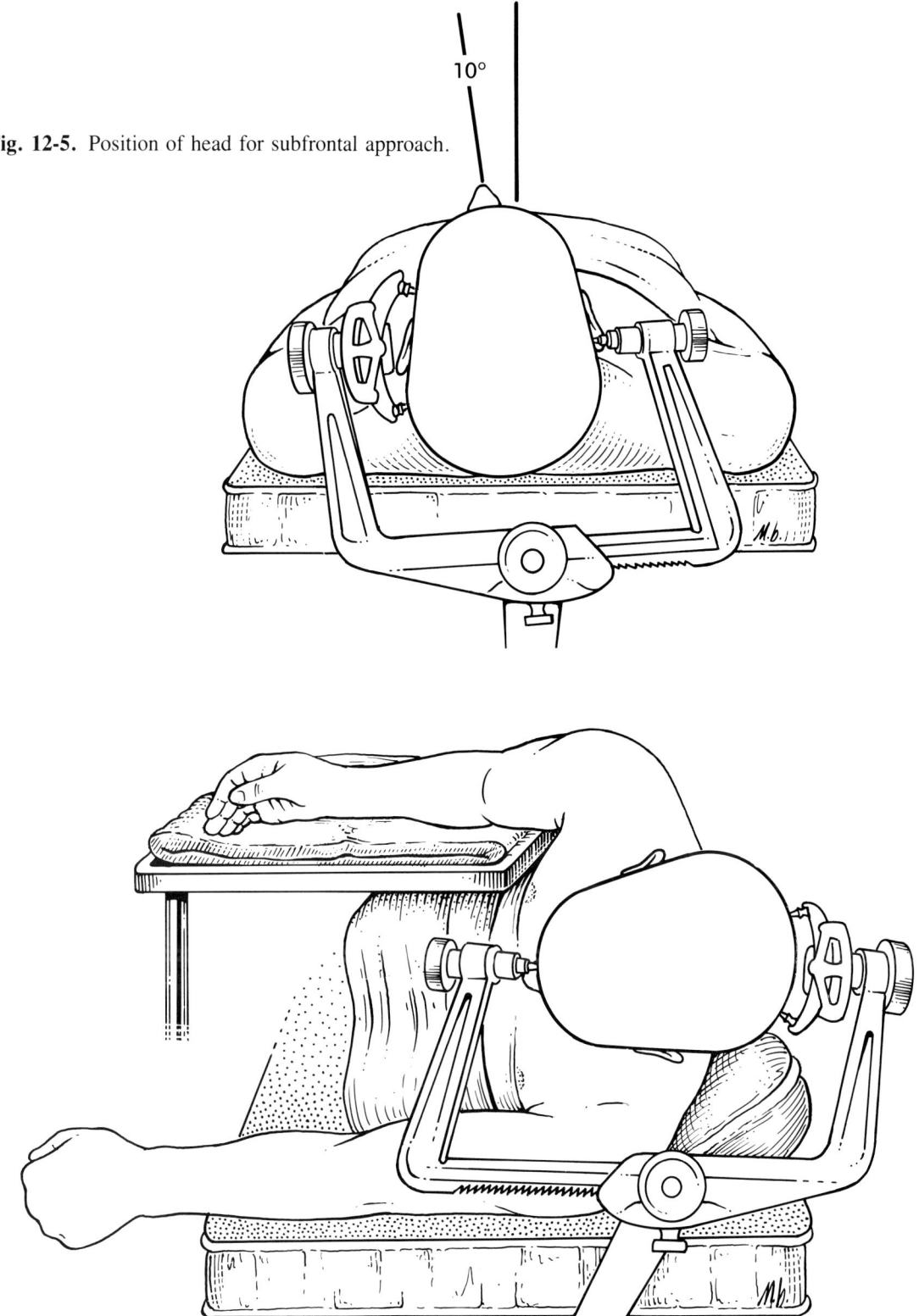

Fig. 12-6. Position of head for subtemporal approach.

358 *Disorders of the pituitary*

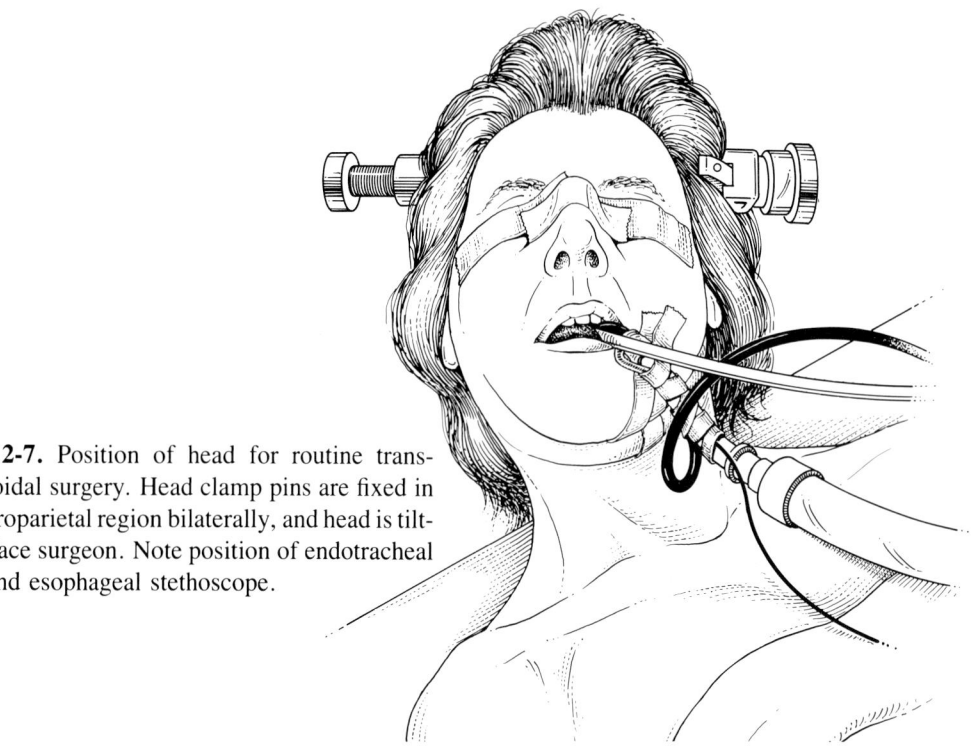

Fig. 12-7. Position of head for routine transsphenoidal surgery. Head clamp pins are fixed in temporoparietal region bilaterally, and head is tilted to face surgeon. Note position of endotracheal tube and esophageal stethoscope.

In transsphenoidal operations, the endotracheal tube, esophageal stethoscope, and temperature probe are taped together and brought out the left side of the mouth. The endotracheal tube must be securely taped to the face. No oral airway is used. In the usual case, the skull clamp is placed with the pins in the temporal bones above the squama just below the parietal bossing (Fig. 12-7). With the metal skull clamp in this position, it is often not possible to obtain an adequate skull x-ray centered on the sella turcica during surgery. Thus if intraoperative x-ray examination or fluoroscopy of the sella is anticipated, such as is the case in most patients with a presellar or conchal type of sphenoid sinus, the clamp should be placed in a position that will not interfere with the x-ray procedure. In this case, the single pin is placed frontally, and the two rear pins are placed in the occipital area to allow free access to intraoperative x-ray examination for localization (Fig. 12-8).

The head is tilted to the patient's left, the face is turned toward the right side, and the head is elevated about 10 degrees from the operating table with the surgeon standing on the patient's right side (Fig. 12-7).

Although we do not routinely use intraoperative x-ray examination or fluoroscopy, many surgeons use a portable image intensifier to verify intraoperative location and to monitor position of instruments in the sella and the suprasellar area. If some doubt about localization exists during the exposure, we do not hesitate to obtain an intraoperative lateral skull x-ray to confirm the bony landmarks.

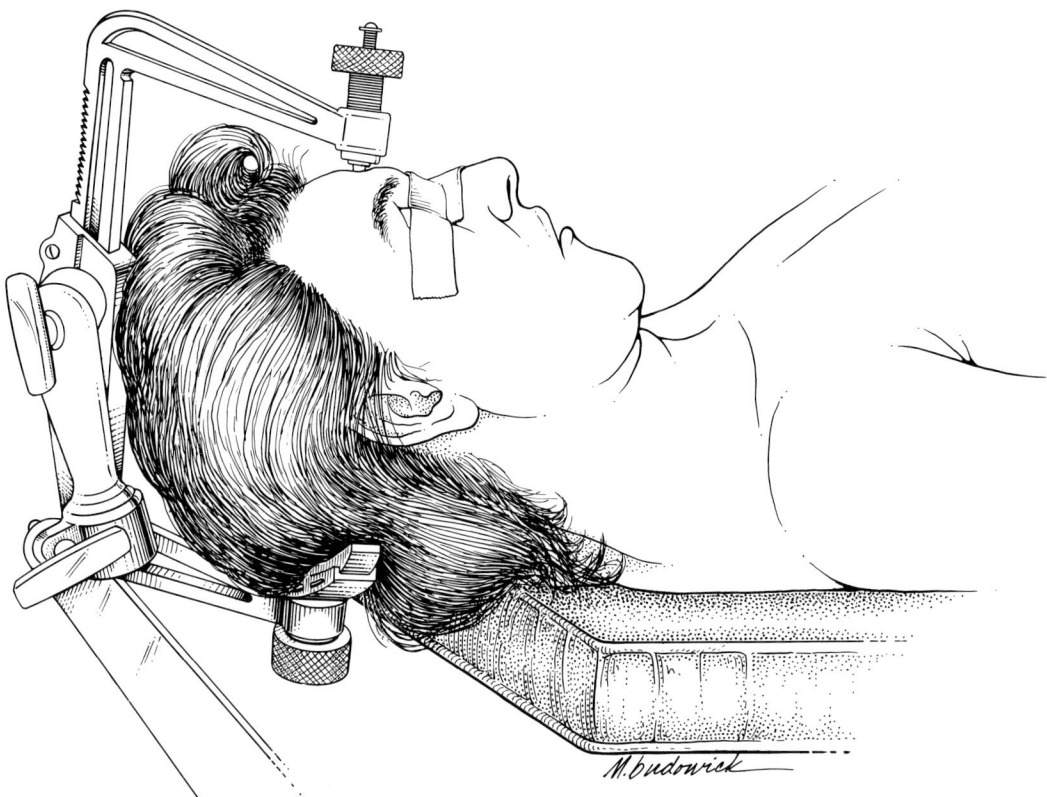

Fig. 12-8. Position of head clamp when intraoperative skull x-ray examination is anticipated. Pins of clamp are placed as shown so that clamp is oriented in an anteroposterior direction and thus will not interfere with obtaining lateral x-ray film of sella and sphenoid sinus.

SURGICAL APPROACHES

No single operation is ideal for all pituitary tumors. Many tumors may be operated adequately with good results by either a transsphenoidal approach or by one of the transcranial operations. Variables involved in determining the most appropriate technique include characteristics of the tumor (e.g., size, extrasellar extensions, and histologic type) and those of the patient (e.g., age, state of health, extent of visual and endocrine impairment, and anatomy of the sella turcica and sphenoid sinus).

In the case of a pituitary tumor that can be safely approached by either a transcranial or transsphenoidal operation, the latter, in our opinion, is the preferred procedure. This provides a more rapid and direct access to the pituitary gland; better differentiation of tumor from gland; less probability of injury to the optic chiasm, nerves, and olfactory tract; and less trauma on the patient. The actual volume of tumor and extrasellar extension is not as important as the shape and direction of growth in determining the most appropriate approach. A large suprasellar extension can usually be adequately handled through a transsphenoidal operation.

TRANSCRANIAL APPROACHES
Indications

One should consider using a transcranial approach when an adenoma has an intracranial extension to the subfrontal, retrochiasmatic, or middle fossa regions (Fig. 12-9).

A transcranial approach is also indicated when the suprasellar portion is separated from the intrasellar tumor by a "bottleneck" constriction (Fig. 12-10) or when a suprasellar mass is associated with a normal-sized sella turcica.

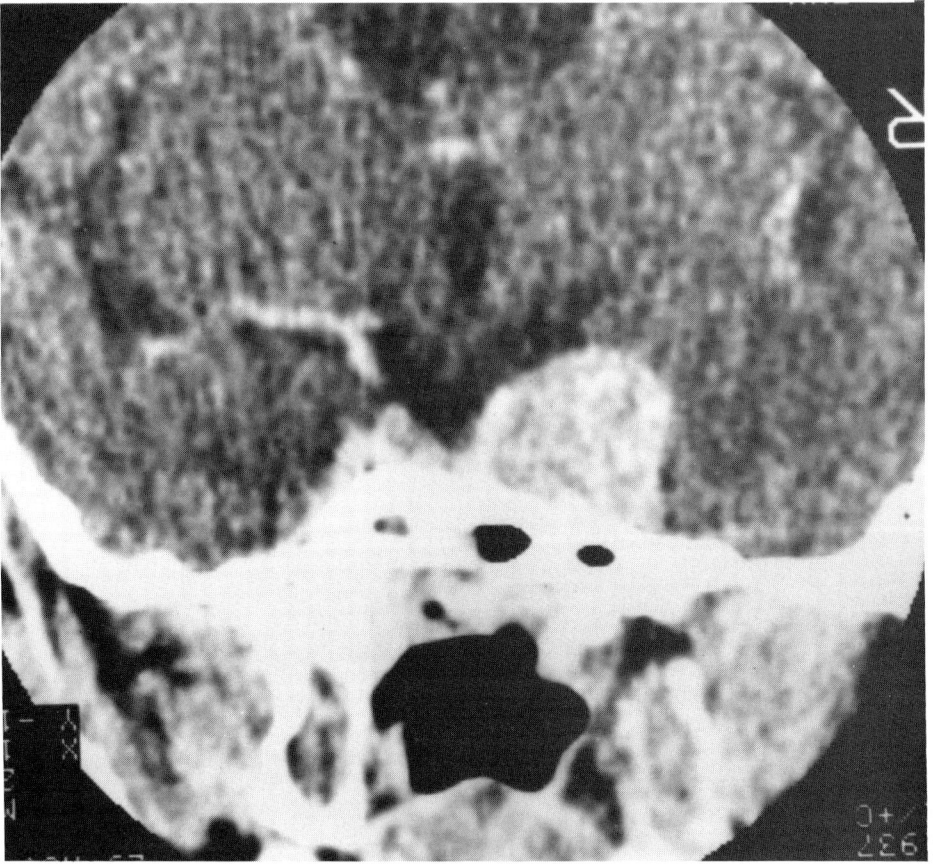

Fig. 12-9. Coronal CT of patient with significant extension of tumor into medial portion of middle cranial fossa.

Three intracranial approaches are used to operate on pituitary tumors, and each one offers a different exposure and certain advantages in particular situations. The subfrontal approach provides a view of both optic nerves, chiasm, carotid arteries, suprasellar cistern, pituitary stalk, and sella. However, if the optic chiasm is prefixed, this structure will obstruct access to the adenoma when using a subfrontal approach. The presence of a prefixed chiasm (see Fig. 1-18) can often be predicted preoperatively by the presence of a bitemporal hemianopic scotoma. When the chiasm is prefixed, the frontotemporal route is preferable; this approach allows access to the space between the optic nerve and tract medially and the internal carotid artery laterally. However, the surgeon's view of the left optic nerve and intrasellar contents is slightly compromised. A subtemporal approach is indicated when tumor has significant retrochiasmatic extension. This exposure will allow decompression of the chiasm but may preclude total removal of intrasellar tumor.

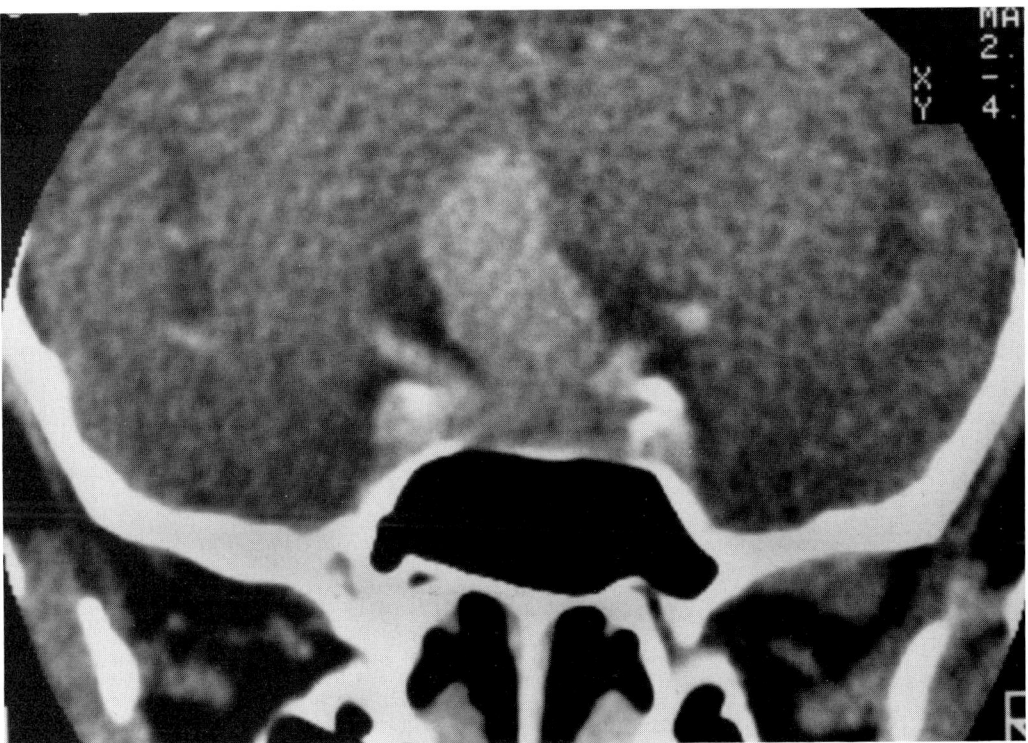

Fig. 12-10. Coronal computed tomography (CT) of patient with ''bottleneck'' type of tumor. Tumor, which is relatively narrow immediately above sella, widens considerably as it extends upward toward third ventricle.

362 *Disorders of the pituitary*

Frontotemporal (pterional) approach

Except under unusual circumstances, all transcranial approaches to pituitary tumors are made from the nondominant side. However, in some patients, the surgeon may choose to operate on the side of poorest vision (see Chapter 11). The usual incision is begun 1 cm anterior to the tragus of the ear at the zygomatic arch and extended up just behind the hairline to the midsagittal plane about 3 cm anterior to the coronal suture (Fig. 12-11). The scalp incision may be varied so as to permit more frontal exposure by bringing it across the center of the head in a curvilinear fashion (cosmetically preferable to curving it down over the forehead in front of the hair line) or more temporal exposure by curving it farther back above the ear and then proceeding in a frontal direction.

It is important to limit dissection in the subgaleal space between the galea and the temporalis fascia anteriorly so as to avoid injuring the frontalis branch of the facial nerve. Using the electrocautery, the temporalis fascia and muscle are incised immediately beneath the scalp incision, and all layers are turned forward as a unit. The temporalis muscle is dissected off the skull far forward to the orbitofrontal angle and the superior orbital ridge and low over the temporal fossa. The muscle can be retracted to achieve maximal exposure with the use of rubber-banded sutures or fishhooks.

While turning the scalp and bone flaps, 30 to 50 g of mannitol (20% solution) are administered IV. If there is a possibility that increased ICP might be a sig-

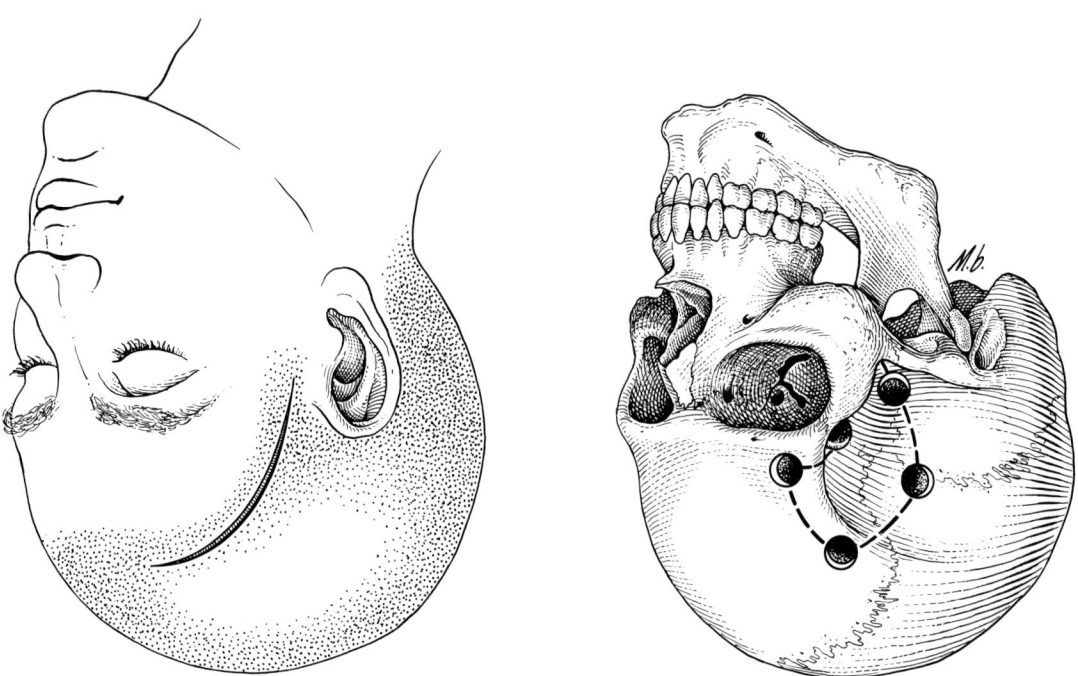

Fig. 12-11. Scalp incision and placement of bone flap for pterional craniotomy.

nificant problem, 40 mg of furosemide may also be given. The arterial pCO_2 is kept in the range of 25 to 30 torr during the procedure, and the patient is paralyzed and mechanically ventilated.

Burr holes are placed as illustrated in Fig. 12-11. If more frontal lobe exposure is needed, then more medially placed burr holes are made. Once the flap is elevated, the dura is tacked up to small holes previously drilled obliquely in the bone edges. Attention is then directed to the sphenoid ridge. The lateral aspect of the sphenoid ridge is drilled away flush with the frontal fossa (Fig. 12-12). This maneuver is combined with a small subtemporal craniectomy. The usual dural opening is shown in Fig. 12-12. The initial opening is curvilinear and situated 1½ to 2 cm back from the sphenoid ridge. The small dural flap is tacked back over the ridge. Several cruciate incisions are made in the dura overlying the frontal and temporal lobes.

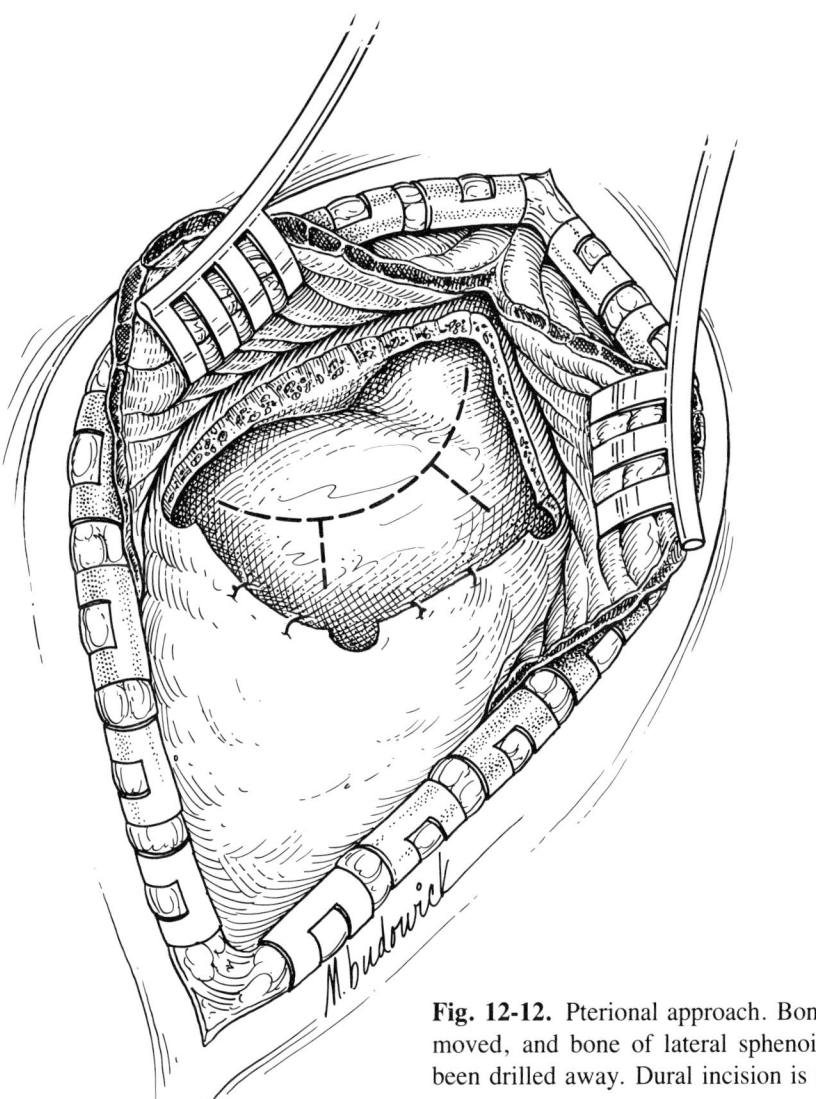

Fig. 12-12. Pterional approach. Bone flap is removed, and bone of lateral sphenoid ridge has been drilled away. Dural incision is indicated.

364 *Disorders of the pituitary*

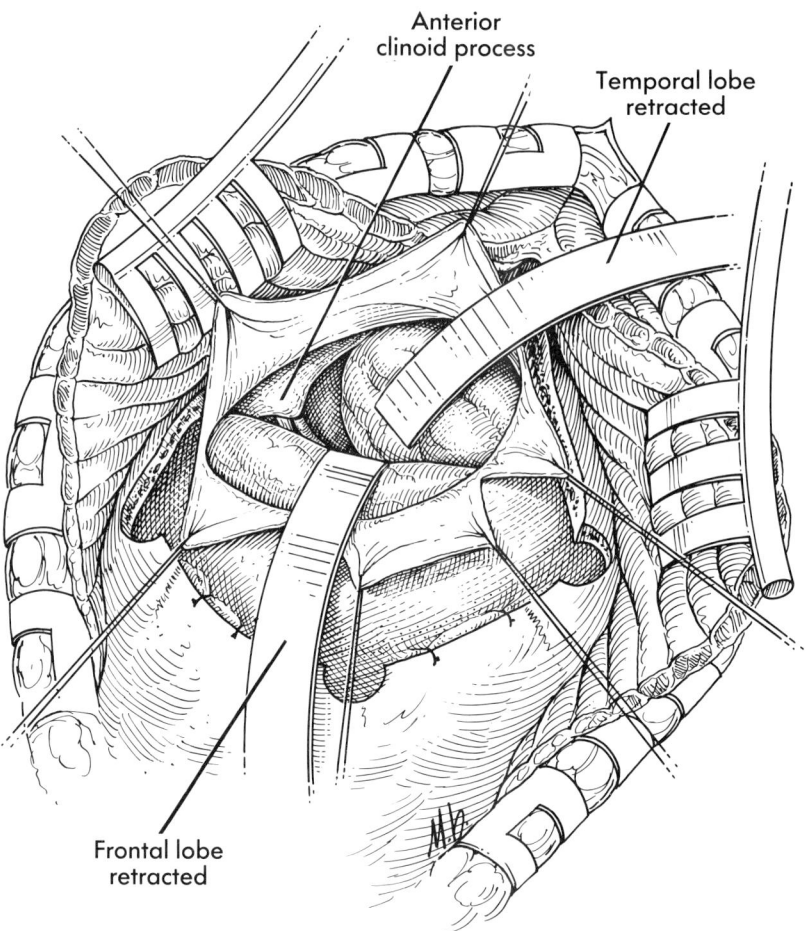

Fig. 12-13. Pterional approach. Subfrontal and temporal self-retaining retractors are in place. Anterior clinoid process, internal carotid artery, and optic nerve can be visualized.

A self-retaining retractor system of the surgeon's choice is set up, and two retractors—a frontal and a temporal—are generally employed. The frontal is usually the wider of the two retractors. The frontal blade is carefully placed beneath the frontal lobe and advanced exposing first the ipsilateral olfactory tract and then the optic nerve at the anterior clinoid. The temporal blade is used for retraction of the anterosuperior temporal lobe (Fig. 12-13). Once the retractors are set as just described, the operating microscope is brought into the field and used throughout the rest of the operation until closure is begun.

Figs. 12-14 and 12-15 illustrate the usual appearance of a pituitary adenoma and its relationship to neighboring anatomic structures as visualized by the transcranial approach. The "capsule" of the tumor is cauterized and incised, and the tumor is removed as thoroughly as possible using blunt curets and enucleators (Fig. 12-15). Since the arterial supply to the chiasm reaches this structure on its inferior aspect, no attempt should be made to remove an adherent capsule from beneath the optic nerves and chiasm, since this manuever may seriously impair vision.

Pituitary surgery **365**

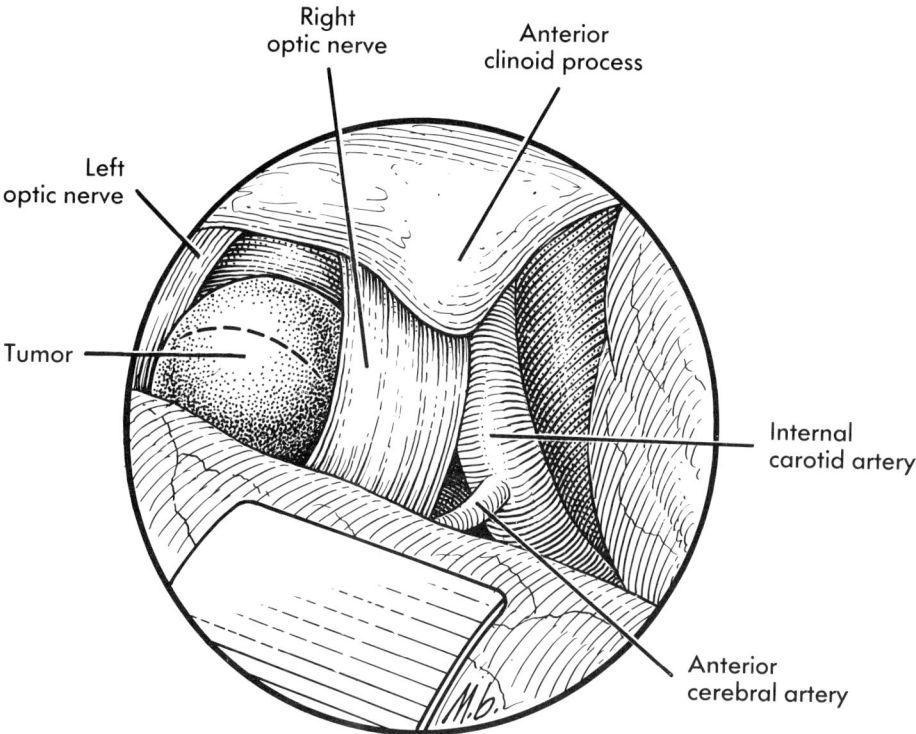

Fig. 12-14. Pterional approach. Further retraction and microdissection exposes tumor situated in space between optic nerves.

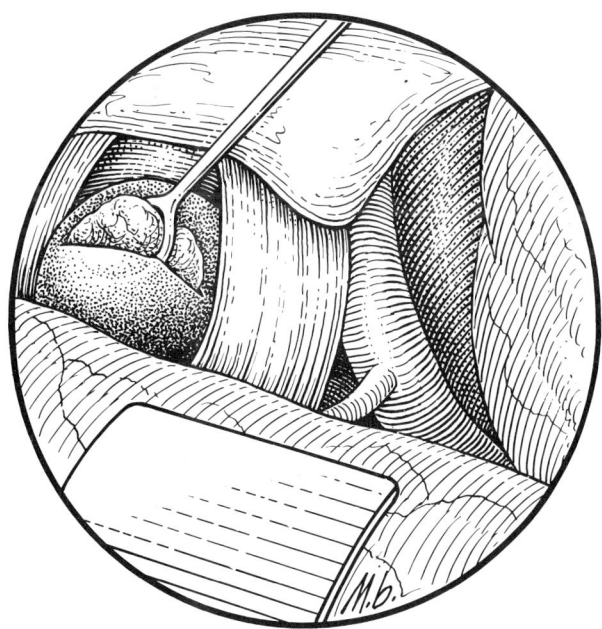

Fig. 12-15. Pterional approach. After cauterizing and opening "capsule," tumor is removed with blunt ring curets.

366 *Disorders of the pituitary*

With completion of definitive removal of the lesion, hemostasis should be meticulously obtained. The anesthesiologist is asked to perform a sustained Valsalva maneuver on the patient to raise venous pressure and to check for hemostasis before closure. The self-retaining retractors are then removed under direct vision, and closure of the wound is performed.

Subfrontal approach

The classic incision for the subfrontal approach begins on the midforehead and extends superiorly to the hairline and laterally within the hairline to the zygoma. A visible forehead scar can be avoided by making a bicoronal scalp incision (Fig. 12-16). The scalp flap is reflected downward to expose the frontal bone to the superior orbital ridge and midline. The crucial burr hole is the anterior medial one, which should be placed close to the midline and far forward (Fig. 12-16). The frontal sinus should be avoided, but if large, the trephine will often enter the sinus. In this situation, the sinus is exenterated as well as possible and the open sinus then closed with a muscle, adipose tissue, or fascial graft. The posterior medial burr hole is made at approximately the level of the hairline and is usually placed about 1 cm off the midline. The lateral burr holes are placed as indicated in Fig. 12-16 with or without trephines between, depending on the surgeon's preference. The dural opening is based medially and the right frontal

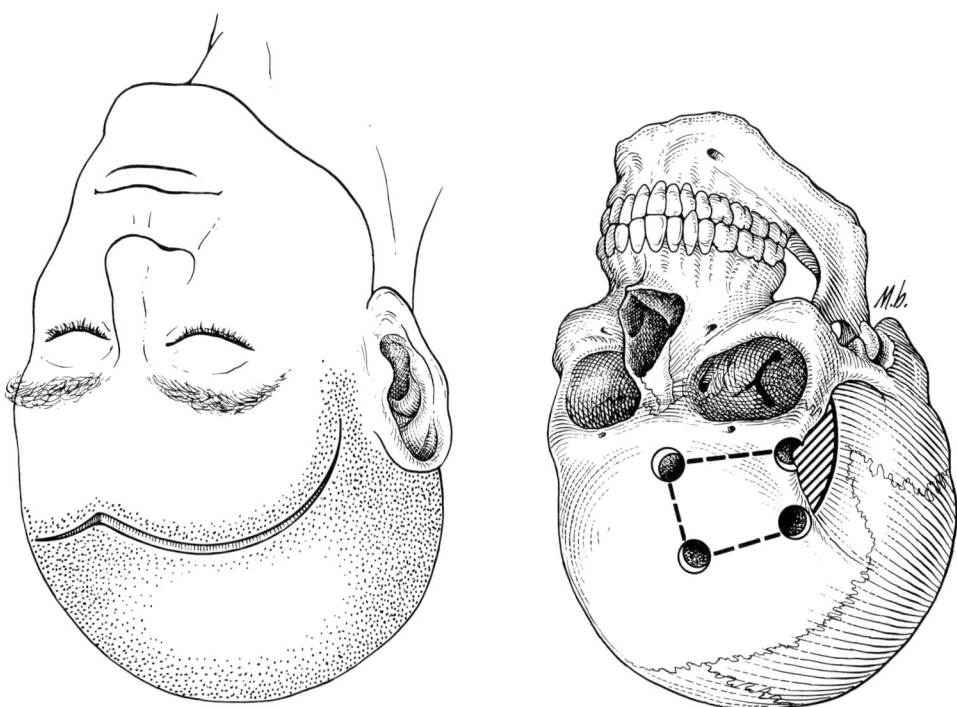

Fig. 12-16. Scalp incision and placement of bone flap for subfrontal approach.

lobe gently elevated and held with a self-retaining retractor. In the process of making a subfrontal exposure, the right olfactory tract is interrupted behind the olfactory bulb. As the frontal lobe is gently elevated and the retractor advanced toward the tuberculum sella, the optic nerves and chiasm are visualized. If the chiasm is prefixed and it appears that the tumor cannot be reached in the space between the anterior chiasm and the tuberculum sella, then the surgeon may choose to drill off the tuberculum sella with a high-speed drill so that the superoanterior portion of the sella can be entered through the superior portion of the sphenoid sinus.[64] This maneuver will diminish the retraction that is necessary to obtain exposure if one encounters a prefixed chiasm. When the sphenoid sinus is opened, care should be taken to seal it off before closure to avoid a postoperative CSF leak.

Subtemporal approach

The subtemporal approach can be made using the incision shown in Fig. 12-17. The incision is extended to the zygomatic arch to perform a temporal craniectomy down to the floor of the middle fossa. It is mandatory that the brain be slack before the temporal lobe is retracted upward to expose the retrochiasmal suprasellar extension of tumor.

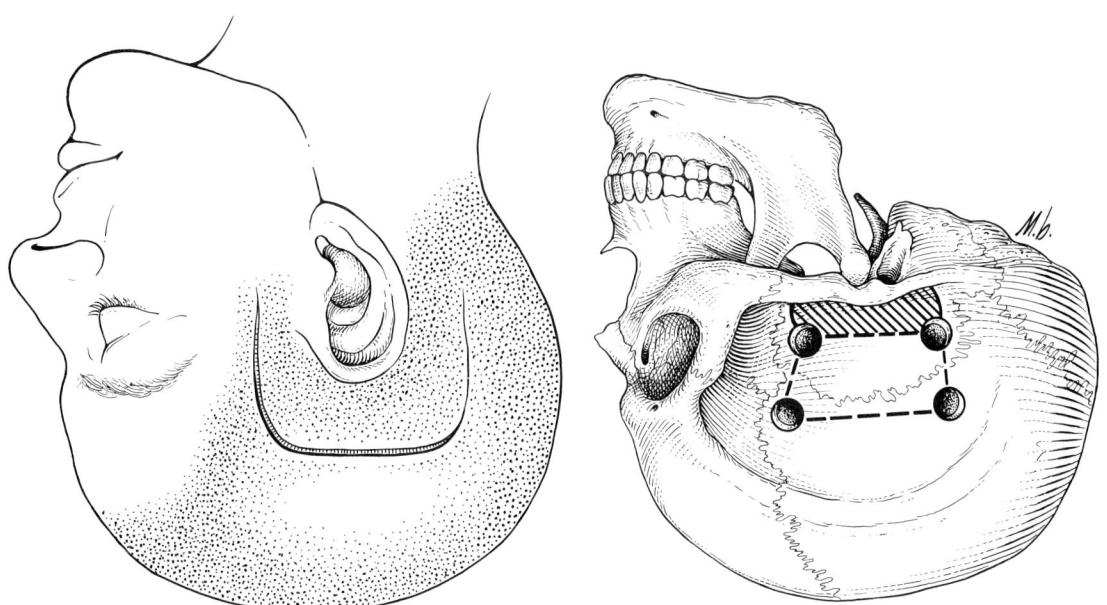

Fig. 12-17. Scalp incision and placement of bone flap for subtemporal approach.

TRANSSPHENOIDAL APPROACHES
Indications

Transsphenoidal surgery is currently the preferred approach for the surgical management of the vast majority of pituitary tumors. Absolute indications for transsphenoidal surgery over transcranial approaches in pituitary tumors include (1) tumor extension into the sphenoid sinus, (2) intrasellar microadenomas, (3) tumor associated with CSF rhinorrhea, (4) tumor invading and destroying the sphenoid bone with multidirectional intracranial extensions, and (5) an intracranial operation that carries an excessive risk for a patient such as an elderly person in poor health or a patient that has severely compromised vision. Occasionally, pituitary apoplexy may fall into this category when the surgeon wishes a relatively rapid decompression of the optic chiasm.

Other indications for this approach include intrasellar craniopharyngioma, hypophysectomy, repair of CSF fistula involving the sphenoid sinus, biopsy and/or excision of lesions in the sphenoid and parasellar area including chordoma, nasopharyngeal carcinoma, sphenoid mucocele, abscess, or cyst.

Contraindications

Transsphenoidal surgery is contraindicated when the patient has an infectious process involving the sphenoid sinus, a suprasellar mass associated with a normal sella turcica, or a "bottleneck" connection between an intrasellar tumor and the dumbbell suprasellar extension (see Fig. 12-10). Also, as mentioned previously, one may want to consider a transcranial approach in patients with significant intracranial extension to the subfrontal, retrochiasmatic, or middle fossa regions (see Fig. 12-9). In our opinion, a conchal sphenoid sinus (Fig. 5-5) is not a contraindication to the transsphenoidal operative approach. With the use of air-driven, high-speed, angled drills, the bone can be removed safely, and the dura mater over the pituitary gland and/or tumor can be exposed.

Sublabial transsphenoidal technique

Antiseptic solution (such as povidone) is applied to the nose and mouth, and the area is draped with sterile towels. The left lower quadrant of the abdomen is prepped and draped to obtain adipose tissue for later insertion into the sella turcica and sphenoid sinus. In young women and girls, an attempt is made to keep this incision low below the "bikini line." A separate set of sterile instruments is used to obtain the adipose tissue graft.

Fig. 12-18 provides an orientation for subsequent illustrations of the transsphenoidal approach. The initial exposure is performed using magnifying loupes and a headlight. The upper lip is elevated by an assistant using a hand-held retractor.

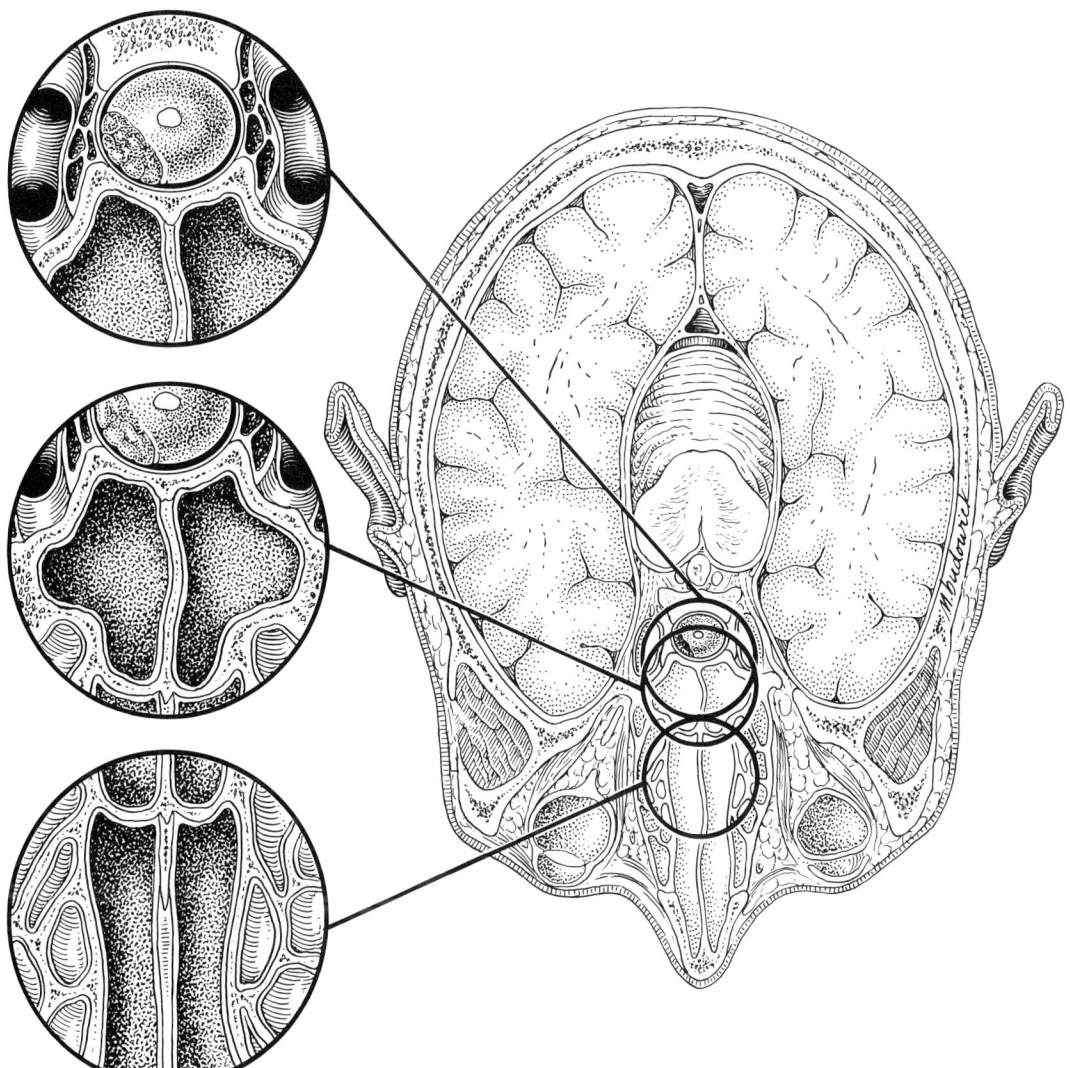

Fig. 12-18. Orientation for illustrations of transsphenoidal approach to pituitary. View is seen from above, and some of the insets that will be used in following illustrations depict steps in the procedure in a horizontal orientation.

370 *Disorders of the pituitary*

A small transverse incision is made in the upper gingival mucosa with a cutting cautery (Fig. 12-19). The use of this instrument considerably minimizes the bleeding that occurs whenever a simple scalpel cut is made in this area. A cuff of mucosa on the inferior gingival edge should be left to be used for later closure.

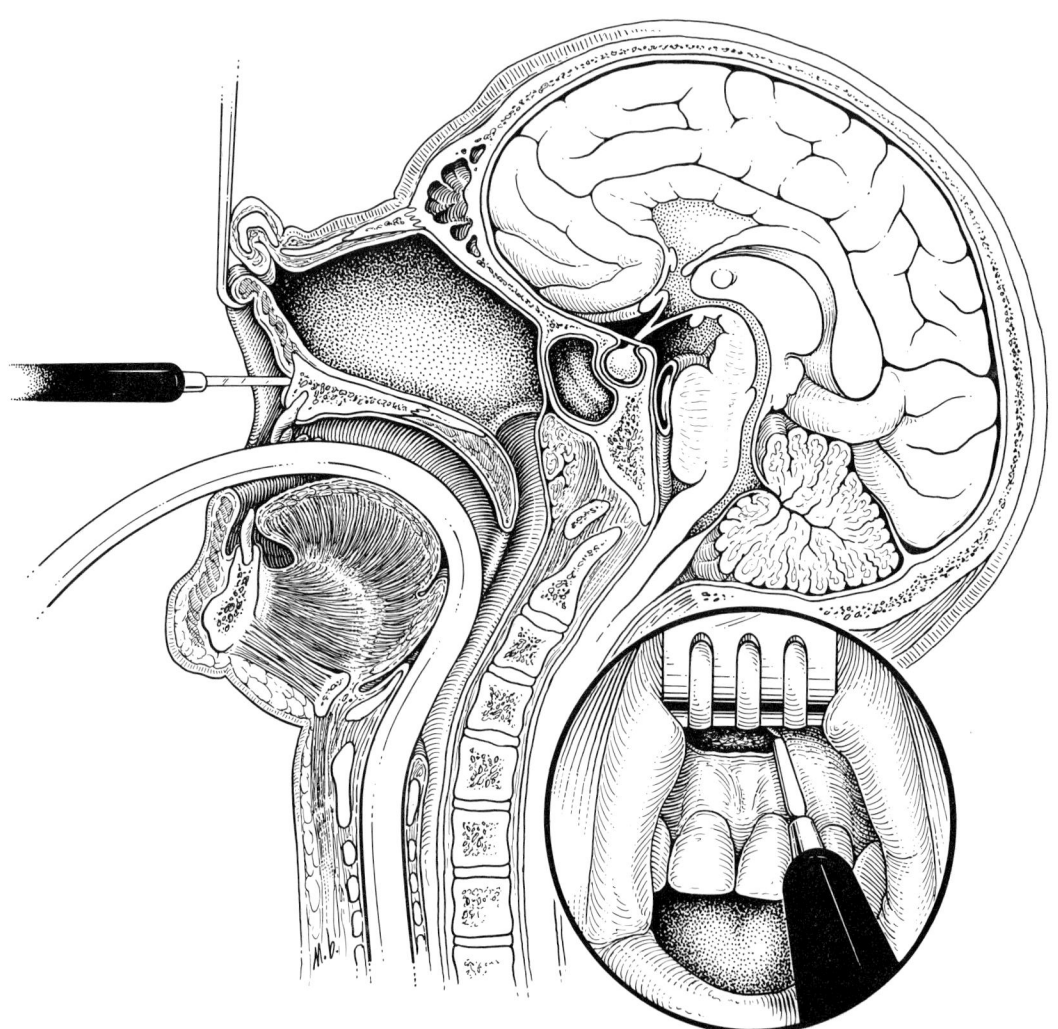

Fig. 12-19. Transsphenoidal approach. Incision in gingival mucosa with electrocautery.

The incision is carried down to the maxilla, and a blunt dissector is used to separate the soft tissue in an upward direction to expose the piriform aperture, the floor of the nares, and the nasal mucosa (Fig. 12-20).

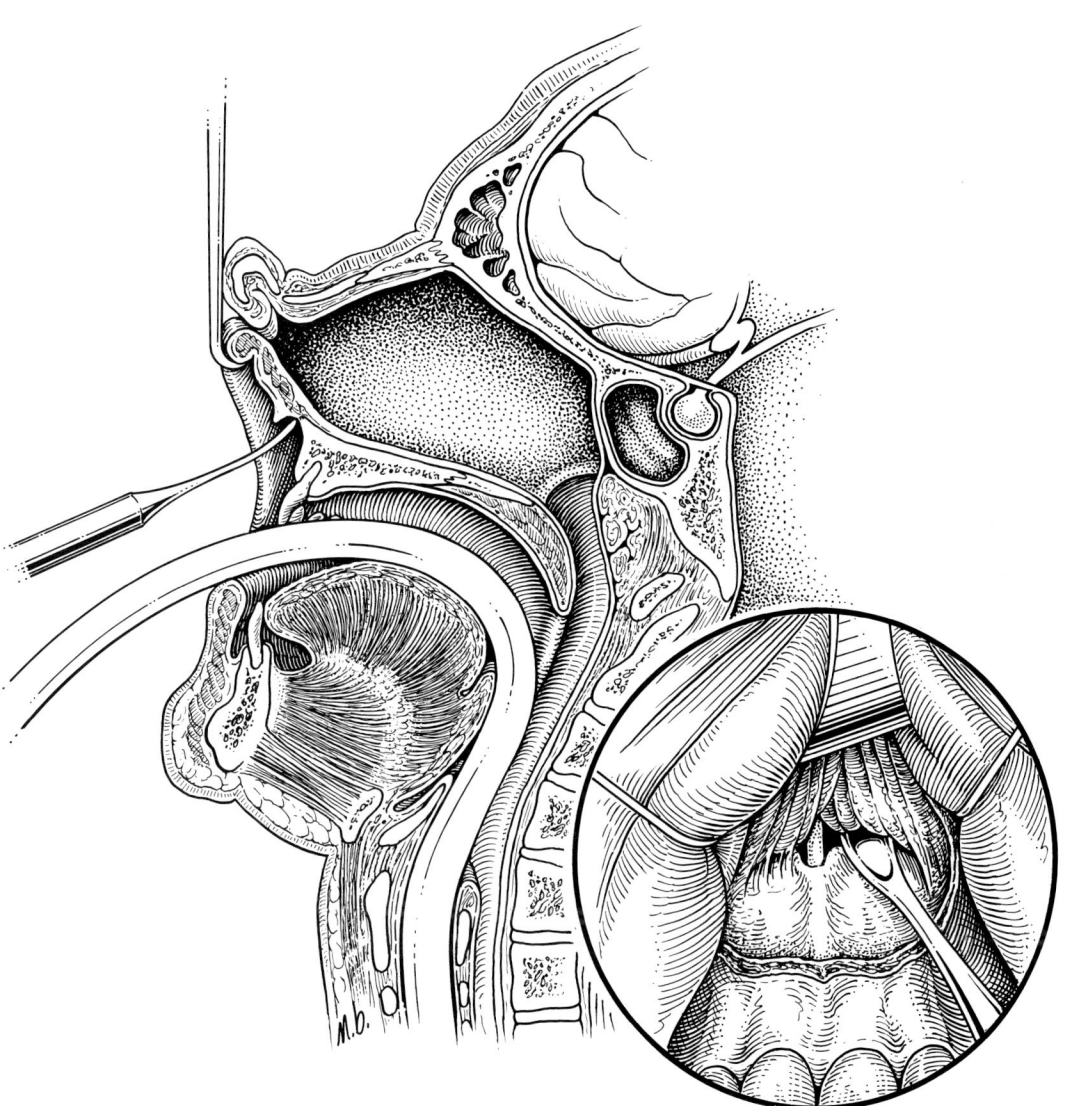

Fig. 12-20. Separation of soft tissue from maxilla to expose floor of nose and nasal mucosa.

With the cutting cautery in contact with a dissector, the tissue over the superior cartilaginous nasal septum is incised (Fig. 12-21). Extending the incision slightly into the cartilage facilitates a subchondral separation of the mucosa from the nasal septum on one side (determined by the surgeon's preference). We prefer using the patient's left side (i.e., separating the mucosa on the left from the left side of the septum).

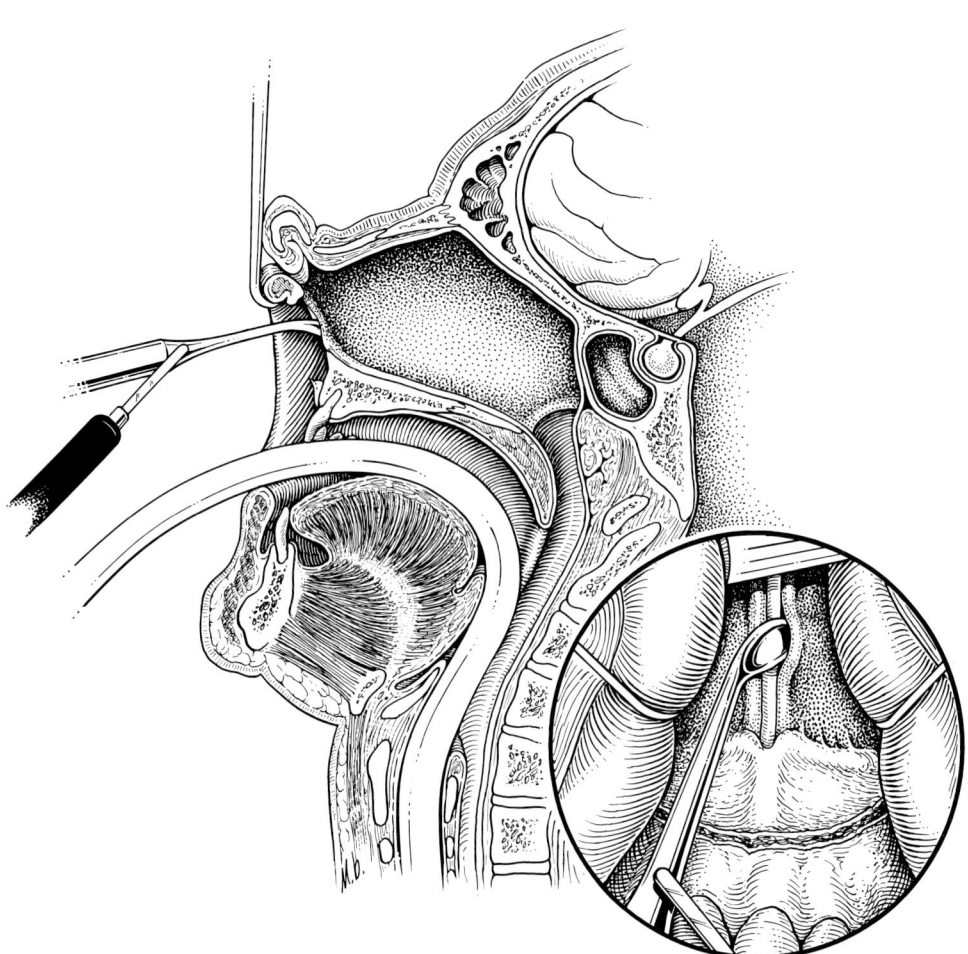

Fig. 12-21. Identification and development of plane between nasal septum and mucosa. Beginning of plane is made by cautery separating mucosa from septal cartilage.

Once the mucoperichondral plane between the septum and nasal mucosa is identified, it is developed inferiorly to the nasal spine using a small suction tip in the left and a dissector in the right hand (Fig. 12-22). At that level, the mucosa is often adherent to the spine, and considerable care should be taken to avoid a tear. The piriform aperture may have to be enlarged inferiorly and laterally with a small Kerrison punch.

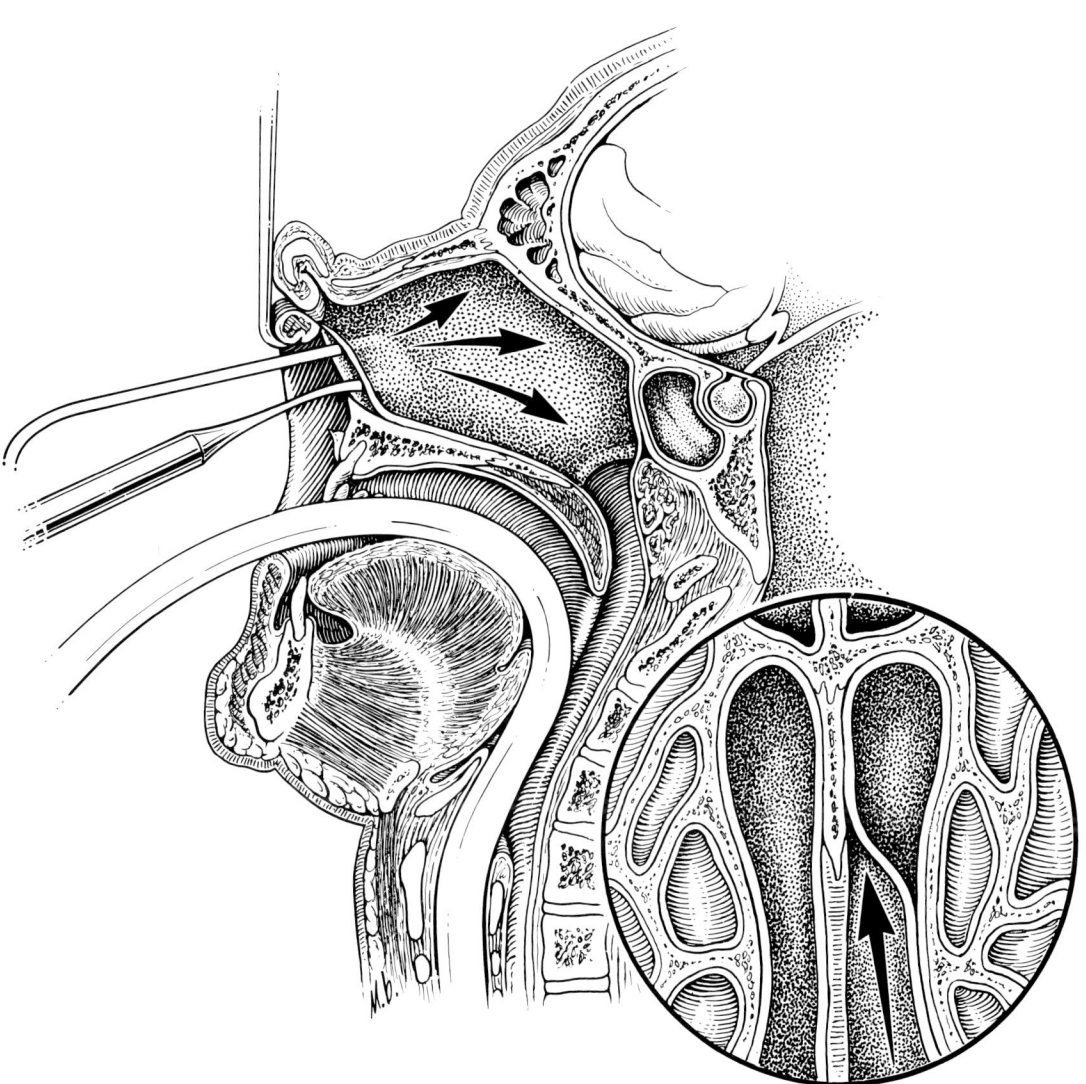

Fig. 12-22. Method of separation of nasal mucosa from septum. Separation is made on only one side (usually left) of septum (unilateral septal approach).

Next, the nasal septum is fractured at its base with a small osteotome, allowing it to be displaced to the opposite side. One of the palatine arteries, which are located anteromedially (see Fig. 1-8), may be the source of troublesome bleeding at this point and may require coagulation. Continued separation of mucosa from the nasal septum in a posterior direction is accomplished by the use of a small sucker held in the right hand and a nasal speculum with long, thin blades held in the left hand (Fig. 12-23). The blades are advanced and opened just enough to admit the tip of the sucker, which performs the actual separation of the mucosa from the nasal septum. As the separation proceeds posteriorly, the dissection becomes easier. At the posterior limit of the cartilaginous septum, a thin bony septum comprised of the superior portion of the vomer and inferior parts of the perpendicular plate of the ethmoid comes into view.

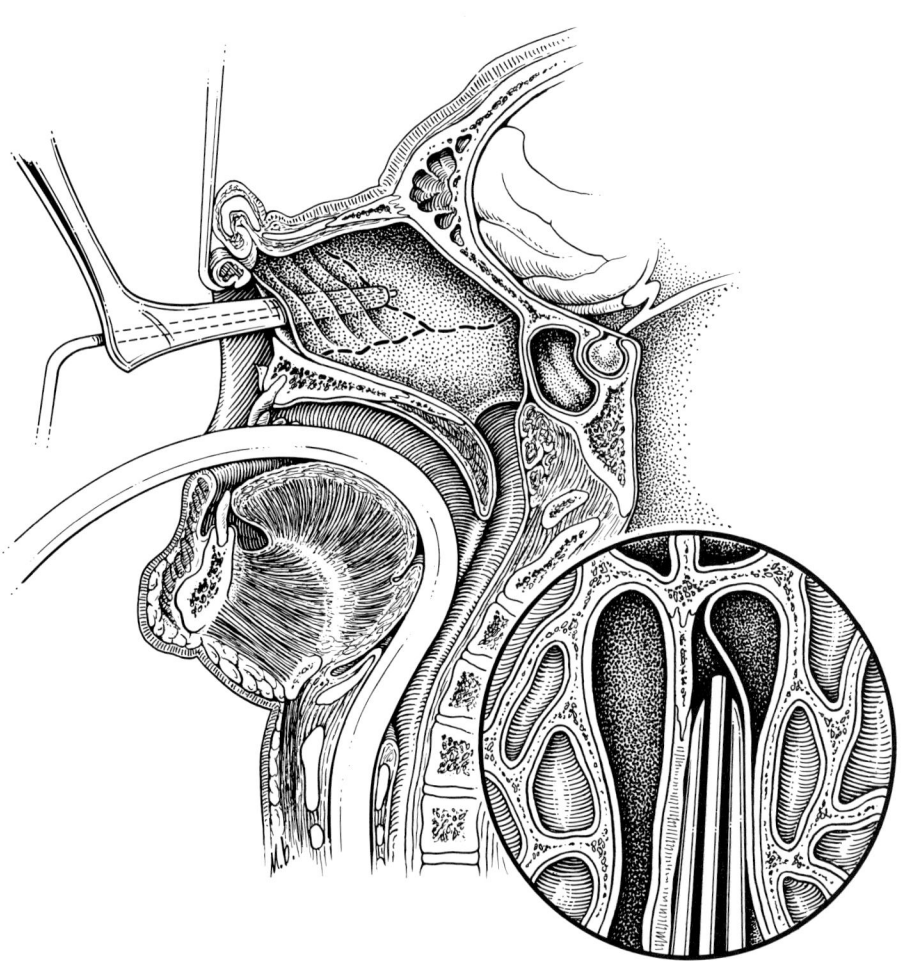

Fig. 12-23. Separation of mucosa from septum posteriorly using sucker tip and long, thin speculum.

Once the bony septum is seen, a speculum (e.g., Hardy type) is introduced between the septum and mucosa and opened (Fig. 12-24). This opening will fracture the thin perpendicular plate of the ethmoid near or at its junction with the sphenoid crest allowing one blade of the speculum to swing across the midline and thus expose both sides of the anterior wall of the sphenoid sinus. The anterior wall of the sphenoid sinus with its characteristic keel appearance is a distinctive structure easily recognized. The Hardy speculum is replaced with a Cushing-Landolt speculum, and its flanged tips are advanced to the anterior wall of the sphenoid sinus. The speculum is then opened exposing the sphenoid. Although the speculum is inserted unilaterally, displacement of the nasal septum to the patient's right side makes the orientation midline (if the surgeon is using the left side). From this point on, the operating microscope is used with a 300 mm objective lens and 12.5× oculars. The anterior wall of the sphenoid sinus is usually thin and can be opened with either Jansen-Middleton rongeurs, osteotomes, or Kerrison punches. The opening into the sinus can be started through the ostia of the sphenoid, located laterally.

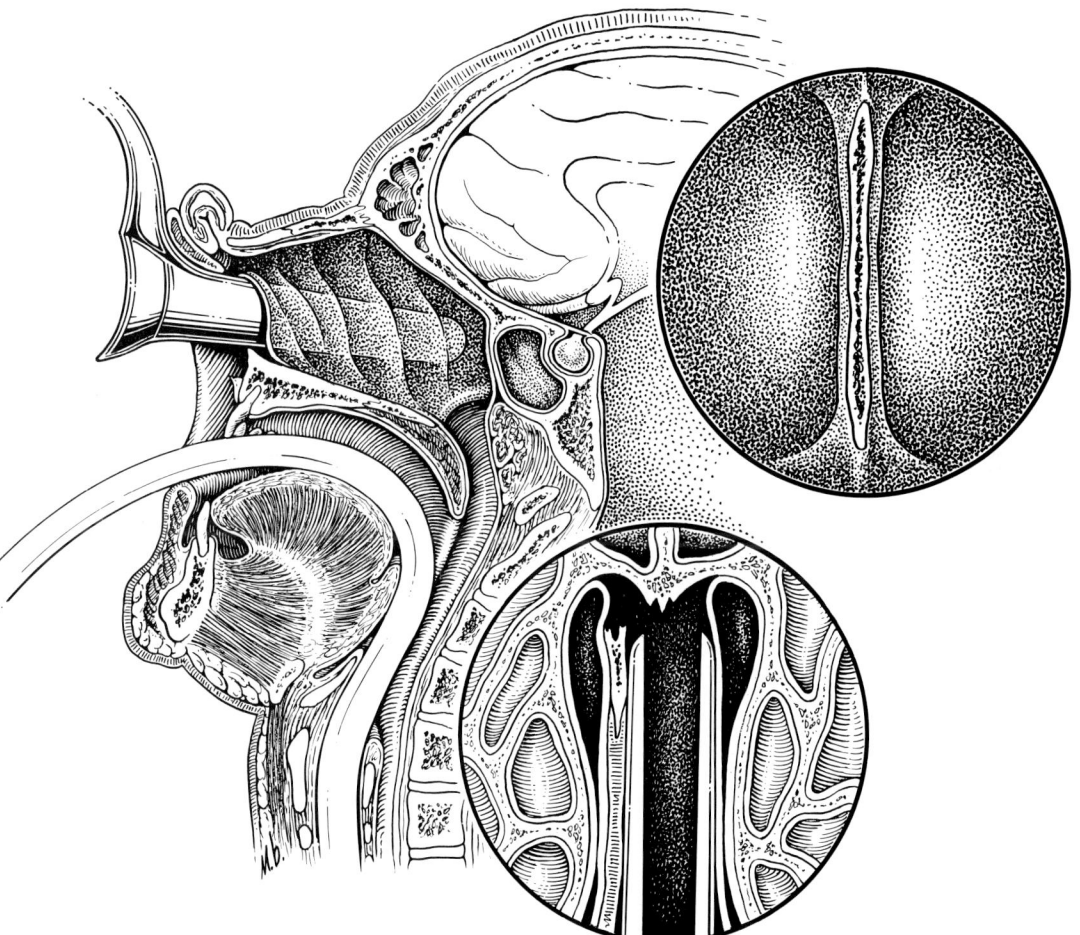

Fig. 12-24. Insertion and opening of bivalved speculum posteriorly fractures thin bony septum near or at sphenoid crest and exposes anterior wall of sphenoid sinus on both sides.

The opening in the sinus is made slightly larger than the speculum blades. The lateral extensions of the sphenoid opening are carried just far enough to visualize the most lateral aspect of the sella. The sphenoid mucosa can be cauterized and shrunk using an insulated suction cautery. The speculum tip is advanced into the sinus and gently opened by hand only. This maneuver brings the surgeon closer to the sella and brings the long axis of the speculum directly in line with the center of the sella turcica (Fig. 12-25). It should be emphasized that although advancing the tips of the speculum into the sinus as just described offers technical advantage, there is also potential danger of fracturing the sphenoid bone if force is used to open the speculum. Thus one should not use excessive force and certainly not a speculum-spreading instrument when the tips of the speculum are positioned within the sphenoid sinus.

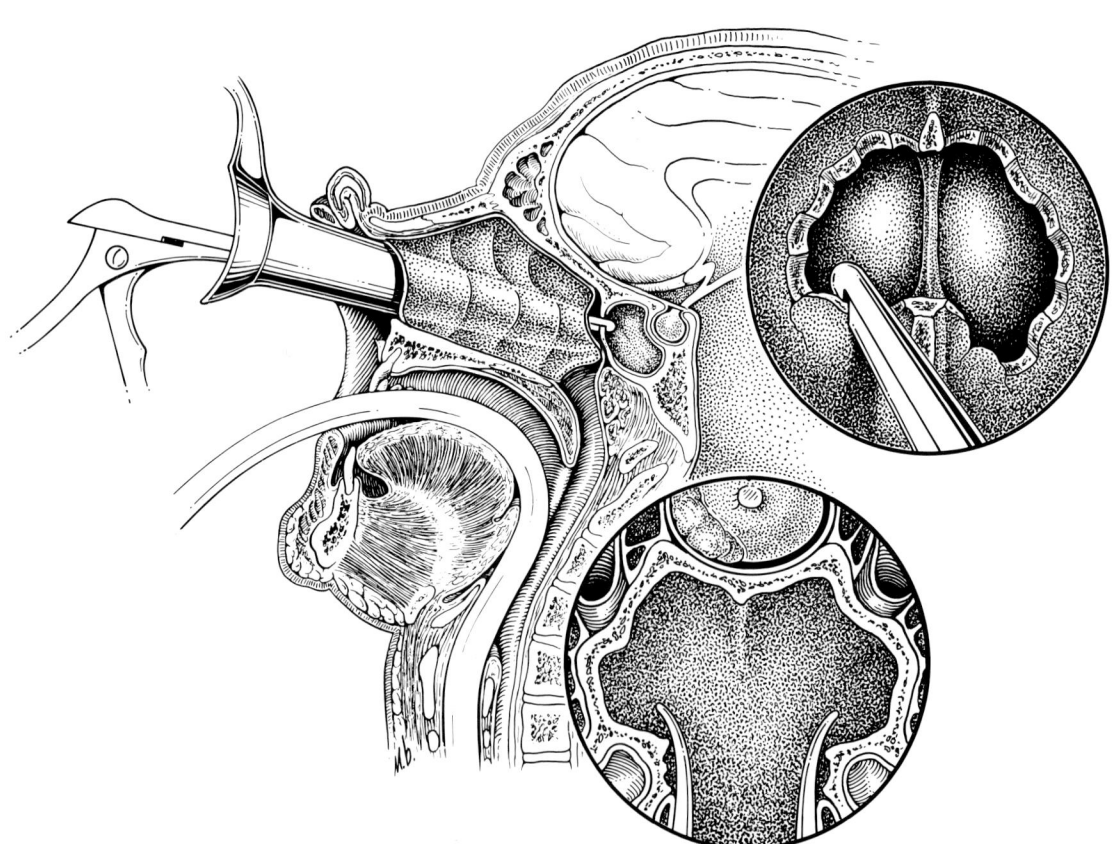

Fig. 12-25. Anterior wall of sphenoid sinus is opened, and flanged tips of the speculum are gently placed within sinus.

Once the surgeon visualizes the interior of the sphenoid sinus, positive identification of the sellar floor should be made. With a fully pneumatized sphenoid sinus (sellar type, see Fig. 5-5), the recognition of the position of the sellar floor is straightforward. However, should any doubt exist in the surgeon's mind, a lateral skull x-ray can be obtained with a metallic marker such as a Kirchner wire lightly impacted into the anticipated position of the sellar floor (Fig. 12-26).

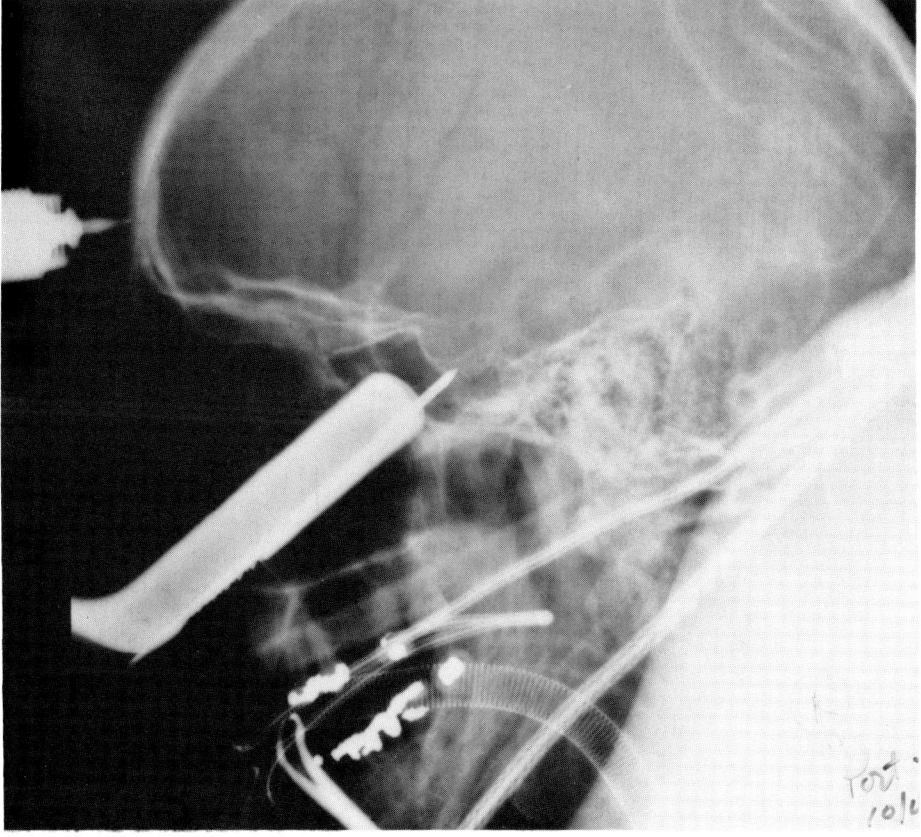

Fig. 12-26. Lateral x-ray film (intraoperative) showing position of metal marker identifying floor of sella.

An opening is made in the anterior wall of the sella with a small osteotome placed on the sellar floor. Light mallet taps on the base of the instrument will fracture the sella floor, thus initiating the opening (Fig. 12-27). The opening is then enlarged with a small punch laterally as far as the cavernous sinus and carotid bulge, inferiorly to the sella floor, and superiorly to the intercavernous sinus (Fig. 12-28). Removing too much bone superiorly and exposing the interface between the frontobasal dura and diaphragm sella increase the chances for a CSF leak from that area. Some surgeons may elect to puncture the sellar contents with a long 18-gauge needle and aspirate before opening the dura although we virtually never perform this maneuver. Using this technique, one can aspirate a cystic adenoma or, more importantly, identify an unsuspected intrasellar aneurysm.

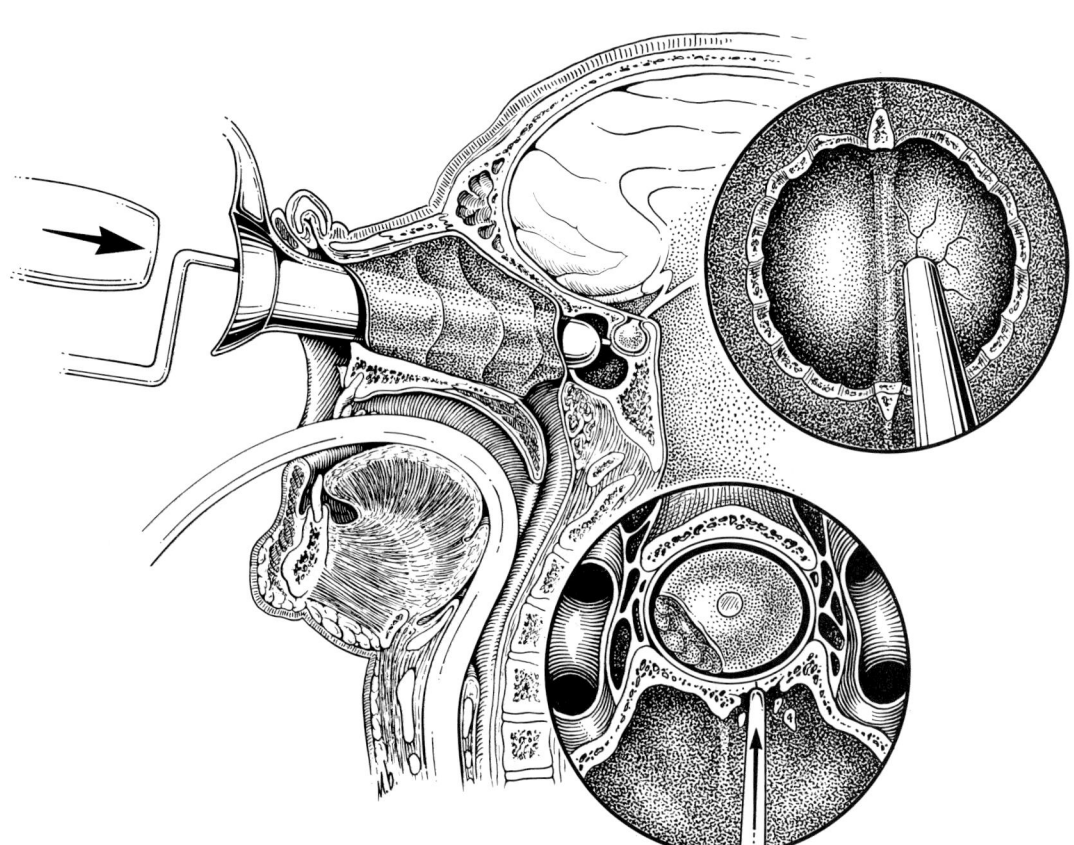

Fig. 12-27. Opening of floor of sella with a small osteotome.

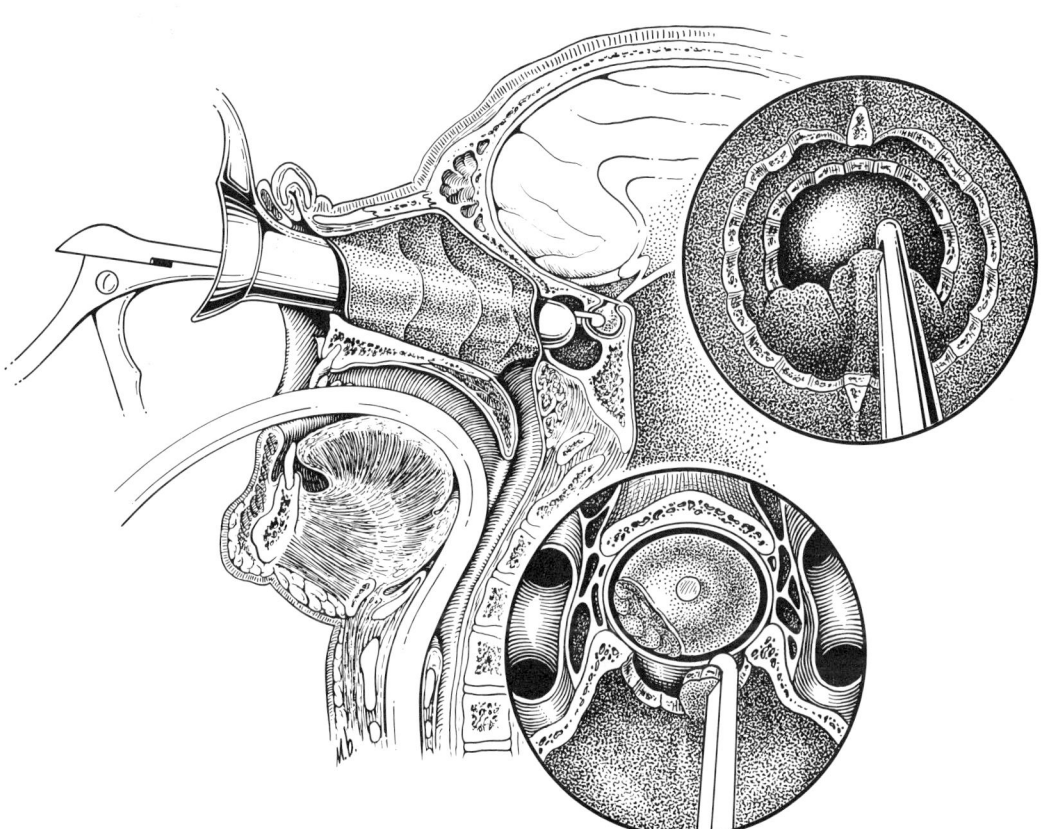

Fig. 12-28. Removal of sella floor with small Kerrison rongeur.

A vertical incision is made in the dura with a bayonet-handled scapel (#11) (Fig. 12-29). The dura is excised in an elliptic manner using angled microscissors (Fig. 12-30). If possible, a blunt hook is used to establish a plane between the dura and pituitary gland or tumor. If a plane is inadvertently developed between the two layers of the dura, especially laterally, one will be in communication with the cavernous sinus and could engender considerable bleeding. Additional radiating cuts can be made to enlarge the dural opening, and the edges can be coagulated with the bipolar cautery.

Since many pituitary tumors are small, it is important to avoid damage to the pituitary gland during dural opening. Lacerations in the gland with consequent subcapsular bleeding obscure the subtle differences that may exist between normal gland and tumor. Usually the tumor is readily visible and is removed easily with blunt ring curets, enucleators, and/or suction (Fig. 12-31 and Plate 3).

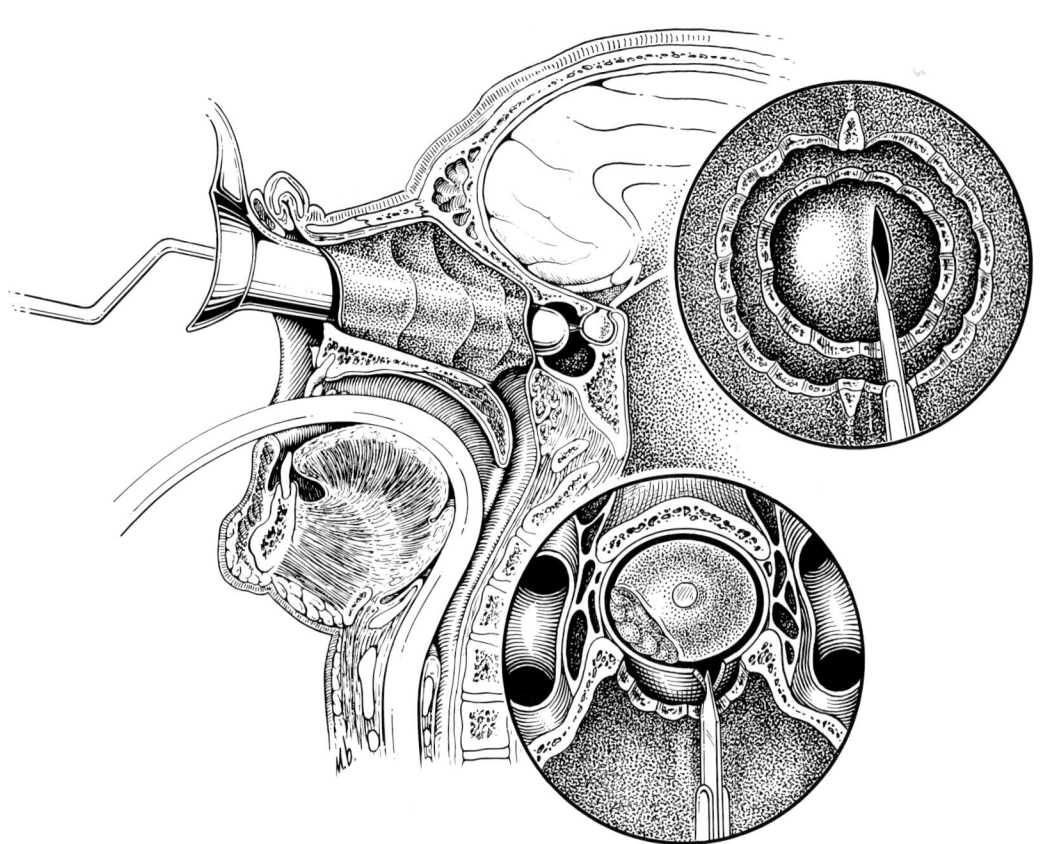

Fig. 12-29. Incision in dura covering pituitary gland.

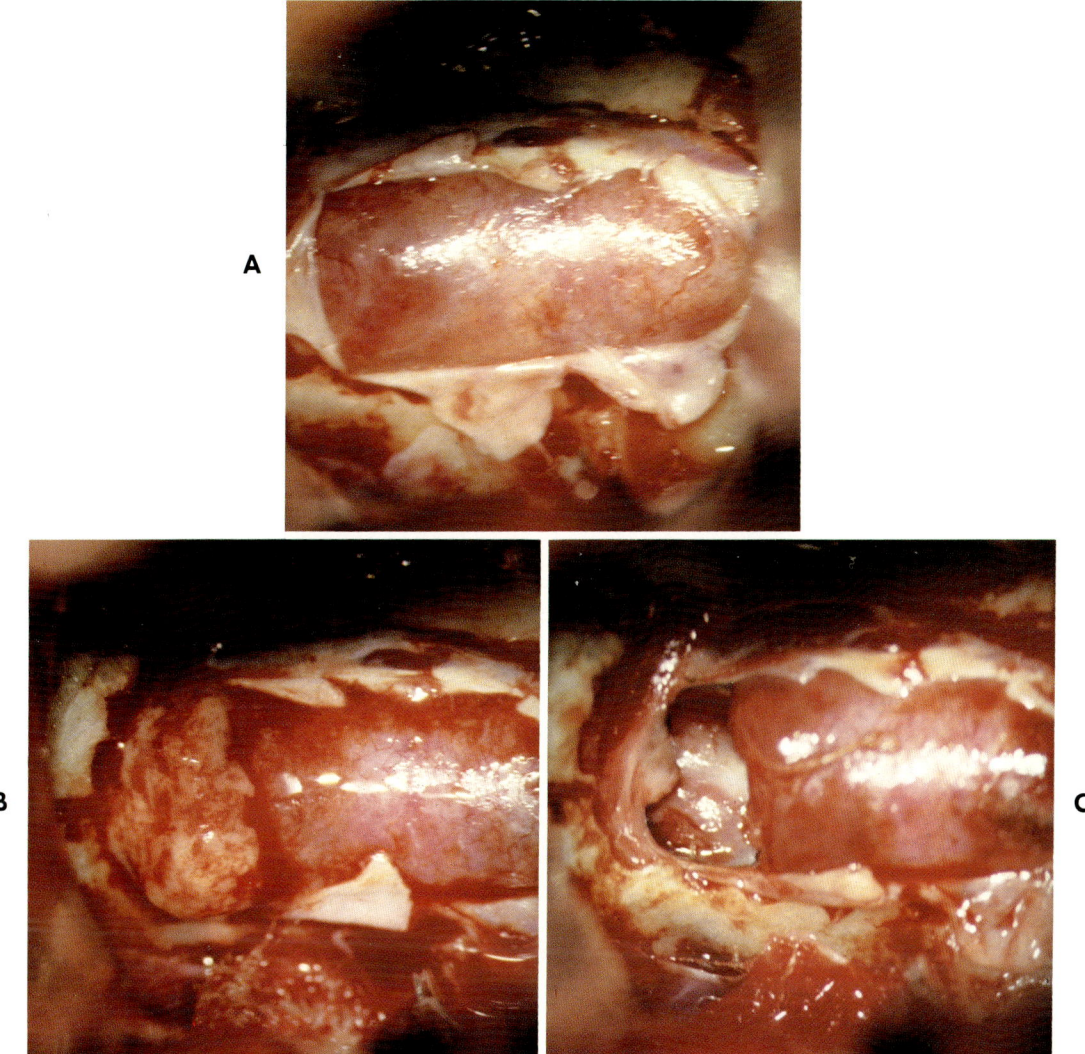

Plate 3. Operative appearance of microadenoma. Operative photo showing appearance of microadenoma in lateral *(left)* portion of normal gland (**A**), tumor separated from gland and ready for excision (**B**), and appearance of normal gland and tumor bed after excision of microadenoma (**C**). Patient was 26-year-old woman with amenorrhea-galactorrhea syndrome. Preoperative serum prolactin was 180 ng/ml.

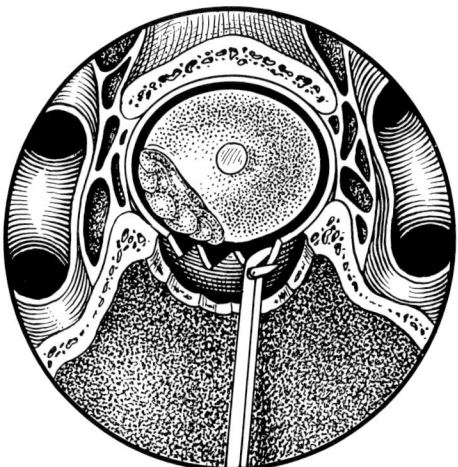 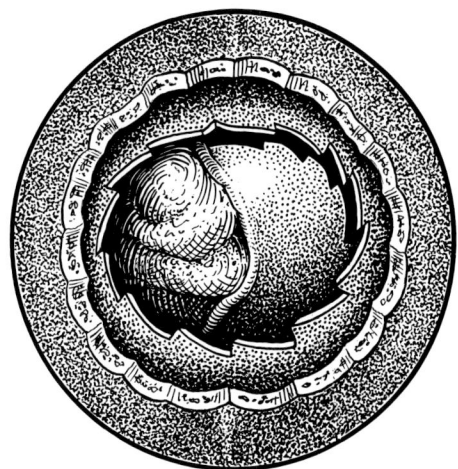

Fig. 12-30. Dura over pituitary gland and adenoma is opened with small angled microscissors.

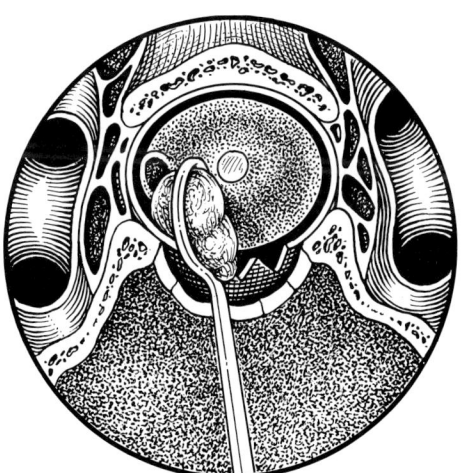 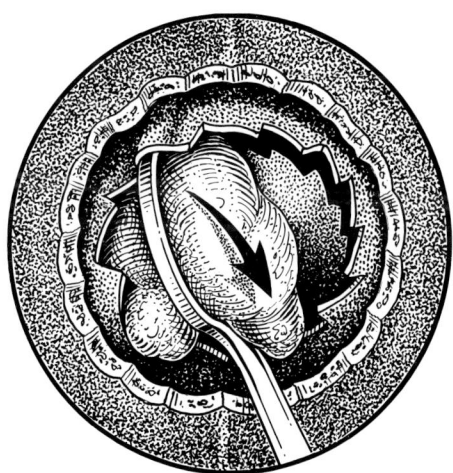

Fig. 12-31. Adenoma (microadenoma) is removed using blunt curets and/or enucleators.

Larger tumors frequently erode the floor of the sella and are encountered in the sphenoid sinus or extrude into the sphenoid on opening the dura. Even with large tumors, a thin, flattened pituitary gland can usually be identified and spared. It is generally displaced posteriorly and superiorly. If the tumor has suprasellar extension, this can be removed after evacuation of the intrasellar portion. In many cases, preserving a cuff of tumor in the anterior and superior aspect of the sella provides a handle to manipulate the remaining suprasellar extension to remove it. The diaphragm sella and tumor capsule can be inverted into the sella by carefully raising ICP using a slow infusion of Ringer's solution through the lumbar subarachnoid catheter. The tumor is then carefully peeled off the diaphragm with gentle suction.

Microadenomas with diameters of 5 mm or less are often not apparent after opening the dura. Exploration of the gutter between the cavernous sinus and lateral lobes with an enucleator will occasionally expose the lesion. If the tumor is still not apparent, lateral vertical incisions will usually expose prolactin and growth hormone-secreting adenomas, whereas ACTH-secreting adenomas are more apt to be midline. Asymmetries and thinning of the sella floor on polytomography or computed tomography (CT) are undependable in determining tumor location. Low-density lesions seen on CT are sometimes of localizing value.

The tumor bed will usually stop bleeding once all neoplasm is removed. After removal of the tumor, in the absence of any CSF leak, absolute alcohol can be applied to the tumor bed for a period of about 5 minutes. This is an optional maneuver designed to destroy remaining tumor cells. One should not use alcohol if there has been a tear in the diaphragm sella. The tumor bed and sphenoid sinus are loosely packed with adipose tissue previously taken from the abdomen, and the speculum is withdrawn (Fig. 12-32). The surgeon may use tissue adhesive (cyanoacrylate) to hold the adipose tissue in place, making sure the speculum is out of the way. One or two absorbable catgut sutures are used to close the gingival mucosa. Soft rubber nasal airway tubes are placed in each nostril to reapproximate the nasal mucosa and are left in place for only 24 hours. The nasopharynx and mouth are suctioned well, and if a lumbar subarachnoid catheter was used, it is removed before awakening the patient.

Hypophysectomy

Exposure of the pituitary gland is performed as described above. After the dura is opened, the gland is freed from any dural attachments. Gentle downward traction is placed on the superior surface of the gland with the suction tip in the left hand, and the stalk is cut with fine alligator-action scissors (Fig. 12-33). The gland is removed from the sella using a pituitary rongeur. The surgeon should make an attempt to remove the gland in one piece. The sella and sphenoid are loosely packed with adipose tissue, and closure is routine as described above.

Pituitary surgery **383**

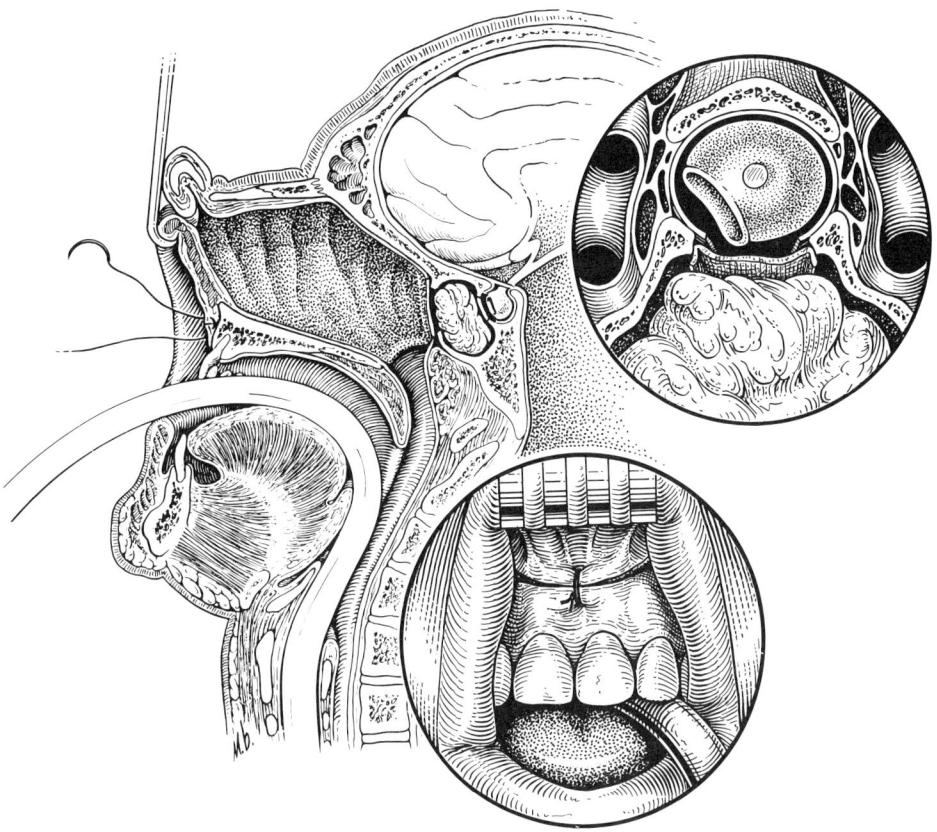

Fig. 12-32. Closure of incision. Sphenoid sinus is lightly packed with adipose tissue, and gingival incision is closed with single absorbable suture.

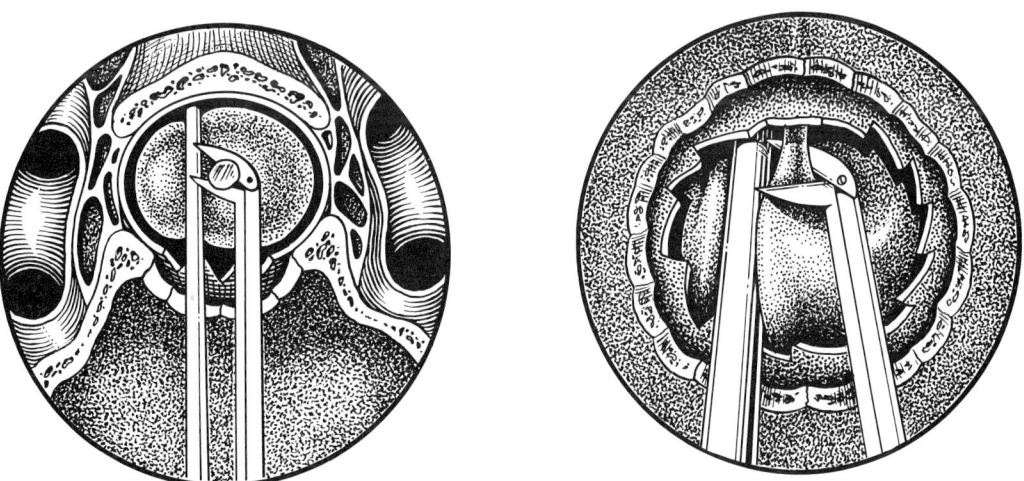

Fig. 12-33. Hypophysectomy technique. Gentle downward traction is placed on superior surface of gland, and stalk is cut at its junction with gland. Entire gland can then be removed from sella.

Variations

Transnasal midline transsphenoidal approach. Some surgeons still employ the transnasal midline bilateral septal transsphenoidal approach used by Halstead and Cushing and modified by Hardy. Although it provides excellent exposure, this technique involves bilateral separation of the mucosa from the nasal septum and removal of the lower portion of the septum. We prefer the unilateral septal technique described earlier because it can be performed in a shorter time period, removes none of the septum, carries less risk of a postoperative nasal septal perforation, and makes reoperation easier, if necessary, in the future.

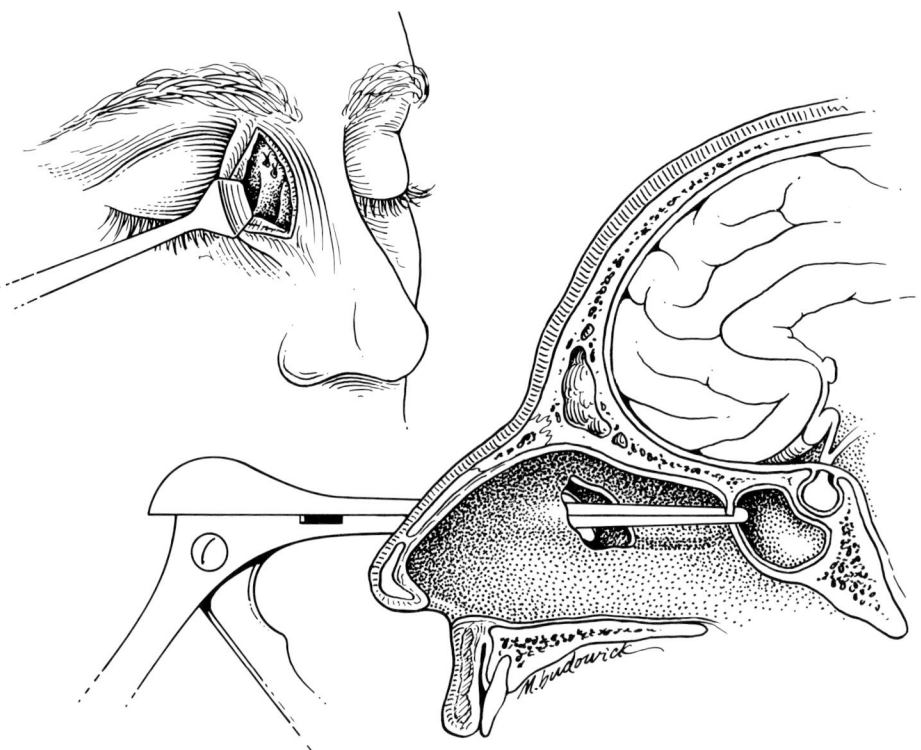

Fig. 12-34. Transethmoidal approach shows skin incision and surgical approach to sphenoid sinus and sella turcica.

Transethmoidal approach. The patient is placed prone with the head elevated about 20 degrees. The eyelids on the operative side are sutured, or plastic eye shields are inserted to protect the globe. A semicircular skin incision is made one half the distance between the dorsum of the nose and the medial canthus (Fig. 12-34). The inner canthal ligament and lacrimal sac are retracted laterally to expose the lacrimal fossa and the anterior and posterior ethmoid arteries. These arteries may be sacrificed, but their position is at the level of the cribriform plate and represents the superior limits of the bone dissection. The posterior ethmoid artery also marks the posterior limit of dissection because the buttress of the optic foramen lies only a few millimeters posteriorly.

Identification of the middle turbinate is accomplished by removing the lamina papyracea of the lacrimal fossa and incising the underlying nasal mucosa. The insertion of the middle turbinate is immediately lateral to the cribriform plate, which is directly parallel with the floor of the anterior fossa. Trauma to this area increases the potential of a postoperative CSF leak. The middle turbinate is removed, but its insertion is preserved as a landmark. The ethmoid air cell mucosa is removed transnasally, and the air cell is opened. A mucosal flap, based inferiorly, exposes the sphenoid ostium. Entrance into the sphenoid sinus is accomplished with small rongeurs and punches either directly through the ethmoidectomy or transnasally while directly observing transethmoidally (Fig. 12-34). The operating microscope is then brought into the field, and the sella is entered. Tumor removal or hypophysectomy is performed as described under the section on the transseptal approach. The pituitary fenestration and sphenoid sinus are obliterated with fat, and the inner canthal incision is closed in two layers.

The advantages of this procedure over the transseptal transsphenoidal approach are the shorter anatomic distance to the sphenoid, allowance for two-plane instrumentation (transnasal and transethmoidal), avoidance of contamination from the oral cavity, and avoidance of devitalization of the teeth. However, this procedure necessitates an external scar, is not a midline approach, and its plane of approach makes it more difficult to visualize the suprasellar area.

Transantral approach. The transantral approach seems to produce considerable blood loss and, like the transethmoidal approach, is not a midline procedure.

An incision is made in the buccal mucosa over the anterior wall of the maxillary sinus, and the underlying bone is removed. The medial bony wall of the sinus is resected to expose the soft nasal wall, which is mobilized. The inferior ethmoid sinus is entered, and the sphenoid sinus is exposed through the combined maxillectomy and inferior ethmoidectomy. The sphenoid sinus is opened to expose the sella turcica, and the remainder of the procedure is performed under magnification as described previously.

COMPLICATIONS

Complications of surgery for pituitary tumors and other parasellar lesions depend on the operative procedure used. Most large series in which a transcranial operation was used for pituitary tumors were reported before the use of modern microsurgical techniques, and thus comparisons with complications incurred during modern transsphenoidal surgery may be misleading. In addition, series that combine both approaches generally include the larger and more extensive lesions in the craniotomy group, thus increasing craniotomy-related complications by selection.

Operative complications—craniotomy

Hemorrhage. Bleeding may occur during any intracranial operation or may present in the postoperative period as an epidural, subdural, intracerebral, or suprasellar clot. During surgery the carotid artery may be torn and produce severe bleeding. The tumor itself may be the source of troublesome bleeding if the neoplasm is not totally removed. Bleeding from the cavernous sinus may occur, especially if the tumor invades this structure. As with other intracranial procedures, the operative site should be completely dry before closure. Postoperative extracerebral hematomas will usually manifest themselves by an altered level of consciousness with focal motor deficits. The relatively high incidence of postoperative hematomas in Cushing's experience (2.3%)[28] was related to his technique of stripping dura from the orbital roof to gain access to the sella, a procedure predisposed to the formation of epidural hematomas.[34] More recent series in which a transdural method is used cite lower incidences of postoperative hematomas. Suprasellar hematomas may not produce alterations in the level of consciousness unless they compress the diencephalon or produce acute hydrocephalus. The clot probably forms as a result of slow oozing from the tumor bed, and the only clinical sign may be a rapid loss of vision.

An intracerebral hematoma is usually the result of too vigorous retraction on either the frontal or temporal lobes. A relatively rapid alteration in the level of consciousness and focal deficits are the usual presenting findings in significant lesions.

Once a postoperative hematoma is suspected, a CT scan should be performed to confirm the suspicion, illustrate its location and amount of mass effect, exclude other complications, and help plan therapy. However, if the patient begins to deteriorate rapidly, it is appropriate to proceed immediately to the operating room for reopening of the wound without losing time waiting for a CT scan. Smaller hematomas without significant mass effect can often be managed medically by controlling intracranial hypertension, but large masses in a deteriorating patient should undergo immediate evacuation. A suprasellar hematoma causing visual loss should be removed. The prognosis for recovery of lost vision in the latter situation is guarded, however, even with prompt re-exploration.[68]

Cerebral edema, infarction, and elevated ICP. Cerebral edema either with or without infarction is usually the result of overzealous retraction of a lobe of the brain. This is more common with large suprasellar extensions where more retraction is needed for visualization. Modern adjuncts such as steroids, osmotic diuretics, controlled ventilation, microsurgery, and self-retaining retractors have diminished but not eliminated the problem. Infarction may occur as a result of damage to small perforating arteries off the internal carotid artery to the internal capsule, basal ganglia, or brainstem.[34]

An unusual and interesting cause of infarction is vasospasm following the removal of a pituitary adenoma. Mawk et al[53] described three cases in which angiographically proven vasospasm followed the removal of large pituitary adenomas, one resulting in death. The release of vasospastic substances from the necrotic tumor was suggested as an etiologic agent. Ono et al[61] believe such vasospasm is the result of bleeding into the basal cisterns during surgery. Should symptomatic proven vasospasm occur, treatment is directed toward maximizing cerebral blood flow through controlled hypertension, volume expansion, and hypervolemic hemodilution to optimize blood rheology.

Infection. Most cases of postoperative meningitis or abscess following craniotomy for parasellar lesions occur in those cases where exposure traverses the frontal sinus. Ray[66] reported an infection rate less than 2% among patients with frontal sinus entry operated on by the transfrontal route. His patients were treated for 10 days with antibiotics, and no fatal meningitis occurred in 168 cases. Based on the results of two large series,[1,9] Horwitz and Rizzoli[34] have estimated the mortality from meningitis following craniotomy for pituitary tumor to be between 1% and 1.5%.

At the earliest suspicion of a septic process, a CT scan should be performed to rule out the presence of mass effect, and a lumbar puncture with CSF examination should follow. The patient is treated with broad-spectrum antibiotics until culture results are available, at which time antibiotic administration is tailored to the specific organism.

Damage to parasellar structures. Any of a variety of intracranial structures are subject to injury during the transcranial removal of sellar lesions. The possibility of hemorrhage resulting from injury to the carotid artery and its branches or the cavernous sinus has been mentioned previously.

Certain cranial nerves are prone to injury. Anosmia can occur following a frontal craniotomy, especially with a direct frontal approach as used by Ray.[65] Unilateral loss of smell occurs in many patients after a standard transfrontal approach and is much reduced with the frontotemporal approach.

Postoperative suprasellar hematoma was mentioned previously as a cause of visual deterioration. Other potential causes for damage to the optic nerves or chiasm include direct damage from surgical instruments[34] and manipulation of these structures, which may produce a permanent worsening of vision probably caused by disruption of the vascular supply.[68] In an anatomic study by Bergland and Ray,[3] the arterial supply to the decussating fibers of the chiasm was shown to be supplied inferiorly by small branches from the circle of Willis. Thus an overly vigorous attempt to remove an adherent capsule from the inferior surface of the chiasm may devascularize this structure that already has marginal perfusion as a result of the mass effect. Old age, large tumors, preoperative visual loss, and prior treatments for the tumor seem to predispose the patient to this unfortunate complication. Visual deterioration resulting from the swelling of oxidized cellulose used to control intraoperative bleeding has been reported.[34,62] In one case, vision was restored after the removal of the substance.[34]

Another cause of visual deterioration following transcranial surgery for pituitary tumors is downward migration of the optic chiasm and/or nerves into a partially empty sella, which in turn results from the removal of a large adenoma. This condition can sometimes be corrected by inserting fat, a silicone sponge,[77] bone, or cartilage[16] into the sella after removing the adenoma, thus providing a prop for the chiasm and optic nerve. Muscle tissue is not a particularly good substance to use for this purpose because it may atrophy, thus allowing prolapse of the visual structures into the sella.[35] Transcranial lysis of adhesions to the chiasm has been reported to be curative of chiasmal migration.[59] Guiot has attributed this same problem to a "pushing" mechanism resulting from hydrocephalus.[17]

The surgeon should monitor the patient's postoperative visual status carefully, and if there is any deterioration, an intense search for a reversible cause should be initiated. A CT scan is valuable in differentiating the various potential causes and in planning definitive therapy.

Those cranial nerves that traverse the cavernous sinus—the oculomotor, trochlear, and abducens nerves and ophthalmic and maxillary divisions of the trigeminal nerves—may be damaged during a transcranial approach. Such damage can occur from manipulation of the extracavernous portion of the nerves or as a result of excessive pressure applied to the cavernous sinus. Fortunately, many of the third and sixth cranial nerve palsies are transient. MacKay and Hosobuchi[51] reported a permanent third cranial nerve palsy after purposely entering the cavernous sinus in an attempt to remove an invasive adenoma.

Either direct surgical manipulation during craniotomy or postoperative hemorrhage may cause injury to the pituitary stalk and/or hypothalamus. Diabetes insipidus is often transient after manipulation of these structures. However, if diabetes insipidus is prolonged or permanent, it can be treated with parenteral vasopressin (Pitressin) replacement or with intranasal desmopressin acetate (DDAVP) (see Chapter 15). Damage to the supraoptic and paraventricular nuclei or their connections to the neural lobe of the pituitary via the pituitary stalk may produce permanent diabetes insipidus. The condition should be suspected if the patient excretes dilute urine (specific gravity 1.005 or less/osmolality below 200 mOsm/kg) in the face of a high serum osmolality (300 mOsm/kg or more). In 100 patients who underwent transcranial surgery for a pituitary tumor reported by Symon and Jakubowski,[73] almost half had transient and 13% had permanent diabetes insipidus.

Damage to the hypothalamus may also produce neurogenic hyperthermia. Erickson[10] described the autopsy findings in 20 patients dying of this condition and found gross lesions in the hypothalamus and brainstem. Patients with damage to these structures lose the ability to dissipate heat and thus become hyperthermic, usually with a failure to regain consciousness or a decline in the level of consciousness if previously awake. Most of the reports of this condition are from the older literature. Three of Cushing's cases died as a result of neurogenic hyperthermia,[28] as did three patients from the series of Grant[13] and Olivecrona.[1]

Laws[46] in 1976, however, reported one such case after a transsphenoidal operation for a pituitary adenoma. Kahn[38] described the pathophysiology as a splanchnic pooling of blood and peripheral vasoconstriction combined with a diminished circulatory volume. He recommends avoidance of cooling, which exacerbates the peripheral vasoconstriction, and advocates volume replacement for the hypovolemia, mild application of heat and friction to promote vasodilatation, application of external cooling only to warm surface areas, and the administration of high-dose intravenous glucocorticoids.[34,38]

Operative mortality—craniotomy. Table 12-1 summarizes the mortality figures associated with craniotomy for pituitary tumors from major published series. There is a wide range in reported mortality with figures ranging from 1.4% (Ray and Patterson)[66] to 24% (Nürnberger and Korey).[57] The mortality figures for craniotomy contrast sharply with those associated with transsphenoidal surgery (see p. 391 and 397).

Operative complications—transsphenoidal approach

One of the first reports of a complication of transsphenoidal adenomectomy was published by Halstead in 1910.[22] In one of two patients operated in 1909 by a sublabial transsphenoidal approach, he described a surgical death with a clinical course suggestive of hypothalamic damage.

Complications of transsphenoidal surgery can be divided anatomically and are listed as follows:

Parasellar
  CSF leakage
  Hypopituitarism
  Diabetes insipidus
  Damage to cavernous sinus
  Intracavernous cranial nerve
    damage
  Intracavernous internal carotid
    artery damage
  Hemorrhage
  False aneurysm
  Carotid-cavernous sinus
    fistula
Intracranial
  Intracranial hemorrhage
  Hypothalamic damage

Intracranial—cont'd
  Meningitis
  Optic chiasm or nerve damage
  Cerebral vasospasm
  Embolization
Sphenoid and nasofacial
  Sinusitis
  Mucocele
  Fracture of hard palate
  Fracture of cribriform plate
  Nasoseptal perforation
  External nasal deformity
  Devascularization or denervation of
    teeth

Table 12-1
Mortality figures for craniotomy for pituitary tumor from major published series

Series, year	Number of cases	Operative mortality (%)
Cushing (Henderson) (1939)[28]	205	2.4
Bakay (1950)[1]	232	6.4*
		35.0†
Horrax et al (1952)[32]	125	14.1
Tönnis (1952)[74]	240	11.2
Nürnberger and Korey (1953)[57]	—	24.0
Tönnis et al (1953)[75]	264	10.4
Gurdjian et al (1955)[21]	38	16.8
Mogensen (1957)[55]	60	12.0
Rand (1957)[63]	67	8.9
Echols (1958)[8]	20	15.0
Guillaume and Caron (1958)[14]	—	12.0
Baker (1960)[2]	150	5.3
Lazorthes et al (1960)[48]	32	9.4
MacCallum (1960)[49]	46	4-10?
Jager and Wijngaarden (1961)[36]	54	13.0
Krayenbühl (1961)[43]	151	8.6
Kunc (1961)[44]	—	14.8
Obrador (1961)[58]	—	20.0
Ray and Patterson (1971)[66]	146	1.4
Clarke et al (1963)[5]	40	2.2
Martins et al (1965)[52]	54	5.0
Svien and Colby (1967)[72]	117	6.8
Elkington and McKissock (1967)[9]	260	10.0
Jefferson (1969)[37]	110	5.4
Stern and Batzdorf (1970)[70]	64	5.9
MacCarty et al (1973)[50]	100	3.0
Fager et al (1973)[11]	197	2.0 (after 1950)
Wirth et al (1974)[79]	157	8.9
Hankinson and Banna (1976)[23]	120	6.7

*Intrasellar adenomas.
†Adenomas with extrasellar extension.
Modified from Stern WE, Batzdorf U: *J Neurosurg* 33:564, 1970; and Post KD: Transfrontal surgery for pituitary tumors, in Post KD, Jackson IMD, Reichlin S (eds): *The Pituitary Adenoma*. New York, Plenum Medical Book Co., 1980.

Table 12-2
Mortality and morbidity for transsphenoidal surgery

Series (author)	City	Number of cases	Deaths		Complications	
			Number	(%)	Number	(%)
Becker	Richmond, Va.	265	4	1.5	35	13
Brodkey	Cleveland, Ohio	360	2	0.5	9	2.5
Ciric	Evanston, Ill.	303	0	0	7	2.3
Collins	New Haven, Conn.	429	3	0.70	8	1.9
Hardy	Montreal, Canada	1102	10	0.90	26	2.4
Kageyama/ Kuwayama	Nagoya, Japan	404	3	0.74	35	8.7
Kelley	Winston-Salem, N.C.	92	0	0	1	1.1
Landolt	Zurich, Switzerland	496	4	0.8	30	6.0
Laws	Rochester, Minn.	1315	6	0.46	67	5.1
Lüdecke	Hamburg, Germany	625	8	1.3	24	3.8
Post	New York, N.Y.	400	0	0	8	2
Rhoton	Gainesville, Fla.	268	1	0.4	6	2.2
Roberts	Salt Lake City, Utah	210	0	0	8	3.8
Tindall	Atlanta, Ga.	709	2	0.3	17	2.4
Van Gilder	Iowa City, Iowa	607	3	0.5	16	2.6
Weiss	Los Angeles, Calif.	658	1	0.15	17	2.6
Wilson	San Francisco, Calif.	1227	3	0.24	25	2.0
Zervas	Boston, Mass.	317	0	0	12	3.8
TOTALS		9787	50	0.5	351	3.6

Data compiled January to March, 1985.

Based on a survey of several pituitary surgeons in early 1985 (see Table 12-2 and the "Operative Mortality" section of this chapter), the overall incidence of nonfatal complications is 3.6%.

Parasellar. The incidence of postoperative CSF leakage following transsphenoidal surgery is dependent on a number of factors, primarily the experience of the surgeon and the intrasellar pathologic findings. Leaks are more frequent following total hypophysectomy than after removal of tumors. As would be expected, CSF leakage is more common if the diaphragm sella is disrupted during tumor removal. However, a postoperative leak may occur following the removal of a microadenoma without evidence of an intraoperative CSF leak. This presumably occurs as a result of postoperative rupture of the diaphragm sella where it herniates into the space left by removal of the microadenoma.

Many substances—cartilage, bone, fascia lata, and lyophilized dura—have been used to reconstruct the floor of the sella and reduce the incidence of CSF leakage. We prefer to fill the intrasellar cavity and sphenoid sinus with fat tissue held in place with tissue adhesive. The fat is loosely packed so as not to produce a mass itself. If the diaphragm sella is torn or is intentionally opened during surgery, hyperventilation of the patient will diminish the intraoperative leakage of CSF and thus allow the surgeon to obtain a watertight seal. In cases of large tumors where the surgeon anticipates an intraoperative leak, the placement of a lumbar subarachnoid drain allows drainage of CSF and reduces the chance of postoperative leakage.

The major complications resulting from a postoperative CSF leak are pneumocephalus and meningitis. There is usually no difficulty diagnosing the presence of CSF rhinorrhea. If only a few drops of clear to yellowish fluid are present, this usually represents nasal secretions or breakdown of the fat graft used for obliteration of the dead space. The use of glucose oxidase test papers is not reliable in determining if a nasal discharge is CSF. There is a 45% to 75% chance of positive results with normal nasal secretions. If an adequate amount of fluid can be collected for quantitative analyses of glucose, a value greater than 30 mg/dl is diagnostic for CSF. Significant leakage of CSF usually manifests itself as a steady dripping of clear fluid, especially when the patient places his head in a dependent position.

Not all CSF leaks persist and require surgical intervention. Many can be treated successfully by lumbar puncture performed on one occasion or serially. Another option is to place the patient on closed drainage of CSF with a lumbar subarachnoid catheter. A potential complication of these forms of CSF diversion is reversing the flow gradient and inducing infection.[60] The head of a patient with a postoperative CSF leak should be elevated to reduce the pressure gradient and retard leakage.

In a patient with a persistent CSF leak, one should not hesitate to reoperate and seal the defect. Again, the preoperative placement of a lumbar subarachnoid drain will reduce leakage during repair, and its continuation in the early postoperative period may reduce the chance of recurrence. One potential cause for a persistent postoperative leak is hydrocephalus that may occur after the initial operation. If suspected, a CT scan should be obtained, and a ventricular shunt may treat both the hydrocephalus and the leak. However, the presence of normal-sized ventricles on a CT scan performed on a patient with steady CSF rhinorrhea does not absolutely rule out hydrocephalus, since the leak may prevent ventriculomegaly.

Our approach to a persistent CSF leak is to manage the patient initially by performing a lumbar puncture and slowly removing CSF to as low a pressure as the patient's headache will tolerate. If the CSF leak persists, an indwelling spinal subarachnoid catheter is inserted percutaneously and left in place for 3 days, during which time the patient remains in bed with the head elevated. The catheter is connected to a sterile reservoir, which is placed no higher than the lumbar puncture site. Should the fluid continue to leak following removal of the catheter, the transsphenoidal wound is reopened, and the sella and sphenoid sinus are repacked with adipose tissue. Reopening the wound after a transsphenoidal operation is relatively easy.

Hypopituitarism may result from damage to or removal of the normal pituitary gland during adenomectomy. Large adenomas will usually thin the gland and flatten it against the posterior-superior aspect of the sella. An experienced transsphenoidal surgeon will usually recognize pituitary tissue by the fine capillary network on its red-orange surface and by the toughness of the structure, which is resistant to the vacuum effect of the sucker. That is to say, tumor tissue is usually removed easily by the sucker, whereas normal pituitary tissue is tougher and cannot be pulled out by the sucker. Postoperative hypopituitarism should be recognized and early treatment instituted with steroid replacement. The subject of hypopituitarism is considered in more detail in Chapter 15.

Hypopituitarism occurs more commonly after removal of large adenomas. To determine the effect transsphenoidal surgery has on pituitary endocrine function, we performed complete endocrine tests before and 10 days after transsphenoidal surgery on 97 women with prolactinomas, 70 of which had microadenomas.[12] Of 65 patients who had normal pituitary endocrine function preoperatively, 50 had normal function postoperatively, 13 had a temporary impairment in one or more axes and fully recovered, and two had permanent damage to one or more axes. Of 32 patients who had impairment of at least one axis preoperatively, 11 showed documented improvement in endocrine function, 19 showed no change, and two were worse. From this data, one can conclude that about 4% (i.e., four out of 97) of patients will incur permanent damage to one or more pituitary-target organ axes following transsphenoidal surgery.[12,54]

Diabetes insipidus may occur transiently following transsphenoidal surgery or may be permanent if there is damage to the posterior lobe or the proximal portion of the pituitary stalk. Severe dehydration and electrolyte imbalance may result if the disorder is not recognized. Options for the management of diabetes insipidus are discussed in Chapter 15.

The intimate anatomic relationship of the cavernous sinuses to the sella renders these venous structures and their contents susceptible to injury during transsphenoidal surgery. Venous hemorrhage may occur from either of the sinuses or from a variety of venous connections between the two sinuses within the dura. Such an opening in the venous system is a potential source for air emboli if the patient's head is positioned significantly above the level of the heart. Vigorous attempts to pack a venous bleeder or removal of tumor from the lateral wall of the sella may cause damage to the cranial nerves traversing the cavernous sinuses. Injury to the third, fourth, fifth, and/or sixth cranial nerves are often transient.

Injury to the carotid artery may result in serious morbidity or death. The position of the intracavernous carotid artery is variable and may extend into the surgical exposure. Based on dissections in cadavers with no intrasellar pathologic findings, Renn and Rhoton[67] reported that the two carotids were occasionally as close as 4 mm to each other. A laceration of the carotid or avulsion of an intracavernous branch produces marked arterial bleeding. Should this occur, the surgeon must resist the temptation to quickly and forcefully pack the sella in an attempt to tamponade the bleeding. This portion of the carotid is relatively immobile, and such pressure may enlarge a small rent in the artery, thus enhancing the bleeding. Instead, one should gently place a piece of fat and/or Avitene over the bleeding site and hold gentle pressure for several minutes. Mild induced hypotension may help stop the bleeding during this time. On rare occasions, the hemorrhage will be so profuse that control may only be gained by proximal ligation of the carotid artery in the neck as a last resort. Once bleeding from the carotid artery is controlled, there exists the potential for the development of a false aneurysm (Fig. 12-35) or a carotid–cavernous sinus fistula.

The patient illustrated in Fig. 12-35 initially had intermittent episodes of massive epistaxis 6 months after transsphenoidal surgery. He was successfully treated by detachable balloon occlusion of the internal carotid artery at the site of the aneurysm following a superficial temporal artery to middle cerebral artery bypass.

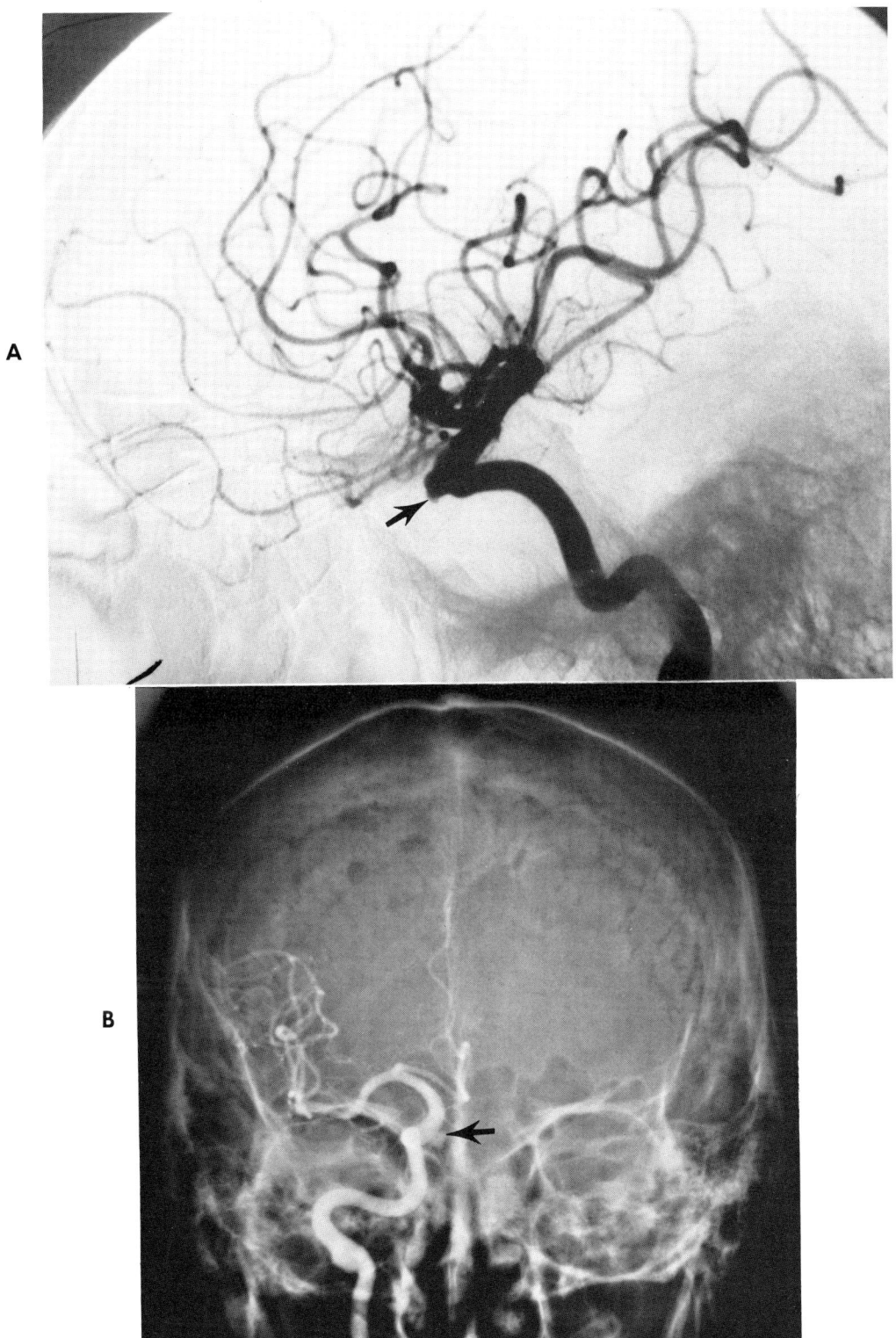

Fig. 12-35. False aneurysm resulting from injury to intracavernous internal carotid artery during transsphenoidal surgery. Patient had intermittent episodes of epistaxis 6 months after surgery. Lateral (**A**) and anteroposterior carotid (**B**) arteriograms show aneurysm (arrows).

Intracranial. Although damage to the hypothalamus is rare, when it occurs, it is a devastating complication of transsphenoidal surgery. This may result from direct trauma through instrumentation of a suprasellar extension of tumor or may result from hemorrhage. Such an injury usually causes a reduction in the level of consciousness and high fever as described previously.

Intracranial hemorrhage may also occur into the frontal or temporal lobes if there is tumor extension into these areas. This can be the result of hemorrhage from portions of the tumor that are inadequately handled transsphenoidally. In such circumstances, a transcranial approach may be a safer operation.

Meningitis may result from the introduction of bacteria into the CSF space during surgery or as a delayed result of postoperative CSF rhinorrhea.

The optic nerves and/or chiasm may be injured in one of several ways. Direct damage to these structures may occur during removal of tumor from the suprasellar region. Attempts to remove adherent tumor or the tumor capsule from the optic apparatus may devascularize the nerves and produce an irreversible visual deficit following infarction. This is probably more common in patients that have been previously treated by craniotomy or radiation and in those patients with poor vision preoperatively. Pressure from a hematoma may cause damage to the optic nerves and/or chiasm and may be reversible following prompt removal of the mass.[17,78] Overpacking of the sella with fat or muscle may cause pressure on the optic nerves and result in visual reduction.[47] Alternatively, the failure to leave a "prop" in the sella following removal of a large intrasellar tumor leaves a cavity that potentially may allow prolapse of the optic nerves and chiasm, thus leading to visual impairment from the traction. Direct damage to the optic nerves can result from a fracture of the optic foramen and orbit produced by over-enthusiastic spreading of the bivalved speculum in the sphenoid sinus.[56]

Once reduction of vision below the preoperative level is recognized, one should immediately obtain a CT scan to search for a remediable cause such as a hematoma or overpacked sella.

Cerebral vasospasm and embolization are rare complications of transsphenoidal surgery. The former may be caused by subarachnoid blood released during surgery or from injured vessels in the circle of Willis. Embolization can occur from thrombus generated within the carotid artery caused by injury to this vessel.

Sphenoid and nasofacial. An occasional patient may develop sinusitis after transsphenoidal surgery. This is usually manifested by headache and tenderness to percussion over the sinuses. This complication is almost always self-limited and only analgesics are required for treatment. Rarely, antibiotics may be required to resolve the condition.

The development of a mucocele has been reported following a transethmoidal approach to the sphenoid.[4] Excessive retraction with the speculum may cause a fracture of the hard palate or cribriform plate. Nasal septal perforations are a known complication of transsphenoidal surgery and can be avoided by careful dissection of the nasal mucosa from the septum. External nasal deformities such as a saddle-nose deformity can occur from the rhinologic portion of the transsphenoidal exposure. This is the result of excessive removal of cartilage or removal of cartilage too high in the nose.

Damage to the branches of the anterior superior dental nerve and/or artery may result in denervation or pulp death of the anterior teeth.[76] This results from excessive bone removal from the piriform rim.

Operative mortality—transsphenoidal approach. In an attempt to determine the incidence of mortality and morbidity associated with modern transsphenoidal surgery, a number of neurosurgeons with extensive experience in pituitary surgery were polled, and the results are shown in Table 12-2. The majority of neurosurgeons to whom this request was addressed responded. A total of 50 deaths were reported out of a total of 9787 operations for pituitary tumor for an incidence of 0.5%. In every case, the neurosurgeon provided details of the fatal cases, and in virtually every instance, there were unusual or extenuating circumstances surrounding the unfortunate outcome.

From these data, it is obvious that the risk of transsphenoidal surgery in terms of operative deaths in the hands of a neurosurgeon experienced in pituitary surgery is very low. It should be emphasized that when an operative death occurs, there are almost always some extenuating circumstances. As already mentioned above, the incidence of nonfatal complications ranges from 1.1% to 13%, with an average of 3.6%. In these series, this was often CSF rhinorrhea and meningitis.

REFERENCES

1. Bakay L: The results of 300 pituitary adenoma operations (Professor Herbert Olivecrona's series). *J Neurosurg* 7:240, 1950.
2. Baker GS: Treatment of pituitary adenomas. *Arch Surg* 81:842, 1960.
3. Bergland R, Ray BS: The arterial supply of the human optic chiasm. *J Neurosurg* 31:327, 1969.
4. Burian K: A two-stage neurorhinosurgical procedure in the treatment of pituitary tumors, in Koos WT, Böck FW, Spetzler RF (eds): *Clinical Microneurosurgery*. Stuttgart, Georg Thieme Verlag, 1976.
5. Clarke HA, Knighton RS, Bebin J: Treatment of pituitary tumors: Analysis of 100 cases. *J Mich Med Soc* 62:1183, 1963.
6. Cushing H: *The Pituitary Body and its Disorders*. Philadelphia, JB Lippincott Co, 1912.
7. Cushing H: Surgical experiences with pituitary disorders. *JAMA* 63:1515, 1914.
8. Echols DH: Experience with surgical treatment in twenty cases of pituitary adenomas. *J Neurosurg* 15:447, 1958.
9. Elkington SG, McKissock W: Pituitary adenoma: Results of combined surgical and radiotherapeutic treatment of 260 patients. *Br Med J* 1:263, 1967.
10. Erickson TC: Neurogenic hyperthermia (a clinical syndrome and its treatment). *Brain* 62:172, 1939.
11. Fager CA, Poppen JL, Takaoka Y: Indications for and results of surgical treatment of pituitary tumors by the intracranial approach, in Kohler PO, Ross GT (eds): *Diagnosis and Treatment of Pituitary Tumors*. International Congress Series No. 303, Amsterdam, Excerpta Medica, 1973.
12. Faria MA Jr, Tindall GT: Transsphenoidal microsurgery for prolactin-secreting pituitary adenomas: Results in 100 women with the amenorrhea-galactorrhea syndrome. *J Neurosurg* 56:33, 1982.
13. Grant FC: Surgical experience with tumors of the pituitary gland. *JAMA* 136:668, 1948.
14. Guillaume J, Caron JP: Remarques cliniques et chirurgicales rélatives aux adénomes hypophysaires. *Neurochirurgie* 4:338, 1958.
15. Guiot G: *Adénomes hypophysaires*. Paris, Masson Editeur, 1958.
16. Guiot G: Transsphenoidal approach in surgical treatment of pituitary adenomas: General principles and indications in nonfunctional adenomas, in Kohler PO, Ross GT (eds): *Diagnosis and Treatment of Pituitary Tumors*. International Congress Series No. 303, Amsterdam, Excerpta Medica, 1973.
17. Guiot G: Considerations on the surgical treatment of pituitary adenomas, in Fahlbusch R, Werder KV (eds): *Treatment of Pituitary Adenomas*. First European Workshop on Treatment of Pituitary Adenomas at Rottach-Egern, Stuttgart, Georg Thieme Verlag, 1978.
18. Guiot G, Derome P: Surgical problems of pituitary adenomas, in Krayenbühl H, Brihaye J, Loew F, et al (eds): *Advances and Technical Standards in Neurosurgery*. New York, Springer-Verlag New York Inc, 1976, vol 3.
19. Guiot G, Rougerie J, Brion S, et al: L'utilisation des amplificateurs de brillance en neuro-radiologie et dans la chirurgie stereotaxique. *Ann Chir* 12:689, 1958.
20. Guiot G, Thibaut B: L'extirpation des adénomes hypophysaires par voie trans-sphénoïdale. *Neurochirurgia* 1:133, 1959.
21. Gurdjian ES, Webster JE, Latimer FR, et al: Recent advances in surgical management of chromophobe tumor of the pituitary. *JAMA* 158:23, 1955.
22. Halstead AE: Remarks on the operative treatment of tumors of the hypophysis: With the report of two cases operated on by an oro-nasal method. *Trans Am Surg Assoc* 28:73, 1910.
23. Hankinson J, Banna M: Pituitary and parapituitary tumours. Philadelphia, WB Saunders Co, 1976.
24. Hardy J: La chirurgie de l'hypophyse par voie transsphénoidale ouverte: Etude comparative de deux modalités techniques. *Ann Chir* 21:1011, 1967.
25. Hardy J: Transphenoidal microsurgery of the normal and pathological pituitary. *Clin Neurosurg* 16:185, 1969.
26. Hardy J: Transsphenoidal hypophysectomy. *J Neurosurg* 34:582, 1971.
27. Hardy J, Wigser SM: Trans-sphenoidal surgery of pituitary fossa tumors with televised radiofluoroscopic control. *J Neurosurg* 23:612, 1965.
28. Henderson WR: The pituitary adenomata: A follow-up study of the surgical results in 338 cases (Dr. Harvey Cushing's series). *Br J Surg* 26:811, 1939.
29. Hirsch O: Endonasal method of removal of hypophyseal tumors. *JAMA* 55:772, 1910.
30. Hirsch O: Ueber Methoden der operativen Behandlung von Hypophysistumoren auf endonasalem wege. *Arch Laryngol Rhinol* 24:129, 1910.
31. Hirsch O: Hypophysentumoren—ein Grenzgebiet. *Acta Neurochir* 5:1, 1957.
32. Horrax G, Hare HF, Poppen JL, et al: Chromophobe pituitary tumors: II. Treatment. *J Clin Endocrinol* 12:631, 1952.

33. Horsley V: On the technique of operations on the central nervous systm. *Br Med J* 2:411, 1906.
34. Horwitz NH, Rizzoli HV: Intracranial neoplasms, in Horwitz, NH, Rizzoli HV (eds): *Post Operative Complications of Intracranial Neurological Surgery*. Baltimore, Williams & Wilkins, 1982.
35. Hudgins WR, Raney LA, Young SW, et al: Failure of intrasellar muscle implants to prevent recurrent downward migration of the optic chiasm. *Neurosurgery* 8:231, 1981.
36. Jager WA, Van Wijngaarden GK: Experiences with the treatment of chromophobec adenoma of the hypophysis. *Tijdschr voor Geneeskd* 105:2496, 1961.
37. Jefferson AA: Chromophobe pituitary adenomata: The size of the suprasellar portion in relation to the safety of operation. *J Neurol Neurosurg Psychiatry* 32:633, 1969.
38. Kahn EA: Some physiologic implications of craniopharyngiomas. *Neurology* 9:82, 1959.
39. Kanavel AB: The removal of tumors of the pituitary body by an infranasal route. *JAMA* 53:1704, 1909.
40. Kanavel AB, Grinker J: Removal of tumors of the pituitary body. *Surg Gynecol Obstet* 10:414, 1910.
41. Killian G: Die submucose Fensterresektion der Nasenscheidewand. *Arch Laryngol Rhinol* 16:362, 1904.
42. Kocher T: Ein Fall von Hypophysis—Tumor mit operativer Heilung. *Dtsch Z Chir* 100:13, 1909.
43. Krayenbühl H: *Hypophysial Adenomas and Craniopharyngiomas*. Abstracts and descriptions of the scientific program of the 2nd International Congress of Neurological Surgery, International Congress Series No. 36, Amsterdam, Excerpta Medica, 1961.
44. Kunc Z: On the current status of surgery in pituitary adenomas. *Cas Lek Cesk* 100:769, 1961.
45. Landolt AM, Strebel P: Technique of trans-sphenoidal operation for pituitary adenomas, in Krayenbühl H (ed): *Advances and Technical Standards in Neurosurgery*. New York, Springer-Verlag, New York Inc, 1980, vol 7.
46. Laws ER Jr, Kern EB: Complications of transsphenoidal surgery. *Clin Neurosurg* 23:401, 1976.
47. Laws ER Jr, Trautmann JC, Hollenhorst RW Jr: Transsphenoidal decompression of the optic nerve and chiasm: Visual results in 62 patients. *J Neurosurg* 46:717, 1977.
48. Lazorthes G, Anduze-Acher H, Espagno J, et al: Statistique opératoire de traitement neurochirurgical par voie frontale des adénomes hypophysaires. *Rev Otoneuroophtalmol* 32:360, 1960.
49. MacCallum PH: Pituitary tumours in the Dunedin Neurosurgical Unit. *NZ Med J* 59:146, 1960.
50. MacCarty CS, Hanson EJ, Randall RV, et al: Indications for and results of surgical treatment of pituitary tumors by the transfrontal approach, in Kohler PO, Ross GT (eds): *Diagnosis and Treatment of Pituitary Tumors*. International Congress Series No. 303, Amsterdam, Excerpta Medica, 1973.
51. MacKay A, Hosobuchi Y: Treatment of intracavernous extensions of pituitary adenomas. *Surg Neurol* 10:377, 1978.
52. Martins AN, Kempe LG, Hayes GJ: Pituitary adenomas: Concepts based on twelve years' experience at Walter Reed General Hospital. *Acta Neurochir* 13:469, 1965.
53. Mawk JR, Ausman JI, Erickson DL, et al: Vasospasm following transcranial removal of large pituitary adenomas: Report of three cases. *J Neurosurg* 50:229, 1979.
54. McLanahan CS, Chirsty JH, Tindall GT: Anterior pituitary function before and after transsphenoidal microsurgical resection of pituitary tumors. *Neurosurgery* 3:142, 1978.
55. Mogensen EF: Chromophobe adenoma of the pituitary gland: A follow-up study on 60 surgical patients with special reference to endocrine disturbances. *Acta Endocrinol* 24:135, 1957.
56. Nicola GC, Giovanelli M: Postoperative course in pituitary surgery: Comparison between transfrontal and transsphenoidal approach. *Minerva Neurochir* 14:89, 1970.
57. Nurnberger JI, Korey SR: *Pituitary Chromophobe Adenomas: Neurology, Metabolism, Therapy*. New York, Springer Publishing Co Inc, 1953.
58. Obrador AS: Adenomas of the pituitary based on a neurosurgical experience of 65 operated patients. *Rev Clin Esp* 81:396, 1961.
59. Olson DR, Guiot G, Derome P: The symptomatic empty sella: Prevention and correction via the transsphenoidal approach. *J Neurosurg* 37:533, 1972.
60. Ommaya AK: Spinal fluid fistulae. *Clin Neurosurg* 23:363, 1976.
61. Ono N, Misumi S, Nukui H, et al: Vasospasm following removal of a large pituitary adenoma by the subfrontal approach: Report of a case and review of the literature. *Neurol Med Chir* 21:609, 1981.
62. Otenasek FJ, Otenasek RJ Jr: Dangers of oxidized cellulose in chiasmal surgery: Report of two cases. *J Neurosurg* 29:209, 1968.
63. Rand CW: Notes on pituitary tumors: Including suggestions of others, and personal experiences in 100 cases. *Clin Neurosurg* 3:1, 1957.

64. Rand RW: Transfrontal transsphenoidal craniotomy in pituitary and related tumors. In Rand RW (ed): *Microneurosurgery*, ed 3. St. Louis, The CV Mosby Co, 1984.
65. Ray BS: Intracranial hypophysectomy. *J Neurosurg* 28:180, 1968.
66. Ray BS, Patterson RH Jr: Surgical experience with chromophobe adenomas of the pituitary gland. *J Neurosurg* 34:726, 1971.
67. Renn WH, Rhoton AL Jr: Microsurgical anatomy of the sellar region. *J Neurosurg* 43:288, 1975.
68. Sanchis J, Bordes M: Immediate visual deterioration after attempts at radical excision of pituitary adenomas. *Acta Neurochir* 38:251, 1977.
69. Schloffer H: Zur Frage der Operationen an der Hypophyse. *Beitr Klin Chir* 50:767, 1906.
70. Stern WE, Batzdorf U: Intracranial removal of pituitary adenomas: An evaluation of varying degrees of excision from partial to total. *J Neurosurg* 33:564, 1970.
71. Sung YF: Anesthetic considerations for patients undergoing transsphenoidal surgery, in Tindall GT, Collins WF (eds): *Clinical Management of Pituitary Disorders*. New York, Raven Press, 1979.
72. Svien HJ, Colby MY: *Treatment for Chromophobe Adenoma*. Springfield, Ill., Charles C Thomas Publishers, 1967.
73. Symon L, Jakubowski J: Transcranial management of pituitary tumours with suprasellar extension. *J Neurol Neurosurg Psychiatry* 42:123, 1979.
74. Tönnis W: Report of 240 adenomata of the hypophysis. *Zentralbl Chir* 77:2103, 1952.
75. Tönnis W, Oberdisse K, Weber E: Bericht über 264 operierte Hypophysenadenome. *Acta Neurochir* 3:113, 1953.
76. Watson SW, Sinn DP, Neuwelt EA: Dental considerations in the sublabial trans-sphenoidal surgical approach to the pituitary gland. *Neurosurgery* 10:236, 1982.
77. Welch K, Stears JC: Chiasmapexy for the correction of traction on the optic nerves and chiasm associated with their descent into an empty sella turcica: Case report. *J Neurosurg* 35:760, 1971.
78. Wilson CB, Dempsey LC: Transsphenoidal microsurgical removal of 250 pituitary adenomas. *J Neurosurg* 48:13, 1978.
79. Wirth FP, Schwartz HG, Schwetschenau PR: Pituitary adenomas: Factors in treatment. *Clin Neurosurg* 21:8, 1974.

CHAPTER 13

Radiation therapy

Physics
    Electromagnetic radiation
    Particulate radiation
        Electrons
        Protons
        Neutrons
        Alpha particles
        Pi-mesons
        Heavy-charged ions
    Absorption of ionizing radiation
    Properties of radiation influencing their biologic effects
Effects of radiation on tissues
    General effects of ionizing radiation
    Effects of radiation on the normal pituitary
    Pathologic effects of radiation on pituitary adenomas
    Effects of radiation on the CNS
        Acute reactions
        Early delayed reactions
        Late delayed reactions
Treatment techniques and tumor dosages
    Conventional megavoltage irradiation
    Proton beam radiotherapy
    Alpha particle radiotherapy
    Internal irradiation (brachytherapy)
Treatment results
    Prolactinomas
    Acromegaly
    Cushing's disease
    Nelson's syndrome
    Nonfunctional adenomas
    Meningiomas
    Craniopharyngiomas
        Primary irradiation
        Secondary irradiation
        Interstitial irradiation
Complications of CNS and pituitary irradiation
    Cerebral radionecrosis
    Optic nerve/chiasm damage
    Hypopituitarism
    Effect on intellectual function
    Soft tissue reaction
    Tumorigenesis
Summary

Radiation therapy was first used to treat a pituitary adenoma by Gramegna[50] in 1907, 1 year after Schloffer pioneered the transsphenoidal operative approach to the pituitary. Gramegna used an intraoral glass applicator to supply radiation to a 45-year-old acromegalic woman, who experienced temporary improvement. In the same year, Béclère[12] using external radiation treated a 16-year-old girl with gigantism. The patient experienced improvement in vision and relief of headache and was reported to be doing well 15 years after therapy. Hirsch, who contributed significantly to the development of an endonasal transsphenoidal route to the pituitary, was also a pioneer in irradiation of pituitary tumors. Between 1910 and 1956 he treated 413 patients with a combination of surgery and local radium capsule implantation.[60] Advocates of the combined use of surgery and radiotherapy point out Henderson's follow-up of Cushing's patients that indicated postoperative radiation raised the recurrence-free rate for pituitary tumors from 32.8% to 65.3% in the transsphenoidally operated patients and from 57.5% to 87.1% in those managed by craniotomy.[58]

Today radiation therapy remains a therapeutic option for many pituitary and parasellar tumors. This chapter presents indications for radiation therapy, results of treatment of pituitary adenomas and other parasellar neoplasms (especially craniopharyngiomas and meningiomas), and complications of this form of therapy. The physics of the various types of available radiation is also briefly presented as a basis for understanding the advantages and disadvantages of each, and the effects of ionizing radiation on both the normal and neoplastic pituitary gland and central nervous system (CNS) are discussed.

PHYSICS

Ionizing radiation produces sufficient energy to eject an electron from an atom or molecule, thus producing ions. This action provides sufficient energy to break chemical bonds, and as will be discussed below, this important property produces many of the final effects of ionizing radiation.

Ionizing radiations can be broadly classified as electromagnetic and particulate radiations. An understanding of the physical properties of these different types of radiation is important in discussing advantages and disadvantages of each as a radiotherapeutic modality.

Electromagnetic radiation

Radio waves, heat waves, light waves, ultraviolet rays, radar, x-rays and gamma rays are all examples of electromagnetic radiation. Of these examples, x-rays and gamma rays are the only ionizing radiations, that is, they have enough energy to produce ionization of radiated biologic tissue by ejecting electrons from the tissues' molecules. X-rays and gamma rays do not differ in their properties, only in the manner in which they are produced.

X-rays are produced whenever a substance is bombarded by high-speed electrons that are accelerated to high energy and then abruptly stopped in a target. All x-ray tubes consist of a cathode and anode assembly placed inside a vacuum tube. When the electrons strike the target, usually made of tungsten or gold, part of the energy of the electrons is converted into x-rays.

Gamma rays are emitted by radioactive isotopes such as radium, cesium, iridium, cobalt, and others. Radioactive isotopes are atoms that are unstable because of an imbalance in the number of protons and neutrons. When this imbalance exists, a particle or particles will be ejected until a stable configuration is achieved. The gamma rays represent excess energy given off as the unstable nucleus breaks up. A photon is defined as a corpuscle of energy, and in this chapter, the term *photon irradiation* is synonymous with electromagnetic irradiation.

Particulate radiation

Through the development of supervoltage machines such as linear accelerators, cyclotrons, betatrons, and synchrotrons, beams of high energy particles can be produced. The type of radiation emanating from these sources include electrons, protons, alpha particles, neutrons, negative pi-mesons, and heavy-charged particles. There has been much interest in the possible use of certain of these high-energy beams in radiotherapy, and some of these particles have been used for pituitary radiation. In the following, the individual particles will be defined and their use in radiation therapy briefly discussed.

Electrons. Electrons are small particles with a negative charge that can be accelerated to a speed near that of light by means of an electrical device such as a betatron. In a betatron, electrons are bent into a circular path by a magnetic field and spiral inward while being accelerated. In this fashion, electrons can either be directed against a target within the betatron to produce an x-ray beam or extracted from the machine to produce an electron beam for therapy.

Protons. Protons differ from electrons in that they are about 2000 times larger and have a positive charge. Because of their relatively large mass, they require more complex and expensive cyclotrons to accelerate them to useful energies. A cyclotron is able to accelerate beams of protons, neutrons, and alpha particles for clinical use. The particles are accelerated in a circle of increasing diameter between the poles of a large direct current magnet connected to a high-frequency, high-voltage oscillator.

Neutrons. Neutrons have a mass similar to protons but are electrically neutral and, for this reason, cannot be accelerated in an electrical device. Neutrons with a wide range of energies are produced as a by-product when heavy radioactive atoms undergo fission inside a nuclear reactor. Also, neutrons can be produced when a charged particle such as a deuteron is accelerated to high energy as in a cyclotron and made to impinge on a suitable target such as beryllium. The proton is "stripped" from the deuteron, leaving a neutron that carries much of the kinetic energy of the original deuteron. A deuteron is the nucleus of a deuterium atom (hydrogen-2) consisting of a proton and a neutron in close association.

Alpha particles. Alpha particles are the nuclei of helium atoms made up of two protons and two neutrons in close association. Alpha particles have a positive charge and can be accelerated in electrical devices similar to those used for protons and deuterons. Alpha particles are also emitted during the decay of certain radioactive isotopes.

Pi-mesons. Pi-mesons, or pions, are particles of intermediate size between electrons and protons. Protons and neutrons are believed to be held together within an atomic nucleus by the mutual exchange of pi-mesons.[52] Pi-mesons may be electrically positive, neutral, or negative and are unstable with a mean lifetime of only 2.54×10^{-8} seconds. Only negative pi-mesons are of interest in radiotherapy. They are produced by a very complex process that requires expensive devices such as a synchrocyclotron or linear accelerator.

Heavy-charged ions. The term *heavy-charged ions* refers to the nuclei of elements after some or all of the electrons have been stripped leaving the particles with a positive charge. Elements used for this purpose include carbon, nitrogen, boron, neon, and argon. To be useful, they must be accelerated to energies of hundreds or thousands of millions of volts.

Absorption of ionizing radiation

Ionizing radiations may be *directly* or *indirectly ionizing*. All of the charged particles described above are *directly* ionizing. Provided the particles have sufficient kinetic energy, they directly disrupt the atomic structure of the absorbing medium and are responsible for the chemical and biologic changes themselves. *Indirectly* ionizing radiation means that the radiation itself does not cause biologic damage but instead gives up energy that when absorbed produces fast-moving charged particles that results in chemical and biologic damage. Electromagnetic radiation (x-ray and gamma ray photons) are indirectly ionizing. Uncharged fast neutrons are also indirectly ionizing but give rise to protons, alpha particles, and other heavy nuclear fragments that directly ionize. X-ray and gamma ray photons are absorbed by two major processes—the *Compton process* and the *photoelectric process*. At high energies used in radiotherapy, the Compton process dominates. In this process, an x-ray or gamma ray photon interacts or collides with an atom of the radiated medium causing the ejection of a loosely bound planetary electron as part of the photon's energy is given to the electron.[52] The photon is deflected and travels with reduced energy. Both the photon and ejected electron may interact with other atoms to cause secondary ionization (Fig. 13-1). In the *photoelectric process,* the photon interacts with a tightly bound electron of an atom of the radiated medium. The photon gives up all of its energy—some to overcome the binding energy of the electron to cause its release and the remainder as kinetic energy. The vacancy caused by the ejection of the electron is filled by an outside electron or one from a lower energy level. The movement of an electron from a loosely to a tightly bound shell involves a decrease in potential energy. The energy change is balanced by the emission of a photon with characteristic electromagnetic radiation (Fig. 13-2).[52]

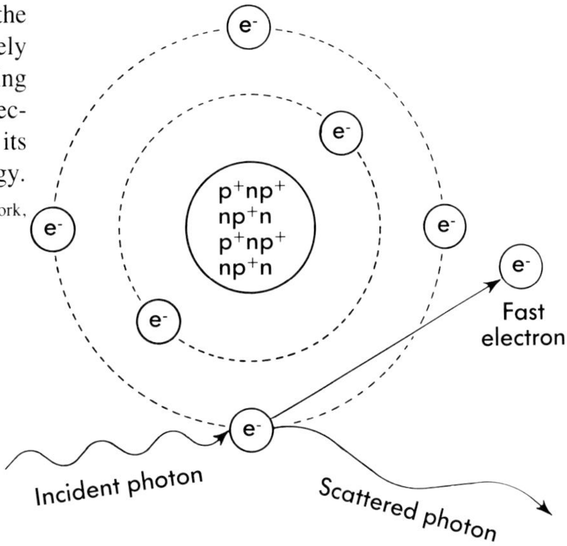

Fig. 13-1. Absorption of an x-ray photon by the Compton process. Photon interacts with loosely bound planetary electron of atom of absorbing material. Part of photon energy is given to electron as kinetic energy. Photon, deflected from its original direction, proceeds with reduced energy.

From Hall EJ: *Radiobiology for the Radiologist*, ed 2. New York, Harper & Row, Publishers Inc, 1978.

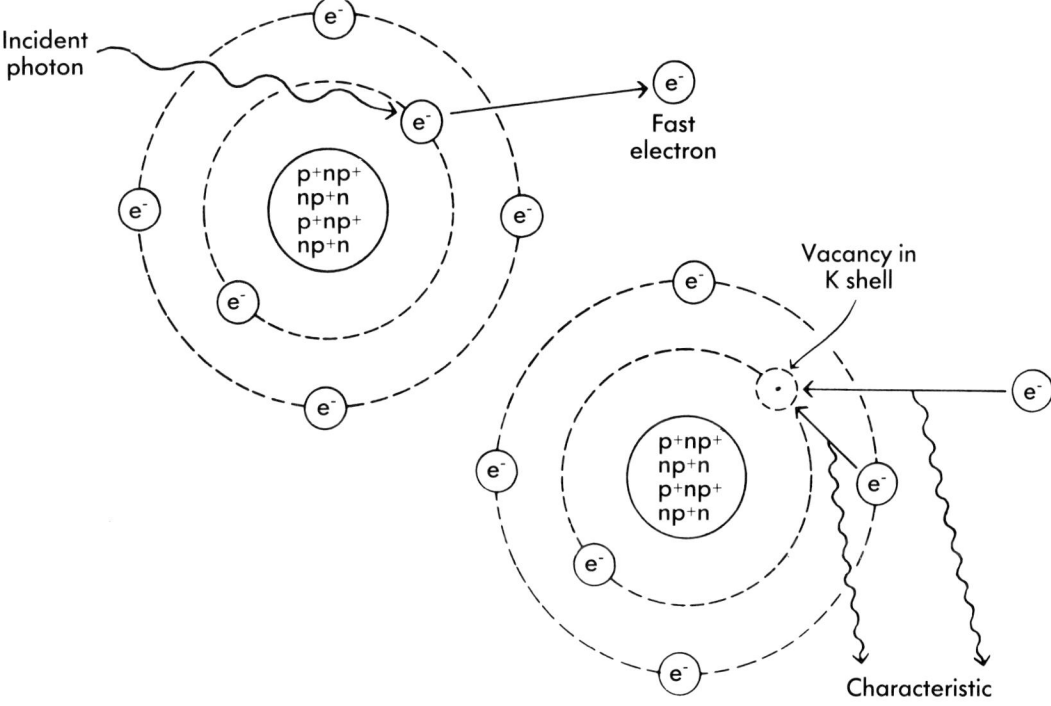

Fig. 13-2. Absorption of photon of x- or gamma-radiation by photoelectric process. Interaction involves photon and "tightly bound" orbital electron of atom of absorber. Photon gives up its energy entirely; electron is ejected with kinetic energy equal to energy of incident photon, less binding energy, which previously held electron in orbit (upper panel). Vacancy caused by ejection of electron is filled either by electron from outer orbit or by "free" electron from outside atom (lower panel). When electron changes energy levels, the difference in energy is emitted as a photon of characteristic x-rays. For tissue, these x-rays are of very low energy.

From Hall EJ: *Radiobiology for the Radiologist*, ed 2. New York, Harper & Row, Publishers Inc, 1978.

It is believed that there are discrete sites within mammalian cells that must be damaged to kill the cell. Although the critical target(s) have not been determined with certainty, it is likely that both nuclear DNA and intracellular membranes represent such targets.[55,151] It has been suggested that lysosomes are the cause of radiation injury in cells,[119,141] but there is not agreement on the significance of lysosomal damage.[4,156]

Properties of radiation influencing their biologic effects

The level of oxygen in irradiated tissue has an influence on the effectiveness of the radiation. Oxygen is a potent radiosensitizer of biologic systems, and conversely, hypoxia has a dramatic protective effect against radiation. Several ingenious approaches have been attempted to overcome the problem of radioinsensitivity of hypoxic cells within radiated tissue. These include the use of high-LET (linear energy transfer) radiations to increase the cytotoxic effect of a given radiation, hyperbaric oxygen, hypoxic cell sensitizers, and hyperthermia.

The protective effect of hypoxia varies with different types of radiation and is expressed as the *oxygen enhancement ratio* (OER). The OER is the ratio of hypoxia to aerated doses of radiation required to achieve the same biologic effect. Therefore, the lower the OER for a given type of radiation, the less effect the state of oxygenation of the radiated tissue will have on the ability of that radiation to kill cells. For sparsely ionizing radiation such as x-rays or gamma rays, the OER is relatively high indicating that the oxygen effect is important. For a densely ionizing radiation such as alpha particles, the survival of cells in the presence or absence of oxygen is the same; the OER is 1, or unity, indicating no oxygen effect. For radiation of intermediate ionizing density such as neutrons, there is an intermediate oxygen effect giving an OER value between that for x-rays and alpha particles.

Linear energy transfer (LET) is a term used to define the energy transferred to the absorbing medium per unit length along the track of radiation.[160] The unit usually used for this quantity is the kilo-electron-volt (KeV) per micron (μ) of unit density. A KeV is the unit of energy equal to the energy possessed by an electron accelerated through 1000 volts. LET is a useful way to indicate the radiation quality of different types of ionizing photons and particles.

LET and radiation effect decrease as the beam penetrates tissues. This physical characteristic of photon beams is responsible for certain inherent characteristics of conventional photon irradiation. For instance, portions of the tumor nearest the radiation source receive a higher dose than those located deeper; furthermore, the dose received by normal tissue between the entrance surface and target can be greater than the dose received by the target itself. Also undesired radiation is absorbed by normal tissues beyond the target, the so-called exit-dose.[106] Exit-dose phenomenon can be overcome by using more than a single field in the treatment of a centrally located tumor.

The LET and ionizing effects achieved with particulate radiation are not constant along their path through an homogenous medium. Instead there is an increase in energy and ionizing effect near the end of the path because of decreased velocity of the particles, allowing nearby atoms to be influenced for a longer period of time. This region of increased LET and ionizing effect is called the *Bragg peak* (Fig. 13-3). There is no Bragg peak observed for electrons, since as electrons slow down, multiple changes in direction occur that smear out the Bragg peak. On the other hand, heavy-charged particles such as protons, pi-mesons, nuclei of helium, carbon, and neon maintain their direction as they pass through a medium, and a Bragg peak is observed.

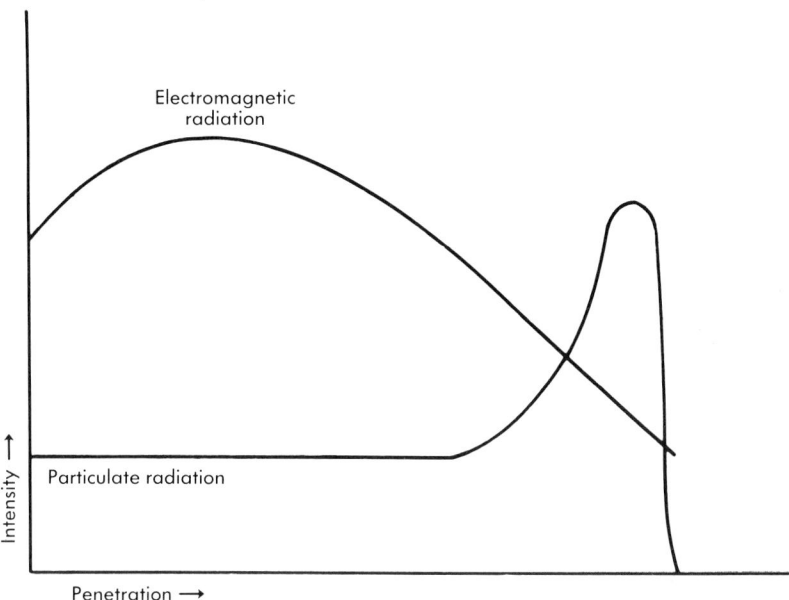

Fig. 13-3. Graph illustrates difference in energy release between electromagnetic (gamma rays, x rays) and particulate (proton beam, alpha particles) radiation. Cyclotron-generated heavy-charged particles (particulate radiation curve) of a specific initial energy share the property of penetrating a uniform absorber at uniform depth and stopping completely. In stopping, ionization intensity is greater than elsewhere along path, and this rise in intensity of radiation is known as the Bragg peak. Ionization curve for electromagnetic radiation is more diffuse, and thus more normal tissue exposure occurs with this form of radiation.

The concept of the Bragg peak has excited many radiotherapists because the dosage of radiation can be concentrated. If the Bragg peak is centered within a tumor, maximal energy is delivered to that area with the surrounding normal tissue receiving considerably less radiation. There is no exit-dose for particulate radiation. Theoretically, these properties make particulate radiation an appropriate therapy for small targets such as the pituitary, and experience has been accumulated with this form of therapy in a number of hyperfunctional pituitary adenomas.

Wilson[157] in 1946 was the first to suggest the use of a proton beam for radiation therapy. He proposed that by using the Bragg peak region of the absorption curve it would be possible to treat a small volume of tumor with several times the dose of radiation given to neighboring tissue. Following Wilson's suggestion, Tobias, Anger, and Lawrence[148] experimented with beams of deuterons and alpha particles. The first human patients treated with this technique underwent radiation hypophysectomy for palliation of metastatic breast cancer in 1954.[101] Subsequently, the use of particulate radiation has been expanded to achieve hypophysectomy for diabetic retinopathy and to treat pituitary adenomas.[76,78,90,92]

Primarily because of availability and lower cost of equipment, electromagnetic radiations are used therapeutically far more often than particulate radiations. Furthermore, because of advances in dosimetry and treatment planning, some of the disadvantages of conventional radiation can be overcome. There are a limited number of institutions that have the capacity to generate high energy beams of particulate radiation for therapeutic purposes. At the present time, it is not possible to choose the ideal form of radiation from among the various heavy particles. Proton and helium beams, however, have been used extensively in the treatment of pituitary disorders. The usefulness of proton beams must rest on the physical properties of protons, since their biologic effects on tissues are virtually indistinguishable from those of x-rays. Protons result in a much more localized dose of radiation within the target volume. Helium ions share all of the advantages of protons as far as distribution of dose is concerned and offer a slightly reduced OER. Neutrons are suitable for radiotherapy with an improved OER over x-rays, although it is far from the ideal value of unity. Neutrons offer no advantage over modern photon beams with respect to dose distribution of radiation. Use of fast neutron radiation is primarily experimental. Negative pi-mesons offer some improvement in both the distribution of radiation in a target and OER. However, protons and helium ions offer most of the same advantages at a fraction of the cost.

EFFECTS OF RADIATION ON TISSUES
General effects of ionizing radiation

For most human neoplasms and normal tissues, there is a particular amount of radiation that has a definite probability of killing a specific percentage of cells of a given type within the volume receiving that dose.[106] This is referred to as a *dose response curve*. In general, the proportion of cells killed by a specific dose increases as the dose increases. The molecular events that occur when a photon or particle collides with an atom of the absorbing medium (Compton process, photoelectric effect) have been discussed previously. Irradiated cells may show (1) no detectable effect; (2) latent chromosomal damage that does not somatically affect the cell but may be expressed in later generations; (3) severe chromosomal damage, which may not lead to cell death immediately but prevents the cell from dividing or kills it when attempting division; and/or (4) immediate death.[42] Certainly intermediate or a combination of these effects can occur.

There are characteristics of both the radiation and the absorbing cells or tissue that influence the effects of radiation. The biologic effects of the radiation are determined by the energy, dose rate, and fractionation of irradiation and the LET and OER.[11,40,42,52] The LET, which is a measure of the density of ionization produced by the radiation along its path, is very important. The oxygen tension of the radiated cells or tissue is one of the most important local factors influencing the radiation effect.[51] Another important factor is the stage in the reproductive cycle a cell is in at the time of radiation.[138,146] Although radiation is able to kill cells in any phase of their cycle, there is greater sensitivity in G_2 and M than in S, with G being relatively radioresistant. Furthermore, cells that are actively dividing are more responsive to radiation than cells that divide only occasionally or not at all. The ability of a cell to repair radiation damage is another important determinant of the effect of radiation. This repairability is more pronounced in normal cells than in neoplastic cells.

Effects of radiation on the normal pituitary

The human pituitary gland has been irradiated under a variety of circumstances.[42] The more common clinical situation consists of exposure of the gland during the course of radiation treatment of pituitary tumors, brain tumors, or other neoplasms (e.g., nasopharyngeal carcinoma). Another situation in which the pituitary gland would be radiated is in an attempt to produce hypophysectomy either as palliation for disseminated breast and prostate cancer or for control of diabetic retinopathy.

The normal pituitary gland is relatively radioresistant, and thus large doses of radiation are necessary to achieve destruction of the gland. An unfractionated dose of 20,000 rad is needed to effectively destroy the gland by external x-ray irradiation.[33] The effects of lower or fractionated doses are less clear. Between 20,000 and 26,000 rad, there is gross damage to the pituitary although it may not be apparent for 5 months, and above 27,000 rad, there is necrosis in all cases.[42] Dosages above 20,000 rad are obtainable only with Bragg peak therapy and with interstitial implantation. Conventional radiation therapy cannot achieve these dosages because of damage to surrounding normal brain tissue.

In an autopsy series of 53 patients who had received 14,000 to 30,000 rad of fractionated protons or alpha particles to the pituitary for control of metastatic cancers, no necrosis was seen below 20,000 rad.[122] With the larger doses, necrosis of 90% of the gland could be seen as early as 5 days following completion of therapy. Necrosis reached up to 98% of the gland in the long-term survivors. This necrosis progressed with time, presumably as a result of ischemia from vascular damage, and no regeneration was observed.[122] The acute necrosis is of the coagulative type in which ghosts of the pre-existing cells can be recognized months after radiation.[42]

Low to moderate therapeutic doses of radiation appear to produce either no significant alterations in the pituitary or nonspecific changes such as degranulation of acidophilic cells.[46] Vacuolization of basophilic cells has been described in humans following atomic bomb casualties.[96]

Functional damage to the neurohypophysis is rare.[139] However, clinical evidence of hypothalamic damage is common after irradiation for carcinoma of the nasopharynx, occurring with an incidence as high as 83% according to some authorities.[127] The radiosensitivity of the hypothalamus may be responsible for much of the clinical hypopituitarism observed following radiation to this area. Additionally, the more focused beam achieved with heavy particle therapy may avoid hypothalamic radiation and account for the somewhat lower incidence of hypopituitarism following these methods of therapy. Hypopituitarism, as a complication of radiation to the sellar region, is considered on p. 428.

Pathologic effects of radiation on pituitary adenomas

Data on the effects of irradiation on pituitary tumors are limited, and pathologic changes appear to be both nonspecific and variable. There are both qualitative and quantitative differences in the pathologic changes induced by different methods of irradiation. Anniko and Wersall[5] compared the morphology of pituitary tumors irradiated by a single dose technique (3000 to 7000 rad) to others undergoing fractionated radiation (2600 to 4500 rad). Hyalinization around blood vessels must have occurred independent of the type of irradiation but required some time to develop, since it was not found in one tumor studied 2 months after a single dose treatment. Single dose treatment caused extensive fibrosis, and few surviving cells were identified in the primary target area. On the other hand, tumors treated with fractionated dose irradiation showed a large number of tumor cells present 6 to 8 years after treatment. Many of these cells were morphologically damaged with intracellular and intercellular vesiculation.

Using an *in vitro* system of irradiating pituitary tumor tissue in organ culture, Anniko[4] was able to study the morphology of irradiated adenoma cells. The irradiation-induced morphologic cell damage in this study was nonspecific, showing vesiculation of cell cytoplasm and organelles, much of which was reversible. A large number of pituitary cells were either devoid of hormone granules or contained only a small number 5 to 12 hours after irradiation. This degranulation occurred before ultrastructural damage could be identified. This finding lends support to the hypothesis that degranulation occurs because of biochemical and/or physiologic alterations in the permeability of the cell membrane.[4]

Postmortem examination of pituitary tumors having undergone helium ion irradiation revealed fibrosis most marked in the central portion of the gland.[158]

Effects of radiation on the CNS

Unfortunately, radiation may cause damage to the normal CNS surrounding an irradiated tumor or within the path of radiation given to extracranial neoplasms. The clinical effects of radiation injury to the brain may be divided into *acute reactions*, which appear during the course of radiation; *early delayed reactions*, occurring from a few weeks to a few months after irradiation; and *late delayed reactions*, with onset from several months to years later.

Acute reactions. Acute reactions are rare events unless extremely large doses are given. These are manifested by such symptoms and signs as lethargy, somnolence, vomiting, ataxia, dysphagia, or dysarthria and are usually transient.[134] With daily doses in the order of 200 rad, total doses as high as 7000 to 8000 rad are tolerated without serious *acute* CNS reactions.[124,137] Some of these acute "reactions" may be an exacerbation of pre-existing signs or symptoms possibly caused by radiation-induced edema and treatable or preventable with steroids.[124,137]

Early delayed reactions. Early delayed reactions, occurring from a few weeks to a few months after irradiation, are believed to result from demyelination. Such an injury from radiation to the spinal cord may result in transient tingling and paresthesias brought on by cord extension (Lhermitte's phenomenon). These symptoms usually disappear within 2 to 36 weeks and are believed to be a result of a transient radiation myelopathy resulting from temporary demyelination of sensory neurons.[68] A similar reaction can affect the brain. Freeman et al[44] described mild to pronounced somnolence in 78% of children receiving 2400 rad over a period of 28 days to the cranium plus intrathecal methotrexate as a CNS prophylaxis for prevention of acute lymphoblastic leukemia. The alteration in level of consciousness appeared 24 to 56 hours after completion of the radiation, lasted 10 to 38 days, and completely recovered in all cases.[44]

Boldrey and Sheline[17] described a series of patients treated with irradiation for low-grade gliomas, meningiomas, and pituitary adenomas that experienced adverse but transient signs and symptoms during the first 10 weeks after therapy. These reactions could not be explained on the basis of the patient's neoplasm, since they were transient with a peak incidence in the second month postirradiation and disappeared within about 6 weeks.

Because the early delayed reactions are almost always nonlethal, little histopathology is available.

One patient with Cushing's disease expired from a cerebral hemorrhage 34 days after receiving 5000 rad to the pituitary gland.[2] Calculations indicated that the location of the hemorrhage received <60% of the pituitary dose. Pathologic examination revealed perivascular round cell infiltration, edema, degenerative nuclear changes of ganglion cells, and thickening of vessel walls.[2] Another patient died 14 weeks after irradiation for a pituitary adenoma and was found to have loss of myelin and axons in the medial temporal white matter.[104] Hoffman et al[61] postulated that demyelination might be the underlying factor in reporting a series of 51 patients with malignant gliomas treated with 5000 rad (170 to 180 rad/day). Seven of the 25 patients that showed deterioration improved spontaneously without change in therapy over a period of time that corresponded to the turnover time for myelin.[61] Reversible anosmia has been reported as an early delayed reaction to pituitary irradiation and was assumed to result from demyelination.[24] Lampert et al[87,88] have described two patients dying 3 months after receiving 5750 and 5700 rad respectively in which disseminated plaques of demyelination with central necrosis and petechial hemorrhages were identified.

Late delayed reactions. Late delayed reactions (radionecrosis) are the major risk of CNS irradiation and are principally dose and fractionation related. The onset is several months to years after treatment and is generally progressive and often fatal. Kramer et al[85] showed that 74% of patients with radionecrosis developed the disorder within 3 years of radiation. These delayed reactions may present with focal neurologic deficits or as diffuse cerebral injury suggestive of cerebral edema with elevated intracranial pressure (ICP). Occasionally, radiation necrosis will present as a space-occupying mass lesion indistinguishable from tumor.[42]

Radionecrosis of the brain occurs most commonly in the cerebral hemisphere, followed by the cerebellum, and occurs infrequently in the brainstem. The delayed lesions are grossly yellow-white or hemorrhagic, poorly defined areas of necrosis generally confined to the white matter.[42] Microscopically, there are large areas of demyelination and coagulation necrosis of white matter. Areas of granular calcium deposits are sometimes seen within the necrotic regions.[20] The necrotic brain is surrounded by gliosis and intact cortical tissue although some glial and axonal alterations occur in the adjacent cortex. There is not a prominent inflammatory infiltrate of lymphocytes or granulocytes except in the Virchow-Robin spaces.[42]

Intracerebral blood vessels are affected by radiation within the areas of necrosis, and these changes may be responsible for some of the damage. The lumen of most medium and large arterioles and arteries are compromised because of severe intimal, endothelial, and/or perimedial proliferation.[42] Many become completely thrombosed. The weight of evidence suggests that demyelination is important in the early delayed reaction and that vascular changes become progressively more important with time.[137]

TREATMENT TECHNIQUES AND TUMOR DOSAGES
Conventional megavoltage irradiation

Given the complications that can arise following irradiation of both central nervous and extracranial tissues, one of the cardinal principles of radiation therapy is to maximize the radiation dose to the neoplasm while keeping normal tissues at or below the limits of dose tolerance. Conventional megavoltage radiotherapy is the most widely used form of irradiation. This refers to the use of photon irradiation (x-rays or gamma rays) with a beam energy of at least 1.2 million electron-volts (MeV). Sources for this type of radiation include cobalt-60 units and linear accelerators, both widely available throughout the United States. Because of certain beam characteristics, treatment with a linear accelerator is usually preferable.[109]

An older technique of using stationary opposed bilateral temporal radiation fields delivers an undesirably high radiation dose to auditory structures and the temporal lobes.[109,133] To protect these and other structures such as the lens and retina, radiotherapists use either rotational or converging three-field (bilateral temporal and single frontal) technique and wedge filters.

The treatment plan should be tailored for each individual patient, taking into consideration previous radiation therapy, tumor size, and any asymmetric extension of tumor.[133] With conventional radiation, it is impossible to protect the normal pituitary. The optic chiasm and hypothalamus are also exposed, especially with the larger tumors.[133]

Pituitary irradiation is usually given as a single course in 4 or 5 fractions per week for 4.5 to 5 weeks. A total tumor dose of 4500 to 5000 rad in 180 rad/day fractions is recommended, although the total may be increased to 5000 to 5500 rad for large and invasive tumors or for craniopharyngiomas.[133]

Proton beam radiotherapy

Protons were first used therapeutically at the University of California in Berkeley.[106] Tobias, Lawrence, and associates reported preliminary results of proton beam pituitary irradiation in 1958. The largest experience in the use of proton beam radiotherapy is that of Kjellberg et al performed at Cambridge, Massachusetts since 1963.[72,73,74,75] These investigators have used protons accelerated in a cyclotron to an energy of 160 MeV. Extreme precision is required for proton beam irradiation since a high radiation dose is delivered to the target and not to adjacent normal tissues. Therefore the patients are placed in a stereotaxic frame, and multiple fields converging on the tumor are irradiated in one session. The procedure requires about 1.5 to 2 hours to complete, and the patient is usually discharged after overnight observation.[75] A dose of 6000 to 10,000 rad at the Bragg peak is used to produce radionecrosis for pituitary ablation, and 2000 to 4000 rad are used to arrest growth of adenomas.[109]

Alpha particle radiotherapy

Since 1958, alpha particles (helium nuclei) have been used at the University of California in Berkeley by Lawrence et al,[90-94] Linfoot et al,[97,98] and Tobias et al[149] for irradiation of pituitary tumors. The alpha particles are accelerated in a cyclotron to an energy of 910 MeV. Like protons, alpha particles have the Bragg peak property; however, some investigators have modified the dose distribution of the alpha particle beam by spreading it out to yield a plateaulike configuration.[149] As with proton beam therapy, accuracy of the alpha particle beam requires that the patient be placed in a stereotaxic mask or frame. For growth hormone (GH)-secreting and nonfunctional adenomas, total dose ranges from 3400 to 10,000 rad divided into three to six equal treatments over a 5- to 12-day period.[93,94,97] Doses of 6000 to 15,500 rad in 5 to 12 days have been used for Cushing's disease, although for this condition Lawrence et al[90,91] now recommend 10,000 to 15,000 rad in 5 days.

Internal irradiation (brachytherapy)

Internal irradiation, or brachytherapy, has been used in the treatment of pituitary adenomas, craniopharyngiomas, and certain brain tumors (gliomas). A center with vast experience in transsphenoidal implantation, begun in 1958, is Hammersmith Hospital in London.[21,43,70,159] Internal irradiation for cystic craniopharyngiomas was first performed by Leksell and Liden[95] in 1953 using stereotaxic injection of ^{32}P chromic phosphate into cysts. Ideal isotopes for internal irradiation must have a short half-life and easy applicability and be a pure beta emitter.[80] Table 13-1 summarizes these qualities in the most commonly used radioisotopes. ^{90}Y is the most suitable radiation source to date.[80] ^{198}Au has enough beta emission that the relative parasellar dosage is higher.

Table 13-1
Radioisotopes used for internal radiation

Feature	^{198}Au	^{32}P	^{90}Y
Physical half-life (days)	2.69	14.2	2.67
Maximal beta energy (MeV)	0.96	1.71	2.27
Mean beta energy (MeV)	0.32	0.69	0.93
Maximal range in soft tissue (mm)	3.8	7.9	11
Half-value depth in soft tissue (mm)	0.4	0.8	1.1
Major gamma energy (MeV)	0.41	—	—

From Kobayashi T, Kageyama N, Ohara K: Internal irradiation for cystic craniopharyngioma. *J Neurosurg* 55:896, 1981.

The Hammersmith group places the radioactive sources in the sella transsphenoidally under general anesthesia following an aspiration biopsy. The dosage of radiation as calculated at the tumor surface varies with the type of neoplasm. Twenty thousand rad have been used for prolactinomas,[70] 10,000 to 50,000 for acromegaly with better results at the upper range,[43,159] and 10,000 to 30,000 rad for Cushing's disease.[21] The higher doses are reserved for those cases in which there is an obviously abnormal sella. Kobayashi et al[80] have used between 9000 and 20,000 rad for internal irradiation of cystic craniopharyngiomas with ^{32}P and ^{198}Au. Strauss et al[144] deliver 20,000 rad to the wall of cystic craniopharyngiomas with stereotaxically placed ^{90}Y.

TREATMENT RESULTS

Evaluating the efficacy of radiation therapy for pituitary adenomas is difficult. The use of radiation as a primary means of therapy was much more common before the modern popularization of transsphenoidal surgery. Therefore much of the literature dealing with the results of radiation therapy was published before the advent of computed tomographic (CT) scanning and radioimmunoassays to determine size and excess hormone production of pituitary adenomas, respectively. Keeping these limitations in mind, the results of radiation therapy in pituitary adenomas will be reviewed.

Prolactinomas

Radiation therapy, as a primary treatment for pituitary adenomas had lost much of its popularity by the time prolactinomas were identified as a pathologic entity. Therefore most of these lesions have been treated surgically, and the literature (Table 13-2) on irradiation is relatively limited.

Table 13-2
Radiation therapy for prolactin-secreting pituitary adenomas (prolactinomas)

Parameter	Antunes et al[6]	Kleinberg et al[79]	De Schryver et al[34]	Gomez et al[48]	Sheline[133]	Kelly et al[70]
Patients treated	8	6	8	6	8	4	21
Treatment	S&RT	RT	RT	RT	RT	S&RT	90Y
Mean prolactin (ng/ml)							
Before	1070	2500	195	300	168	387	427
After	144	165	50	?	64	192	317
Mean decrease (%)	59	87	75	?	62	50	26
Galactorrhea ceased	1/3	2/3	3/8	?	2/8	1/2	9/15
Menses resumed	0/3	1/3	2/6	?	4/?	0/3	5/18
Follow-up (months)	3-39	13-72	—	—	6-57	1-16	—

S&RT, Surgery and postoperative radiation.
RT, Radiation therapy.
90Y, Yttrium[90] implantation.

Antunes et al[6] reported six patients with prolactinomas that received conventional irradiation as the sole means of therapy. The mean prolactin levels declined to 12% of the initial value with no patient achieving a normal prolactin level. Galactorrhea improved in three of the six, and menses returned in only one patient. In this same study, a rapid reduction in prolactin level was achieved only with surgery. Prolactin declined to a mean of 20% of preoperative levels in the 16 patients undergoing transsphenoidal surgery alone and was normalized in seven. Four of their patients received irradiation after transsphenoidal surgery with a mean decline of prolactin to 27% of initial value. Levels declined to a mean of 15% of pretreatment values in four patients managed by craniotomy and radiation.

Kleinberg et al[79] reported a mean prolactin reduction to 26% of pretreatment values in eight patients who underwent irradiation compared to a mean prolactin decline to 16% of initial values among 15 patients undergoing surgery. None of the eight irradiated patients became pregnant, and none of the six amenorrheic patients had a resumption of menses although galactorrhea disappeared in three following radiation.

De Schryver et al[34] reported six women presumed to have prolactinomas that were treated with irradiation. They were referred for sella enlargement, prolactin levels of 300 ng/ml or more, ophthalmologic symptoms, primary resistance to bromocriptine, or any combination of these factors. Three of the six patients achieved normal prolactin levels following irradiation, but all were given postoperative bromocriptine indefinitely. In one patient, visual deterioration after radiation and bromocriptine therapy led to surgery.

Kelly et al[70] of the Hammersmith Hospital group reported on the implantation of ^{90}Y into the pituitaries of 21 women with prolactinomas, all of whom had radiographically abnormal sellae and amenorrhea, galactorrhea, or infertility. In these patients, the mean prolactin for the group showed an average reduction of 26% (427 ng/ml to 317 ng/ml) and only three of the 21 (14%) achieved normal levels. Nine of 15 (60%) had some improvement in galactorrhea, five of 18 (28%) resumed menstruation after therapy, and three of the 21 (14%) became pregnant after radiation implantation alone.

Gomez et al[48] presented the results of radiation therapy in eight patients with microprolactinomas. Prolactin levels were measured immediately after radiotherapy in three patients. Significantly, in each there was a marked drop in the prolactin level followed within a few months by a rebound to pretreatment levels. Prolactin remained normalized in only one patient, menses resumed in four, and galactorrhea ceased in two.

In general, the results of irradiation for prolactinomas can be characterized as *unimpressive and inconclusive*.[109]

Acromegaly

In those studies carried out before the availability of GH assays, the results of treating acromegaly with radiation were evaluated on the basis of improvement in endocrine activity and mass effects. Evaluation of endocrine activity was generally based on metabolic rate, carbohydrate tolerance, serum phosphorus level, 17-ketosteroid and 17-hydroxysteroid excretion, and growth of skeletal and soft tissues.[136] The disease was considered to be controlled if there were reversal of chemical abnormalities, arrest of soft tissue changes, improvement in visual fields, cessation of headaches, and no further expansion of the sella. Table 13-3 summarizes the results of conventional radiation in the treatment of acromegaly before the availability of GH assays. In these three studies, the criteria cited above were used in assessing the results. Table 13-4 shows the effect of radiation on GH levels as measured after treatment, and Table 13-5 outlines those studies where GH levels were measured before and after irradiation.

Eastman et al[37] reported beneficial therapeutic results in 47 acromegalic patients treated with 4000 to 5000 rad of conventional supervoltage therapy and followed for a period of 10 years after treatment. In the majority, GH levels continued to fall over the 10-year interval and were <10 ng/ml in 81% and <5 ng/ml in 69% of the patients. Also the subjective (acral and facial changes) and the objective (metabolic) effects of GH excess all showed significant improvement over time with the improvement roughly paralleling the fall in plasma GH levels. After therapy, no patient developed extrasellar extension, and headaches improved in the majority of patients. On the negative side, the prevalence of hypopituitarism, which was low before treatment, increased progressively during the 10-year follow-up period and was documented in nine of 19 patients 10 years after therapy. These results certainly indicate that conventional radiation therapy is an effective mode of treatment for pituitary tumors causing acromegaly.

Table 13-3
Conventional radiation therapy for acromegaly before availability of GH assay

Parameter	Sheline et al[135]	Pistenma et al[115]		Kramer[81]
Dose (rad)	3500	3500	5800	4500
Patients treated	19	18	19	29
Visual field defects	8 (42%)	8 (44%)	6 (32%)	NA
Controlled by initial treatment	5 (26%)	14 (78%)	17 (90%)	25 (86%)
Controlled by re-treatment	7/9	—	—	—
Total controlled	12/19 (64%)	14/18 (78%)	17/19 (90%)	25/29 (86%)
Hypophysectomy for failure	2	1	2	4
Induced hypothyroidism		0	1	2
Major complications		3 (8%)*	NA	3 (10%)†
Follow-up (years)		1-18	1-18	NA

NA, Not available.
*1 breakdown of skin in external auditory canals.
 1 sarcoma.
 1 paranasal sinus carcinoma.
†2 radiation-induced optic nerve lesions.
 1 marked memory loss.

Table 13-4
Conventional radiation therapy for acromegaly after availability of GH assay—post-treatment GH only

Parameter	Lawrence et al[89]	Kramer et al[81]
Patients treated	16	8
Dose (rad)	1680-6600	5000
GH < 10 ng/ml	13/16 (81%)	7/8 (87%)
GH < 5 ng/ml	6/16 (37%)	7/8 (87%)

Table 13-5
Conventional radiation therapy for acromegaly after availability of GH assay—pretreatment and post-treatment GH levels

Parameter	Lawrence[89] et al	Gordon and Roth[49]	Kramer[81]	Sheline and Wara[136]*	Eastman et al[37]
Follow-up (years)	1-27	1-2	3-6	1-5	NA	2-10
Patients treated	12	30	16	8	18	47
Dose (rad)	3500-6500	4000-5000		4000-5000	4000	4000-5000
Mean pre-treatment GH (ng/ml)	84.75	58		26	52	62
Mean post-treatment GH	26	22	13	10.6	22	12
Reduction in GH (%)	69%	62	78	60	58	80
GH < 10 ng/ml	9/12 (75%)	13/30 (43%)	11/16 (69%)	7/8 (87.5%)	11/18 (61%)	(81%)†
GH < 5 ng/ml	7/12 (58%)	3/30 (1%)	5/16 (31%)	4/8 (50%)	7/18 (50%)	(69%)†

*Combined data from Radiation Therapy Oncology Group (RTOG).
†Results in the 16 patients followed >10 years.

Table 13-6
Conventional radiation therapy for surgical failures in acromegaly

Author	Surgery	Interval from irradiation (years)	Number with normal GH
Sheline[133]	Cryohypophysectomy	1	2/7
		2	4/7
	Transcranial	2	3/4
Williams et al[155]	Transsphenoidal	—	4/6
Eastman et al[37]	Transcranial	2	4/5
TOTAL			15/22 (68%)

Radiation therapy appears to be useful in treating acromegaly that persists after surgery. Table 13-6 shows the results of the small series available.

The experiences of both Kjellberg and Kliman[77] and Lawrence et al[90] indicate that good control of acromegaly can also be achieved by using heavy particle radiation therapy with an acceptable incidence of side effects. Kjellberg treated 431 acromegalic patients with proton beam radiotherapy and obtained a "remission" (GH <10 ng/ml) rate of 80% 4 years after therapy was administered.[77] He had a failure rate of 10%, and approximately 10% of his series developed hypopituitarism from the treatment and required replacement thyroid and/or steroid medication.[75] Lawrence et al[90] obtained levels of GH <10 ng/ml in 90% of 258 acromegalic patients within 5 years of heavy particle therapy.

Interstitial therapy has also been used in acromegaly, and Table 13-7 summarizes the results of Wright et al[159] and Fraser et al[43] who used ^{198}Au and ^{90}Y implantation, respectively. In general, the results are poor both in terms of clinical response and reduction of GH below 5 or 10 ng/ml. Additionally, there appears to be a significant incidence of complications associated with the technique.

Table 13-7
Results of implantation of ^{198}Au and ^{90}Y for treatment of acromegaly

Parameter	Wright et al[159]	Fraser et al[43]
Patients treated	80 (93 implants)	109 (125 implants)
Dose (rad)	10,000-50,000	≤50,000
Satisfactory clinical response*	53% (at 1 year)	21%
Improvement in visual field defects	5/5 (100%)	NA
Mean fall in GH†	54% (34 patients)	63% (45 patients)
GH ≤ 10 (ng/ml)	10/34 (29%)	11/45 (24%)
GH ≤ 5 (ng/ml)	6/34 (18%)	5/45 (11%)
Complications		
Deaths	3/93 (3%)	3/125 (2%)
Local infection	11/93 (12%)	—
Cerebrospinal fluid (CSF) rhinorrhea	12/93 (13%)	11/125 (9%)
Hypopituitarism	26/93 (28%)	42/125 (33%)
Diabetes insipidus	16/93 (17%)	3/125 (2%)
Visual loss or paresis	—	5/125 (4%)

NA, Not available.
*Satisfactory response means full relief of symptoms, visible regression of signs of acromegaly, return to normal of the insulin resistance index, and/or improvement in glucose tolerance.
†Mean serum GH during oral glucose tolerance test.

Table 13-8

Conventional radiation therapy for Cushing's disease

Parameter	Dohan et al[35]		Heuschele and Lampe[59]	Orth and Liddle[111]	Edmonds[38]
Dose (rad)	400-1570	3800-5200	4000	4000-5000	3500-5000
Patients	6	6	16	44	15
Cure	—	—	—	10 (23%)	9 (60%)
Control*	0 (0%)	5 (83%)	10 (62.5%)	23 (52%)	10 (67%)
Failures	6	1	1	21	5
Recurrences		0	5	0	0
Complications		0	—	0	0
Follow-up (years)		5.5-7	3-7	1-14 (mean 9)	—

*Criteria for control or cure:
  Disappearances of physical stigmata, improved glucose metabolism, lowered blood pressure (Dohan, et al).
  Criteria not given (Heuschele, Lampe).
  Urinary 17-hydroxycorticosteroid excretion 7 mg/g creatinine + Mean plasma cortisol 10 μg/100 ml (Orth, Liddle).

Cushing's disease

The first patient to benefit from pituitary irradiation for Cushing's syndrome was described by Cushing[31] in 1932. Most reports (Table 13-8) of the use of radiation for this disease include only small numbers of patients and use differing criteria for cure. It can be seen that conventional irradiation usually controls the disease to the point where no additional therapy is needed in 50% to 80%, the latter figure possibly being somewhat high. The response to radiation appears to be higher for children with Cushing's disease than for adults[59,67] (Table 13-9). The interval between therapy and clinical or biochemical remission varies from months to a year but is shorter than that required to control GH in irradiated acromegalic patients. With long follow-up periods, recurrences and complications of radiation are rare.

Table 13-9

Conventional radiation therapy for Cushing's disease in children

Dose (rad)	3500-4950
Patients treated	15
Cures*	12 (80%)
Failures	3
Recurrences	0
Complications	0
Follow-up (years)	1-19 (mean 8)

Modified from Jennings AS, Liddle GW, Orth, DN: Results of treating childhood Cushing's disease with pituitary irradiation. N Engl J Med 297:957, 1977.
*Cure defined as mean plasma cortisol <10 μg/dl with a 24-hour urinary 17-hydroxycorticosteroid excretion of 7 mg/g creatinine.

Of 124 patients treated by Kjellberg and Kliman[76,77] with proton beam radiation, about 65% underwent complete remission with restoration of normal clinical and laboratory findings. Another 20% were improved to the point that no further therapy was considered necessary. The 15% that were failures were treated by adrenalectomy or open hypophysectomy. Thirteen of their patients required replacement hormonal therapy. Temporary oculomotor disturbances occurred in 1% to 4% of patients, and one patient developed a visual field defect.

Fraser et al[43] and Burke et al[21] have reported the experience at the Hammersmith Hospital in treating 55 patients with Cushing's disease by implantation of ^{198}Au and ^{90}Y seeds. Table 13-10 summarizes the results in the 46 patients followed for 5 years. Thirty (55%) of the 55 treated patients required some form of hormone replacement, 14% had transient diabetes insipidus, 10% required reoperation for cerebrospinal fluid (CSF) leak, and 7% developed meningitis.

Table 13-10

^{198}Au or ^{90}Y implantation for Cushing's disease—results of 5-year follow-up in 55 patients

Sella	Abnormal	Possibly abnormal	Normal
Patients treated	12	6	28
Complete remission	2 (17%)	4 (67%)	11 (61%)
Partial remission	0	0	2 (28%)
Failure	3 (25%)	0	3 (17%)
Dead	7 (58%)	2 (33%)	2 (11%)

From Burke CW, Doyle FH, Joplin GF, et al: Cushing's disease: Treatment by pituitary implantation of radioactive gold or yttrium seeds, *Quart. J. Med.* 42:693, 1973.

Nelson's syndrome

Radiation therapy has been used both to prevent Nelson's syndrome and to treat the disorder once it is established. The role of radiation in each of these situations is disputed. Nelson's syndrome is a relatively uncommon disorder with meager data concerning its prevention and treatment. Table 13-11 summarizes the literature concerning the occurrence of this disorder and its prevention by pituitary radiation in patients undergoing adrenalectomy for Cushing's disease. Orth and Liddle[111] found no instance of Nelson's syndrome among 43 patients treated with pituitary radiation for Cushing's disease, 20 of which also had bilateral adrenalectomies. Moore et al,[105] however, studied 120 patients who underwent adrenalectomy for Cushing's disease and found about the same incidence of Nelson's syndrome regardless of whether or not they received pituitary radiation.

Table 13-11
Incidence of Nelson's syndrome in patients treated for Cushing's disease

Author	Treatment for Cushing's disease	Mean observation (years)	Number developing Nelson's syndrome
Orth and Liddle[111]	PRT	9	0/23
	PRT + A	8	0/20
Moore et al[105]	A	6	7/100
	PRT + A	12.5	2/20
Wild et al[154]	PRT + A	2	2/?
Hopwood and Kenny[62]	A	3	8-18*/30
Jennings et al[67]	PRT	8	0/11
	PRT + A	12	0/4

A, Adrenalectomy.
PRT, Pituitary radiation therapy.
*Eight patients had Nelson's syndrome, whereas 10 others developed hyperpigmentation but incomplete radiologic studies of the sella to determine if a tumor was present.

In childhood Cushing's disease, Hopwood and Kenny[62] found that at least eight of 30 patients treated with total adrenalectomy without pituitary radiation developed Nelson's syndrome and at least 10 others developed hyperpigmentation but did not have serial x-ray examinations to document changes in the size of the sella. This finding underscores the significance of the absence of Nelson's syndrome in the 15 children reported by Jennings et al[67] treated with pituitary irradiation, although only four had adrenalectomies. These data indicate that although pituitary irradiation does not prevent Nelson's syndrome in all patients, it probably reduces the incidence significantly.[133]

As a treatment for established Nelson's syndrome, radiotherapy has been used both as primary therapy and as an adjunct to surgery. Available data on the results of irradiation for Nelson's syndrome are relatively meager and inconclusive. For instance, Moore et al treated seven patients, five with irradiation alone and two with partial surgical excision plus irradiation. Six patients were alive and "clinically stable" for an average of 9.4 years after discovery of the tumor. Although limited, the data suggest that irradiation alone controls many patients with this disorder and that it may be of value when pituitary surgery fails to cure the disease.[133]

Nonfunctional adenomas

An analysis of the literature on radiation therapy of nonfunctional pituitary adenomas is complicated by several factors. Most of the available reports were published before the use and/or availability of laboratory and histologic techniques used in modern classifications of pituitary adenomas (e.g., electron microscopy, radioimmunoassay (RIA), immunocytochemistry). Certainly, many of the adenomas included in the large series of "nonfunctional" tumors were prolactin-secreting tumors, and others may have been unrecognized hyperfunctional tumors of various types. In the larger series that compare the results of radiation and surgery, craniotomy rather than transsphenoidal adenomectomy was the surgical procedure performed. Both presentation of the tumors and results of treatment were judged grossly by the appearance of mass effects rather than by more precise parameters such as CT. The postoperative use of radiation was either as an immediate adjunct or for clear surgical failures that developed mass effects (usually visual loss) as opposed to following the tumor postoperatively by CT to document a recurrence before symptoms and signs appear. In many of the reports, patients with lesser deficits were more likely to be treated by radiation alone. On the other hand, poor surgical risks would likewise be treated by radiation alone.

Table 13-12 summarizes several of the larger series in which radiation therapy was used alone or in combination with surgery for the treatment of nonfunctional pituitary adenomas. From this table, it is apparent that the control rate is about equal between radiation alone and surgery plus radiation, both of which are superior to the control rates obtained with surgery alone.

Table 13-12

Conventional radiation therapy for nonfunctional pituitary adenomas

Authors	Year	Percentage of control rate			Duration of follow-up (years)
		RT	S & RT	S	
Horrax et al[63]	1955	88	72	—	1-6
Correa and Lampe[30]	1962	79	76	—	1-5
Emmanuel[41]	1966	75	92	—	4+
Bouchard[18]	1966	71	82	—	5-20
Hayes et al[57]	1971	78	74	45	2-16
Bloom[13]	1973	92.6	91.6	—	5+
Kramer[82]	1973	82	90	—	1-6
Pistenma et al[114]	1975	89.6	84.9	—	5+
Urdaneta et al[150]	1976	86	86	—	5+
Sheline[133]	1979	93	96	38	5+
Salmi et al[125]	1982	—	80	—	0.5-6
MEANS OF TOTALS		85	85	41	

RT, Radiation therapy.
S&RT, Surgery and postoperative radiation.
S, Surgery alone.

Surgery provides a definitive diagnosis and debulking of the tumor for rapid decompression. If a complete resection cannot be accomplished, radiation therapy will usually increase the recurrence-free survival rate. The advent of modern transsphenoidal surgery and CT scanning has raised the question whether such radiation should be administered in the immediate postoperative period or after tumor recurrence is documented on CT. At the present time, data to answer this question are unavailable.

Meningiomas

Total surgical excision of a meningioma including the dural site of origin is curative but is not always possible. Although the role of radiation therapy in the management of meningiomas is not clearly established and many authors have stressed the radioinsensitivity of these tumors,[36,45,102,129] some reports have spoken to the value of radiation therapy for certain meningiomas.[19,23,71,153]

In the series of Wara et al,[153] there were no recurrences among 84 patients treated by gross total removal alone. However, of 58 patients treated by subtotal removal, 43 (74%) had recurrences. Of 34 patients given postoperative radiation to a dose of at least 5000 rad following subtotal resection, only 10 (29%) had recurrences. In addition, the irradiated patients tended to have longer intervals to recurrence.

Carella et al[23] reported 68 patients that underwent radiation therapy for meningiomas. These authors divided their patients into three groups. Group A included 43 patients who underwent operation followed by radiation therapy. Group B was 14 patients that had radiation for recurrence after operation, and Group C included 11 patients that had radiation as a primary treatment. Forty-one of the 43 Group A patients were alive and only two deteriorated during a follow-up period of 1 to 10 years. Five of the 14 Group B patients showed neurologic improvement, and seven showed deterioration, including five who died of their tumor. All 11 of the Group C patients were alive after follow-up periods of 3 to 6 years, and nine of the patients showed improvement in neurologic condition. Eleven of their patients had malignant meningiomas, of whom eight were alive and stable at the time of the report.

Based on their study, Carella et al[23] recommended the following guidelines:
1. Postoperative radiation is not recommended if resection is complete and the meningioma is not malignant.
2. In cases of malignant meningioma, postoperative radiation should be given whether or not the resection was complete.
3. Postoperative radiation should generally be given if resection is known to be incomplete. In older patients with small residual tumor, radiation can be withheld until regrowth is documented by CT.
4. For recurrent meningiomas, particularly in the younger age group, radiation therapy should be given either postoperatively or as the primary mode of therapy, particularly if the initial operation was difficult.
5. Radiation therapy should be considered as the primary treatment for certain basilar meningiomas where the neurologic deficit will not be improved by surgery in the absence of mass effects and in other situations where surgery would be dangerous or cause permanent neurologic damage.

Recommended radiation doses for meningiomas range from 4500 to 6500 rad.[19,23,71,153] In the series of Carella et al,[23] dose ranged from 5200 to 7495 rad, and no correlation between doses and tumor control could be found. These authors recommend 5000 to 5500 rad in 5.5 to 6 weeks using a small field beam-directed technique.[23]

Craniopharyngiomas

Irradiation treatment for craniopharyngioma was first described by Carpenter et al[25] in 1937. Since then, there have been steady improvements and refinements in this treatment modality. As discussed in Chapter 11, we divided irradiation therapy into two categories—primary, or definitive, and secondary, or adjunctive. Primary, or definitive, radiotherapy is that administered as the main treatment modality to a patient with a craniopharyngioma and includes those patients treated in this fashion either with no biopsy or in those in whom the only surgery was to establish a tissue diagnosis. Secondary, or adjunctive, radiotherapy is that delivered to patients in whom surgery was used as the primary treatment modality but in whom only a partial resection was accomplished or in whom a symptomatic recurrence has developed.

Primary irradiation. The two major advocates of primary irradiation are Kramer and Bloom, who recommend "radical" radiotherapy following establishment of a positive tissue diagnosis by "conservative" surgery. On the basis of his experience, Kramer concludes that adequate irradiation can arrest the growth of craniopharyngiomas and, if applied properly, carries a minimal risk for the patient.[83,84,86] He also believes that recurrence is common even after total surgical excision and for this reason recommends that irradiation should always be a part of the management of these patients.

Bloom gives survival figures following radiation of new cases (i.e., those treated before recurrence following previous surgery).[14-16] Seventy-four percent of 46 children and 60% of 66 adults are listed as surviving 10 years following irradiation treatment.

Secondary irradiation. The results of secondary radiotherapy were discussed by Richmond et al[121] who reported a retrospective study of 32 children treated for craniopharyngiomas using a variety of treatment modalities. They found that the group receiving radiation therapy after known subtotal resection did as well as the group with estimated total removal. Furthermore, the authors obtained an excellent response in eight patients with "conservative" surgery followed by irradiation, a finding that the authors believe provides further evidence of the efficiency of adjunctive radiotherapy.

Cabezudo et al[22] conducted a retrospective study in 45 patients with craniopharyngioma treated by three different therapeutic approaches—total excision, subtotal excision, and surgery followed by a course of irradiation. Their results indicate that adjunctive radiotherapy can yield beneficial results.

Of particular interest in regard to the neurologic and psychophysiologic sequelae in patients treated by different modalities was the recent report by Cavazzuti et al.[26] They compared patients treated with radiation alone or by radiation plus conservative surgical procedures (e.g., biopsy, cyst aspiration, shunting) with a group in whom radical tumor resection was attempted by craniotomy (subfrontal approach). The authors make a case for treatment with radiotherapy, although they admit that late unfavorable outcomes may occur as a result of the delayed effects of radiotherapy. Therefore long-term follow-up review of these cases is indicated.

For further analysis of the results of irradiation in craniopharyngiomas and especially the complications of this form of therapy, the reader is referred to Chapter 11.

Interstitial irradiation. Another form of therapy available for treatment of certain craniopharyngiomas is interstitial, or implanted, irradiation. This is also discussed in Chapter 11.

The advantages of intracyst isotope radiotherapy are that relatively large doses of radiation can be delivered to the entire cyst capsule with theoretically, little exposure to adjacent neural structures (provided beta emission is used).[28] The optimal candidates are those patients with large, uncontrollable cysts invading a vital area or patients with multiple or recurrent cysts.[65]

COMPLICATIONS OF CNS AND PITUITARY IRRADIATION

Although therapeutic radiation of the brain and pituitary carry the same potential risks, the incidence of complications is much lower with pituitary irradiation. This is thought to be a result of the smaller volumes of tissue irradiated with pituitary tumors and the advances in treatment planning resulting in dosages to surrounding normal tissue below that required for significant necrosis of brain tissue. The major risks of radiation to the brain or hypothalamic-pituitary region include radionecrosis, damage to the optic nerves or chiasm, hypopituitarism, impairment of intellectual function, soft tissue reactions, and radiation-induced tumorigenesis.

Cerebral radionecrosis

The incidence of radiation-induced brain injury, or cerebral radionecrosis, is difficult to establish and is dependent on the dosage of radiation given, the volume of tissue treated, the technique of delivery of irradiation (multiple versus single field), and the period of time over which the brain is irradiated. The incidence is probably underestimated because autopsy confirmation is often lacking and the assumption is often made that patients deteriorate or die as a result of progression of their disease (i.e., brain tumor).[99] Bouchard[18] indicates that the limit of tolerance of the adult brain to radiation is 6500 rad/50 days, but brain necrosis may occur following lower dosages.[20] For the smaller volumes needed for pituitary tumors, higher dosages (6500 rad in 7 weeks for a child or 7000 rad in 7 weeks for an adult) can usually be tolerated,[42] especially if multiple treatment fields are used to keep the dose of irradiation to surrounding normal tissue within established tolerances.

The incidence varies widely among different authors. For instance, Marks et al[99] reported pathologically documented cerebral radionecrosis in seven, or 5%, of 139 patients receiving 4500 rad or greater (180 to 200 rad fractions) for brain and pituitary tumors. This incidence of 5% may be higher because two additional patients were suspected of having radionecrosis on clinical grounds. In this report, 20 patients were radiated for pituitary tumors, and one developed pathologically documented cerebral radionecrosis. Although the risk of radionecrosis was greatest with higher doses, these authors were unable to correlate risk with shorter time, larger fractions, or larger field size. They did find that radionecrosis did not occur below dosages equivalent to 5400 rad in 30 fractions over 42 days. On the basis of a literature search, Sheline et al[137] concluded that radiation dosages of 5200 rad/5 weeks (200 rad fractions) are associated with a very low incidence of delayed reactions. These authors found 20 patients reported in the literature that developed radiation injury to the brain following radiation therapy for pituitary or parapituitary tumors. Radiation lesions were described in the hypothalamus in five patients, temporal lobe(s) in eight, frontal lobe(s) in seven, parapituitary or walls of the third ventricle in three, and brainstem in one.[137] By assuming that all 20 of these patients with necrosis were from a total irradiated pool of 5000 and that all instances of necrosis were reported, Sheline et al[137] estimated the incidence of necrosis in pituitary-craniopharyngioma patients to be 0.4%. Of 464 patients irradiated for pituitary adenomas in the combined series of Sheline et al,[133,136] Kramer,[81] Pistenma et al,[114] and Emmanuel,[41] there were no cases of radiation-induced brain necrosis. Martins et al[100] reported brain necrosis in two patients following radiation of pituitary adenomas, but these patients received doses of 6600 and 6700 rad, well above doses presently used.

Despite the theoretic physical advantages of particulate irradiation over conventional photon radiation, there are complications with the former. The brains of eight patients treated with a single proton beam dose ranging from 10,000 to 18,000 rad with a 7-mm diameter portal for pituitary ablation were studied histologically by Neilson et al.[108] These patients, none of whom had clinically evident neurologic injury attributed to radiation, all died within 3 to 49 months after radiation from progression of their primary disease. Five of the eight brains contained areas of radiation necrosis in the medial temporal lobes, and four were found to have areas of radiation injury in the ventral hypothalamus. The pituitaries contained a large central necrotic zone and were completely fibrotic. Radiation dose to the medial temporal region was estimated to be 3500 to 5000 rad.

A similar study was performed by the same authors on the brains of six patients treated with proton beam radiotherapy for malignant gliomas and four for pituitary adenomas.[107] Survivals ranged from 1 to 28 months after radiation, and doses ranged from 3970 to 10,500 rad delivered through multiple ports ranging from 16 to 51 mm in diameter. The causes of death were not reported. Histologic evidence of radiation injury was seen in all patients and increased in severity as the dose increased. The hypothalamus, medial thalamus, and tegmentum of the upper brainstem were found to be more vulnerable than the corpus striatum, cerebral cortex, or basis pontis.

Optic nerve/chiasm damage

Aristizabal et al[7] found 14 patients in the literature with radiation damage to the CNS (including the optic pathways) after irradiation for pituitary tumors. These authors indicated that patients received "moderate doses" of radiation although lack of information regarding size of irradiated populations prevented determinations of incidence rates. Aristizabal et al[8] had previously reported four optic nerve or chiasmal injuries attributed to pituitary irradiation from a total of 122 patients (3%) treated at Vanderbilt University, Nashville, Tennessee, between 1952 and 1971. No visual complications occurred in patients receiving <5000 rad. When daily doses were <220 rad, the visual complication rate was 2% but rose to 13% for daily fractions >220 rad. Harris and Levene[54] reported five cases of radiation-induced optic nerve damage among 55 patients treated for pituitary adenomas, each injury associated with a daily fraction of 250 rad or greater. Three of 42 patients with acromegaly treated by Kramer with a total dose of 5000 rad in 5 weeks had damage to the optic nerves or chiasm.[133] Since reducing the dose to 4500 rad, there were no further injuries nor were any identified among 190 patients treated with 4500 rad in 4.5 weeks for "chromophobic" adenomas.[133] Sheline reports that only one patient out of 181 treated for pituitary adenomas between 1934 and 1975 had radiation-induced blindness.[133] That particular patient received a daily dose of 225 rad.

Temporary oculomotor disturbance has in some instances been associated with heavy particle irradiation, with an incidence of about 6% in a group of 50 acromegalic patients treated with protons[72] and 3.5% of 140 patients treated with alpha particles.[90]

Hypopituitarism

The incidence of radiation-induced hypopituitarism as a function of radiation dose is unknown, but most studies indicate that there is both a latent period of several years and a dose effect relationship.[120,137] The incidence is reflected in the diligence of the search for endocrine deficiencies. Although all serum hormone levels may be depressed by irradiation of the pituitary-hypothalamic axis, GH production is the most sensitive, and children seem to be more susceptible.[53,56,69,130,131] This is most likely a result of hypothalamic damage, although higher doses can produce direct pituitary deficiency.[126] Both gonadotropin deficiency[118] and hyperprolactinemia[27,128] have been documented following radiation therapy of the pituitary region.

Some reports indicate that the incidence of overt clinical pituitary deficiency is rare following radiation for extrahypophysial lesions.[39,139] Of 810 patients receiving up to 14,000 rad for nasopharyngeal carcinoma, only one (a 12-year-old girl treated with 9000 rad) developed growth deficiency.[139,145] However, if more extensive and sensitive endocrine testing is done, then endocrine deficiencies can be identified at lower radiation doses.[46] Samaan et al[127] observed 65 patients for

3 to 20 years after photon irradiation (500 to 8500 rad) for neoplasms in the nasopharynx, orbit, or paranasal sinuses and studied hormone levels by radioimmunoassay. The patients ranged from 14 to 76 years of age. In 60 (92%), the retrospectively calculated radiation dose to the hypothalamic-pituitary region was between 4000 and 8500 rad. They detected evidence of hypothalamic dysfunction in 54 patients (83%) and primary deficiency of pituitary hormones in 25 (38.5%). In a later article, Samaan et al[128] expanded their series to 110 patients and follow-up of one to 26 years following radiotherapy. Evidence of endocrine deficiencies were identified in 91 (83%) of the 110 patients, 76 showing some evidence of hypothalamic lesions and 43 having a primary pituitary deficiency. Richards et al[120] reported four children irradiated for nonpituitary, nonhypothalamic neoplasms of the brain that developed GH deficiencies. One of the four also developed deficiency of thyroid-stimulating hormone (TSH), adrenocorticotropic hormone (ACTH), and gonadotropins. Pituitary doses were between 4000 and 5200 rad given in 160 to 180 rad/day fractions.

The incidence of clinically apparent pituitary deficiency following radiation for pituitary adenomas is apparently low. Jenkins et al[66] studied endocrine function in 22 patients treated with radiation for pituitary adenomas. One patient developed hypoadrenalism and hypothyroidism but had some evidence of pituitary-adrenal deficiency before radiation. Eastman et al[37] reported 47 patients with acromegaly treated by irradiation and found the incidence to increase from 9% before therapy to 19% at 10 years. Hypoadrenalism was found in 6% before treatment and rose to 30% at 5 years and 38% at 10 years. These patients were given between 4000 and 5000 rad to the pituitary region in daily fractions of <200 rad. Halse et al[53] studied the effect of pituitary irradiation (4500 rad over 4 weeks) on the thyrotropin-releasing hormone (TRH)-stimulation test in 14 patients, all but one with prior transcranial surgery. No change in the TSH response to TRH was observed either during or after a 4-week treatment period, indicating a relative resistance of the pituitary against irradiation.

Diabetes insipidus has occurred in about 14% of patients treated by internal irradiation (i.e., brachytherapy)[21,159] and in less than 2% of patients treated by proton beams[72] and has not been reported following alpha particles or conventional radiotherapy.[109]

Effect on intellectual function

More difficult to quantitate is the effect of cranial irradiation on intellectual function. After prophylactic irradiation for acute lymphocytic leukemia in children with 1200 to 2400 rad, psychometric tests failed to demonstrate any loss of function.[140] Impairment of intellectual function in patients with brain tumors has ranged from minimal to major after cranial irradiation (400 to 6000 rad).[10,32,110,117,143] These patients may have had preirradiation neurologic damage, however, from tumor, elevated ICP, or surgery.[26,137]

Soft tissue reactions

During cranial irradiation, the soft tissues external to the brain are at risk for radiation-induced reactions. Baglan and Marks[9] evaluated the soft tissue reactions that occurred in 199 patients who received radiation therapy for primary brain or pituitary tumors. The most common soft tissue effect, complete epilation, was defined as total and permanent loss of hair (except villus hair); it occurred in 40% of the patients, whereas 21% of patients experienced some other soft tissue reaction as outlined in Table 13-13.[9] The single most important parameter correlating with the incidence of these reactions was the radiation dose calculated at 5 mm below the skin surface. Patients with pituitary lesions were treated with small fields to a low dose at 5 mm and consequently had the lowest rate of soft tissue reactions.[9]

Table 13-13
Soft tissue reactions from cranial irradiation

	Incidence (%)
Scalp	
Complete epilation	40
Swelling	6
Suturosis	3.5
Folliculitis	2
Wet desquamation	1.5
Infection	0.5
Skull	
Lost skull flap	1
Bone exposure	1
Ear	
External otitis	6
Otitis media	5
Swelling	4
Chondritis	1
Jaw	
Temporomandibular joint tenderness	0.5
Trismus	0.5
Radiation caries	0.5
Soft tissue effects other than complete epilation	21

Modified from Baglan RJ, and Marks JE: Soft-tissue reactions following irradiation of primary brain and pituitary tumors, *Int J Radiat Oncol Biol Phys* 7:455, 1981.

Tumorigenesis

It is well established on an epidemiologic basis that radiation can induce secondary neoplasia such as thyroid and breast carcinomas, leukemia, multiple myeloma, and sarcomas.[42,112] There appear in the literature a number of well-documented cases of secondary CNS neoplasms following radiation therapy to the brain or sellar region. However, a causal relationship should be considered critically, and to establish such a relationship, certain criteria should be met.[42] First, the secondary neoplasm should occur in the irradiated field. Next, it should appear after a latency sufficient to indicate that the lesion was not present at the time of irradiation, and lastly, the neoplasms should appear more frequently among irradiated patients than among matched controls. The establishment of a dose-response relationship and existence of an animal model provide important supporting evidence.[42] Not all of this evidence is present for each of the reported cases of secondary CNS neoplasms occurring after radiation therapy.

Terry et al[147] first reported the combination of fibrosarcoma and pituitary adenoma arising in three patients with previously irradiated pituitary neoplasms. Waltz and Brownell[152] reviewed the literature and found eight fibrosarcomas and one osteosarcoma reported in radiated tissues following radiation therapy for pituitary tumors. These authors also reported two of their cases that developed fibrosarcomas following radiation doses of 3500 and 4500 rad and one osteosarcoma after 6000 rad.[152] Subsequent cases of fibrosarcoma have been reported by others.[113,116,123] In most reported cases, the tumors consisted of a combination of fibrosarcoma and pituitary adenoma,[113] exceptions being an anaplastic sarcoma with no residual pituitary tissue,[47] a fibrosarcoma alone,[1] and an osteogenic sarcoma with extrasellar extension.[3] Other tissues in the irradiation path are also subject to oncogenesis, and several cases of osteogenic sarcoma of the skull have been reported following radiotherapy for benign pituitary adenomas.[103,142,152] The documented postirradiation pituitary sarcomas have generally presented after a long latent interval since radiation (2.5 to 21 years), have grown to a large size, and have failed to metastasize.[113] The doses of radiation in these cases range from 2400 and 11,400 rad. An intrasellar and parasellar fibrosarcoma was diagnosed 7 years after proton irradiation (10,000 rad) for acromegaly.[29]

Radiation-associated gliomas have also been reported following CNS and sellar radiotherapy. Piatt et al[112] reported two patients that developed a glioblastoma multiforme 14 and 10 years, respectively, after pituitary irradiation for acromegaly with dosages of 4900 rad over 5.5 weeks and 4500 rad over 5 weeks. These authors found 16 other cases of radiation-associated gliomas in the literature.[112]

The evidence for the radiation-induction of meningiomas was reviewed by Iacono et al,[64] who demonstrated a relationship between dose and latency. The average time from radiation to diagnosis among patients receiving more than 2300 rad for various malignancies was 20.8 years, whereas the average latency for the entire series including patients irradiated with low dosages for tinea capitis in childhood, was 31.3 years.[64]

SUMMARY

Although irradiation is an effective mode of therapy in patients with pituitary tumors and certain parasellar neoplasms, it usually does not provide definitive cures and does carry some risks. Therefore it should only be used after thoughtful consideration on an individualized basis. In general, although it is sometimes recommended as primary treatment in certain special situations (e.g., medically unstable acromegalic patients), in our opinion, the attitude toward irradiation is that it should be considered an important *adjunctive* therapeutic tool.

REFERENCES

1. Ahmad K, Fayos JV: Pituitary fibrosarcoma secondary to radiation therapy. *Cancer* 42:107, 1978.
2. Almquist S, Dahlgren S, Notter G, et al: Brain necrosis after irradiation of the hypophysis in Cushing's disease. *Acta Radiol Ther* 2:179, 1964.
3. Amine ARC, Sugar O: Suprasellar osteogenic sarcoma following radiation for pituitary adenoma: Case report. *J Neurosurg* 44:88, 1976.
4. Anniko M: Early morphological changes following gamma irradiation: A comparison of human pituitary tumours and human acoustic neurinomas (schwannomas). *Acta Pathol Microbiol Scand* 89:113, 1981.
5. Anniko M, Wersall J: Morphological effects in pituitary tumours following radiotherapy. *Virchows Arch Pathol Anat* 395:45, 1982.
6. Antunes JL, Housepian EM, Frantz AG, et al: Prolactin-secreting pituitary tumors. *Ann Neurol* 2:148, 1977.
7. Aristizabal S, Boone MLM, Laguna JF: Endocrine factors influencing radiation injury to central nervous tissue. *Int J Radiat Oncol Biol Phys* 5:349, 1979.
8. Aristizabal SA, Caldwell WL, Avila J: The relationship of time-dose fractionation factors to complications in the treatment of pituitary tumors by irradiation. *Int J Radiat Oncol Biol Phys* 2:667, 1977.
9. Baglan RJ, Marks JE: Soft-tissue reactions following irradiation of primary brain and pituitary tumors. *Int J Radiat Oncol Biol Phys* 7:455, 1981.
10. Bamford FN, Morris-Jones P, Pearson D, et al: Residual disabilities in children treated for intracranial space-occupying lesions. *Cancer* 37:1149, 1976.
11. Barendsen GW, Walter HMD: Effects of different ionizing radiations on human cells in tissue culture: IV. Modification of radiation damage. *Radiat Res* 21:314, 1964.
12. Béclère A: The radio-therapeutic treatment of tumours of the hypophysis, gigantism, and acromegaly. *Arch Roentgen Ray* 14:142, 1909.
13. Bloom HJG: Radiotherapy of pituitary tumors, in Jenkins JS (ed): *Pituitary Tumors*. New York, Appleton-Century-Crofts, 1973.
14. Bloom HJG: Combined modality therapy for intracranial tumors. *Cancer* 35:111, 1975.
15. Bloom HJG: Recent concepts in the conservative treatment of intracranial tumours in children. *Acta Neurochir* 50:103, 1979.
16. Bloom HJG, Harmer CL: Craniopharyngioma: General aspects and treatment, in Bucalossi P, Veronesis U, Emanuelli H, et al (eds): *I Tumori Infantili*. Milan, Case Editrice Ambrosiana, 1976.
17. Boldrey E, Sheline G: Delayed transitory clinical manifestations after radiation treatment of intracranial tumors. *Acta Radiol* 5:5, 1966.
18. Bouchard J: *Radiation Therapy of Tumors and Diseases of the Nervous System*. Philadelphia, Lea & Febiger, 1966.
19. Bouchard J: Central nervous system, in Fletcher GH (ed): *Textbook of Radiotherapy*, ed 3. Philadelphia, Lea & Febiger, 1980.
20. Burger PC, Mahaley MS Jr, Dudka L, et al: The morphologic effects of radiation adminis-

tered therapeutically for intracranial gliomas: A postmortem study of 25 cases. *Cancer* 44:1256, 1979.
21. Burke CW, Doyle FH, Joplin GF, et al: Cushing's disease: Treatment by pituitary implantation of radioactive gold or yttrium seeds. *Q J Med* 42:693, 1973.
22. Cabezudo JM, Vaquero J, Areitio E, et al: Craniopharyngiomas: A critical approach to treatment. *J Neurosurg* 55:371, 1981.
23. Carella RJ, Ransohoff J, Newall J: Role of radiation therapy in the management of meningioma. *Neurosurgery* 10:332, 1982.
24. Carmichael KA, Jennings AS, Doty RL: Reversible anosmia after pituitary irradiation. *Ann Intern Med* 100:532, 1984.
25. Carpenter RC, Chamberlin GW, Frazier CH: The treatment of hypophyseal stalk tumors by evacuation and irradiation. *AJR* 38:162, 1937.
26. Cavazzuti V, Fischer EG, Welch K, et al: Neurological and psychophysiological sequelae following different treatments of craniopharyngioma in children. *J Neurosurg* 59:409, 1983.
27. Clark AJL, Mashiter K, Goolden AW, et al: Hyperprolactinaemia after external irradiation for acromegaly. *Clin Endocrinol* 17:291, 1982.
28. Cobb CA, Youmans JR: Brain tumors of disordered embryogenesis in adults, in Youmans JR (ed): *Neurological Surgery*, ed 2. Philadelphia, WB Saunders Co, 1982, vol 5.
29. Coppeto JR, Roberts M: Fibrosarcoma after proton-beam pituitary ablation. *Arch Neurol* 36:380, 1979.
30. Correa JN, Lampe I: The radiation treatment of pituitary adenomas. *J Neurosurg* 19:626, 1962.
31. Cushing H: The basophil adenomas of the pituitary body and their clinical manifestations (pituitary basophilism). *Bull Johns Hopkins Hosp* 50:137, 1932.
32. Danoff BF, Cowchock FS, Kramer S: Childhood craniopharyngioma: Survival, local control, endocrine and neurologic function following radiotherapy. *Int J Radiat Oncol Biol Phys* 9:171, 1983.
33. De Schryver A, Ljunggren JG, Bååryd I: Pituitary function in long-term survival after radiation therapy of nasopharyngeal tumours. *Acta Radiol Ther* 12:497, 1973.
34. De Schryver A, VandeKerckhove D, Debruyne G: Prolactin-secreting pituitary adenoma: Observations in irradiated patients. *Acta Radiol Oncol* 19:169, 1980.
35. Dohan FC, Raventos A, Boucot N, et al: Roentgen therapy in Cushing's syndrome without adrenocortical tumor. *J Clin Endocrinol Metab* 17:8, 1957.
36. Dyke G, Davidoff LM: *Roentgen Treatment of Diseases of the Nervous System*. Philadelphia, Lea & Febiger, 1942.
37. Eastman RC, Gorden P, Roth J: Conventional supervoltage irradiation is an effective treatment for acromegaly. *J Clin Endocrinol Metab* 48:931, 1979.
38. Edmonds MW, Simpson WJK, Meakin JW: External irradiation of the hypophysis for Cushing's disease. *Can Med Assoc J* 107:860, 1972.
39. Einhorn J, Einhorn N: Effects of irradiation of the endocrine glands. *Front Rad Ther Oncol* 6:386, 1972.
40. Ellis F: Dose, time and fractionation: A clinical hypothesis. *Clin Radiol* 20:1, 1969.
41. Emmanuel IG: Symposium on pituitary tumours: Historical aspects of radiotherapy, present treatment technique and results. *Clin Radiol* 17:154, 1966.
42. Fajardo LF: Pathogenesis of radiation injury, in Fajardo LF: *Pathology of Radiation Injury*. New York, Masson Publishing USA Inc, 1982.
43. Fraser R, Doyle F, Joplin GF, et al: The assessment of the endocrine effects and the effectiveness of ablative pituitary treatment by ^{90}Y and ^{198}Au implantation, in Kohler PO, Ross GT (eds): *Diagnosis and Treatment of Pituitary Tumors*. International Congress Series No. 303, Amsterdam, Excerpta Medica, 1973.
44. Freeman JE, Johnston PGB, Voke JM: Somnolence after prophylactic cranial irradiation in children with acute lymphoblastic leukaemia. *Br Med J* 4:523, 1973.
45. Freid JR: Treatment of central nervous system neoplasms with irradiation: General considerations, in Pack GT, Ariel IM (eds): *Treatment of Cancer and Allied Diseases*. New York, Paul B Hoeber, Inc., 1959, vol 2.
46. Fuks Z, Glatstein E, Marsa GW, et al: Long-term effects of external radiation on the pituitary and thyroid glands. *Cancer* 37:1152, 1976.
47. Goldberg MB, Sheline GE, Malamud N: Malignant intracranial neoplasms following radiation therapy for acromegaly. *Radiology* 80:465, 1963.
48. Gomez F, Reyes FI, Faiman C: Nonpuerperal galactorrhea and hyperprolactinemia: Clinical findings, endocrine features and therapeutic responses in 56 cases. *Am J Med* 62:648, 1977.
49. Gorden P, Roth J: The treatment of acromegaly by conventional pituitary irradiation, in Kohler PO, Ross GT (eds): *Diagnosis and Treatment*

of *Pituitary Tumors*. International Congress Series No. 303, Amsterdam, Excerpta Medica, 1973.
50. Gramegna A: Un cas d'acromegalie traité par la radiothérapie. *Rev Neurol* 17:15, 1909.
51. Gray LH, Conger AD, Ebert M, et al: The concentration of oxygen dissolved in tissues at the time of radiation as a factor in radiotherapy. *Br J Radiol* 45:81, 1982.
52. Hall EJ: *Radiobiology for the Radiologist*. New York, Harper & Row Publishers Inc, 1973.
53. Halse J, Larsen IF, Rootwelt K: Pituitary function during x-ray treatment of the hypothalamic-pituitary region as evaluated by the TRH test response. *Acta Med Scand* Suppl. 645:109, 1981.
54. Harris JR, Levene MB: Visual complications following irradiation for pituitary adenomas and craniopharyngiomas. *Radiology* 120:167, 1976.
55. Harris JW: Effects of ionizing radiation on lysosomes and other intracellular membranes. *Adv Biol Med Phys* 13:273, 1970.
56. Harrop JS, Davies TJ, Capra LG, et al: Hypothalamic-pituitary function following successful treatment of intracranial tumours. *Clin Endocrinol* 5:313, 1976.
57. Hayes TP, Davis RA, Raventos A: The treatment of pituitary chromophobe adenomas. *Radiology* 98:149, 1971.
58. Henderson WR: The pituitary adenomata: A follow-up study of the surgical results in 338 cases (Dr. Harvey Cushing's series). *Br J Surg* 26:811, 1939.
59. Heuschele R, Lampe I: Pituitary irradiation for Cushing's syndrome. *Radiol Clin Biol* 36:27, 1967.
60. Hirsch O: Hypophysentumoren—ein Grenzgebiet. *Acta Neurochir* 5:1, 1957.
61. Hoffman WF, Levin VA, Wilson CB: Evaluation of malignant glioma patients during the postirradiation period. *J Neurosurg* 50:624, 1979.
62. Hopwood N, Kenny F: Increased incidence of post-adrenalectomy Nelson's syndrome in pediatric vs adult Cushing's disease: A nationwide study. *Pediatr Res* 9:290, 1975.
63. Horrax G, Smedal MI, Trump JG, et al: Present-day treatment of pituitary adenomas: Surgery versus x-ray therapy. *N Engl J Med* 252:524, 1955.
64. Iacona RP, Apuzzo MLJ, Davis RL, et al: Multiple meningiomas following radiation therapy for medulloblastoma. *J Neurosurg* 55:282, 1981.
65. Ingraham FD, Scott HW: Craniopharyngiomas in children. *J Pediatr* 29:95, 1946.
66. Jenkins JS, Ash S, Bloom HJG: Endocrine function after external pituitary irradiation in patients with secreting and non-secreting pituitary tumours. *Q J Med* 41:57, 1972.
67. Jennings AS, Liddle GW, Orth DN: Results of treating childhood Cushing's disease with pituitary irradiation. *N Engl J Med* 297:957, 1977.
68. Jones A: Transient radiation myelopathy (with reference to Lhermitte's sign of electrical paraesthesia). *Br J Radiol* 37:727, 1964.
69. Kaplan SL, Grumbach MM: Pathophysiology of GH deficiency and other disorders of GH metabolism, in La Cauza C, Root AW (eds): *Problems in Pediatric Endocrinology*. Proceedings of the Serono Symposia, London, Academic Press Inc, 1980, vol 32.
70. Kelly WF, Mashiter K, Doyle FH, et al: Treatment of prolactin-secreting pituitary tumours in young women by needle implantation of radioactive yttrium. *Q J Med* 47:473, 1978.
71. King DL, Chang CH, Pool JL: Radiotherapy in the management of meningiomas. *Acta Radiol Ther* 5:26, 1966.
72. Kjellberg RN: A system of therapy of pituitary tumors—Bragg peak proton hypophysectomy, in Seydel HG (ed): *Tumors of the Nervous System*. New York, John Wiley & Sons Inc, 1975.
73. Kjellberg RN, Kliman B: Proton-beam therapy. *N Engl J Med* 284:333, 1971.
74. Kjellberg RN, Kliman B: A system for therapy of pituitary tumors, in Kohler PO, Ross GT (eds): *Diagnosis and Treatment of Pituitary Tumors*. International Congress Series No. 303, Amsterdam, Excerpta Medica, 1973.
75. Kjellberg RN, Kliman B: Bragg peak proton treatment for pituitary-related conditions. *Proc R Soc Med* 67:32, 1974.
76. Kjellberg RN, Kliman B: Lifetime effectiveness—A system of therapy for pituitary adenomas, emphasizing Bragg peak proton hypophysectomy, in Linfoot JA (ed): *Recent Advances in the Diagnosis and Treatment of Pituitary Tumors*. New York, Raven Press, 1979.
77. Kjellberg RN, Kliman B: Proton radiosurgery for functioning pituitary adenomas, in Tindall GT, Collins WF (eds): *Clinical Management of Pituitary Disorders*. New York, Raven Press, 1979.
78. Kjellberg RN, Shintani A, Frantz AG, et al: Proton-beam therapy in acromegaly. *N Engl J Med* 278:689, 1968.

79. Kleinberg DL, Noel GL, Frantz AG: Galactorrhea: A study of 235 cases, including 48 with pituitary tumors. *N Engl J Med* 296:589, 1977.
80. Kobayashi T, Kageyama N, Ohara K: Internal irradiation for cystic craniopharyngioma. *J Neurosurg* 55:896, 1981.
81. Kramer S: Indications for, and results of, treatment of pituitary tumors by external radiation, in Kohler PO, Ross GT (eds): *Diagnosis and Treatment of Pituitary Tumors*. International Congress Series No. 303, Amsterdam, Excerpta Medica, 1973.
82. Kramer S: Treatment of pituitary tumors by radiation therapy, in Seydel HG (ed): *Tumors of the Nervous System*. New York, John Wiley & Sons Inc, 1975.
83. Kramer S: Radiation therapy in the management of craniopharyngiomas, in Deeley TJ (ed): *Central Nervous System Tumours*. Kent, England, Butterworth & Co Ltd, 1974.
84. Kramer S: Craniopharyngioma: The best treatment is conservative surgery and postoperative radiation therapy, in Morley TP (ed): *Current Controversies in Neurosurgery*. Philadelphia, WB Saunders Co, 1976.
85. Kramer S, Southard ME, Mansfield CM: Radiation effect and tolerance of the central nervous system. *Front Radiat Ther Oncol* 6:332, 1972.
86. Kramer S, Southard M, Mansfield CM: Radiotherapy in the management of craniopharyngiomas: Further experiences and late results. *AJR* 103:44, 1968.
87. Lampert PW, Davis RL: Delayed effects of radiation on the human central nervous system: "Early" and "late" delayed reactions. *Neurology* 14:912, 1964.
88. Lampert P, Tom MI, Rider WD: Disseminated demyelination of the brain following Co^{60} (gamma) radiation. *Arch Pathol* 68:322, 1959.
89. Lawrence AM, Pinsky SM, Goldfine ID: Conventional radiation therapy in acromegaly. *Arch Intern Med* 128:369, 1971.
90. Lawrence JH, Born JL, Linfoot JA, et al: Heavy particle radiation treatment of pituitary tumors. *JAMA* 214:2061, 1970.
91. Lawrence JH, Chong CY, Lyman JT, et al: Treatment of pituitary tumors with heavy particles, in Kohler PO, Ross GT (eds): *Diagnosis and Treatment of Pituitary Tumors*. International Congress Series No. 303, Amsterdam, Excerpta Medica, 1973.
92. Lawrence JH, Okerlund MD, Linfoot JA, et al: Heavy-particle treatment of Cushing's disease. *N Engl J Med* 285:1263, 1971.
93. Lawrence JH, Tobias CA, Linfoot JA, et al: Successful treatment of acromegaly: Metabolic and clinical studies in 145 patients. *J Clin Endocrinol Metab* 31:180, 1970.
94. Lawrence JH, Tobias CA, Linfoot JA, et al: Heavy-particle therapy in acromegaly and Cushing disease. *JAMA* 235:2307, 1976.
95. Leksell L, Lidén K: A theropeutic trial with radioactive isotopes in cystic brain tumor, in *Radioisotope Techniques,* vol 1, *Medical and Physiological Applications*. London, Her Majesty's Stationery Office, 1953.
96. Leroy GV: The medical sequelae of atomic bomb explosion. *JAMA* 134:1143, 1947.
97. Linfoot JH, Chong CY, Garcia JF, et al: Heavy particle therapy for acromegaly, Cushing's disease, Nelson's syndrome and nonfunctioning pituitary adenomas, in Lawrence JH (ed): *Progress in Atomic Medicine: Recent Advances in Nuclear Medicine*. New York, Grune & Stratton Inc, 1971.
98. Linfoot JA, Lawrence JH, Tobias CA, et al: Progress report on the treatment of Cushing's disease. *Trans Am Clin Climatol Assoc* 81:196, 1969.
99. Marks JE, Baglan RJ, Prassad SC, et al: Cerebral radionecrosis: Incidence and risk in relation to dose, time, fractionation and volume. *Int J Radiat Oncol Biol Phys* 7:243, 1981.
100. Martins AN, Johnston JS, Henry JM, et al: Delayed radiation necrosis of the brain. *J Neurosurg* 47:336, 1977.
101. McCombs RK: Proton irradiation of the pituitary and its metabolic effects. *Radiology* 68:797, 1957.
102. McWhirter R, Dott NM: Tumours of the brain and spine cord, in Carling ER, Windeyer BW, Smithers DW (eds): *British Practice in Radiotherapy*. Kent, England, Butterworth & Co Ltd, 1955.
103. Meredith JM, Mandeville FB, Kay S: Osteogenic sarcoma of the skull following roentgenray therapy for benign pituitary tumor. *J Neurosurg* 17:792, 1960.
104. Monro P, Mair WGP: Radiation effects on the human central nervous system 14 weeks after x-radiation. *Acta Neuropathol* 11:267, 1968.
105. Moore TJ, Dluhy RG, Williams GH, et al: Nelson's syndrome: Frequency, prognosis, and effect of prior pituitary irradiation. *Ann Intern Med* 85:731, 1976.
106. Munzenrider JE, Shipley WU, Verhey LJ: Future prospects of radiation therapy with protons. *Semin Oncol* 8:110, 1981.
107. Nielsen SL, Kjellberg RN, Asbury AK, et al:

Neuropathologic effects of proton-beam irradiation in man: I. Dose-response relationships after treatment of intracranial neoplasms. *Acta Neuropathol* 20:348, 1972.
108. Nielsen SL, Kjellberg RN, Asbury AK, et al: Neuropathologic effects of proton-beam irradiation in man. II. Evaluation after pituitary irradiation. *Acta Neuropathol* 21:76, 1972.
109. Noell KT: Prolactin- and other hormone-producing pituitary tumors: Radiation therapy. *Clin Obstet Gynecol* 23:441, 1980.
110. Obetz SW, Smithson WA, Groover RV, et al: Neuropsychological follow-up study of central nervous system (CNS) function in children with acute lymphocytic leukemia (ALL). *Proc Am Assoc Cancer Res Am Soc Clin Oncol* 20:342, 1979.
111. Orth DN, Liddle GW: Results of treatment in 108 patients with Cushing's syndrome. *N Engl J Med* 285:243, 1971.
112. Piatt JH Jr, Blue JM, Schold SC Jr, et al: Glioblastoma multiforme after radiotherapy for acromegaly. *Neurosurgery* 13:85, 1983.
113. Pieterse S, Dinning TAR, Blumbergs PC: Post-irradiation sarcomatous transformation of a pituitary adenoma: A combined pituitary tumor. Case report. *J Neurosurg* 56:283, 1982.
114. Pistenma DA, Goffinet DR, Bagshaw MA, et al: Treatment of chromophobe adenomas with megavoltage irradiation. *Cancer* 35:1574, 1975.
115. Pistenma DA, Goffinet DR, Bagshaw MA, et al: Treatment of acromegaly with megavoltage radiation therapy. *Int J Radiat Oncol Biol Phys* 1:885, 1976.
116. Powell HC, Marshall LF, Ignelzi RJ: Post-irradiation pituitary sarcoma. *Acta Neuropathol* 39:165, 1977.
117. Raimondi AJ, Tomita T: The disadvantages of prophylactic whole CNS postoperative radiation therapy for medulloblastoma, in Paoletti P, Walker MD, Butti G, et al (eds): *Multidisciplinary Aspects of Brain Tumor Therapy*. Amsterdam, North-Holland Publishing Co, 1979.
118. Rappaport R, Brauner R, Czernichow P, et al: Effect of hypothalamic and pituitary irradiation on pubertal development in children with cranial tumors. *J Clin Endocrinol Metab* 54:1164, 1982.
119. Rene AA, Darden JH, Parker JL: Radiation induced ultrastructural and biochemical changes in lysosomes. *Lab Invest* 25:230, 1971.
120. Richards GE, Wara WM, Grumach MM, et al: Delayed onset of hypopituitarism: Sequelae of therapeutic irradiation of central nervous system, eye, and middle ear tumors. *J Pediatr* 89:553, 1976.
121. Richmond IL, Wara WM, Wilson CB: Role of radiation therapy in the management of craniopharyngiomas in children. *Neurosurgery* 6:513, 1980.
122. Rubin P, Casarett GW: *Clinical Radiation Pathology*. Philadelphia, WB Saunders Co, 1968, vol 2.
123. Rubinstein LJ: *Atlas of Tumor Pathology*, Second Series, Fascicle 6, *Tumors of the Central Nervous System*. Washington, D.C., Armed Forces Institute of Pathology, 1972.
124. Salazar OM, Rubin P, McDonald JV, et al: High dose radiation therapy in the treatment of glioblastoma multiforme: A preliminary report. *Int J Radiat Oncol Biol Phys* 1:717, 1976.
125. Salmi J, Grahne B, Valtonen S, et al: Recurrence of chromophobe pituitary adenomas after operation and postoperative radiotherapy. *Acta Neurol Scand* 66:681, 1982.
126. Samaan NA, Bakdash MM, Caderao JB, et al: Hypopituitarism after external irradiation: Evidence of both hypothalamic and pituitary origin. *Ann Intern Med* 83:771, 1975.
127. Samaan NA, Maor M, Sampiere VA, et al: Hypopituitarism after external irradiation of nasopharyngeal cancer, in Linfoot JA, (ed): *Recent Advances in the Diagnosis and Treatment of Pituitary Tumors*. New York, Raven Press, 1979.
128. Samaan NA, Vieto R, Schultz PN, et al: Hypothalamic, pituitary and thyroid dysfunction after radiotherapy to the head and neck. *Int J Radiat Oncol Biol Phys* 8:1857, 1982.
129. Schulz MD, Wang CC, Zinninger GF, et al: Radiotherapy of intracranial neoplasms: With a special section on the radiotherapeutic management of central nervous system tumors in children. *Prog Neurol Surg* 2:318, 1968.
130. Shalet SM, Beardwell CG, Morris-Jones PH, et al: Pituitary function after treatment of intracranial tumours in children. *Lancet* 2:104, 1975.
131. Shalet SM, Beardwell CG, Pearson D, et al: The effect of varying doses of cerebral irradiation on growth hormone production in childhood. *Clin Endocrinol* 5:287, 1976.
132. Sheline GE: Treatment of chromophobe adenomas of the pituitary gland and acromegaly, in Kohler PO, Ross GT (eds): *Diagnosis and Treatment of Pituitary Tumors*. International Congress Series No. 303, Amsterdam, Excerpta Medica, 1973.

133. Sheline GE: Conventional radiation therapy in the treatment of pituitary tumors, in Tindall GT, Collins WF (eds): *Clinical Mangement of Pituitary Disorders.* New York, Raven Press, 1979.
134. Sheline GE: Irradiation injury of the human brain: A review of clinical experience, in Gilberg HA, Kagan AR (eds): *Radiation Damage to the Nervous System.* Raven Press, New York, 1980.
135. Sheline GE, Goldberg MB, Feldman R: Pituitary irradiation for acromegaly. *Radiology* 76:70, 1961.
136. Sheline GE, Wara WM: Radiation therapy of acromegaly and nonsecretory chromophobe adenomas of the pituitary, in Seydel HG (ed): *Tumors of the Nervous System.* New York, John Wiley & Sons Inc, 1975.
137. Sheline GE, Wara WM, Smith V: Therapeutic irradiation and brain injury. *Int J Radiat Oncol Biol Phys* 6:1215, 1980.
138. Sinclair WK, Morton RA: X-ray sensitivity during the cell generation cycle of cultured Chinese hamster cells. *Radiat Res* 29:450, 1966.
139. Sommers SC: Effects of ionizing radiation upon endocrine glands, in Berdjis CC (ed): *Pathology of Irradiation.* Baltimore, Williams & Wilkins, 1971.
140. Soni SS, Martin GW, Pitner SE, et al: Effects of central-nervous-system irradiation on neuropsychologic functioning of children with acute lymphocytic leukemia. *N Engl J Med* 293:113, 1975.
141. Sottocasa GL, Glass G, de Bernard B: The effect of x-irradiation on the activities of some lysosomal hydrolases of heart tissue. *Radiat Res* 24:32, 1965.
142. Sparagana M, Eells RW, Stefani S, et al: Osteogenic sarcoma of the skull: A rare sequela of pituitary irradiation. *Cancer* 29:1376, 1972.
143. Spunberg JJ, Chang CH, Goldman M, et al: Quality of long-term survival following irradiation for intracranial tumors in children under the age of two. *Int J Radiat Oncol Biol Phys* 7:727, 1981.
144. Strauss L, Sturm V, Georgi P, et al: Radioisotope therapy of cystic craniopharyngiomas. *Int J Radiat Oncol Biol Phys* 8:1581, 1982.
145. Tan BC, Kunaratnam N: Hypopituitary dwarfism following radiotherapy for nasopharyngeal carcinoma. *Clin Radiol* 17:302, 1966.
146. Terasima T, Tolmach LJ: X-ray sensitivity and DNA synthesis in synchronous populations of HeLa cells. *Science* 140:490, 1963.
147. Terry RD, Hyams VJ, Davidoff LM: Combined nonmetastasizing fibrosarcoma and chromophobe tumor of the pituitary. *Cancer* 12:791, 1959.
148. Tobias CA, Anger HO, Lawrence JH: Radiological use of high energy deuterons and alpha particles. *AJR Rad Ther Nucl Med* 67:1, 1952.
149. Tobias CA, Lyman JT, Lawrence JH: Some considerations of physical and biological factors in radiotherapy with high-LET radiations including heavy particles, pi mesons, and fast neutrons, in Lawrence JH (ed): *Progress in Atomic Medicine: Recent Advances in Nuclear Medicine.* New York, Grune & Stratton Inc, 1971.
150. Urdaneta N, Chessin H, Fischer JJ: Pituitary adenomas and craniopharyngiomas: Analysis of 99 cases treated with radiation therapy. *Int J Radiat Oncol Biol Phys* 1:895, 1976.
151. Wallach DFH, Weidekamm E: Radiation effects in biomembranes. *Klin Wochenschr* 51:419, 1973.
152. Waltz TA, Brownell B: Sarcoma: A possible late result of effective radiation therapy for pituitary adenomas. Report of two cases. *J Neurosurg* 24:901, 1966.
153. Wara WM, Sheline GE, Newman H, et al: Radiation therapy of meningiomas. *AJR Rad Ther Nucl Med* 123:453, 1975.
154. Wild W, Nicolis GL, Gabrilove JL: Appearance of Nelson's syndrome despite pituitary irradiation prior to bilateral adrenalectomy for Cushing's syndrome. *Mt Sinai J Med* 40:68, 1973.
155. Williams RA, Jacobs HS, Kurtz AB, et al: The treatment of acromegaly with special reference to trans-sphenoidal hypophysectomy. *Q J Med* 44:79, 1975.
156. Wills ED, Wilkinson AE: Release of enzymes from lysosomes by irradiation and the relation of lipid peroxide formation to enzyme release. *Biochemistry* 99:657, 1966.
157. Wilson RR: Radiological use of fast protons. *Radiology* 47:487, 1946.
158. Woodruff KH, Lawrence JH, Tobias CA, et al: Delayed lesions in pituitary glands irradiated with helium ions. *Radiat Oncol Biol Phys* 7:1285, 1981.
159. Wright AD, Hartog M, Palter H, et al: The use of ytrrium 90 implantation in the treatment of acromegaly. *Proc R Soc Med* 63:221, 1970.
160. Zirkle RE: The radiobiological importance of linear energy transfer, in Hollaender A (ed): *Radiation Biology.* New York, McGraw-Hill Inc, 1954, vol 1.

CHAPTER 14

Hypophysectomy

Beneficial results
Selection of breast cancer patients for hypophysectomy
   Previous response to castration
   Previous response to hormone therapy
   Presence of estrogen and progesterone receptors
   Duration of free interval
   Age
   Site of metastases
   Levodopa test
Selection of prostate cancer patients for hypophysectomy
Criteria for remission
Incidence of remission in breast cancer
Incidence of remission in prostate cancer
Indications for and timing of hypophysectomy
   Breast cancer
   Prostate cancer
Hypophysectomy for diabetic retinopathy
Choice of hypophysectomy over adrenalectomy
Techniques
Postoperative considerations
Medical alternatives to surgical hypophysectomy
Summary

The beneficial influence of endocrine manipulation on certain breast cancers has been known since 1896, when Beatson[2] showed that some patients with disseminated disease achieved regression following oophorectomy. Hypophysectomy, as a method for achieving palliation of malignant disease, was first reported during the early 1950s by Perrault et al[25] in a case of breast cancer with pulmonary metastases and by Shimkin et al[34] in a man with malignant melanoma. In 1962 Scott and Schirmer[33] recount that hypophysectomy was actually first performed in September 1948 in a patient with disseminated prostatic cancer. The procedure proved unsuccessful, and the patient died 11 days after surgery. In 1953 Luft and Olivecrona[14] cited their experiences with hypophysectomy in 26 cases for a variety of conditions including Cushing's syndrome, diabetes mellitus, and cancer of the breast and prostate gland. These workers, who performed hypophysectomy via a transcranial approach, concluded that the procedure was well tolerated by patients and that when total pituitary ablation was accomplished, cancer regression was possible. Subsequently several others showed that hypophysectomy is a worthwhile palliative operation in metastatic breast* and prostate gland cancer.†

In 1953 Poulsen[26] described a patient who later experienced a 15-year regression[27] of diabetic retinopathy following the development of Sheehan's syndrome in 1945. This report along with the pioneering work by Luft and Olivecrona[14,15] stimulated interest in hypophysectomy as a treatment for diabetic retinopathy. By 1972 over 1000 patients had been treated by pituitary ablation for this condition.[46] Although results were generally favorable in certain patients, the interest in pituitary ablation for diabetic retinopathy has decreased significantly in recent years with the advent of photocoagulation.

Originally hypophysectomy was accomplished by performing a craniotomy. Although beneficial effects resulted, many physicians considered this operative approach too extensive and risky for many patients with diabetes mellitus and advanced breast and prostatic cancer, particularly elderly patients with prostatic cancer. Fortunately, easier and safer methods for performing hypophysectomy (e.g., cryohypophysectomy, radiofrequency coagulation, and transsphenoidal surgical removal of the pituitary gland) were developed. As a result, hypophysectomy currently can be recommended to a greater number of patients than would be the case if craniotomy were the only option for performing this palliative procedure.

In this chapter, we will present the indications and contraindications for and the benefits of hypophysectomy in breast and prostatic cancer and diabetic retinopathy. Additionally, factors influencing responsiveness to hypophysectomy in breast and prostate cancer, evaluation and management, and procedures available for performing hypophysectomy will be discussed.

BENEFICIAL RESULTS

Remission of breast cancer following hypophysectomy is probably best explained by the suppression of estrogen production by the gonads and adrenal glands because of the removal of gonadotropins and ACTH, respectively. Although estrogenic substances appear to be the chief hormones influencing breast cancer, others, including growth hormone and prolactin, could conceivably exert a direct or indirect role in tumor growth.

In patients with prostatic cancer who relapse after castration, it is likely that the adrenal glands have begun to produce a significant amount of extragonadal androgen. Thus in this situation, hypophysectomy removes the source of ACTH, thereby abolishing androgen production by the adrenal glands. However, the mechanism for tumor regression following hypophysectomy may be more com-

---

*See references 3-5, 9, 10, 12, 24, 29-31, 36, 39, and 42.
†See references 6, 16, 21, 33, 35, 37-39, and 43.

plex than simply removing the stimulus for androgen production. For instance, prolactin and growth hormone may synergize the action of testosterone and thereby could have a stimulating effect on this tumor. As with breast cancer, the possible effects of hormones other than those elaborated by the gonads on tumor growth remain unknown.

It is well recognized and will be further discussed later in this chapter that a significant number of patients with breast and prostate cancer who undergo hypophysectomy may obtain gratifying relief of pain, particularly osseous pain, even if disease remission does not occur. As a matter of fact, pituitary ablation has been reported to provide pain relief in patients with a wide variety of metastatic cancers,[11,40] some of them not generally classified as endocrine-sensitive neoplasms. Pain relief may be noticed within 2 to 4 hours of the operative procedure and may last indefinitely. Temporal aspects of the pain relief are evidence against a placebo effect, effect of steroids, or regressive changes in the tumor. Conceivably, certain pituitary trophic hormones (i.e., gonadotropins, growth hormone, and prolactin) may influence the pain associated with cancer. In recent years, peptides, including enkephalins and alpha and beta endorphins—all of which have significant pain relieving properties, have been discovered in the brain and the pituitary gland of several mammals including man. It is interesting to speculate that pituitary ablation in humans may stimulate an inappropriate release of these peptides, which act in some as yet unknown manner to alleviate pain.

The mechanism by which hypophysectomy brings about an arrest of the angiopathy and visual impairment of diabetic retinopathy is unknown. The role of growth hormone in aggravating diabetes makes it reasonable to suspect that elimination of this hormone or some other unidentified diabetogenic pituitary substance may be a factor in this response.

SELECTION OF BREAST CANCER PATIENTS FOR HYPOPHYSECTOMY

In patients with breast cancer, the following factors may be helpful in predicting whether a patient will achieve an objective remission following hypophysectomy.

Previous response to castration

The most reliable index for predicting a satisfactory remission from hypophysectomy is a previous favorable response to oophorectomy in the premenopausal patient. For instance, Pearson and Ray[23,24] contend that about 90% of patients who have shown remission after oophorectomy obtain objective improvement from hypophysectomy, and Conway and Collins[4] noted similar results in 100 cases, obtaining a remission in 86%.

Previous response to hormone therapy

Several series have shown that postmenopausal women who have exhibited a good response to hormone manipulative therapy stand a better chance of obtaining disease remission from hypophysectomy than those women who have not demonstrated such a response.[4]

Presence of estrogen and progesterone receptors

The presence of estrogen receptors (i.e., specific estrogen-binding protein, which can be demonstrated from excised malignant tissue) forecasts a good chance of an objective remission from surgical ablation of either the pituitary or adrenal glands.[17] If estrogen receptors are not demonstrable, there is little chance (<10%) of obtaining objective disease remission from hypophysectomy. There is some evidence that the presence of both estrogen and progesterone receptors in the tumor tissue indicates an even greater possibility for objective remission from hypophysectomy.

An interesting observation was reported by Lippman et al[13] relative to estrogen receptors and response to chemotherapy. They found that 34 (76%) of 45 patients with low or absent estrogen receptor values had objective responses to chemotherapy, whereas only 3 (12%) of 25 with higher estrogen receptor values responded. These findings, which were not affected by the type of chemotherapy used, indicate that estrogen receptor values might well become an important predictor of response to cytotoxic chemotherapy in metastatic breast cancer.

Duration of free interval

The free interval is defined as the period of time between the original treatment of the breast cancer and the discovery of the first metastasis. A comparatively long (i.e., >3 years) free interval is a relatively good prognostic sign in terms of a favorable hypophysectomy response.

Age

The incidence of remission after hypophysectomy in older (i.e., >60 years) postmenopausal women is higher than in younger (i.e., <40 years) premenopausal women.

Site of metastases

Although most authorities agree that the best response is obtained in patients with bony metastases, patients with visceral involvement also can be considered for hypophysectomy. Contrary to popular belief, the presence of liver metastases does not prognosticate a poor response to hypophysectomy. Indeed, in Conway and Collins' series,[4] 37% of 30 patients with liver metastases had a remission after pituitary ablation.

Levodopa test

Therapeutic doses of levodopa alleviate bone pain in a significant number of patients with metastatic breast cancer. Encouraged by the results in a relatively small number of patients, Minton et al[18,19] concluded that the responsiveness of the tumor to ablative therapy could be predicted on the basis of the response to levodopa (i.e., patients showing relief of bone pain would be expected to respond objectively and subjectively to either hypophysectomy or adrenalectomy). However, this study was not conclusive in that 20 of the 30 who did not respond to levodopa were never subjected to any type of ablative procedure. Consequently, the value of this drug in predicting an objective remission remains unproved.

Since the majority of patients with severe bone pain are relieved of their pain by transsphenoidal hypophysectomy (perhaps 85% to 90%), the results of a predictive test to determine the effects of an endocrine ablative procedure on pain is not needed. For these reasons, we do not recommend the use of a levodopa test for predicting the response of breast cancer patients to hypophysectomy.

The ideal breast cancer patients to undergo hypophysectomy are older postmenopausal women with a long free interval and an estrogen receptor positive tumor or premenopausal women who have responded to oophorectomy and who have estrogen receptor positive tumor tissue.

SELECTION OF PROSTATE CANCER PATIENTS FOR HYPOPHYSECTOMY

Factors that predict a favorable response to hypophysectomy in patients with disseminated carcinoma of the prostate are not as evident as in patients with breast cancer. In general, the clinical results following orchiectomy and/or estrogen therapy bear no consistent relationship to the outcome following hypophysectomy. Consequently, hypophysectomy can be recommended in all patients with proven progressive prostatic cancer who have previously undergone orchiectomy and estrogen therapy regardless of the response to these two methods of treatment.

However, patients with prostatic cancer tend to be elderly and to present more problems from the standpoint of general health than the relatively younger patients with breast cancer. For these reasons, hypophysectomy would be contraindicated in patients with prostatic cancer who demonstrate debilitation, poor general health, significant hematologic disorders (e.g., coagulopathies, thrombocytopenia), or unreliability from the standpoint of taking replacement medications.

CRITERIA FOR REMISSION

Subjective remission is assessed by relief of pain, correction or improvement of anemia, gain in weight, and improvement in appetite. An objective remission is measured by a decrease in lesion size following hypophysectomy without advance of other lesions or development of new lesions, disappearance of a neurologic deficit, increase in function of an obstructed organ (e.g., ureter), and/or a significant decrease in serum acid and/or alkaline phosphatase activity. Most authorities believe that the objective remission should last a minimum of 3 months to be considered a positive response.

INCIDENCE OF REMISSION IN BREAST CANCER

Following hypophysectomy, approximately 75% of patients with severe pain resulting from metastatic breast cancer obtain gratifying relief of pain, particularly bone pain.[39] Consequently, in considering candidates with breast cancer for hypophysectomy, selection of patients need not be restricted to those who have shown a previous remission from oophorectomy and/or hormone therapy because significant pain relief, and at times objective remission, may occur in candidates who have not responded to either of these therapies.

Table 14-1
Results of hypophysectomy in patients with disseminated cancer of the breast

Series	Number of patients	Patients achieving remission		Average survival after hypophysectomy (months)	
		Number	Percentage	Patients with remission	Patients without remission
Kennedy and French[12]	71	39	55	28	6.2
Stevens[36]	50	29	58	20	5
Kapur and Dalton[10]	63	29	46	—	—
Conway and Collins[4]	100	40	40	20.3	4.4
Collins[3]	394	184	47	—	—
Ray[29]	630	264	42	24.5	5.6

A comprehensive survey of hypophysectomy results for breast cancer is beyond the scope of this chapter. A summary (Table 14-1) of several selected large series* indicates that objective remission occurs in nearly one half of women who undergo hypophysectomy. Furthermore, the period of survival in those who respond to hypophysectomy is significantly increased over those who do not respond. Conway and Collins[4] obtained a remission in 40% of 100 patients undergoing cryohypophysectomy. Of this number, 13 patients were alive and in remission 14 to 30 months (mean 18.6 months) after hypophysectomy; two living patients had remissions of 9 and 12 months, respectively; and 25 patients were dead after remissions of 3 to 28 months (mean 11.3 months). The latter group survived for periods ranging from 5 to 40 months (mean survival 20.3 months). Ray[29,30] obtained an objective remission in 42% of 630 patients. For those having a remission longer than 6 months, the average duration was more than 17 months. In this same group, the average survival after hypophysectomy exceeded 24.5 months, with some still living after 3 to 5 years. In those patients who failed to obtain a remission, the average survival was only 5.6 months.

The remission statistics from many reports in the literature represent data from unselected series of cases. Consequently, it is not surprising that the overall incidence of objective remission is just under 50%. The importance of selection is emphasized in a report by Collins[3] summarizing his personal experience with hypophysectomy for breast cancer. He obtained a 27% response rate in 156 unselected women compared to a 57% response in 238 selected cases. Thus a higher response rate can be expected in those patients who have met one or more of the previously discussed criteria predisposing to a positive response.

---

*See references 3, 4, 10, 12, 29, and 36.

INCIDENCE OF REMISSION IN PROSTATE CANCER

The incidence of pain relief in prostatic cancer following hypophysectomy varies among the reported series but usually is significantly higher than the incidence of objective remission of disease. As with breast cancer, pain relief occurs in many patients who fail to achieve an objective remission. In the series of 53 patients treated at our institution, the remarkably high incidence (91%) of pain relief probably reflects the completeness of pituitary ablation accomplished via the transsphenoidal surgical method.

The percentage of patients with carcinoma of the prostate gland who obtain an objective remission following hypophysectomy is not completely clear. This is partly because there is a wide variation among reports in terms of criteria for objective remission and types of surgical procedures performed and also because most series report relatively small numbers of cases. Realistically, it appears that somewhere between 20% and 40% of the patients with carcinoma of the prostate undergoing hypophysectomy achieve objective remission of disease.[16,35,39]

INDICATIONS FOR AND TIMING OF HYPOPHYSECTOMY
Breast cancer

Hypophysectomy can be recommended for most patients with widespread and advancing cancer of the breast whose recurrent disease is not suitable for either local excision or radiation therapy. In premenopausal patients, oophorectomy should be considered as the initial palliative procedure. An oophorectomy failure does not necessarily contraindicate hypophysectomy, however. In postmenopausal patients, the effects of androgen/estrogen therapy should be evaluated before performing hypophysectomy. It is still uncertain whether a trial of chemotherapy should precede or follow hypophysectomy in patients who have failed previous endocrine therapy. Hypophysectomy should be considered relatively early in the course of metastatic breast cancer because when this is performed as a last resort procedure in a patient with uncontrolled extensive metastatic disease, relatively poor results in terms of a useful remission can be expected.

The results of hypophysectomy in alleviating pain in patients with disseminated breast cancer have been so gratifying that the presence of severe pain, particularly osseous pain, constitutes one of the principal indications for hypophysectomy in this disease.

Prostate cancer

Hypophysectomy can be recommended in all patients with proven progressive prostatic cancer who have previously undergone orchiectomy and estrogen therapy regardless of the response to these two methods of treatment. However, bearing in mind that many patients are elderly, that the majority have been through several treatment programs, that the incidence of objective remission (20% to 40%) from hypophysectomy is relatively low, and that a few patients are in marginal general health, one could reasonably question if hypophysectomy is an appropriate palliative operative procedure in patients with disseminated carcinoma (stage IV) of the prostate.

Nevertheless, hypophysectomy can be performed on elderly individuals without significant risk, provided they are in reasonably good general health and do not have extensive, widespread metastatic disease. Although an objective remission rate of 20% to 40% is not comparable with the higher remission rate that is usually achieved in certain patients with disseminated carcinoma of the breast, some patients may choose to proceed with the operation knowing that their chances of obtaining an objective remission are relatively low. The most significant benefit of hypophysectomy and one that does appear to justify the operation is the dramatic pain relief that follows the procedure in the majority of patients. For this reason, we believe that hypophysectomy is an appropriate procedure, especially in patients with severe osseous pain who are in reasonably good health.

HYPOPHYSECTOMY FOR DIABETIC RETINOPATHY

Hypophysectomy definitely has a beneficial effect in certain cases of diabetic retinopathy.[41] Candidates for this procedure would include patients who have progressive proliferative retinopathy with impending blindness and no serious cardiovascular or renal disease. The results of hypophysectomy in properly chosen candidates indicate that the procedure arrests the progression of proliferative retinopathy in more than 60% of diabetic patients. At least one form of diabetic retinopathy (florid retinopathy) has been shown to respond considerably better to hypophysectomy than to photocoagulation. However, with the advent of photocoagulation, the number of patients being referred for hypophysectomy for treatment of diabetic retinopathy has decreased considerably, and currently, hypophysectomy is rarely performed for this disorder.

CHOICE OF HYPOPHYSECTOMY OVER ADRENALECTOMY

Hypophysectomy and adrenalectomy are effective endocrine ablative procedures for disseminated carcinoma of the breast and prostate gland when the procedure is performed by a competent and experienced surgeon. Judging from reports in the literature, there does not appear to be a clear advantage of either operative procedure over the other in terms of objective remission rate for breast cancer.[1,7,44] In our opinion, adequate data are not available on the use of the two operative procedures for prostatic cancer to make a comparative analysis. When craniotomy was the method for performing hypophysectomy, the risks and magnitude of the two operative approaches for achieving endocrine ablation were approximately equal. However, present-day techniques for performing hypophysectomy (e.g., cryohypophysectomy, transsphenoidal surgery[8]) are considerably simpler and less troublesome to patients than bilateral adrenalectomy. Currently, an experienced neurosurgeon can perform a transsphenoidal hypophysectomy within a relatively short period of time with extremely low mortality. In premenopausal women, bilateral oophorectomy is also necessary when adrenalectomy is performed. Perhaps the major advantage of hypophysectomy over adrenalectomy other than simplicity is the higher incidence of significant pain relief achieved with hypophysectomy. In patients having adrenalectomy, pain relief occurs only when the patient acquires an objective remission, whereas hypophysectomy produces pain relief even when an objective remission fails to occur.

TECHNIQUES

Originally, hypophysectomy required a craniotomy. Although beneficial effects resulted, many physicians considered this operative approach too extensive and risky for many patients with metastatic cancer and diabetes mellitus. Because of the relative resistance of the normal pituitary gland to irradiation, x-ray therapy directed at the sella turcica for purposes of pituitary destruction is not a reasonable option. Transsphenoidal stereotaxic insertion of either yttrium or other radioactive substances is not recommended because of the relatively high complication rate that usually develops several weeks or months following placement of the radioactive material.

Procedures that are effective and relatively safe include stereotaxic cryohypophysectomy,[4,16,28] stereotaxic radiofrequency lesioning,[45] and open transsphenoidal surgical removal of the gland.[8] In experienced hands, any one of these three procedures yields good results in properly chosen patients. Although safe and well tolerated, neither cryohypophysectomy nor radiofrequency lesioning accomplishes complete pituitary destruction or at least complete ablation of all intrasellar pituitary tissue. However, whether it is absolutely necessary to produce total destruction of the pituitary gland to achieve remission in a significant number of patients is a controversial issue. Currently, the open transsphenoidal surgical operation described by Hardy[8] is probably the most commonly used procedure for performing hypophysectomy. It is the only one that consistently accomplishes complete ablation of the gland. The results with the open transsphenoidal surgical technique are comparable with any other method for performing hypophysectomy in terms of achieving objective remission and are probably superior to other methods in alleviating pain, a factor most likely related to the completeness of pituitary ablation.

Transnasal alcohol injection into the pituitary has been reported to be effective in relieving pain and occasionally in obtaining remission in patients with breast and prostate cancer.[11,20] The procedure, which has been variously termed "neuroadenolysis" and "chemoadenolysis," has also been used in patients with pain caused by a variety of malignant tumors with generally good results in terms of pain relief. The procedure is usually performed in the x-ray department using televised fluoroscopy to ensure correct position of the needle tip in the sella turcica. From 1 to 2.5 cc of alcohol are usually injected.

There are no special anesthetic techniques required for patients undergoing hypophysectomy. It is necessary to administer hydrocortisone 100 mg IV immediately before and during the operative procedure. The question of prophylactic antibiotics during operation (particularly via the transsphenoidal approach) and during the postoperative course is not a settled issue. Currently, we prefer *not* to use prophylactic antibiotics. Some authorities believe that the prolonged use of antibiotics encourages the overgrowth of opportunistic micro-organisms.

POSTOPERATIVE CONSIDERATIONS

During the immediate postoperative period, the primary concerns are adequate corticosteroid coverage and fluid balance. The patient receives hydrocortisone 100 mg IV immediately before and during the operative procedure. Postoperatively, hydrocortisone is administered in a dosage of 50 mg IV or PO every 8 hours for the first 2 days, and the dosage is then tapered over several more days to a maintenance dose of 20 mg in the morning and 10 mg in the afternoon, which is continued indefinitely. The physician must be alert for early signs of cortisone deficiency, postural hypotension being a simple bedside maneuver to test for this possibility. Thyroid supplementation is begun within a week after surgery and is also continued indefinitely. We use levothyroxine sodium (Synthroid, Flint Laboratories, Deerfield, Illinois) 0.05 mg PO daily for the first week, 0.10 mg PO daily for the second week, and 0.15 mg daily thereafter. (The complications of hypophysectomy and their management are considered in detail in Chapter 12.)

MEDICAL ALTERNATIVES TO SURGICAL HYPOPHYSECTOMY

Over the past several years, many investigators have attempted to develop medical alternatives to surgical ablative procedures for the treatment of patients with endocrine dependent malignancies. One approach has been to interfere with hormone action through the use of antiestrogens and to inhibit estrogen synthesis with enzyme antagonists. Tamoxifen citrate, a nonsteroidal antiestrogen, was first introduced into clinical studies in 1969 and is now widely used either singly or in combination with cytotoxic agents in patients with advanced breast cancer.[22] The overall objective response rate when tamoxifen is used singly in breast cancer is 32%, and side effects are generally mild. Although effective use of tamoxifen in patients with prostatic carcinoma is not as well documented as it is for patients with breast cancer, objective remissions have also been reported.

Another approach has been through the use of adrenal cortical inhibition. Aminoglutethimide, a blocker of steroidogenesis in the adrenal gland, has been used to accomplish "medical adrenalectomy" in patients with breast cancer. Although its use is occasionally associated with relatively unpleasant side effects, one report showed a 53% objective response rate in patients with breast cancer treated with aminoglutethimide and hydrocortisone, and the authors of this report concluded that medical adrenalectomy is at least as satisfactory as surgical adrenalectomy in the treatment of women with advanced breast cancer.[32] With the recent success of these medical forms of treatment, relatively few patients with endocrine-dependent cancers are now being referred for surgical hypophysectomy.

SUMMARY

Hypophysectomy is a useful, gratifying, palliative operative procedure in patients with disseminated breast and prostatic cancer. Objective remission occurs in nearly 50% of patients with breast cancer and approximately 20% to 40% of patients with prostatic cancer. In women with breast cancer who have shown a positive response to previous oophorectomy, the remission rate following hypophysectomy may be as high as 80% to 85%. In a significant number of patients with breast and prostate cancer, a remission follows hypophysectomy despite the fact that a previous castration procedure and/or endocrine manipulation did not effect regression of the tumor. The relief of pain, particularly osseous pain, is one of the principal benefits of hypophysectomy and occurs in the majority of patients with breast and prostatic cancer, irrespective of whether there is other evidence of remission of the lesion. Hypophysectomy has also been shown to be a beneficial surgical procedure in selected cases of diabetic retinopathy.

The procedures of choice for performing hypophysectomy include stereotaxic cryohypophysectomy, stereotaxic radiofrequency lesioning, and the open transsphenoidal surgical technique. All three operations yield comparable results in terms of objective remission of disease, and all are considerably safer and less troublesome to the patient than craniotomy. The open transsphenoidal technique appears to provide pain relief in a higher percentage of patients than the stereotaxic methods. Most likely, this is because the majority of patients achieve complete pituitary ablation with the open transsphenoidal operation, and this does not invariably occur with stereotaxic methods.

As a result of many advances in pituitary surgery in recent years, all of which have resulted in safer procedures, we conclude that hypophysectomy should be given early and serious consideration in patients with disseminated breast and prostatic cancer. When this operation is delayed until after extensive chemotherapy, irradiation treatment, and other methods have been exhausted, hypophysectomy becomes a "last resort" procedure; in this situation, it is likely that unsatisfactory results will be obtained in many, if not most, of the patients.

REFERENCES

1. Atkins H, Falconer MA, Hayward JL, et al: The timing of adrenalectomy and of hypophysectomy in the treatment of advanced breast cancer. *Lancet* 1:827, 1966.
2. Beatson GT: On the treatment of inoperable cases of carcinoma of the mamma: Suggestions for a new method of treatment, with illustrative cases. *Lancet* 2:104, 162, 1896.
3. Collins WF: Hypophysectomy: Historical and personal perspective. *Clin Neurosurg* 21:68, 1974.
4. Conway LW, Collins WF: Results of trans-sphenoidal cryohypophysectomy for carcinoma of the breast. *N Engl J Med* 281:1, 1969.
5. Edelstyn G, Gleadhill C, Lyons A: Total hypophysectomy for advanced breast cancer. *Clin Radiol* 19:426, 1968.
6. Fergusson JD, Phillips DEH: A clinical evaluation of radioactive pituitary implantation in the treatment of advanced carcinoma of the prostate. *Br J Urol* 34:485, 1962.
7. Fracchia AA, Farrow JH, Miller TR, et al: Hypophysectomy as compared with adrenalectomy in the treatment of advanced carcinoma of the breast. *Surg Gynecol Obstet* 241, 1971.
8. Hardy J: Transsphenoidal hypophysectomy. *J Neurosurg* 34:582, 1971.
9. Harrold BP, Cates JE, James JA: Treatment of advanced breast cancer by trans-sphenoidal hypophysectomy. *Br J Cancer* 22:19, 1968.
10. Kapur TR, Dalton GA: Trans-sphenoidal hypophysectomy for metastatic carcinoma of the breast. *Br J Surg* 56:332, 1969.
11. Katz J, Levin AB: Treatment of diffuse metastatic cancer pain by instillation of alcohol into the sella turcica. *Anesthesiology* 46:115, 1977.
12. Kennedy BJ, French L: Hypophysectomy in advanced breast cancer. *Am J Surg* 110:411, 1965.
13. Lippman ME, Allegra JC, Thompson EB, et al: The relation between estrogen receptors and response rate to cytotoxic chemotherapy in metastatic breast cancer. *N Engl J Med* 298:1223, 1978.
14. Luft R, Olivecrona H: Experiences with hypophysectomy in man. *J Neurosurg* 10:301, 1953.

15. Luft R, Olivecrona H, Sjögren B: Hypophysectomy in man: Experiences in severe diabetes mellitus. *J Clin Endocrinol Metab* 15:391, 1955.
16. Maddy JA, Winternitz WW, Norrell H: Cryohypophysectomy in the management of advanced prostatic cancer. *Cancer* 28:322, 1971.
17. McGuire WL, Horwitz KB, Pearson OH, et al: Current status of estrogen and progesterone receptors in breast cancer. *Cancer* 39:2934, 1977.
18. Minton JP: The response of breast cancer patients with bone pain to L-dopa. *Cancer* 33:358, 1974.
19. Minton JP, Bronn DG, Kibbey WE: L-Dopa effect in painful bony metastases. *N Engl J Med* 294:3210, 1976.
20. Morrica G: Chemical hypophysectomy for cancer pain, in Bonica JJ (ed): *Advances in Neurology*, vol 4, *Pain*. New York, Raven Press, 1974.
21. Murphy GP, Boctor ZN, Gailani S, et al: Hypophysectomy for disseminated prostatic carcinoma. *J Surg Oncol* 1:81, 1969.
22. Patterson JS, Battersby LA: Tamoxifen: An overview of recent studies in the field of oncology. *Cancer Treat Rep* 64:775, 1980.
23. Pearson O: Endocrine treatment of breast cancer. *Cancer* 26:165, 1976.
24. Pearson OH, Ray BS: Hypophysectomy in the treatment of metastatic mammary cancer. *Am J Surg* 99:544, 1960.
25. Perrault M, Lebeau J, Klotz B: L'hypophysectomie totale dans le traitement du cancer sein: Premier cas français. Avenir de la method. *Therapie* 7:290, 1952.
26. Poulsen JE: Recovery from retinopathy in a case of diabetes with Simond's disease. *Diabetes* 2:7, 1953.
27. Poulsen JE: Diabetes and anterior pituitary insufficiency: Final course and postmortem study of a diabetic patient with Sheehan's syndrome. *Diabetes* 15:73, 1966.
28. Rand RW, Dashe AM, Paglia DE, et al: Stereotactic cryohypophysectomy. *JAMA* 189:255, 1964.
29. Ray BS: Hypophysectomy as palliative treatment. *JAMA* 200:974, 1967.
30. Ray BS: Hypophysectomy by craniotomy, in Youmans, JR (ed): *Neurological Surgery*. Philadelphia, WB Saunders Co, 1973, vol 3.
31. Robin PE, Powell DJ, Waterhouse JAH, et al: Transsphenoidal hypophysectomy in disseminated carcinoma of the breast. *Br J Surg* 62:85, 1975.
32. Santen RJ, Worgul TJ, Samojlik E, et al: A randomized trial comparing surgical adrenalectomy with aminoglutethimide plus hydrocortisone in women with advanced breast cancer. *N Engl J Med* 305:545, 1981.
33. Scott WW, Schirmer HKA: Hypophysectomy for disseminated prostatic cancer, in Haddow A (ed): *On Cancer and Hormones: Essays on Experimental Biology*. Chicago, University of Chicago Press, 1962.
34. Shimkin MB, Boldrey EB, Kelley KH, et al: Effects of surgical hypophysectomy in a man with malignant melanoma. *J Clin Endocrinol Metab* 12:439, 1952.
35. Silverberg GD: Hypophysectomy in the treatment of disseminated prostate carcinoma. *Cancer* 39:1727, 1977.
36. Stevens D: Hypophysectomy: A report on 50 operations for metastasizing breast cancer. *J Laryng* 82:73, 1968.
37. Straffon RA, Kiser WS, Robitaille M, et al: Yttrium hypophysectomy in the management of metastatic carcinoma of the prostate gland in 13 patients. *J Urol* 99:102, 1968.
38. Thompson JB, Greenberg E, Pazianos A, et al: Hypophysectomy in metastatic prostate cancer. *NY State J Med* 74:1006, 1974.
39. Tindall GT, Ambrose SS, Christy JH, et al: Hypophysectomy in the treatment of disseminated carcinoma of the breast and prostate gland. *South Med J* 69:579, 1976.
40. Tindall GT, Nixon DW, Christy JH, et al: Pain relief in metastatic cancer other than breast and prostate gland following transsphenoidal hypophysectomy: A preliminary report. *J Neurosurg* 47:659, 1977.
41. Tindall GT, Tindall SC: Hypophysectomy—Current status, in Tindall GT, Collins WF (eds): *Clinical Management of Pituitary Disorders*. New York, Raven Press, 1979.
42. VanGilder JC, Goldenberg IS: Hypophysectomy in metastatic breast cancer. *Arch Surg* 110:293, 1975.
43. West CR, Murphy GP: Pituitary ablation and disseminated prostatic carcinoma. *JAMA* 225:253, 1973.
44. Wilson RE, Piro AJ, Aliapoulios MA, et al: Evaluation of adrenalectomy and hypophysectomy in the treatment of metastatic cancer of the breast. *Cancer* 24:1322, 1969.
45. Zervas NT: Sterotaxic radiofrequency surgery of the normal and the abnormal pituitary gland. *N Engl J Med* 280:429, 1969.
46. Zimmerman BR, Molnar GD: Prolonged follow-up in diabetic retinopathy treated by sectioning the pituitary stalk. *Mayo Clin Proc* 52:233, 1977.

CHAPTER 15

Pituitary deficiency states

Hypopituitarism
  Etiology
    Postsurgical
    Tumor involvement
    Postirradiation
    Infarction
    Infectious and granulomatous lesions
      Histiocytosis X
      Pituitary abscess
      Tuberculosis and syphilis
      Sarcoidosis
      Hemochromatosis
    Trauma
    Hypothalamic lesions
  Clinical features of hypopituitarism
  Diagnostic evaluation
  Treatment of hypopituitarism
    Adrenal replacement
    Thyroid replacement
    Androgen replacement in men
    Estrogen replacement in women
Diabetes insipidus
  Etiology
    Idiopathic
    Familial or congenital
    Post-traumatic
    Neoplastic and granulomatous
    Histiocytosis X
    Vascular lesions
  Clinical and laboratory findings
  Management
    Chlorpropamide
    Clofibrate
    Carbamazepine
    Synthetic 8-lysine vasopressin
    1-Desamino-8-D-Arginine Vasopressin (DDAVP)
    Injectable vasopressin
Inappropriate secretion of ADH (Schwartz-Bartter syndrome)
  Etiology
  Clinical manifestations
  Pathophysiology
  Diagnosis and management

Anterior pituitary deficiency states, or hypopituitarism, result from a variety of causes with neoplasms and surgery accounting for the majority of cases. It is important that the clinician be aware of these conditions because of the potential dangers of certain deficiency states and the fact that appropriate replacement therapies are available and can be instituted. Posterior pituitary disorders are expressed as alterations in fluid homeostasis, and the principal clinical manifestations are diabetes insipidus (DI) and the syndrome of inappropriate antidiuretic hormone secretion (SIADH). We will discuss various aspects of hypopituitarism, DI, SIADH, and certain hypothalamic syndromes.

HYPOPITUITARISM
Etiology

The various causes of hypopituitarism are listed as follows*:

Pituitary tumors
  Functional
  Nonfunctional
Vascular disorders
  Intracranial aneurysm
  Sheehan's syndrome
  Arteritides, including polyarteritis nodosa and systemic lupus erythematosus
  Wernicke's encephalopathy
  Atheroma
Physical agents
  Trauma, head injury
  Radiation
  Surgery
  Alcohol injection
Infectious and granulomatous processes
  Tuberculosis, mycoses, syphilis, virus infections
  Sarcoidosis
  Histiocytosis X
  Demyelinating conditions
Hypothalamic and parasellar tumors
  Craniopharyngioma
  Glioma, including optic nerve glioma
  Meningioma
  Pinealoma
  Metastasis, especially breast and lung
  Leukemia, lymphoma
  Hamartoma
Congenital-familial
  DI
  Hypogonadotrophic hypogonadism
  Isolated growth hormone (GH) deficiency
  Prader-Willi syndrome
  Laurence-Moon-Biedl syndrome
Miscellaneous
  Idiopathic DI
  Iron overload, hemochromatosis, multiple transfusions
  "Empty sella" syndrome

---

*Modified from Belchetz PE: Hypopituitarism. In Belchetz PE (ed): *Management of pituitary disease*. New York, John Wiley & Sons, 1984.

Although the most common causes of pituitary endocrine deficiency are those related either to involvement of the normal gland by a pituitary tumor or to the surgery for such lesions, there are a variety of other causes for this deficiency state. Familiarity with these conditions is essential to achieve early recognition and institute proper therapeutic management. The normal pituitary gland has considerable reserve function, and probably as much as 50% of the gland can be destroyed or removed before significant hypopituitarism develops either clinically or by laboratory criteria.

Postsurgical. Both the incidence and degree of hypopituitarism following pituitary surgery will vary considerably and depend on a variety of factors. These will include the surgical approach (transsphenoidal as opposed to transcranial), the experience and skill of the surgeon, and the size and type of the tumor being treated. In many of the larger tumors, a mild degree of hypopituitarism already exists and surgical manipulation of the compromised pituitary gland may serve to increase the deficiency. Hypopituitarism may result from damage to or removal of functional adenohypophysial tissue, injury to the pituitary stalk, or a combination of both. We determined the incidence of postoperative pituitary endocrine deficiency in a series of 100 patients who underwent transsphenoidal removal of a prolactinoma.[10] Complete preoperative and postoperative baseline endocrine studies were available for comparison in 97 of these 100 cases. Preoperatively, all three pituitary–target organ axes (pituitary-thyroidal, -adrenal, and -gonadal) were intact in 65 patients, and one or more axes were deficient in 32 patients. Postoperatively, 50 of the 65 with intact pituitary function remained completely normal immediately (7 to 10 days) following surgery. Although 15 of the 65 showed a deficiency in one or more axes, it was usually temporary, and only two of the 15 required any type of endocrine replacement more than 6 months following surgery. Of the 32 patients who had a preoperative deficiency in one or more axes, it is significant that 11 (34%) cases showed an improvement in the deficiency(-ies) following surgery. Thus from these data, it appears that the incidence of *permanent* pituitary endocrine deficiency in patients is low (only four of 97 or 4%), and furthermore, there is the distinct possibility that preoperative pituitary endocrine deficiency(-ies) may improve as a result of surgery.

These findings, along with the necessity to recognize and treat postoperative pituitary endocrine deficiencies, underscore the importance of obtaining both preoperative and postoperative studies of pituitary–target organ function (see Chapter 4). Only by a comparison of these two sets of values can one objectively measure and determine any pituitary endocrine deficit present preoperatively and postoperatively and thus plan an appropriate replacement regimen.

Tumor involvement. Varying degrees of hypopituitarism can result from compression of the gland and/or stalk from a gradually expanding tumor. Most commonly, the tumor responsible for the deficiency is a pituitary adenoma. The size of the tumor is the major determinant of the degree and incidence of hypopituitarism. For instance, in 15 patients with microprolactinomas, we found that only three (20%) had compromised function of one or more pituitary–target organ axes, whereas in 25 patients with macroadenomas, the incidence of impaired function was 56% (14 patients).[21] As already discussed in the preceding section, it is important to obtain baseline pituitary endocrine studies so that the effects of any type of treatment, especially surgical, can be accurately assessed.

In addition to pituitary adenomas, other intrasellar or parasellar neoplasms may compromise pituitary endocrine function. These other tumors (which include metastatic neoplasms, craniopharyngioma, and meningioma among others) impair pituitary function by involvement of the hypophysial stalk and/or gland. The frequency, extent, and mechanism(s) for pituitary endocrine deficiency resulting from craniopharyngiomas are discussed in Chapter 11.

Postirradiation. Both conventional and heavy particle irradiation can cause varying degrees of hypopituitarism, and as with surgery, the incidence varies with a number of factors, the most significant being the dosage of irradiation administered.[9,13,20,25,30] When caused by irradiation, the endocrine deficiencies begin to appear approximately 18 months following completion of the course of treatment, although this time interval can vary from 6 to 8 months up to several years. The hypopituitarism as a consequence of irradiation is more likely a result of hypothalamic damage as opposed to pituitary damage, since the gland is relatively radioresistant.[6,26] A more detailed discussion of these issues is provided in Chapter 13.

Infarction. Pituitary infarction occurs with postpartum hemorrhage, diabetes mellitus, sickle cell disease, and other conditions. It is seen most commonly in association with postpartum uterine hemorrhage, and the resulting hypopituitarism is referred to as Sheehan's syndrome.[28,29] The pathogenesis of Sheehan's syndrome likely results from the pregnancy-induced pituitary hypertrophy, which makes the pituitary more vulnerable to changes in the circulatory status than would be the case with a normal gland. Postpartum hemorrhage with its attendant shock and associated coagulation abnormalities is the precipitating cause of the ischemic necrosis. Sheehan postulated that vasospasm (probably in response to the shock) developed in the arterial supply to the hypophysial portal system. The vasospasm leads to pituitary ischemia and thrombosis. Later, when the vasospasm clears and the circulatory status returns to normal, pituitary hemorrhage develops into the hyperplastic gland.[29] The posterior lobe is usually spared because it is less dependent on the portal system for its blood supply.

Infectious and granulomatous lesions

Histiocytosis X. Histiocytosis X is a granulomatous disease of unknown origin and highly variable course, characterized by solitary or multiple lesions that can involve virtually any tissue in the body and can occur at any age, although it is most common in childhood. Histiocytosis X includes several clinical varieties now believed by most pathologists to be different manifestations of a single underlying pathogenetic defect. The most common variety is Hand-Schüller-Christian disease. The typical lesions are granulomatous, containing histiocytes, eosinophils, and occasional multinucleated giant cells. The part of the brain involved most frequently is the hypothalamus.[4,18,32]

DI is the most frequent endocrine manifestation of histiocytosis X and occurs in somewhat less than half of the cases. It is often seen in partial form, and can present as the earliest sign of the disease in the absence of any other manifestations. Other endocrine abnormalities, of much less frequency, are impaired growth, hypogonadism, and partial or complete hypopituitarism. The lesion in the basal hypothalamus usually consists of a localized granulomatous lesion of histiocytic character with eosinophilic elements.

Pituitary abscess. Slightly more than 50 cases of pituitary abscess, a relatively rare entity, have been reported. Before the antibiotic era, almost all pituitary abscesses were found at autopsy in patients who had died of generalized sepsis. The extension of contiguous infections from purulent sphenoid sinusitis, meningitis, or cavernous sinus thrombophlebitis have all been reported as causes, but a clearly definable source of infection is often not apparent. On occasions, an abscess may develop within a primary pituitary tumor or cyst. Tumors may be more vulnerable to infection because of impaired circulation or areas of necrosis. A common clinical presentation in these patients is meningitis, and in fact, the presence of the latter in a patient with an enlarged or eroded sella or in a patient known to harbor a pituitary tumor is a clinical situation in which the diagnosis of pituitary abscess should be considered. Another clinical finding that should evoke suspicion of a pituitary abscess is the presence of visual field defects in a patient with meningitis. The overall mortality of a pituitary abscess unaccompanied by meningitis is estimated to be 28%, whereas a pituitary abscess associated with meningitis carries a 45% mortality.[8]

The range of micro-organisms causing pituitary abscesses reported in the literature is diverse.[17] Lindholm et al reviewed 20 cases and found that in nine of 17 cases where the results of bacteriologic studies were given, the abscess was "sterile." Among reports that cited a definitive micro-organism, *Staphylococcus aureus* and *Diplococcus pneumoniae* were the most commonly encountered.

Tuberculosis and syphilis. Tuberculosis and syphilis are rarely implicated in the pathogenesis of hypopituitarism. Isolated cases have been reported in which mycoses, brucellosis, and other infections have led to hypopituitarism.

Sarcoidosis. Sarcoidosis is a noncaseating granulomatous disease of undetermined cause and pathogenesis that can involve any part of the body. The central nervous system (CNS) is involved in less than 10% of cases. Mayock et al[19] found involvement of the CNS in 10 (7%) of 145 patients with sarcoidosis. DI caused by sarcoid was first described by Tilligren in 1935.[31] The pathologic process causing the DI and/or hypopituitarism in sarcoid consists of a granulomatous process in the basilar meninges with involvement of the stalk and infiltrative nodules in the hypothalamus and the pituitary gland. Other clinical findings that may be seen in CNS sarcoid include somnolence and hyperphagia from hypothalamic involvement, optic atrophy and visual field defects from local pressure on the visual apparatus, and unilateral or bilateral cranial nerve palsies resulting from extension of the granulomatous process along the base of the brain.

Hemochromatosis. Hemochromatosis is characterized pathologically by excessive deposits of iron in the body and clinically by hepatomegaly with eventual hepatic insufficiency, skin pigmentation, diabetes mellitus, and frequently cardiac failure. It is a rare disease and probably has several causes. Rarely, pituitary infiltration by the hemosiderin-laden macrophages can produce hypopituitarism in adults.

Trauma. Despite the frequency of CNS trauma, significant degrees of hypopituitarism as a sequel to moderate or severe head injury is relatively uncommon. Nevertheless, studies in patients experiencing prolonged coma as a result of severe head injury have revealed reduced pituitary-hypothalamic function. Fleischer et al[11] found levels of thyroid-stimulating hormone (TSH), thyroxine (T_4), free T_4, triiodothyronine (T_3), luteinizing hormone (LH), follicle-stimulating hormone (FSH), and testosterone to be subnormal in 15 patients with traumatic coma lasting longer than 2 weeks. Interestingly, the reduction in testosterone and T_4 were proportional to both the severity of coma and depletion of cerebrospinal fluid (CSF) $3',5'$-cyclic adenosine monophosphate (cyclic AMP). In those patients who regained consciousness, the endocrine deficits improved partially or completely. Thus these studies suggested that even if profound pituitary deficiency states accompany severe head injury, they are apt to improve concomitant with clinical improvement. Generally, any head injury severe enough to damage the hypothalamus or disrupt the stalk or gland will either be fatal or produce a neurovegetative survival.[11]

Hypothalamic lesions. In addition to its role in the regulation of the anterior and posterior pituitary gland, the hypothalamus controls water balance and body temperature and has a significant influence on consciousness, sleep, emotion, and behavior. Despite its small size, a large number of complex functions are included or integrated in the hypothalamus; consequently, a variety of neurologic abnormalities, altered physiologic body functions, and endocrinopathies can result from lesions involving various areas of this important CNS structure.[3]

The neurologic manifestations of nonendocrine hypothalamic disease are extensive*:

Disorders of temperature regulation	Disorders of psychic function
Hyperthermia	Rage behavior
Hypothermia	Hallucinations
Poikilothermia	Periodic diseases of hypothalamic origin
Disorders of food intake	Diencephalic epilepsy
Hyperphagia (bulimia)	Kleine-Levin syndrome
Anorexia, aphagia	Periodic discharge syndrome of Wolff
Disorders of water intake	Disorders of the autonomic nervous system
Compulsive water drinking	Pulmonary edema
Adipsia	Cardiac arrhythmias
Essential hypernatremia	Sphincter disturbance
Disorders of sleep and consciousness	Hereditary hypothalamic disease
Somnolence	Laurence-Moon-Biedl syndrome
Sleep-rhythm reversal	Miscellaneous
Akinetic mutism	Prader-Willi syndrome
Coma	Diencephalic syndrome of infancy
	Cerebral gigantism

These nonendocrine neurologic manifestations have been covered extensively in other publications and except for a tabulation of the symptoms and signs of hypothalamic disease shown in Table 15-1 will not be discussed further in this book.

Generally, the causes listed previously involving the pituitary gland and/or stalk that result in hypopituitarism are also those that can involve the hypothalamus with a similar result (i.e., pituitary endocrine deficiency).

---

*From Martin JB, Reichlin S, Brown GM: *Clinical Neuroendocrinology,* Philadelphia, FA Davis Co, 1977.

Table 15-1

Symptoms and signs of hypothalamic disease

Symptoms and signs	Number of cases
Sexual abnormalities (hypogonadism or precocious puberty)	43
Diabetes insipidus	21
Psychic disturbance	21
Obesity or hyperphagia	20
Somnolence	18
Emaciation, anorexia	15
Thermodysregulation	13
Sphincter disturbance	5

*Modified from Bauer HG: Endocrine and other clinical manifestations of hypothalamic disease: A survey of 60 cases with autopsies. *J Clin Endocrinol Metab* 14:13, 1954.

From an anatomic standpoint, hypothalamic lesions that involve the region of the median eminence either destroy the ability to synthesize new hypophysiotropic hormones or impair the transport of these hormones to the pituitary gland. Thus lesions in this region commonly produce endocrine disorders including DI, hypogonadism, hypothyroidism, and abnormalities of secretion of ACTH, GH, and prolactin. Intrinsic lesions such as trauma, irradiation damage, or tumors (such as gliomas) that extend into this area (median eminence) or extrinsic lesions such as a craniopharyngioma or a large intracranial aneurysm that damage the median eminence by compression can be expected to cause varying degrees of hypopituitarism. In practice, the most commonly encountered lesion that results in endocrine deficiency states by involvement of the hypothalamic-stalk system is a craniopharyngioma.

Clinical features of hypopituitarism

The clinical features of hypopituitarism depend on the degree of the deficiency and which particular pituitary hormone or hormones are undersecreted. Most patients with pituitary endocrine deficiency caused by one or more of the factors listed previously will have relative degrees of panhypopituitarism, which may vary from impairment or loss of reserve in one pituitary hormone to complete loss of all pituitary endocrine function. In current practice, the situation associated with partial loss of adenohypophysial function that is commonly encountered is a patient with a pituitary adenoma that compromises pituitary function or a patient who has had an adenomectomy and in whom the surgery itself created an impairment in one or more pituitary–target organ axes.

Complete loss of pituitary gland function without replacement therapy is not compatible with survival in humans because of failure to sustain function of the adrenal cortex. Currently, the clinical situation associated with a total loss of adenohypophysial function that is most commonly encountered is a patient who has had a surgical hypophysectomy. Cases of metastatic breast cancer, prostate cancer, and diabetic retinopathy and the patient with Cushing's disease in whom an adenoma is not found at surgical exploration are those clinical situations in which a total hypophysectomy may be performed.

When the clinical features are well established, the patient with hypopituitarism has a characteristic appearance.[5] Because of a general decrease in pigmentation, the skin develops a pale, waxy character, and the patient may show fine wrinkles about the eyes and mouth, giving an appearance of premature aging. Axillary and pubic hair becomes increasingly sparse, and in men, the rate of beard growth decreases. A moderate anemia may occur and reflects a decrease in bone marrow function in patients with hypopituitarism.

The clinical features of specific pituitary endocrine deficiencies are listed as follows:

> Adenohypophysial (anterior lobe) deficiency
>   Pituitary-adrenal axis
>   Nausea
>   Vomiting
>   Asthenia
>   Postural hypotension
>   Hyperthermia
>   Vascular collapse, death, if deficiency state is severe
>   ? Hyponatremia
>   Pituitary-thyroidal axis
>   Inactivity, sluggishness (torpor)
>   Cold intolerance
>   Skin dryness
>   Myxedema
>   Reduced basal metabolism
>   Pituitary-gonadal axis
>   Gonadal atrophy
>   Decrease in libido and potency
>   Amenorrhea in women
>   Disappearance of sperm in men
>   Other clinical findings
>   Waxy, pale character of skin
>   Decrease in pigmentation
>   Decrease in general body hair
>   Moderate anemia (normocytic, normochronic)
> Neurohypophysial (posterior lobe) deficiency
>   Diabetes insipidus

Impairment in the pituitary adrenal axis is typified by nausea, vomiting, postural hypotension, hyperthermia, and (if the deficiency is severe) eventual collapse. Moderate hypotension present in the early phase may become more pronounced and, unless corrected, can lead to an extreme medical situation. The clinical course of a patient with impairment of the pituitary adrenal axis is clearly related to adrenal cortical insufficiency.

The clinical findings of hypothyroidism usually begin to appear 4 to 8 weeks after acute loss of pituitary function, although in some patients undergoing a transsphenoidal hypophysectomy, we have noted the onset of these symptoms and/or signs as early as 10 days after pituitary ablation. Clinical features resulting from deficiency of the pituitary-thyroidal axis consist of relative inactivity, sluggishness, cold intolerance, dryness of the skin, and myxedema.

Deficiency of pituitary gonadotropin leads to gonadal atrophy. In women, amenorrhea occurs, libido decreases, and the uterus and vagina atrophy. In men, the testes become soft and atrophic, both libido and potency decrease, and sperm disappears from the semen.

Diagnostic evaluation

The diagnosis of hypopituitarism is based on the presence of clinical features of the disorder and characteristic laboratory findings. After establishing a clinical diagnosis, studies should be initiated to determine the cause and extent of the disorder. Endocrine testing to establish the diagnosis of pituitary endocrine deficiency is discussed in Chapter 4. Endocrine tests and routine neuroradiologic studies will serve to determine the cause in most cases, whereas in others, the diagnostic workup may require special procedures (e.g., metrizamide computed tomographic (CT) cisternography, magnetic resonance imaging [MRI]), to be determined on an individualized basis.

Treatment of hypopituitarism

Hypopituitarism is generally treated with hormonal preparations that replace the secretions of the adrenals, thyroid, and gonads rather than replacing with pituitary hormones themselves. The clinical response to such hormonal therapy of the patient with hypopituitarism is most gratifying. Hormonal therapy should be tailored to the individual patient, since isolated hormonal deficiencies may exist and are treated differently than panhypopituitarism. Additionally, there are varying degrees of hypopituitarism requiring individualized dosage schedules.

Adrenal replacement. Corticosteroid deficiency is a life-threatening disorder and must be treated in patients with hypopituitarism. If pituitary function is absent, replacement treatment with physiologic doses of corticosteroids is man-

Table 15-2
Relative potencies and equivalent doses of corticosteroids

Agent	Relative anti-inflammatory potency	Relative sodium-retaining potency	Duration of action*	Approximate equivalent dose†(mg)
Cortisol (Hydrocortisone)	1	1	Short	20
Tetrahydrocortisol	0	0	—	—
Prednisone (Δ^1-Cortisone)	4	0.8	Intermediate	5
Prednisolone (Δ^1-Cortisol)	4	0.8	Intermediate	5
6α-Methylprednisolone	5	0.5	Intermediate	4
Fludrocortisone (9α-Fluorocortisol)	10	125	Short	—
11-Desoxycortisol	0	0	—	—
Cortisone (11-Dehydrocortisol)	0.8	0.8	Short	25
Triamcinolone (9α-Fluoro-16α-hydroxyprednisolone)	5	0	Intermediate	4
Betamethasone (9α-Fluoro-16β-methyl-prednisolone)	25	0	Long	0.75
Dexamethasone (9α-Fluoro-16α-methyl-prednisolone)	25	0	Long	0.75

Modified from Haynes RC Jr, Murad F: Adrenocorticotrophic hormone; Adrenocortical steroids and their synthetic analogs; Inhibitors of adrenocortical steroid biosynthesis, in Gilman AG, Goodman LS, Gilman A (eds): *The Pharmacological Basis of Therapeutics*, ed 6, New York, MacMillan Publishers Co, Inc, 1980.
*Short, 8- to 12-hour biologic half-life; *intermediate*, 12- to 36-hour biologic half-life; *long*, 36- to 72-hour biologic half-life.
†These dose relationships apply to oral or intravenous administration.

datory. If pituitary dysfunction is mild, patients may only require therapy during periods of physiologic stress such as fever, infections, or surgical procedures. Any pituitary-adrenal deficiency existing before surgery for hypothalamic or pituitary disease should be corrected and additional corticosteroid given to cover the stress of surgery. An adult usually requires 30 mg/day of hydrocortisone (20 mg in the morning and 10 mg in the evening) for replacement therapy. Equivalent dosages of other analogues are appropriate (Table 15-2). There is usually no need to prescribe mineralocorticoids routinely if the patient has a normal salt intake.

Thyroid replacement. Most clinicians recommend a gradual restoration of thyroid replacement. An initial dose of 30 mg of desiccated thyroid (0.05 mg of L-thyroxine) should be gradually increased over a 1- to 2-month period to a full maintenance dose of 120 to 180 mg (0.2 to 0.3 mg L-thyroxine). The preoperative treatment of a pituitary-thyroidal deficiency is desirable but not mandatory as in the case of corticosteroids.

Androgen replacement in men. Androgen replacement therapy in men with hypopituitarism will usually restore libido and potency. Adequate treatment involves daily oral methyltestosterone in doses of 20 to 30 mg or the intramuscular injection of a slowly absorbed preparation such as testosterone enanthate, 200 mg every 3 to 4 weeks.

Estrogen replacement in women. Estrogen therapy may be indicated in young women to correct vaginal mucosal atrophy, for its beneficial extragenital action on skin, and possibly to diminish the incidence of osteoporosis.

Restoration of fertility is possible by replacement with human pituitary gonadotropins. FSH-containing preparations obtained from human pituitaries or postmenopausal human urine is given to women for 10 to 14 days to stimulate follicular development. The administration of human chorionic gonadotropin will then cause ovulation.

In addition to adenohypophysial deficiencies, patients undergoing total hypophysectomy or patients with suprasellar tumors that involve the hypophysial portal system (e.g., craniopharyngiomas) will usually exhibit some degree of posterior lobe (neurohypophysial) deficiency in the form of DI.

DIABETES INSIPIDUS

DI is a disorder of excessive renal water loss because of a deficiency in production or release of vasopressin, the antidiuretic hormone (ADH) produced in the supraoptic and paraventricular nuclei of the hypothalamus and transported within the axons of neurosecretory neurons down the stalk to the neurohypophysis.

A discussion of the normal physiology of ADH secretion and its extreme sensitivity to alterations in osmolality, blood volume, or blood pressure is included in Chapter 2. In brief review, the normal human subject synthesizes ADH in neurons of the supraoptic and paraventricular nuclei of the hypothalamus from which it gains access to the neurohypophysis by way of axons extending down the supraopticoneurohypophysial tract. From these axons, ADH is released, after proper stimulation, into the bloodstream and carried to the kidneys where it acts to conserve water and concentrate urine by enhancing the reabsorption of water from the collecting tubules into the medullary interstitium.

In the kidney, the ADH molecule attaches to a specific vasopressin receptor on the contraluminal side of the renal medullary tubular cell. A resultant activation of renal medullary adenylate cyclase stimulates the production of cyclic AMP, which activates a protein kinase on the luminal side of the cell. Phosphorylation of membrane proteins results in increased permeability of the cell to water. Water is thus transported from the collecting tubules into the intercellular spaces, renomedullary circulation, and the systemic circulation. Additionally, a number of drugs effecting ADH release are as follows:

>   ADH stimulators
>   Nicotine
>   Morphine
>   Barbiturates
>   Vincristine
>   Cyclophosphamide
>   Tricyclic antidepressants
>   Certain anticonvulsants
>   ADH inhibitors
>   Chlorpromazine
>   Reserpine
>   Diphenylhydantoin (Dilantin)
>   Ethanol

Etiology

DI may result from a variety of lesions at any of a number of sites along the pathway including ADH production, transport, release into the bloodstream, and action on the kidney. Therefore ADH production may be deficient or absent or synthesis may be intact, but the ability to release ADH following appropriate stimulation may be impaired. ADH release may occur but only after plasma osmolality has reached extremely high levels. Nephrogenic DI or a renal resistance to the action of ADH may also occur. A particularly useful etiologic classification with two major categories—primary and secondary—was proposed by Randall et al*:

>   Primary DI
>   Idiopathic
>   Familial or congenital
>   Secondary DI
>   Posttraumatic—head injury (e.g., basal skull fractures), neurosurgical operations
>   Neoplastic
>   Infectious and granulomatous lesions—sarcoidosis, tuberculosis, cryptococcosis, meningovascular syphilis, pyogenic meningitis
>   Histiocytosis X
>   Vascular lesions

---

*Modified from Randall RV, Clark EC, Bahn RC: Classification of the causes of diabetes insipidus. *Proc Mayo Clinic* 34:299, 1959.

Idiopathic. Idiopathic DI is a disease of unknown cause that accounts for approximately half of the acquired cases. It may occur at any age and can affect either sex. The disorder is characterized by the typical clinical features of DI (see p. 464) in the absence of other signs of hypothalamic or pituitary dysfunction.

Familial or congenital. Familial or congenital DI is a very rare disease constituting about 1% or less of all cases. The affliction occurs in infancy or childhood and affects either sex. Failure of development of the supraoptic or paraventricular neurons with subsequent reduction in posterior pituitary size appears to be the cause.

Post-traumatic. Trauma has become a common cause of DI as a result of the increasing number of head injuries caused by automobile accidents and surgical procedures in the neurohypophysial region. During a deceleration injury, the pituitary stalk may be compressed or sheared by the edge of the diaphragm sella resulting in either temporary or permanent DI. Traumatic cases may follow a classic three-stage response caused by damage to the neural mechanisms controlling ADH release. This pattern begins with severe DI that abates as the neurohypophysis degenerates and releases excessive ADH into the bloodstream, predisposing to hyponatremia. In the third stage, permanent DI usually follows, although varying degrees of water imbalance may result. This latter fact underscores the importance of periodic re-evaluation of patients with post-traumatic (and postsurgical) DI.

Neoplastic and granulomatous. Neoplastic and granulomatous DI is usually caused by destruction of the upper pituitary stalk and median eminence, where the neurohypophysial neurons converge in a relatively superficial position on their way to the neural lobe. Almost any tumor metastatic to the brain may occur in the infundibulum or upper stalk and cause DI. As mentioned elsewhere in this book, breast cancer has a special predilection for metastatic involvement of the hypothalamic-pituitary region, and carcinoma of the lung is notorious in this regard. Sarcoidosis is the most common of the granulomatous lesions causing DI, but tuberculosis, syphilis, cryptococcosis, and meningovascular syphilis may also produce the disorder.

Histiocytosis X. As with the granulomatous and neoplastic disorders, histiocytosis X may produce DI when the disease involves the hypothalamus, infundibulum, and/or upper pituitary stalk.

Vascular lesions. Vascular lesions can cause DI in a variety of ways. Intracranial aneurysms, particularly of the anterior communicating artery, can cause the condition either from mass effect as a result of progressive enlargement of the lesion or from rupture with resultant subarachnoid hemorrhage. The latter catastrophe may damage the hypothalamic nuclei or the infundibulum either during the acute bleed or later as a result of ischemia caused by the vasospasm that often follows aneurysmal subarachnoid hemorrhage. Postpartum pituitary necrosis (Sheehan's syndrome) occasionally causes DI in addition to adenohypophysial deficiency, presumably through vascular damage to the upper stalk. Interestingly, however, damage to or the removal of the adenohypophysis in a patient with DI greatly reduces the severity of the latter condition. The apparent amelioration of DI in hypopituitarism may result from the low rate of glomerular filtration resulting from both GH and adrenal steroid deficiencies and increased tubular reabsorption of water caused by adrenal insufficiency.

Clinical and laboratory findings

The patient with DI will have polyuria and polydipsia usually with a urine specific gravity below 1.005. In patients with large volumes of dilute urine, hypercalcemia, hypokalemia, or drug toxicity (as occurs with lithium) should be considered. Those with unexplained hypotonic polyuria should have plasma osmolality or sodium determinations. If low, the patient is water overloaded, and if high, the patient has DI. Central and nephrogenic DI are distinguished by the response or lack thereof to any form of administered ADH. Barlow and de Wardener[2] found that the plasma osmolalities of patients suffering from DI average 295 ± 15 mOsm/kg, whereas that for normal subjects averaged 280 ± 16 mOsm/kg. As this difference is associated with considerable overlap, the determination of plasma osmolality is of little help diagnostically in certain individual cases. As long as the patient maintains normal thirst mechanisms, the total solute concentration of the body fluids will be preserved close to the normal limits, albeit accompanied by the polydipsia and polyuria associated with this condition. However, the clinical situation may become catastrophic if there is a defect in the normal thirst mechanism (e.g., unconsciousness from trauma or anesthesia, destruction of thirst center) in a patient with DI. The resulting dehydration with accompanying hypovolemia and hyperosmolality can lead to fever, stupor, coma, and even prove fatal unless the underlying clinical condition is recognized and corrected. If the patient with hypotonic polyuria has a normal random plasma osmolality or sodium, dehydration tests should be done.

The water deprivation test will determine whether the patient can respond to an osmotic stimulus by elaboration of a concentrated urine. In the test, water intake is restricted, and changes in urine volume and plasma concentration are measured for a period of 6 to 8 hours. In normal individuals, water deprivation causes a dehydration that produces a fall in urine volume and a rise in urine osmolality. After 6 to 8 hours of fluid deprivation, the urine flow reduces to <0.5 ml/min, urine osmolality plateaus anywhere between 500 and 1400 mOsm/kg, and plasma osmolality rises to the range of 288 to 291 mOsm/kg. The subcutaneous administration of 5 u of aqueous vasopressin will not cause a further increase in urine osmolality, indicating that the maximal ability of the kidney to concentrate the urine has been realized.

The patient with severe DI is only able to concentrate the urine to <200 mOsm/kg after dehydration, and plasma osmolality may rise as high as 320 to 330 mOsm/kg. The administration of 5 u of aqueous pitressin will cause the urine osmolality to approximately double, indicating that the inability to concentrate the urine results from a deficiency of circulating ADH.

Patients with milder DI will exhibit levels of plasma and urine osmolalities of intermediate volumes following dehydration. Vasopressin will, however, cause a further increase in urine osmolality, indicating a limited capacity for ADH release. In severe dehydration, even DI patients may show a modest increase in urine concentration and a decline in urinary volume caused by contraction of blood volume with decreased renal plasma flow. One of the more difficult diagnostic problems can be differentiating the compulsive water drinker from the patient with DI. In this situation, it may be necessary to extend the dehydration period for as long as 18 hours, by which time compulsive water drinkers are always able to concentrate their urine.

Another situation where errors can be made in interpreting the results of a dehydration test is in a patient with mild DI that is able to secrete enough ADH to prevent diuresis but only at the expense of a higher than normal plasma osmolality. After dehydration occurs and the urine osmolality plateaus, plasma osmolality will be elevated and vasopressin administration will not cause a further concentration of urine. This patient's response to the water deprivation test will appear to be normal unless the plasma osmolality is measured and found to be high. Therefore the determination of plasma osmolality should be made after the urine osmolality plateaus and before giving vasopressin.

In patients with severe polyuria and polydipsia, a water deprivation test should not be carried out overnight because of the risk of severe dehydration and hypovolemic shock. Instead, these patients should begin water deprivation in the morning with urine collected hourly until the osmolality plateaus as determined by three consecutive samples. Plasma osmolality is then measured, and 5 u aqueous vasopressin is administered subcutaneously. Urine is collected at two consecutive 30-minute intervals and urine osmolality measured in each. Patients with DI will show an increase in urine osmolality of 9% or more after the administration of vasopressin.

Other tests for DI are available and include the hypertonic saline infusion test and the nicotine test.[16] In the former, the patient is hydrated initially with an infusion of dextrose and water at a rate (approximately 10 cc/min) to induce diuresis (>5 cc/min). The intravenous solution is then switched to a 2.5% solution of NaCl at a rate of 0.25 cc/min/kg body weight and continued for 45 minutes. Urine flow is measured by voiding every 15 minutes. If both neurohypophysial and renal function are normal, urine flow may be expected to fall sharply with the infusion of hypertonic saline, whereas in DI, urine flow is unaffected. Nicotine, which causes ADH release in normal subjects by its stimulating action on the supraoptic neurons, can be used to assess neurohypophysial function. The test is performed by inducing a water diuresis and then administering nicotine intravenously. In normal subjects, a sharp fall in urine flow will occur, whereas in DI little or no antidiuresis will be observed.

Management

Patients with mild to moderate DI who have an intact thirst mechanism and a readily available supply of water are usually in no danger and are treated mainly from the standpoint of convenience. The marked polydipsia and polyuria are annoying and usually prevent sleep at night. Thus for reasons of convenience, therapy usually is justified.

In clinical practice, there are varying degrees of ADH impairment, and treatment must be tailored for the individual patient. In institutions where a large volume of pituitary surgery is performed, varying degrees of DI will frequently be encountered. Postoperatively, in patients with pituitary tumors, the condition is usually transient; whereas in patients undergoing ablative hypophysectomy, as many as 70% or more will experience postoperative DI, many of which will be permanent.

A number of effective therapeutic preparations are available for treating DI[22] (Table 15-3). As with other peptide hormones, the oral administration of vasopressin is ineffective. Oral treatment with nonhormonal drugs may be efficacious in patients who have some residual capacity to release ADH.

Table 15-3

Agents used to treat diabetes insipidus

Agent	Usual dose	Duration of action	Clinical indication
Hormone replacement			
8-Lysine vasopressin (lypressin) (5 ml bottle, 50 U/ml)	10-20 U IN	4-6 hr	Severe, transient or permanent DI
1-Deamino-8-D-Arginine Vasopressin (DDAVP) (2.5 ml bottle, 160 μg/ml)	10-20 μg IN	12-24 hr	Severe, transient or permanent DI
Aqueous vasopressin (10-20 U/ampule (0.5-1 ml))	5-10 U SC	3-6 hr	DI in unconscious patient
Vasopressin tannate in oil (5 U/ml ampule)	5 U IM	24-72 hr	Severe idiopathic DI
Nonhormonal agents			
Chlorpropamide (100 & 250 mg tablets)	200-500 mg/day	24 hr	Some residual ADH function
Clofibrate (500 mg capsules)	500 mg q.i.d.	24 hr	Some residual ADH function
Carbamazepine (200 mg tablets)	400-600 mg/day	24 hr	—
Thiazide diuretics			
Hydrochlorothiazide (50 mg tablets)	50-100 mg/day	24 hr	Nephrogenic DI

Modified from Moses AM: Diabetes insipidus and ADH regulation. In Krieger DT, Hughes JC (eds): *Neuroendocrinology.* Sunderland, Mass, Sinauer Assoc, Inc, 1980.
IN, intranasal.
IM, intramuscular.
SC, subcutaneous.

Chlorpropamide. Chlorpropamide induces an antidiuresis in patients with DI in proportion to their ability to release ADH. A dose of 200 to 500 mg once daily is usually sufficient for 24 hours. The drug also facilitates the action of ADH on the kidney by increasing the ADH-induced activation of adenylate cyclase. It is not effective in patients with nephrogenic DI. A potential side effect of chlorpropamide administration is hypoglycemia, which can be avoided by eating regular meals.

Clofibrate. Clofibrate is another oral agent effective in the treatment of DI that acts centrally by releasing ADH from the neurohypophysis. It does not have any intrinsic ADH activity of its own and does not potentiate the peripheral action of ADH, so it is only useful in patients with some ADH reserve. The usual dosage is 500 mg four times a day. Some patients who do not respond to chlorpropamide or clofibrate alone will respond to a combination of the two drugs. In this situation, a regimen of chlorpropamide, 100 to 150 mg twice daily, and clofibrate, 1.5 to 2 g in daily divided doses, is used.

Carbamazepine. Carbamazepine, a tricyclic anticonvulsant, also stimulates endogenous ADH. It will induce a diuresis in patients with partial DI at doses of 400 to 600 mg daily. Because of its potential toxicity, it is not used as frequently as the other oral agents.

Synthetic 8-lysine vasopressin. Synthetic 8-lysine vasopressin is available as a nasal spray but has several disadvantages. A single application produces antidiuresis for only 4 to 6 hours, and its absorption is impaired under various circumstances including allergic rhinitis, respiratory infections, transsphenoidal surgery, and other conditions that produce edema of the nasal mucosa.

1-Desamino-8-D-Arginine Vasopressin. 1-Desamino-8-D-Arginine-Vasopressin (DDAVP), which is the synthetic analogue of vasopressin, is more satisfactory than synthetic 8-lysine vasopressin. It is also available as a nasal spray and has an antidiuretic effect for 12 to 24 hours, with no pressor activity.

Injectable vasopressin. Injectable vasopressin is available in an aqueous solution or as pitressin tannate in oil. The short duration of aqueous pitressin is advantageous in treating patients receiving intravenous fluids, especially unconscious patients, because it minimizes the risk of water intoxication. In patients with an altered level of consciousness with DI from head trauma or neurosurgery, we treat with aqueous pitressin administered intramuscularly or subcutaneously in doses of 5 to 10 u. Pitressin tannate in oil is used in similar doses for more chronic treatment of DI.

The only useful treatment of nephrogenic DI is the use of a thiazide diuretic with sodium restriction. Although this appears paradoxical, the drugs cause a depletion of sodium, which decreases the delivery of sodium to the ascending limb of the loop of Henle and causes a consequent reduction in the ability to dilute the urine. The glomerular filtration rate is reduced, and reabsorption of fluid in the proximal nephron is enhanced.

INAPPROPRIATE SECRETION OF ADH (SCHWARTZ-BARTTER SYNDROME)

The syndrome of inappropriate secretion of antidiuretic hormone (SIADH), first described by Schwartz et al[27] results from continued (and inappropriate) secretion of ADH despite a low serum osmolarity and an expanded extracellular fluid volume. Thus the term *inappropriate antidiuresis* is used, for under these conditions the hypothalamic neurons should be inhibited and the secretion of ADH suppressed. In this syndrome, however, ADH excess induces water retention by the kidney to the point of hyponatremic expansion of the extracellular fluid volume and a secondary natriuresis.

Etiology

Dilutional hyponatremia as a result of excessive water retention is a common disorder seen in many unrelated clinical states. The main causes of SIADH follow*:

    Central hypersecretion of ADH
      Hypothalamic disorders
        Trauma
        Surgery
        Metabolic encephalopathy
        Acute intermittent porphyria
        Myxedema
        Subarachnoid hemorrhage
        Vascular lesions
      Suprahypothalamic disorders
        Cerebral infarcts
        Subdural hematoma
        Infections, meningitis (tuberculosis)
    Peripheral hypersecretion
      Excessive stimulation in recumbent posture (coma)
    Excessive production from nonhypothalamic sites (ectopic ADH)
      Pulmonary infections—tuberculosis
      Tumors—lung, etc.
    Drugs
      Vincristine
      Chlorpromazine
      Chlorothiazide
      Cyclophosphamide
      Carbamazepine
      Clofibrate

---

*From Martin JB, Reichlin S, Brown GM: *Clinical Neuroendocrinology*. Philadelphia, FA Davis Co, 1977.

Other causes include (1) suprahypothalamic brain disease causing excessive release of ADH from the neurohypophysial system; (2) hypothalamic disturbances or damage that leads to "leakage" of ADH from the supraoptic neurons; (3) ADH release caused by persistent drive from baroreceptors or volume receptors, as a result of diseases in the heart or chest or of prolonged recumbent posture; (4) ectopic production of ADH by neoplastic tissue. (The most common malignancy causing SIADH is the oat cell tumor of the lung); and (5) administration of drugs that stimulate ADH release (see Table 15-3).

It has been well recognized that patients with various unrelated intracranial disorders are prone to develop SIADH. Subarachnoid hemorrhage, head injury, brain tumors, cerebral infarction, and meningitis are among the long list of CNS disorders associated with the syndrome. Fox et al[12] showed that 30% of neurosurgical patients developed SIADH at some time during hospitalization. The large variety and lack of anatomic specificity of lesions associated with SIADH have not been adequately explained. The assumption that an insult to the suprahypothalamic brain reduces the normal predominately inhibitory effect of these centers on ADH secretion has not been supported by experimental studies.

Clinical manifestations

The signs and symptoms of SIADH are related to the water retention and correlate to some extent with the degree of resultant hyponatremia and the rapidity with which it develops. A slow drop of serum sodium to a value near 125 mEq/liter results in nonspecific symptoms such as anorexia, nausea, vomiting, diffuse weakness, and mental alteration.[1] A more rapid fall in sodium to levels below 120 mEq/liter may be associated with seizures, stupor, or coma.[1] Patients with underlying neurologic disease may have symptoms at higher sodium levels than patients with normal brains. Focal signs such as pseudobulbar palsy, reflex changes, Babinski's sign, or extrapyramidal signs may be associated with hyponatremia.

Pathophysiology

Some investigators believe that water retention and hyponatremia produce a cytotoxic cerebral edema that is responsible for the neurologic manifestations. Severe hyponatremia and water intoxication, however, are not associated with a significant increase in intracranial pressure, and corticosteroids have no effect on the condition. Dila and Pappius[7] have investigated changes in cerebral electrolyte values in a rat model of SIADH and found diminished levels of potassium and sodium with the potassium depletion related to the level of consciousness. This work was expanded by Holliday et al,[14] who found that brain potassium depletion was associated with hyponatremia but not with acute changes in brain intracellular volume.

Diagnosis and management

Hyponatremia may be a result of sodium depletion as seen in prolonged vomiting, adrenal insufficiency, or the cerebral salt wasting syndrome (see below). These disorders require distinctly different treatments. The laboratory criteria for SIADH are (1) a serum sodium <135 mEq/liter; (2) urinary sodium >25 mEq/liter; (3) serum osmolality <280 mOsm/kg; and (4) urine osmolality inappropriately concentrated compared to serum osmolality. To make the diagnosis of SIADH the patient must be in a normal state of hydration; not be on diuretics; and have normal renal, thyroid, and adrenal function. In this syndrome, blood volume and peripheral circulation (pulse and blood pressure) are normal. Hyponatremia resulting from sodium depletion is accompanied by contraction of blood volume and decreased renal blood flow with elevation of blood urea nitrogen and creatinine (prerenal azotemia).

Since water retention is the source of symptoms and signs in SIADH, fluid restriction is the mainstay of therapy. For mild symptoms, daily water restriction of 400 to 800 ml is usually adequate. For more severe symptoms (i.e., seizures or coma) the use of 3% saline (500 ml over 6 to 8 hours) plus a forced diuresis with furosemide (20 to 40 mg) eliminates free water and rapidly corrects the hyponatremia. Because furosemide induces a natriuresis, urinary electrolytes become important, and sodium losses may need to be replaced. Once the hyponatremia has been corrected, institution of fluid restriction is important in preventing recurrence of water intoxication.

Certain drugs that inhibit the secretion or action of ADH have been used to treat SIADH. Dilantin and alcohol both inhibit ADH release but large doses are usually required. Lithium carbonate inhibits the action of ADH at the kidney but is not used frequently because of potential renal toxicity. Demethyl chlortetracycline, a tetracycline antibiotic, has been used more widely in dosages from 600 to 1200 mg/day for the same pharmacologic property of ADH inhibition at the kidney.

Nelson et al[23] have described 10 of 12 unselected neurosurgical patients with intracranial diseases who fulfilled the laboratory criteria for SIADH but had significant decreases in their red blood cell mass, plasma volume, and total blood volume. These authors believe this finding indicates that there is a spectrum of abnormalities in the hyponatremic, natriuretic patient from true SIADH to a "cerebral salt wasting syndrome." The latter disorder may result from an inability of the kidney to conserve sodium, perhaps because of an undefined natriuretic factor in the brain.[15] Blood volume determinations are necessary to differentiate the two causes of hyponatremia, since fluid restriction would exacerbate a cerebral salt wasting syndrome associated with volume depletion. This group of patients requires volume replacement with packed red blood cells and colloids to replace both the volume and sodium deficits.

REFERENCES

1. Arieff AI, Llach F, Massry SG: Neurological manifestations and morbidity of hyponatremia: Correlation with brain water and electrolytes. *Medicine* 55:121, 1976.
2. Barlow ED, de Wardener HE: Compulsive water drinking. *Q J Med* 28:235, 1959.
3. Bauer HG: Endocrine and other clinical manifestations of hypothalamic disease: A survey of 60 cases with autopsies. *J Clin Endocrinol Metab* 14:13, 1954.
4. Cureton RJR: A case of intracerebral xanthomatosis with pituitary involvement. *J Pathol Bacteriol* 61:533, 1949.
5. Daughaday WH: The adenohypophysis, in Williams RH (ed): *Textbook of Endocrinology*, ed 5. Philadelphia, WB Saunders Co, 1974.
6. De Schryver A, Ljunggren JG, Båryd I: Pituitary function in long-term survival after radiation therapy of nasopharyngeal tumours. *Acta Radiol Ther* 12:497, 1973.
7. Dila CJ, Pappius HM: Cerebral water and electrolytes: an experimental model of inappropriate secretion of antidiuretic hormone. *Arch Neurol* 26:85, 1972.
8. Dominigue JN, Wilson CB: Pituitary abscesses: Report of seven cases and review of the literature. *J Neurosurg* 46:601, 1977.
9. Fajardo LF: Endocrine organs, in Fajardo LF: *Pathology of Radiation Injury*. New York, Masson Publishing USA Inc, 1982.
10. Faria MA Jr, Tindall GT: Transspehnoidal microsurgery for prolactin-secreting pituitary adenomas: Results in 100 women with the amenorrhea-galactorrhea syndrome. *J Neurosurg* 56:33, 1982.
11. Fleischer AS, Rudman DR, Payne NS, et al: Hypothalamic hypothyroidism and hypogonadism in prolonged traumatic coma. *J Neurosurg* 49:650, 1978.
12. Fox JL, Falik JL, Shalhoub RJ: Neurosurgical hyponatremia: The role of inappropriate antidiuresis. *J Neurosurg* 34:506, 1971.
13. Fuks Z, Glatstein E, Marsa GW, et al: Long-term effects of external radiation on the pituitary and thyroid glands. *Cancer* 37:1152, 1976.
14. Holliday MA, Kalayyi MN, Harrah J: Factors that limit brain volume changes in response to acute and sustained hyper- and hyponatremia. *J Clin Invest* 47:1916, 1968.
15. Klahr S, Rodriguez HJ: Natriuretic hormone. *Nephron* 15:387, 1975.
16. Leaf A, Coggins CH: The neurohypophysis, in Williams RH (ed): *Textbook of Endocrinology*, ed 5, Philadelphia, WB Saunders Co, 1974.
17. Lindholm J, Rasmussen P, Korsgaard O: Intrasellar or pituitary abscess. *J Neurosurg* 38:616, 1973.
18. Martin JB, Reichlin S, Brown GM: *Clinical Neuroendocrinology*. Philadelphia, FA Davis Co, 1977.
19. Mayock RL, Bertrand P, Morrison CE, et al: Manifestations of sarcoidosis: Analysis of 145 patients, with a review of nine series selected from the literature. *Am J Med* 35:67, 1963.
20. McCombs RK: Proton irradiation of the pituitary and its metabolic effects. *Radiology* 68:797, 1957.
21. McLanahan CS, Christy JH, Tindall GT: Anterior pituitary function before and after transsphenoidal microsurgical resection of pituitary tumors. *Neurosurgery* 3:142, 1978.
22. Moses AM: Diabetes insipidus and ADH regulation, in Krieger DT, Hughes JC (eds): *Neuroendocrinology*. Sunderland, Mass., Sinauer Associates Inc, 1980.
23. Nelson PB, Seif SM, Maroon JC, et al: Hyponatremia in intracranial disease: Perhaps not the syndrome of inappropriate secretion of antidiuretic hormone (SIADH). *J Neurosurg* 55:938, 1981.
24. Randall RV, Clark EC, Bahn RC: Classification of the causes of diabetes insipidus. *Proc Mayo Clin* 34:299, 1959.
25. Rubin P, Casarett GW: *Clinical Radiation Pathology*. Philadelphia, WB Saunders Co, 1968, vol 2.
26. Samaan NA, Maor M, Sampiere VA, et al: Hypopituitarism after external irradiation of nasopharyngeal cancer, in Linfoot JA (ed): *Recent Advances in the Diagnosis and Treatment of Pituitary Tumors*. New York, Raven Press, 1979.

27. Schwartz WB, Bennett W, Cinelop S, et al: A syndrome of renal sodium loss and hyponatremia probably resulting from inappropriate secretion of antidiuretic hormone. *Am J Med* 23:529, 1957.
28. Sheehan HL: Post-partum necrosis of the anterior pituitary. *J Pathol Bacteriol* 45:189, 1937.
29. Sheehan HL, Stanfield JP: The pathogenesis of post-partum necrosis of the anterior lobe of the pituitary gland. *Acta Endocrinol* 37:479, 1961.
30. Sommers SC: Effects of ionizing radiation upon endocrine glands, in Berdjis LL (ed): *Pathology of Irradiation*. Baltimore, Williams & Wilkins, 1971.
31. Tillgren J: Diabetes insipidus as a symptom of Schaumann's disease. *Br J Dermatol* 47:223, 1935.
32. Vogel JM, Vogel P: Idiopathic histiocytosis: A discussion of eosinophilic granuloma, the Hand-Schüller-Christian syndrome, and the Letterer-Siwe syndrome. *Semin Hematol* 9:349, 1972.

CHAPTER 16

The "empty sella" syndrome

Classification
Definition
Etiology
Clinical features
Diagnostic evaluation
Treatment
Surgical approach
Summary

The term *"empty sella" syndrome* (ESS) refers to an anatomic entity in which the subarachnoid space herniates into the sella turcica. The entity is usually associated with radiographic changes of the sella and is often discovered by chance as when a skull film is taken for unrelated reasons. Although most individuals who have an empty sella are asymptomatic, some have clinical symptoms and signs. Although therapeutic intervention is rarely required for this disorder, treatment of complications of the empty sella such as cerebrospinal fluid (CSF) rhinorrhea or progressive visual loss is required.

CLASSIFICATION

Schaeffer[28] in 1924 described the anatomic appearance of the diaphragm sella in 125 autopsies and made the observation that these structures varied from a very dense and complete roof transmitting the infundibulum to a mere peripheral rim with a huge infundibular foramen. The term *empty sella* was first used by Busch[7] in 1951 to describe the autopsy finding of an incomplete diaphragm sella associated with a grossly invisible pituitary gland when the sella turcica was viewed from above. Busch examined 788 sellae of cadavers free of known pituitary pathologic findings and distinguished three main types of diaphragm sellae. In type 1, the diaphragm was a complete covering transmitting the hypophysial stalk. In the type 2 variety, there was a 3-mm or less space around the stalk. In type 3 the diaphragm was only a ring 2 mm or less in width. Occasionally, the last type was associated with a pituitary gland compressed forward to the bottom of the sella, a situation that gave the appearance of an empty sella at first glance. The incidence of the type 3 diaphragm was 5.5%, and 34 (85%) out of the 40

474 *Disorders of the pituitary*

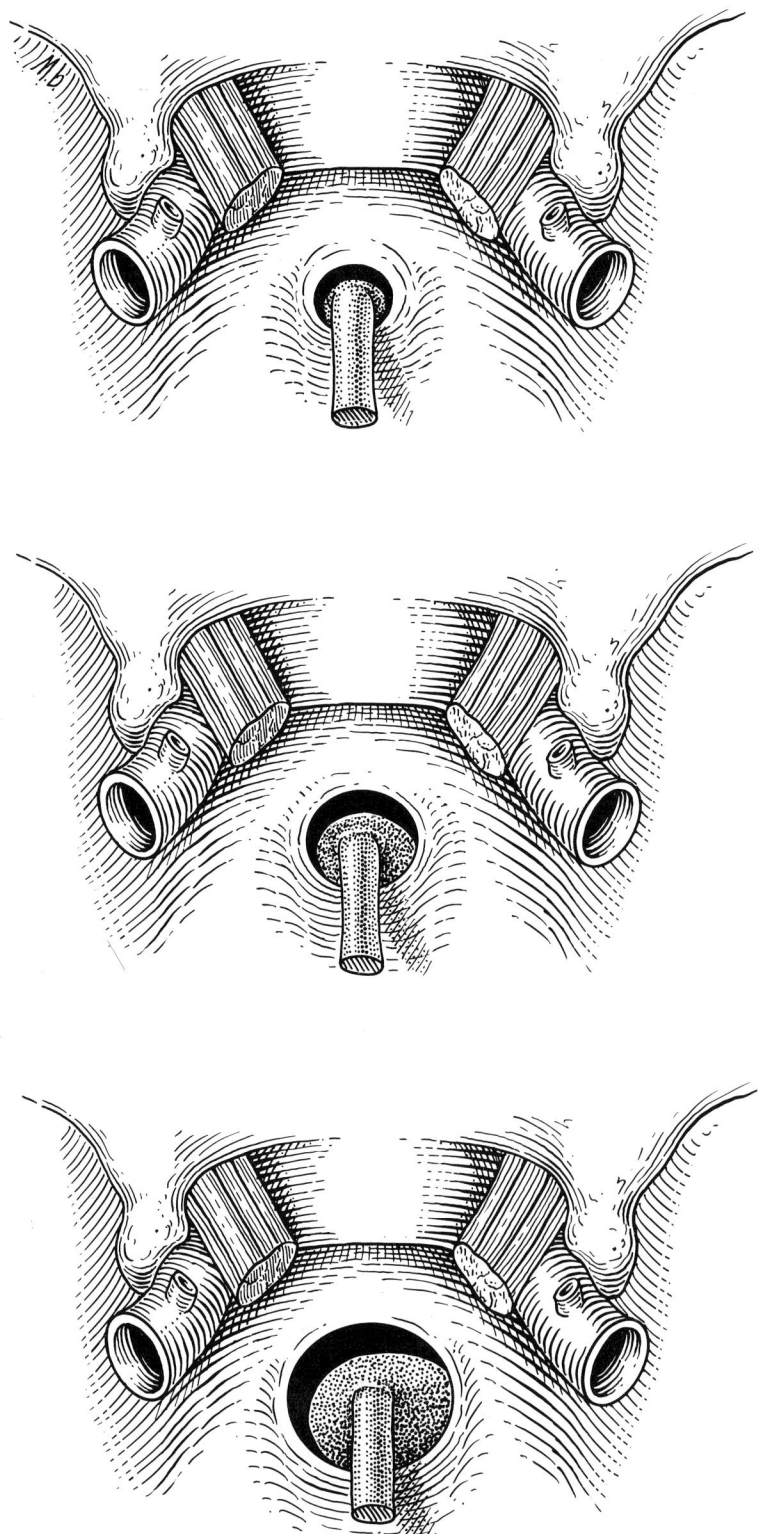

Fig. 16-1. Variations in opening of diaphragm sella.

cases observed were women. The anatomic variations in the size of the opening are illustrated in Fig. 16-1. These important observations by Busch were later confirmed by Bergland et al,[2] who made a detailed autopsy study of 225 cases and found that in 39% of the diaphragms examined, the opening for the stalk was greater than 5 mm in diameter. In 10% of the cases, the diaphragms were too thin to be considered as reliable barriers against inadvertent penetration during transsphenoidal operations. The incidence of a subarachnoid space that lay within the sella turcica that could have been outlined in a lateral pneumoencephalogram exceeded 20%. This is in agreement with the radiologic finding of DiChiro and Nelson[10] that the pituitary gland completely filled the sella in 79% of their cases.

Robertson[27] in 1957 demonstrated air within the sella on pneumoencephalograms, and Engels[12] in 1958 showed intrasellar invagination of the subarachnoid space in a patient who had contrast material that extended into the intracranial cavity and spilled into the sella following cervical myelography.

ESS is now generally accepted as a distinct radiologic and anatomic entity in which the subarachnoid space extends into the sella turcica. There is usually, although not necessarily, an associated enlargement of the sella and compression and remodeling of the pituitary gland. Other terms used to describe the empty sella include *intrasellar arachnoid diverticulum, intrasellar cistern,* and *deficient sellar diaphragm.*

DEFINITION

The ESS is divided into primary and secondary types. Primary empty sella refers to the condition in which there is a significant intrasellar herniation of the subarachnoid space in the absence of previous pituitary surgery or radiation directed to the sellar area. Secondary empty sella refers to those cases in which the extension of the suprasellar cistern into the sella turcica occurs following either pituitary surgery or irradiation.

Our discussion will focus on the *primary ESS*. The term refers to volumetric enlargement of the sella turcica not caused by a pituitary tumor but associated with a significant extension of the subarachnoid space into the sella through an incompetent diaphragm sella. The term further implies that the pituitary gland is flattened, compressed, and displaced posteriorly and inferiorly with resultant elongation of the pituitary stalk.

ETIOLOGY

Several theories have been advanced to explain the cause of primary ESS. Although entities such as pituitary infarction, pituitary apoplexy, and rupture of an intrasellar cyst have all been invoked as potential causes for the entity, the most likely explanation is that the condition arises in a patient who has had either a transient or a chronic elevation in intracranial pressure (ICP) and who also has an incompetent diaphragm sella allowing the subarachnoid space to be forced into the sella by the hydrostatic pressure and pulsatile movements of the CSF. Whether this incompetence of the sellar diaphragm is congenital or acquired is difficult to establish. Thus the pituitary gland and sella turcica are subjected directly to the pulsatile CSF pressure, which eventually leads to flattening and compression of the gland and remodeling of the sella turcica (Fig. 16-2). Primary ESS is more common in obesity and hypertension, both of which are likely to be associated with some degree of chronic elevation of ICP. The not uncommon association of ESS with pseudotumor cerebri, which also occurs predominantly in obese women, further supports the importance of chronically elevated ICP in the development of this condition.[14,35]

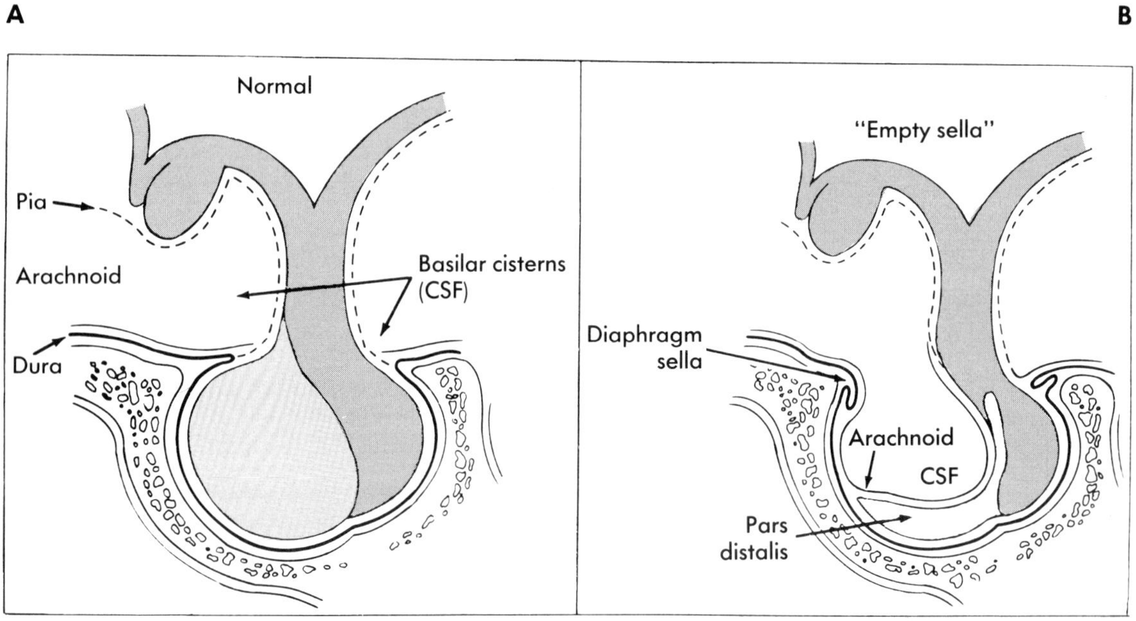

Fig. 16-2. Sagittal illustration of (**A**) normal relationship of diaphragm sella, small opening in diaphragm sella, and normal shaped pituitary gland and stalk, and (**B**) wide opening in diaphragm sella in ESS with prominent intrasellar cistern, elongated stalk, and inferiorly displaced and flattened pituitary gland.

From Jordan RM, Kendall JW, Kerber CW: The primary empty sella syndrome: Analysis of the clinical characteristics, radiographic features, pituitary function and cerebrospinal fluid adenohypophysial hormone concentrations. Am J Med 62:569, 1977.

CLINICAL FEATURES

Although the majority of patients with primary ESS have been middle-aged, obese women who are frequently hypertensive and multiparous, no well-defined clinical entity is characteristic of ESS. Headache is the most common symptom and is usually long-standing, varying in severity and pattern. An empty sella is most frequently detected in an otherwise asymptomatic patient after a skull x-ray is obtained for the evaluation of headache. The physical examination is usually normal with the exception of obesity and possibly hypertension. Papilledema and diplopia may be observed in patients with concomitant pseudotumor cerebri. Visual field defects, although not uncommon with secondary empty sella, are rare in patients with primary ESS.[5,17,18,24] Visual field abnormalities may show considerable variance from enlarged blind spots to bitemporal hemianopsia and may be accompanied by optic atrophy and diminished visual acuity.[3,23,39] Trigeminal neuralgia and atypical facial pain with sensory loss over the face have also been reported.[3,8,24,32]

One of the most striking clinical findings in a patient with ESS is CSF rhinorrhea. This complication was first reported by Ommaya et al[25] in 1968. Brisman et al[6] in 1969 further contributed to the recognition and understanding of this complication. It is relatively rare and may be etiologically related to intracranial hypertension, which frequently is associated with ESS. For instance, in patients with ESS in whom CSF pressure has been measured, pressure elevations have been recorded in as many as 65% of cases.[14] Intermittent elevations of ICP are suspected in the majority of the patients with headaches and ESS. This was documented in a patient with ESS and CSF rhinorrhea in whom continuous ICP monitoring was performed. Transient elevations of ICP were observed, which were abolished with the insertion of a lumboperitoneal shunt.[9] The site of the CSF leak is usually into the sphenoid sinus through the eroded sella floor.

Although it is generally considered that some degree of hypopituitarism is present in approximately 30% of the patients with primary ESS[30], no clinically significant endocrinopathy is found in the majority of the cases.[17,18,24,26] The most frequently reported endocrine abnormalities have consisted of altered biochemical responses of the pituitary gland to various provocative tests. A blunted response of growth hormone (GH) to insulin-induced hypoglycemia is the most commonly reported abnormal test.[5,13,24,36] GH appears to be the pituitary hormone primarily affected.[13] Scepticism about the validity of the studies was raised by Neelon et al,[24] since obesity itself may occasionally blunt the GH response and failure to lower the level of glucose with insulin may also produce false-negative results.[36] Gonadotropin deficiency may be observed,* and reduced adrenocorticotropic hormone (ACTH) and thyroid-stimulating hormone (TSH) reserves have been recorded.[13,24] Global hypopituitarism has also been reported.[4,24,29] These biochemical abnormalities suggest a disturbance in the hypothalamic-pituitary axis and

---

*See references 4, 5, 8, 24, 31, and 34.

would seem most likely to be a result of impairment (i.e., stretching) of the pituitary stalk. This supposition is supported by reports of diabetes insipidus in three patients with primary ESS.[21,29]

Endocrinopathies such as acromegaly are results of a coexisting hyperfunctional microadenoma. The occasional exception is hyperprolactinemia, which may result from pituitary stalk impairment and a prolactin-secreting microadenoma. The association of an ESS and hypersecreting microadenoma is probably coincidental. The cases reported in the literature include microadenomas causing amenorrhea-galactorrhea,[11,18,29,32,33] acromegaly,† and Cushing's disease.[15,16,32] The disproportionately high incidence of GH-secreting tumors associated with ESS may possibly be caused by the higher tendency of these adenomas to undergo infarction,[11] or the high incidence may result from chance alone.

As already mentioned, hyperprolactinemia may also be caused by stretching of the stalk, a situation that impairs normal delivery of prolactin-inhibiting factor (PIF) thus allowing the normal gland to oversecrete prolactin. Galactorrhea and/or amenorrhea may or may not be present.[1] Among 53 patients with amenorrhea-galactorrhea and an enlarged sella turcica reported by Kleinberg et al,[19] 5 were found to have an ESS. Domingue et al[11] found a partial ESS in 17.3% of their patients with amenorrhea-galactorrhea and in 10% of those with acromegaly.

DIAGNOSTIC EVALUATION

Currently, the diagnostic evaluation consists of a lateral skull x-ray, high-resolution computed tomographic (CT) scan, and occasionally, a metrizamide cisternogram. Radiologically, the empty sella presents a diverse picture. As discussed and illustrated in Chapter 5, the lateral skull x-ray often shows enlargement of the sella turcica with erosion of the lamina dura. The dorsum sella retains its normal curvature, and there is apparent approximation of the anterior and posterior clinoids.

Before the advent and widespread use of high-resolution CT scanning, the diagnosis of ESS was radiologically confirmed by pneumoencephalography. The entry of significant quantities of air into the sella revealing the characteristic compressed pituitary gland displaced posteriorly and inferiorly was diagnostic of this condition (Fig. 16-3). Currently, because of the accuracy of CT scanning, there is no need for a pneumoencephalogram to diagnose ESS (Fig. 16-4, *A*). In cases with either an equivocal or nondiagnostic CT scan, metrizamide cisternography (see Chapter 5) should be performed to confirm the diagnosis (Fig. 16-4, *B*). In the future, magnetic resonance imaging (MRI) may become the procedure of choice in confirming this diagnosis.

---

†See references 11, 20, 22, 24, 32, 33, and 40.

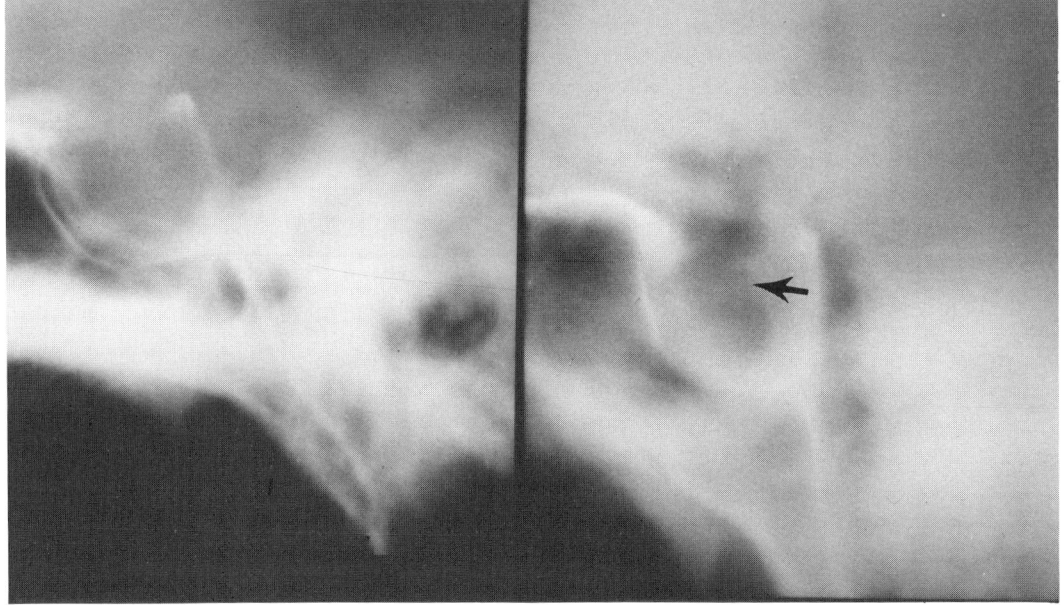

Fig. 16-3. Lateral skull x-ray (**A**) and pneumoencephalogram (**B**) in patient with ESS. The sella is grossly enlarged, and there is a significant amount of air in the intrasellar cistern (arrow) on the pneumoencephalogram.

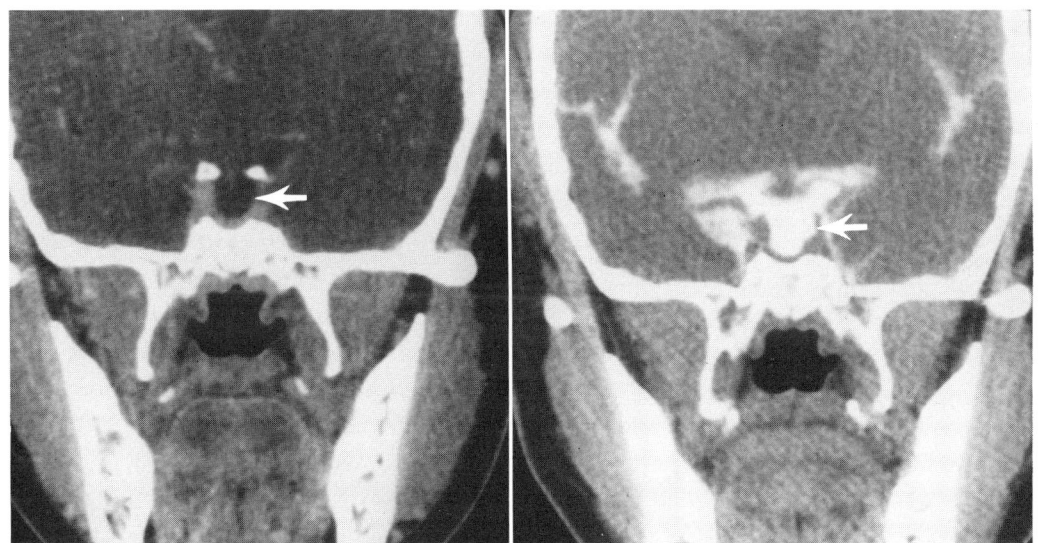

Fig. 16-4. High-resolution coronal CT scan shows intrasellar low-density area (arrow) consistent with ESS (**A**). Pituitary stalk and compressed gland can be visualized. Metrizamide instilled into lumbar subarachnoid space has filled the sella (arrow) confirming diagnosis of ESS (**B**).

TREATMENT

The uncomplicated primary ESS requires no treatment. The patient is usually investigated because of the possibility of a pituitary tumor or other structural lesion of the sella.

Before the use of high-resolution CT scans and metrizamide cisternograms, it was not unusual for patients to occasionally undergo transsphenoidal surgery for a presumed adenoma only to find on exposure that the condition was in reality an ESS. Also on unusual occasions, an ESS can be associated with a microadenoma causing endocrinopathy. The operative appearance of an ESS exposed via the transsphenoidal approach is shown in Plate 4, A.

The intrasellar cistern, which is located anteroinferiorly in the sella, will usually be opened simultaneously with opening of the dura, particularly anteriorly. Thus CSF will be encountered and will continue to leak throughout the remainder of the surgical procedure. The operative appearance after entering an ESS is shown in Plate 4, B. Characteristically, the elongated stalk can be seen entering the sella and passing down to the inferiorly located and flattened pituitary gland. The flow of CSF can be controlled by a catheter placed in the subarachnoid space. Obviously, the latter needs to be in place before starting surgery. Thus, if it is anticipated that an ESS will be encountered, it is advisable to insert a lumbar subarachnoid catheter immediately before beginning surgery. The major advantage of this catheter is to provide a "dry" field at the time of repair of the ESS, thus ensuring a more secure sella closure and thus avoiding a postoperative CSF leak.

SURGICAL APPROACH

The method of surgical management of an ESS is to gently mobilize the flattened gland and push it upward into the large empty space anteriorly that was occupied by the intrasellar cistern. A piece of adipose tissue can then be inserted into the inferior sella to keep the gland propped up. The fat is held in position by wedging a thin plate of bone (taken from the nasal septum) into the open bony floor of the sella. Tissue adhesive applied to the thin plate of bone will serve to seal it in position. At this time, it is important to stop the flow of CSF by opening the subarachnoid catheter and allowing egress of CSF through the catheter. This maneuver will stop the flow of CSF from the intrasellar cistern and "dry" up the operative field so that a good seal can be obtained.

The presence of a spontaneous CSF leak in association with and as a result of the ESS is usually an indication for surgery. The site of the leak can usually be accurately localized by using metrizamide cisternography as described in Chapter 5. The transsphenoidal approach is recommended for the repair of a leak through the floor of the sella into the sphenoid sinus.[37]

In the relatively rare situation in which the optic chiasm sags into an empty sella and the patient has documented and related visual abnormalities, a transsphenoidal chiasmopexy may be a worthwhile procedure. This situation probably occurs more often in the secondary ESS. Transsphenoidal chiasmopexy in this situation has been reported to improve vision.[38,39]

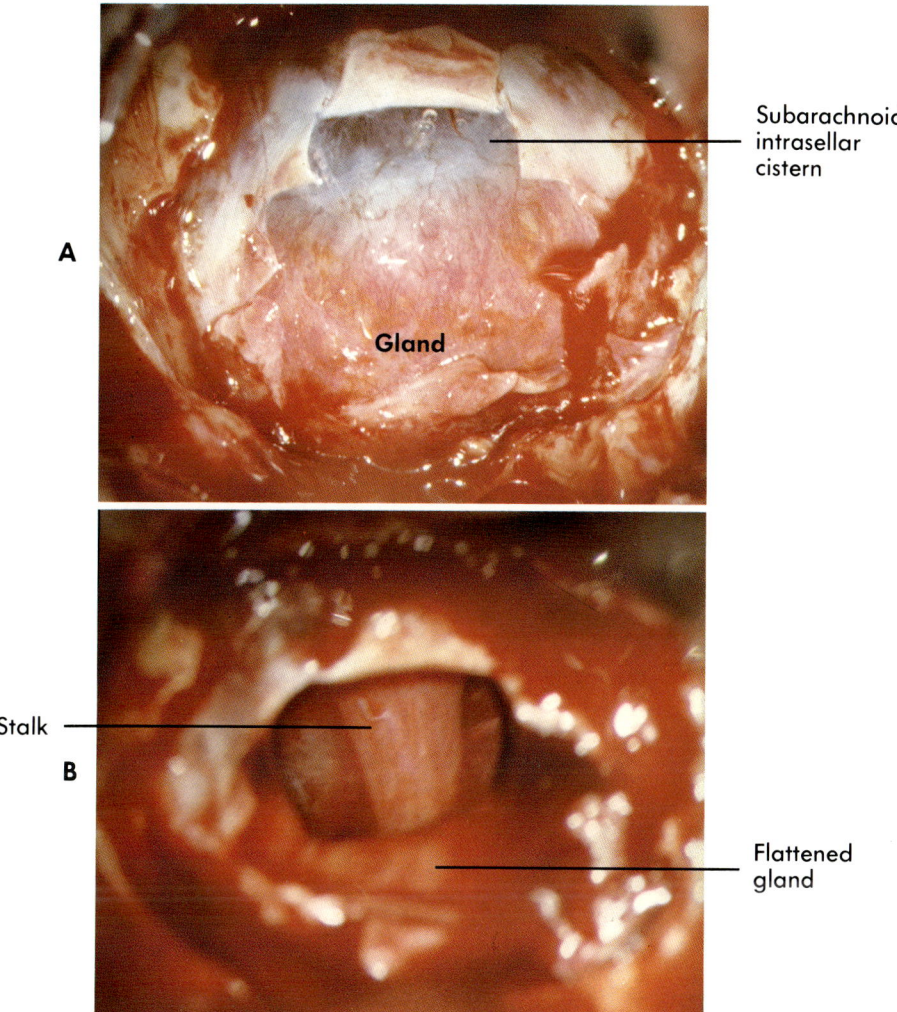

Plate 4. Transsphenoidal operative appearance of "empty sella" syndrome. **A,** Appearance before opening dura and entering intrasellar cistern. Intrasellar cistern filled with cerebrospinal fluid, which appears as light blue, can be seen through intact dura. **B,** Dura and intrasellar cistern have been opened and interior of "empty sella" can be seen. Elongated stalk can be seen passing down to flattened gland situated in inferior portion of sella.

SUMMARY

The primary ESS is an entity characterized by incompetence of the diaphragm sella with extension of the subarachnoid space into the sella turcica. In association with elevated ICP, this anatomic condition is likely to lead to remodeling of the pituitary gland and the pituitary fossa. These patients usually have an enlarged sella on skull film, and the entity is usually discovered during investigation of headaches, following head trauma or some other condition. Subsequent investigation usually concentrates on excluding the diagnosis of a pituitary tumor. Although the majority of patients are overweight, hypertensive women, there is no specific syndrome associated with the empty sella that sets it aside as a distinct entity. Among the complications of the condition, the most serious are visual abnormalities and CSF rhinorrhea, both of which are rare. The definitive diagnostic study is high-resolution CT scanning, and occasionally, this may need to be combined with metrizamide cisternography to confirm the diagnosis. There is no specific treatment for ESS unless one of the uncommon complications occurs. The association of an ESS with a pituitary microadenoma has to be regarded as an incidental occurrence.

REFERENCES

1. Bar RS, Mazzaferri EL, Malarkey WB: Primary empty sella, galactorrhea, hyperprolactinemia and renal tubular acidosis. *Am J Med* 59:863, 1975.
2. Bergland RM, Ray BS, Torack RM: Anatomical variations in the pituitary gland and adjacent structures in 225 human autopsy cases. *J Neurosurg* 93, 1968.
3. Berke JP, Buxton LF, Kokemn E: The "empty" sella. *Neurology* 25:1137, 1975.
4. Bernasconi V, Giovanelli MA, Papo I: Primary empty sella. *J Neurosurg* 36:157, 1972.
5. Brisman R, Hughes JEO, Holub DA: Endocrine function in nineteen patients with empty sella syndrome. *J Clin Endocrinol* 34:570, 1972.
6. Brisman R, Hughes JEO, Mount LA: Cerebrospinal fluid rhinorrhea and empty sella. *J Neurosurg* 31:538, 1969.
7. Busch W: Die Morphologie der Sella Turcica und ihre Beziehangen zur Hypophyse. *Arch F Path Anat* 320:437, 1951.
8. Caplan RH, Dobben GD: Endocrine studies in patients with the empty sella syndrome. *Arch Intern Med* 123:611, 1969.
9. Davis S, Kaye AH: A dynamic pressure study of spontaneous CSF rhinorrhea in the empty sella syndrome: Case report. *J Neurosurg* 52:103, 1980.
10. Di Chiro G, Nelson KB: The volume of the sella turcica. *AJR* 87:989, 1962.
11. Domingue JN, Wing SD, Wilson CB: Coexisting pituitary adenomas and partially empty sellas. *J Neurosurg* 48:23, 1978.
12. Engels EP: Roentgenographic demonstration of a hypophysial subarachnoid space. *AJR* 80:1001, 1958.
13. Faglia G, Ambrosi B, Beck-Peccoz P, et al: Disorders of growth hormone and corticotropin regulation in patients with empty sella. *J Neurosurg* 38:59, 1973.
14. Foley KM, Posner JB: Does pseudotumor cerebri cause the empty sella syndrome? *Neurology* 25:565, 1975.
15. Ganguly A, Stanchfield JB, Roberts TS, et al: Cushing's syndrome in a patient with an empty sella turcica and a microadenoma of the adenohypophysis. *Am J Med* 60:306, 1976.
16. Gutin PH, Cushard WG, Wilson CB: Cushing's disease with pituitary apoplexy leading to hypopituitarism, empty sella, and spontaneous fracture of the dorsum sellae: Case report. *J Neurosurg* 51:866, 1979.
17. Hodgson SF, Randall RV, Holman CB, et al: Empty sella syndrome: Report of 10 cases. *Med Clin North Am* 56(4):897, 1972.
18. Jordan RM, Kendall JW, Kerber CW: The primary empty sella syndrome: Analysis of the clinical characteristics, radiographic features, pituitary function and cerebrospinal fluid adenohypophysial hormone concentrations. *Am J Med* 62:569, 1977.
19. Kleinberg DL, Noel GL, Frantz AG: Galactorrhea: A study of 235 cases, including 48 with pituitary tumors. *N Engl J Med* 296:589, 1977.
20. Login I, Santen RJ: Empty sella syndrome: Sequela of the spontaneous remission of acromegaly. *Arch Intern Med* 135:1519, 1975.

21. Matisonn R, Pimstone B: Case reports: Diabetes insipidus associated with an empty sella turcica. *Postgrad Med J* 49:274, 1973.
22. Molitch ME, Hieshima GB, Marcovitz S, et al: Coexisting primary empty sella syndrome and acromegaly. *Clin Endocrinol* 7:261, 1977.
23. Mortara R, Norrell H: Consequences of a deficient sellar diaphragm. *J Neurosurg* 32:565, 1970.
24. Neelon FA, Goree JA, Lebovitz HE: The primary empty sella: Clinical and radiographic characteristics and endocrine function. *Medicine* 52:73, 1973.
25. Ommaya AK, Di Chiro G, Baldwin M, et al: Non-traumatic cerebrospinal fluid rhinorrhoea. *J Neurol Neurosurg Psychiatry* 31:214, 1968.
26. Ridgway EC, Kourides IA, Kliman B, et al: Thyrotropin and prolactin pituitary reserve in the "empty sella syndrome." *J Clin Endocrinol Metab* 41:968, 1975.
27. Robertson EG: *Pneumoencephalography.* Springfield, Ill., Charles C Thomas Publisher, 1957.
28. Schaeffer JP: Some points in the regional anatomy of the optic pathway, with especial reference to tumors of the hypophysis cerebri and resulting ocular changes. *Anat Rec* 28:243, 1924.
29. Schaison G, Metzger J: The primary empty sella: An endocrine study on 12 cases. *Acta Endocrinol* 83:483, 1976.
30. Schwartz TB, Ryan WG: *Year Book of Endocrinology.* Chicago, Year Book Medical Publishers Inc, 1978.
31. Shore RN, DeCherney AH, Stein KM, et al: The empty sella syndrome: Virilization in a 59-year-old woman. *JAMA* 227:69, 1974.
32. Spaziante R, de Divitiis E, Stella L, et al: The empty sella. *Surg Neurol* 16:418, 1981.
33. Sutton TJ, Vezina JL: Co-existing pituitary adenoma and intrasellar arachnoid invagination. *AJR* 122:508, 1974.
34. Thomas HM Jr, Lufkin EG, Ellis GJ III, et al: Hypogonadotropism and "empty sella": Improvement in 2 cases with clomiphene citrate. *Fertil Steril* 24:252, 1973.
35. Weisberg LA, Housepian EM, Saur DP: Empty sella syndrome as complication of benign intracranial hypertension. *J Neurosurg* 43:177, 1975.
36. Weisberg LA, Zimmerman EA, Frantz AG: Diagnosis and evaluation of patients with an enlarged sella turcica. *Am J Med* 61:590, 1976.
37. Weiss MH, Kaufman B, Richards DE: Cerebrospinal fluid rhinorrhea from an empty sella: Transsphenoidal obliteration of the fistula. *J Neurosurg* 39:674, 1973.
38. Welch K, Stears JC: Chiasmapexy for the correction of traction on the optic nerves and chiasm associated with their descent into an empty sella turcica: Case report. *J Neurosurg* 35:760, 1971.
39. Wood JH, Dogali M: Visual improvement after chiasmapexy for primary empty sella turcica. *Surg Neurol* 3:291, 1975.
40. Zatz LM, Janon EA, Newton TH: The enlarged sella and the intrasellar cistern. *Radiology* 93:1085, 1969.

Index

A

Abscess, pituitary, 112
   causing hypopituitarism, 455
   radiologic studies of, 194
Acetylcholine
   in Alzheimer's disease, 52
   in brain, concentration of, 49
   and oxytocin secretion, 46
   and vasopressin release, 46
Acidophil stem cell adenomas, 206-207
Acidophilic adenomas, 72
Acidophilic cells of anterior pituitary, histology of, 65
Acidophilic stem cell adenomas, pathology of, 78, 79
Acromegaly, 203-225
   acral enlargements in, 210-212
   arthralgias, 212
   burned-out, 209-210
   clinical features of, 209-213
   diagnostic evaluation of, 215-217
   effects of radiation therapy on, 416-419
   electromagnetic irradiation for, 220
   endocrine testing for, 215
   etiology of, 205-209
   facial enlargement in, 210-212
   fugitive, 209
   irradiation for, 220
   medical conditions and metabolic disturbances associated with, 213-214
   menstrual disturbances in, 213
   myopathy in, 213
   pathophysiology of, 205
   persistent or recurrent, following therapy, 222
   pharmacotherapy for, 220-221
   preoperative assessment of patient with, 354
   prognosis for, 214
   radiologic studies in, 216-217
   skin changes in, 212
   special endocrine testing for, 135-136
   surgery for, 218-220
   therapeutic decision making in, 221-224
   treatment of, 217-221
Acroparesthesias in acromegaly, 212
ACTH; *see* Adrenocorticotropin
Adenohypophysis, 9, 27-29
   histology of, 65-66
Adenoma(s)
   acidophil stem cell, 206-207
      pathology of, 78, 79
   acidophilic, 72
   basophilic, 72
   chromophobic, 72; *see also* Nonfunctional pituitary adenomas
   corticotroph cell, pathology of, 80-83
   follicle-stimulating hormone–secreting, 130, 305-306
   gonadotroph cell, pathology of, 84-85
   gonadotropin-secreting, 305-306
   growth hormone cell, 206-207
      pathology of, 75-76
   growth hormone cell–prolactin cell, 77-78, 206, 207
   luteinizing hormone–secreting, 130, 305-306
   mammosomatotroph cell, 207
      pathology of, 79-80
   null cell, pathology of, 88-90
   peripheral nerve entrapments, 212
   pituitary; *see* Pituitary adenomas
   plurihormonal, 207
      pathology of, 86-87
   prolactin cell, pathology of, 72-74
   thyroid-stimulating hormone–secreting, 130, 302-305
   thyrotroph cell, 305
      pathology of, 85-86
   undifferentiated cell; *see* Adenoma, null cell
Adrenal axis, endocrinologic testing of, 133
Adrenal replacement for hypopituitarism, 460-461
Adrenal toxins for Cushing's disease, 242-243
Adrenalectomy
   bilateral, for Cushing's disease, 241
   choice of hypophysectomy over, 446-447
Adrenergic drugs and vasopressin release, 46
Adrenocorticotropic hormone, 35, 49
   concentration of, in brain, 49
   evolutionary aspects of, 50
   measurement of, 133
   plasma levels of, determination of, in Cushing's disease, 139

Breast cancer—cont'd
　remission in, after hypophysectomy, 443-444
Bromocriptine
　for acromegaly, 220-221
　　preoperative, 222, 224
　for Cushing's disease, 244
　for macroprolactinoma, 272, 273
　for prolactinomas, 264, 265-267
　　preoperative, 274-276
Bromocriptine-induced changes in pituitary adenomas, 92, 93
Brookes' carmoisine to differentiate acidophilic cells, 65
Burned-out acromegaly, 209, 210

C

Calcification in pituitary adenoma, 92
Calcitonin, 49
Calcospherites, 92
Canal
　optic, 1, 2, 5
　pharyngeal, 3
　pterygoid, 3, 7
Cancer
　breast; see Breast cancer
　prostate; see Prostate cancer
Carbamazepine for diabetes insipidus, 466, 467
Carcinoma, 94
　embryonal cell, undifferentiated, 312
　growth hormone cell, 207
　pituitary, primary, 306
Cardiomegaly and acromegaly, 213-214
Cardionatrins, 45
Carmoisine, Brookes', to differentiate acidophilic cells, 65
Carnosine, 49
Carotid artery
　damage to, during transsphenoidal surgery, 394, 395
　internal, 21
Carotid bulge, 5
Carotid sulcus, 2, 3
Cartilage, septal, 9
Cavernous hemangioma, 111
Cavernous sinus, 20-22
　cranial nerves in, 20
　transverse or coronal view of, 18
　venography of, 160, 161
Cavity, nasal, 7-9
　roof, floor, and lateral wall of, 7, 8
Cell(s)
　acidophilic, of anterior pituitary, histology of, 65
　basophilic, of anterior pituitary, histology of, 65
　chromophobic
　　of anterior pituitary, histology of, 65
　　histology of, 65
　corticotroph, electron microscopy of, 68
　gonadotroph, electron microscopy of, 69
　growth hormone
　　electron microscopy of, 67
　　immunologic staining of, 70
　magnocellular, of neurohypophysis, 40

Cell(s)—cont'd
　neurosecretory, 25-26
　　activity of, monoamines and, 46-47
　prolactin, electron microscopy of, 66
　secretory, 24
　thyrotroph, electron microscopy of, 68
Central nervous system
　effects of radiation on, 410-412
　irradiation of, complications of, 426-432
　peptide concentrations in, 49
Cerebral angiography; see Angiography
Cerebral aqueduct, 13
Cerebral artery, anterior, 21
Cerebral edema, postoperative, 386
Cerebral radionecrosis, 426-427
Cerebral salt wasting syndrome, 470
Cerebral vasospasm from transsphenoidal surgery, 396
Cerebrospinal fluid
　leakage of, after transsphenoidal surgery, 391-393
　neuropeptides in, 55-56
Cerebrospinal fluid rhinorrhea in "empty sella" syndrome, 199, 417
Chemoadenolysis, 447
Chiasm, optic; see Optic chiasm
Chiasmatic groove, 1
Chiasmatic sulcus, 2
Chiasmopexy, transsphenoidal, 480
Chlorpromazine stimulation test for prolactinomas, 141-142
Chlorpropamide for diabetes insipidus, 466, 467
Cholecystokinin, 49
　in Alzheimer's disease, 52
　concentration of, in central nervous system, 49
　evolutionary aspects of, 50
　measurement of, 51
　in Parkinson's disease, 55
Cholesteatomas, 104, 315
Choline acetyltransferase in Alzheimer's disease, 52
Chondromas, 108
Chordoma, 313-315
　pathology of, 103-104
　radiologic studies of, 188-189
Choriocarcinoma, 312
Choristomas, 95, 315
Choroid plexus, 13
Chromophobe adenoma; see Nonfunctional pituitary adenomas
Chromophobe cells
　of anterior pituitary, histology of, 65
Chromophobic adenomas, 72
Cistern, intrasellar; see "Empty sella" syndrome
Cisternography
　metrizamide; see Metrizamide cisternography
　in craniopharyngioma, 329
Clinical and endocrinologic evaluation of patients with pituitary tumors, 123-142
Clinoid process
　anterior, 2, 7
　middle, 1, 3
　posterior, 2, 3

Clivus, 2, 3
Clofibrate for diabetes insipidus, 466, 467
"Collar button" tumor, 361
Commissure, posterior, 13
Compression of optic chiasm by pituitary tumor, 128
Compton process of absorption of x-ray photons, 404, 405
Computed tomography (CT), 154-156
　for acromegaly, 216-217
　for aneurysm, 193
　for arachnoid cyst, 191
　for chordoma, 188, 189, 313
　for craniopharyngioma, 176-177, 328, 329, 333, 335
　for Cushing's disease, 239
　for ectopic pituitary adenoma, 307
　for "empty sella" syndrome, 198, 478, 479
　in histiocytosis X, 197
　of hypothalamic and optic gliomas, 185
　for meningioma, 180-182
　for nonfunctional pituitary adenomas, 284-287
　for pituitary abscess, 194
　for pituitary adenomas, 163, 166-170, 174
　for pituitary metastasis, 308-309
　for Rathke's pouch cyst, 190
　for sarcoidosis, 195
Concha(e)
　nasal, 7, 8
　sphenoid, 3
Conchal type of sphenoid sinus, pneumatization of, 152, 153
Congenital diabetes insipidus, 463
Corticotroph cell, electron microscopy of, 68
Corticotrophs, histology of, 65
Corticotropin; see Adrenocorticotropin
Corticotropin-releasing factor (hormone), 35, 49
　and ACTH, 232
Cortisol
　free, measurement of, in Cushing's disease, 137
　measurement of, 133
　secretion of, physiology of, 232
Cosyntropin-stimulating test, 133
Cranial nerves in cavernous sinus, 20
Craniopharyngeal duct, 9
Craniopharyngioma(s), 96-100, 321-346
　calcification of, 92
　clinical features of, 323-326
　"conservative" approach to, results of, 337-338
　diagnostic evaluation of, 326-329
　effect of radiation therapy on, 425-426
　embryogenesis of, 322-323
　endocrine involvement in, 325-326
　endocrinologic testing in, 327
　hypothalamic involvement in, 326
　irradiation for, 339-341
　neuro-ophthalmologic evaluation in, 326
　pathology of, 323
　postoperative management of, 338-339
　psychiatric manifestations of, 323-324
　"radical" approach to, results of, 336-337
　radiologic studies of, 174-178, 327-329
　surgery for, 330-335
　　results of, 336-338

Craniopharyngioma—cont'd
　therapeutic decision making for, 341-346
　treatment and results of, 329-330
　visual symptoms associated with, 325
Craniotomy
　frontotemporal (pterional), positioning for, 356
　for nonfunctional pituitary adenoma, 290, 293
　operative, complications of, 385-389
　operative mortality with, 389, 390
　subfrontal, 366-367
　subtemporal, 367
Crest
　infraorbital, 3
　sphenoid, 3, 4
CRF; see Corticotropin-releasing factor (hormone)
CRH; see Corticotropin-releasing factor (hormone)
Cribriform plate of ethmoid, 8
Crooke's hyalin change in corticotroph cell adenomas, 82, 83
Cryohypophysectomy, stereotaxic, 447
Cushing's disease (syndrome), 72, 80, 82, 83, 94
　clinical features of, 236-238
　diagnostic evaluation of, 238-239
　effect of radiation therapy on, 420-421
　endocrine tests for, 238
　establishing diagnosis of, 137
　history of, 232-233
　identifying source of, 137-140
　irradiation for, 241-242
　laboratory findings in, 138
　medical conditions and metabolic disturbances associated with, 236
　and Nelson's syndrome, 231-249
　pathophysiology of, 234-235
　pharmacotherapy for, 242-244
　from pituitary tumors, 130, 131
　preoperative assessment of patient with, 354
　prognosis for, 238
　radiologic studies in, 238-239
　special endocrinologic testing for, 137-140
　surgery for, 240-241
　therapeutic decision making in, 244-245
　treatment of, 239-245
Cushing's syndrome; see Cushing's disease (syndrome)
Cyproheptadine
　for Cushing's disease, 234-235, 243-244
　for Nelson's syndrome, 247
Cyst
　arachnoid
　　pathology of, 111
　　radiologic studies of, 191
　　sellar, 315, 316
　benign, of sellar and parasellar areas, 315-316
　dermoid, sellar, 315
　　pathology of, 104-106
　epidermoid, sellar, 315
　　pathology of, 104-106
　leptomeningeal, 316
　　pathology of, 111
　non-neoplastic, radiologic studies of, 190-191
　Rathke's cleft, 315-316
　　pathology of, 109-110

Cyst—cont'd
  Rathke's pouch, radiologic studies of, 190
  sellar and suprasellar, pathology of, 109-111

D

DA; *see* Dopamine
Dementia
  Alzheimer's, 52
  of Parkinson's disease, 55
Demethyl chlortetracycline to inhibit ADH release, 470
Dermoid cysts
  pathology of, 104-106
  sellar, 315
1-Desamino-8-D-Arginine Vasopressin for diabetes insipidus, 466, 467
Deuteron, 403
Dexamethasone suppression test in Cushing's disease, 137, 138-139
Diabetes insipidus, 43, 461-467
  clinical and laboratory findings in, 464-465
  etiology of, 462-464
  familial or congenital, 463
  granulomatous, 463
  idiopathic, 463
  management of, 465-467
  neoplastic, 463
  from pituitary tumors, 129
  post-traumatic, 463
  radiation-induced, 429
  after transsphenoidal surgery, 393
Diabetic retinopathy, hypophysectomy for, 446
Diaphragm, sella, deficient; *see* "Empty sella" syndrome
Diaphragm sella, 1, 11
  opening of, variations in, 474
Digital intravenous angiography, 157
  for craniopharyngioma, 178
  for meningioma, 183
  for nonfunctional pituitary adenomas, 287
  for pituitary adenoma, 171, 174
Dilantin to inhibit ADH release, 470
Directly ionizing radiation, 404
Disease
  Alzheimer's, postmortem studies, 52
  Ayala's, 114
  Cushing's; *see* Cushing's disease (syndrome)
  Hand-Schüller-Christian, 114
  Huntington's, postmortem studies of, 53-54
  Letterer-Siwe, 114
  Parkinson's, postmortem studies of, 54-55
Diuresis, stress-induced, 46
Diverticulum, arachnoid, intrasellar; *see* "Empty sella" syndrome
Dopamine, 35, 36
  and activity of neurosecretory cells, 46
  in brain, concentration of, 49
  function of, 40
  to innervate hypothalamus, 38
  in Parkinson's disease, 54-55
  as prolactin-inhibiting factor, 38
Dopamine-β-hydroxylase, 39
Dorsomedial nucleus, 15

Dorsum sella, 2, 3
Dose response curve, 406
Double floor, false, in skull films, 148, 149
Duct, craniopharyngeal, 9

E

Ectopic pinealoma, 106
Ectopic pituitary adenomas, 94, 306-307
Edema, cerebral, complicating craniotomy, 386
Electromagnetic radiation, 402-403
  clinical use of, 408
Electron microscopy of pituitary gland and sellar region, 66-67
Electrons, 403
Embolization from transsphenoidal surgery, 396
Embryologic aspects of neuropeptides, 50
Embryonal cell carcinoma, undifferentiated, 312
Eminence, median, 11
"Empty sella" syndrome, 12, 150, 473-481
  classification of, 473-475
  clinical features of, 477-478
  definition of, 475
  diagnostic evaluation of, 478, 479
  etiology of, 476
  radiologic studies of, 198-199
  surgical approach to, 480
  treatment of, 480
Endocrine function, postoperative assessment of, 135
Endocrine involvement in craniopharyngioma, 325-326
Endocrine secretory cells, 24
Endocrine testing; *see also* Endocrinologic testing
  for acromegaly, 215
  for Cushing's disease, 238
  in nonfunctional pituitary adenomas, 282-283
  special, 135-142
Endocrinologic and clinical evaluation of patients with pituitary tumors, 123-142
Endocrinologic studies
  of nonfunctional pituitary adenomas, 282-283
  of prolactinomas, 259
Endocrinologic testing, 132-142; *see also* Endocrine testing
  in craniopharyngioma, 327
Endocrinopathy with pituitary tumors, 130-131
Endogenous opioids, 47
  discovery of, 48
β-Endorphin, 47, 49
  discovery of, 48
  evolutionary aspects of, 50
Endorphins
  and neurohypophysial neurons, 47
  and vasopressin secretion, 47
Endotoxin and vasopressin release, 45
Energy transfer, linear, 406-407, 409
Enkephalins
  discovery of, 48
  leucine, 49
  methionine, 49
Eosinophilic granuloma, 113
Ependymal zone, inner, of median eminence, 32, 33

Epidermoid cysts
  pathology of, 104-106
  sellar, 315
Epinephrine
  to innervate hypothalamus, 39
  and vasopressin release, 46
Ergot alkaloids for prolactinomas, 264
Erythrosin, Herlant's, to differentiate acidophilic cells, 65
Estradiol, measurement of, 134
Estrogen replacement for hypopituitarism in women, 461
Ethmoid, cribriform plate of, 8
Ethmoid sinus, 4
Ethmoid spine of sphenoid bone, 1, 2
Exit-dose of radiation, 406
Exocrine secretory cells, 24
Extrahypothalamic regulation of hypothalamic-adenohypophysial system, 36-37
Extraocular muscles, paralysis of, from pituitary tumors, 128

F

False double floor in skull films, 148, 149
Familial diabetes insipidus, 463
Fibers, Rosenthal, 102
Fibroblastic meningiomas, pathology of, 102
Fibrosarcomas, 94
Films, skull; see Skull films
Fissure, orbital, superior, 2
Follicle-stimulating hormone, 35
  measurement of, 134
Follicle-stimulating hormone–secreting adenoma, 130, 305-306
Foramen
  interventricular, 13
  optic, 1
  sphenopalatine, 8
Foramen ovale, 2, 6
Foramen rotundum, 2, 3, 6
Foramen spinosum, 2, 6
Fornix, 13, 16
  column of, 13
Fossa
  hypophysial, 2
  pterygoid, 7
Free cortisol, measurement of, in Cushing's disease, 137
Frontotemporal approach, 362-366
Frontotemporal craniotomy, positioning for, 356
Frozen section diagnosis, 70-71
FSH; *see* Follicle-stimulating hormone
Fugitive acromegaly, 209

G

GABA; *see* Gamma amino butyric acid
Gagel's granuloma, 114
Gamma amino butyric acid concentration in brain, 49
Gamma rays, 403
Gangliocytomas, 108
Gastrin, 49

Gastrointestinal peptides, list of, 49
Germinoma
  hypothalamic, 310
  pathology of, 106-107
  sellar, 312-313
GH; *see* Growth hormone
GHRH; *see* Growth hormone–releasing hormone
Gigantism, etiology of, 205-209
Gland, pituitary; *see* Pituitary gland
Glandular secretion, neural control of, 24-26
Glioblastoma multiforme, 102, 310
Gliomas
  hypothalamic and optic
    pathology of, 102-103
    radiologic studies of, 184-187
  optic pathway, 310-312
Glucagon, 49
Glucagon stimulation test, 134
Glucocorticoids and vasopressin secretion, 44
Glutamate, concentration of, in brain, 49
Glycine, concentration of, in brain, 49
GnRH; *see* Luteinizing hormone–releasing hormone
Gold-198 for internal radiation, 414
  for acromegaly, 419
  for Cushing's disease, 421
Gonadal axis, endocrinologic testing of, 134
Gonadotroph cell
  electron microscopy of, 69
  histology of, 65
Gonadotroph cell adenomas, pathology of, 84-85
Gonadotropin-releasing hormone, 23, 49
Gonadotropin-secreting adenomas, 305-306
Gonadotropins, serum, measurement of, 134
Granular cell tumors, 95-96, 315
Granule, Langerhans', Birbeck's, or X, 114
Granuloma
  eosinophilic, 113
  Gagel's, 114
Granulomatous diabetes insipidus, 463
GRF; *see* Growth hormone–releasing factor
Groove
  chiasmatic, 1
  nasopalatine, 9
  trigeminal, 2
Growth hormone, 35, 36, 49
  basal levels of, measurement of, in acromegaly, 136
  elevated, causes of, 206
  endocrinologic testing of, 134
  measurement of, 134
  physiology of, 204-205
  secretion of, regulation of, 204-205
Growth hormone cell
  adenomas of, 206-207
    pathology of, 75-76
  carcinoma of, 207
  electron microscopy of, 67
  hyperplasia of, 207
  immunologic staining of, 70
Growth hormone cell–prolactin cell adenoma, 206, 207
  mixed, pathology of, 77-78

Growth hormone–glucose suppression test for acromegaly, 136
Growth hormone release-inhibiting factor (hormone), 35
Growth hormone–releasing factor (hormone), 23, 35, 49, 204, 205
  levels of, in acromegaly, 136
Growth hormone releasing factor test, 134

H

Haloperidol for Huntington's chorea, 53
Hamartomas, hypothalamic, 310
Hamulus, 3
Hand-Schüller-Christian disease, 114
Headache
  in acromegaly, 212
  mass effect of, 124
  from pituitary tumors, 128-129
Heavy-charged ions, 404
Heavy particle irradiation for acromegaly, 220
Hemangioblastomas, 108
Hemangioma, cavernous, giant, 111
Hematomas complicating craniotomy, 386
Hemianopsia, bitemporal, from pituitary tumor, 125, 126
Hemochromatosis causing hypopituitarism, 456
Hemorrhage
  complicating craniotomy, 385-386
  intracranial, during transsphenoidal surgery, 396
  in pituitary adenoma, 92
  venous, after transsphenoidal surgery, 394
Herlant's erythrosin to differentiate acidophilic cells, 65
Histiocytosis X, 113-114
  and diabetes insipidus, 463
  causing hypopituitarism, 454-455
  radiologic studies in, 196-197
Histology of pituitary gland and sellar region, 65-66
Homovanillic acid in Parkinson's disease, 54
Horizontal plate of palatine, 8
Hormone
  adrenocorticotropic; see Adrenocorticotropic hormone
  antidiuretic; see Vasopressin
  corticotropin-releasing, 35
    and ACTH, 232
  follicle-stimulating, 35
    measurement of, 134
  gonadotropin-releasing, 23, 35, 49
  growth; see Growth hormone
  growth hormone release inhibiting, 35
  growth hormone–releasing, 34
  hypophysiotropic, of hypothalamus, 34-36
  hypothalamic releasing, list of, 49
  luteinizing, 35, 49
    measurement of, 134
  luteinizing hormone–releasing, 34, 35
  melanocyte-stimulating, 49
  neurohypophysial, 42-43
    list of, 49
  pituitary, reserve of, assessment of, 132-135

Hormone—cont'd
  thyrotropin-releasing, 23, 34, 35, 49
    as brain-gut peptide, 48
5-HT; see Serotonin
Huntington's disease, postmortem studies of, 53-54
Hydrocephalus
  obstructive
    increased intracranial pressure caused by, in craniopharyngiomas, 326
    nonfunctional pituitary adenoma causing, 296, 297
  shunting for, 334
Hydrochlorothiazide for diabetes insipidus, 466
17-Hydroxycorticosteroids in Cushing's disease, 138, 140
5-Hydroxytryptamine; see Serotonin
Hypercortisolism; see Cushing's disease (syndrome)
Hyperplasia, growth hormone cell, 207
Hyperprolactinemia, 253, 255
  causes of, 255-256
  in "empty sella" syndrome, 478
  medical problems associated with, 256-257
  from pituitary tumors, 130, 131
  recurrent, after treatment, 270-271
Hypertonic saline infusion test, 134
  for diabetes insipidus, 465
Hypnotics and vasopressin secretion, 47
Hypophysectomy, 439-449
  beneficial results of, 440-441
  for breast cancer, indications for and timing of, 445
  choice of, over adrenalectomy, 446-447
  for Cushing's disease, 241
  for diabetic retinopathy, 446
  history of, 439-440
  medical alternatives to, 448
  postoperative considerations after, 448
  for prostate cancer, indications for and timing of, 445-446
  remission of breast cancer after, 443-444
  remission of cancer symptoms after, 443
  remission of prostate cancer after, 445
  selection of breast cancer patients for, 441-443
  selection of prostate cancer patients for, 443
  surgical procedure for, 382-383
  techniques for, 447
Hypophysial artery
  inferior, 11, 12, 27
  superior, 11, 12, 27
Hypophysial fossa, 2
Hypophysial tract, supraoptic, 15-16
Hypophysial vein, long, 11
Hypophysiotropic hormones of hypothalamus, 34-36
Hypophysis; see Pituitary gland
Hypophysitis, lymphocytic, 114
Hypopituitarism, 452-461
  clinical features of, 458-459
  diagnostic evaluation of, 460
  in "empty sella" syndrome, 477
  etiology of, 452-458
  mass effects of, 125
  from pituitary tumors, 129

Hypopituitarism—cont'd
  postsurgical, 453
  preoperative assessment of patient with, 354
  radiation-induced, 428-429
  after transsphenoidal surgery, 393
  treatment of, 460-461
Hypothalamic-adenohypophysial system, 29
  extrahypothalamic regulation of, 36-37
Hypothalamic gliomas
  pathology of, 102-103
  radiologic studies of, 184-187
Hypothalamic involvement in craniopharyngioma, 326
Hypothalamic lesions causing hypopituitarism, 456-458
Hypothalamic-neurohypophysial system, 29
Hypothalamic nuclei, 14-15
  anterior, 15
  lateral, 16
  posterior, 15, 16
  ventromedial, 16
Hypothalamic-pituitary axis, coronal section of, 29
Hypothalamic-pituitary unit, 26-30
  history of study of, 26-27
Hypothalamic regions, 15
Hypothalamic releasing hormones, list of, 49
Hypothalamic sulcus, 13
Hypothalamic tumors, 310
Hypothalamus, 13-16, 30-36
  aminergic innervation of, 38-40
  damage to, during transsphenoidal surgery, 396
  gross anatomy of, 30
  hypophysiotropic hormones of, 34-36
  median sagittal section of, 13
Hypothesis, portal vessel-chemotransmitter, 27

I

Idiopathic diabetes insipidus, 463
Imaging, magnetic resonance; *see* Magnetic resonance imaging
Immunocytochemistry for peptide measurement, 51
Immunologic staining of pituitary gland and sellar region, 67, 70
Immunoperoxidase method of staining, 67
Inappropriate secretion of antidiuretic hormone, 468-470
Infarction
  complicating craniotomy, 386
  in pituitary adenoma, 92
Infection complicating craniotomy, 387
Inferior hypophysial artery, 11, 12, 27
Inferior orbital fissure, 6
Inflammatory disorders, 112-114
Infraorbital crest, 3
Infundibulum, 10, 11, 13, 30; *see also* Median eminence
Inner ependymal zone of median eminence, 32
Inner palisade zone of median eminence, 32
Insulin, 49
  concentration of, in brain, 49
  evolutionary aspects of, 50
Insulin tolerance test, 133, 134
Intellectual function, effect of radiation on, 429
Internal carotid artery, 21

Internal irradiation, 414
Interstitial irradiation for craniopharyngioma, effects of, 426
Interventricular foramen, 13
Intoxication, water, 45, 47
Intracranial hemorrhage during transsphenoidal surgery, 396
Intracranial pressure, elevated, complicating craniotomy, 386
Intrasellar arachnoid diverticulum; *see* "Empty sella" syndrome
Intrasellar cistern; *see* "Empty sella" syndrome
Intravenous angiography, digital; *see* Digital intravenous angiography
Invasive pituitary adenomas, 92, 94
Ionizing radiation
  absorption of, 404-406
  directly ionizing, 404
  general effects of, 406-407
  physics of, 402-408
Ions, heavy-charged, 404
Irradiation
  for acromegaly, 220
  of central nervous system and pituitary, complications of, 426-432
  for craniopharyngioma, 339-341
  for Cushing's disease, 241-242
  hypopituitarism after, 454
  internal, 414
  megavoltage, conventional, 412-413
  for Nelson's syndrome, 246-247
  for nonfunctional pituitary adenomas, 293-295
  for prolactinomas, 268

J

Junctional scotoma
  with craniopharyngioma, 325
  from pituitary tumor, 125, 127

K

Kassinin, 50
"Knee, von Willebrand's," 125

L

Lamina terminalis, 13
Langerhans' granule, 114
Lateral hypothalamic nucleus, 16
Lateral pterygoid plate, 7
Leptomeningeal cysts, 316
  pathology of, 111
Lergotrile for acromegaly, 220
Lesions
  hypothalamic, causing hypopituitarism, 456-458
  parasellar, uncommon, 310-317
  pituitary and parasellar, uncommon, 301-317
  vascular, and diabetes insipidus, 463-464
Letterer-Siwe disease, 114
Leucine enkephalin, 49
Levodopa
  for Parkinson's disease, 54
  for prolactinoma, 264
Levodopa test to predict responsiveness to hypophysectomy, 442-443

Levothyroxine sodium after hypophysectomy, 448
LH; *see* Luteinizing hormone
LHRH; *see* Luteinizing hormone–releasing hormone
Light microscopy of pituitary adenoma, 90, 91
Linear energy transfer, 406-407, 409
Lingula, 2, 3
Lipomas, pathology of, 107
Lithium carbonate to inhibit ADH release, 470
Lobe
    anterior, of pituitary gland, 11, 12
    posterior, of pituitary gland, 10, 11
Luteinizing hormone, 35, 49
    measurement of, 134
Luteinizing hormone–releasing hormone, 34, 35
    measurement of, 51
Luteinizing hormone–secreting adenoma, 130, 305-306
Lymphocytic hypophysitis, 114
Lymphoproliferative disorders, 108
Lysine vasopressin, 50
8-Lysine vasopressin, synthetic, for diabetes insipidus, 466, 467

M

Macroprolactinoma, 271-274
Magnetic resonance imaging, 161-162
    for chordoma, 188, 313, 314
    for "empty sella" syndrome, 478
    for hypothalamic and optic gliomas, 184, 185, 186, 187
    of optic nerve glioma, 311
    of pituitary adenomas, 171, 172
Magnocellular cells of neurohypophysis, 40
Magnocellular pathways, diagram of, 41
Malformations, vascular, 111
Malignant sarcomas, 306
Malignant tumors of pituitary, primary, 94
Mammillary bodies, 13, 15
Mammilloinfundibular nuclei, 15
Mammosomatotroph cell adenomas, 207
    pathology of, 79-80
Marcus Gunn sign, 132, 311
Maxilla, palatine process of, 9
Meatus, nasal, 8
Medial pterygoid plates, 3, 7
Median eminence, 11, 14, 30-33; *see also* Infundibulum
    anterior and posterior, 13
    basic structural arrangement and cellular composition of, 31
    terminals projecting into, 33
    of tuber cinereum, 13
    zones of, 32
Megavoltage irradiation, conventional, 412-413
Melanocyte-stimulating hormone, 49
Melanoma of pituitary, primary, 107-108
Meningioma(s)
    angioblastic, pathology of, 102
    effects of radiation therapy on, 424-425
    fibroblastic, pathology of, 102
    meningothelial, pathology of, 101
    olfactory groove, 316-317
    parasellar, 316-317

Meningioma(s)—cont'd
    pathology of, 100-102
    psammomatous, pathology of, 102
    radiation-induced, 432
    radiologic studies of, 179-183
    syncytial, pathology of, 101
    transitional, pathology of, 102
    tuberculum sella, 316
Meningioma-en-plaque, 101
Meningitis
    complicating craniotomy, 387
    from transsphenoidal surgery, 396
Meningothelial meningioma, pathology of, 101
Metastases to pituitary, 108, 109, 308-309
Met-enkephalin
    in Huntington's disease, 53
    measurement of, 51
    in Parkinson's disease, 55
Metergoline for Cushing's disease, 242
Methionine enkephalin, 49
Metrizamide cisternography, 158-159
    for arachnoid cyst, 191
    for craniopharyngioma, 178, 329
    for ectopic pituitary adenoma, 307
    for "empty sella" syndrome, 199, 478
    for histiocytosis X, 197
    for hypothalamic and optic gliomas, 187
    for meningioma, 183
    for pituitary metastasis, 308-309
    for Rathke's pouch cyst, 190
    for sarcoidosis, 196
Metyrapone for Cushing's disease, 243
Metyrapone test, 133
    for Cushing's disease, 140
Microadenomas, therapy for, 268-271
Microprolactinomas, therapy for, 268-271
Middle clinoid processes, 1, 3
"Milk let-down" reflex, 46
Mitotane for Cushing's disease, 242-243
Mixed prolactin cell–growth hormone cell adenomas, pathology of, 77-78
Monitoring during surgery, 355
Monoaminergic pathways in mammalian brain, 37
Monoamines and activity of neurosecretory cells, 46-47
Morphine and vasopressin, 47
Motilin, 49
Mucoceles
    pathology of, 110
    sellar, 315, 316
    following transsphenoidal surgery, 397
Muscles, extraocular, paralysis of, from pituitary tumors, 128

N

Nasal bone, 7, 8
Nasal cavity, 7-9
    roof, floor, and lateral wall of, 7, 8
Nasal conchae, 7, 8
Nasal meatus, 8
Nasal septum, 3, 7-9
    arterial supply to, 8

Nasal septum—cont'd
  nerve supply of, 9
  sagittal view of, 8
Nasal spine, posterior, 8
Nasopalatine groove, 9
Nausea and vasopressin release, 45
NE; see Norepinephrine
"Nebenkern" formations in prolactin cell adenomas, 74
Nelson's syndrome, 72, 80, 81, 245-248
  clinical features of, 245
  and Cushing's syndrome, 231-249
  diagnostic evaluation of, 246
  effects of radiation therapy for, 421-422
  irradiation for, 246-247
  pharmacology for, 247
  from pituitary tumors, 130
  surgery for, 246
  therapeutic decision making for, 247-248
  treatment of, 246-247
Neoplasms, astrocytic, 102
Neoplastic diabetes insipidus, 463
Neoplastic disorders
  of nonpituitary origin, 100-108
  of pituitary origin, 71-100
Nerve(s)
  cranial, in cavernous sinus, 20
  oculomotor, 13
  optic; see Optic nerve
Nerve tract
  paraventricular-hypophysial, 40
  supraoptic-hypophysial, 40
Neural control of glandular secretion, 24-26
Neural reflexes and vasopressin secretion, 45
Neuroadenolysis, 447
Neuroblastomas, olfactory, 108
Neuroendocrine reflexes, 36, 43
Neuroendocrine transducer, 26
Neuroendocrinology, 23-56
Neurohypophysial hormones, 42-43
  list of, 49
Neurohypophysial neurons, 40-41
  endorphins and, 47
Neurohypophysis, 9, 12, 27, 28, 40-42
  histology of, 65
  physiology of, 40-47
  secretion of, 25-26
Neuron(s)
  neurohypophysial, 40-41
    endorphins and, 47
    supraoptic, excitatory and inhibitory cholinergic receptors in, 46
  tuberoinfundibular, 33, 34
Neuronal secretory cells, 24
Neuro-ophthalmologic testing, 131-132
  in craniopharyngioma, 326
Neuropathy, peripheral, 56
Neuropeptide Y, 49
  concentration of, in central nervous system, 49
Neuropeptides
  in cerebrospinal fluid, 55-56
  evolutionary and embryologic aspects of, 50

Neuropharmacology
  of anterior pituitary regulation, 37-40
  of vasopressin, 46-47
Neurophysin(s), 49
Neurophysin I, 42
Neurophysin II, 42
Neuroradiologic evaluation of nonfunctional pituitary adenomas, 283-287
Neuroradiologic studies, 146-162
  in acromegaly, 216-217
  of prolactinomas, 259
Neuroradiology, 145-199
Neurosecretion, 24-26
Neurosecretory cells, 25-26
  activity of, monoamines and, 46-47
Neurotensin, 49
  measurement of, 51
Neutrons, 403
Nicotine and vasopressin release, 46
Nicotine test for diabetes insipidus, 465
Noncavernous angioma, 111
Nonfunctional pituitary adenomas, 281-298
  classification of, 282
  clinical features of, 282
  definition of, 281
  diagnostic evaluation, 282-283
  effects of radiation therapy on, 422-423
  invasive, causing visual loss, 295
  irradiation for, 293-295
  neuroradiologic evaluation of, 283-287
  causing obstructive hydrocephalus, 296, 297
  with pituitary apoplexy, 295-296
  surgery for, 287-293
  therapeutic decision making with, 295-296
  treatment of, 287-295
Non-neoplastic cysts, radiologic studies of, 190-191
Non-neoplastic disorders, pathology of, 109-111
Nonpituitary origin, neoplastic disorders of, 100-108
Norepinephrine
  and activity of neurosecretory cells, 46
  in brain, concentration of, 49
  functions of, 40
  to innervate hypothalamus, 38-39
  and vasopressin release, 46
Nucleus
  anterior, 15
  arcuate, 15
  dorsomedial, 15
  hypothalamic; see Hypothalamic nuclei
  mammilloinfundibular, 15
  paraventricular, 11, 15, 40
  posterior, 15
  preoptic, 15
  suprachiasmatic, 15, 40
  supraoptic, 11, 15, 40
  tuberal, 14, 16
  ventromedial, 15
Null cell adenoma, pathology of, 88-90

O

Obstructive hydrocephalus
  increased intracranial pressure caused by, in craniopharyngioma, 326

Obstructive hydrocephalus—cont'd
  nonfunctional pituitary adenoma causing, 296, 297
Oculomotor nerve, 13
Olfactory groove meningiomas, 316-317
Olfactory neuroblastomas, 108
Oncocytes, 89
Oncocytic transformation of null cell adenoma, 89-90
Oncocytoma, 89-90
Opioids, endogenous, 47
  discovery of, 48
Optical canal, 1, 2, 5
Optic chiasm, 11, 13, 18-20
  compression of, by pituitary tumor, 128
  damage of
    from radiation, 428
    during transsphenoidal surgery, 396
  postfixed, 19, 20
  prefixed, 19, 20
  superior view of, 19
Optic disc pallor from pituitary tumor, 125
Optic foramen, 1
Optic gliomas, 310-312
  pathology of, 102-103
  radiologic studies of, 184-187
Optic nerve, 5, 16-18
  damage to
    from radiation, 428
    during transsphenoidal surgery, 396
Orbital fissure
  inferior, 6
  superior, 2, 6
Osmolarity and ADH secretion, 43-44
Osmoreceptors, 43
"Osmotic set point" and vasopressin secretion, 44
Ostia, sphenoid, 3
Oxygen enhancement ratio, 406, 408, 409
Oxytocin, 12, 25-26, 40, 41, 42-43, 49
  chemical structure of, 42
  secretion of, acetylcholine and, 46

P

Palatine, horizontal plate of, 8
Palatine process of maxilla, 8
Palisade zone of median eminence, 32
Pallor, optic disc, from pituitary tumor, 125
Pancreatic polypeptide, 49
Papilledema from pituitary tumor, 125
Paraganglioma, 108
Paralysis of extraocular muscles from pituitary tumors, 128
Parasellar anatomic structures, 16-22
Parasellar area, gross abnormalities in, skull films to determine, 150-151
Parasellar lesions, uncommon, 310-317
Parasellar and pituitary lesions, uncommon, 301-317
Parasellar region, superior view of, 17
Parasellar structures, damage to, complicating craniotomy, 387-389
Paraterminal body, 13
Paraventricular-hypophysial nerve tract, 40
Paraventricular nucleus, 11, 15, 40

Parkinson's disease, postmortem studies of, 54-55
Pars distalis, 9-10, 12, 28-30
  electron microscopy of, 66
Pars intermedia, 10, 12, 29
  histology of, 65
Pars tuberalis, 10, 12, 29
  histology of, 65
Particulate radiation, 403-404
Pathology of pituitary gland and sellar region, 64-114
"Pearly" tumor, 104, 105, 315
Peptide(s)
  in brain, concentration of, 49
  brain-gut, 47-56
    listing of, 49
  cerebrospinal fluid, 55-56
  embryologic origins of, 50
  gastrointestinal, list of, 49
  measurements of, validity of, 51
  pituitary, list of, 49
  regulatory, 47-56
  sleep, 49
  vasoactive intestinal, 49
Peptide histidine isoleucine, 35
Peripheral neuropathy, 56
Persistent acromegaly, 222
Petrosal sinus sampling, 21, 160
Pharyngeal canal, 3
Pharyngeal pituitary, 9
Phenylthylamine N-methyl transferase, 39
Phenytoin and vasopressin secretion, 47
PHI; see Peptide histidine isoleucine
Phosphorus-32 for interstitial radiation, 414
Photoelectric process of absorption of radiation, 404, 405
Photon irradiation; seeElectromagnetic irradiation
Phyllomedusin, 50
Physalemin, 50
"Physaliphorous" tumors, 104
Physics of radiation, 402-408
PIF; see Prolactin release-inhibiting factor
Pilocytic astrocytoma, 102, 310
Pi-mesons, 404
Pineal body, 13
Pinealoma, ectopic, 106
Pions, 404
Pitressin tannate in oil for diabetes insipidus, 467
Pituitary adenoma, 72-91
  alpha subunit secreting, 302
  amyloid in, 92
  bromocriptine-induced changes in, 92, 93
  calcification in, 92
  classification of, 72
  ectopic, 94, 306-307
  hemorrhage and infarction in, 92
  invasive, 92, 94
  light microscopy, 90, 91
  nonfunctional; see Nonfunctional pituitary adenomas
  pathologic effects of radiation on, 410
  radiologic findings in, 163-174
  secondary changes in, 92-94

Pituitary apoplexy, 92, 129-130
   mass effects of, 124
   nonfunctional pituitary adenoma with, 295-296
   treatment of, 287
Pituitary deficiency states, 451-470
Pituitary endocrine deficiency from pituitary tumors, 129
Pituitary gland, 9-12, 13, 27-30
   abscess of, 112
      causing hypopituitarism, 455
      radiologic studies of, 194
   anterior lobe of, 11, 12
      regulation of, neuropharmacology of, 37-40
   carcinoma of, primary, 306
   in craniopharyngioma, 325-326
   embryogenesis of, 10
   irradiation of, complications of, 426-432
   metastases to, 108, 109
   normal, effects of radiation on, 409-410
   pharyngeal, 9
   primary melanoma of, 107-108
   posterior lobe of, 10, 11
      electron microscopy of, 69
      endocrinologic testing of, 134
   primary malignant tumors of, 94
   sagittal diagram of, 11
   within sella turcica, diagram of, 28
Pituitary gland and sellar region
   electron microscopy of, 66-67
   histology of, 65-66
   immunologic staining of, 67, 70
   pathology of, 64-114
Pituitary hormone reserve, assessment of, 132-135
Pituitary metastases, 308-309
Pituitary and parasellar lesions, uncommon, 301-317
Pituitary peptides, list of, 49
Pituitary stalk, 9-12
   in craniopharyngioma, 325-326
Pituitary surgery, 349-397; *see also* Surgery
Pituitary tumors
   clinical and endocrinologic evaluation of patients with, 123-142
   clinical features of, 124-131
   endocrinopathy with, 130-131
   uncommon, 301-309
Plexus, choroid, 13
Plurihormonal adenomas, 207
   pathology of, 86-87
Pneumatization of sphenoid sinuses, skull films to determine, 151-153
Pneumoencephalography, 160
   for "empty sella" syndrome, 478
PNMT; *see* Phenethylamine N-methyl transferase
Polypeptide, pancreatic, 49
Polytomography
   of pituitary adenomas, 163
   sellar, 154
Pons, 13
Portal system
   primary, 11
   secondary, 11
Portal vessel chemotransmitter hypothesis, 27
Portal vessels, 27

Positioning for surgery, 356-359
Positive contrast cisternography in craniopharyngioma, 329
Posterior clinoid process, 2, 3
Posterior commissure, 13
Posterior hypothalamic nucleus, 15, 16
Posterior lobe of pituitary gland, 10, 11
   electron microscopy of, 69
Posterior median eminence, 13
Posterior pituitary, endocrinologic testing of, 134
Postoperative assessment of endocrine function, 135
Postsurgical hypopituitarism, 453
Post-traumatic diabetes insipidus, 463
Pouch, Rathke's, 9-10
Pregnancy, women with microprolactinomas desiring, 269
Preoperative assessment of surgical patients, 354-355
Preoptic nucleus, 15
Presellar type of sphenoid sinus, pneumatization of, 152, 153
PRF; *see* Prolactin-releasing factor
Primary malignant tumors of pituitary, 94
Primary melanoma of pituitary, 107-108
Primary pituitary carcinoma, 306
Primary portal system, 11
PRL; *see* Prolactin
Prolactin, 35, 36, 49
   measurement of, 134
   physiology of, 254-255
Prolactin cell adenoma, pathology of, 72-74
Prolactin cell–growth hormone cell adenomas, 206, 207
   mixed, pathology of, 77-78
Prolactin cells, electron microscopy of, 60
Prolactin inhibiting factor, 254
Prolactin-releasing factor, 35, 36, 254
Prolactin-secreting tumors; *see* Prolactinoma
Prolactinoma, 131, 253-278
   calcification in, 92
   clinical features of, 257-258
   diagnostic evaluation of, 258-259
   effects of radiation therapy on, 415-416
   endocrinologic studies of, 259
   irradiation of, 268
   pathology of, 72-74
   pathophysiology of, 255-256
   pharmacotherapy for, 264-267
   radiologic studies of, 259
   recurrent, after surgery, 271
   special endocrine testing for, 141-142
   surgery for, 261-264, 271
      bromocriptine before, 274-276
   therapeutic decision making for, 268-278
   treatment of, 259-268
Prooxyphysin, 42
Propressophysin, 42
Proptosis from pituitary tumors, 128
Prostate cancer
   hypophysectomy for, 440-441
      indications for and timing of, 445-446
   patients with, selection of, for hypophysectomy, 443

Prostate cancer—cont'd
  remission of, after hypophysectomy, 445
Proton beam radiotherapy, 413
Protons, 403
Psammomatous meningiomas, pathology of, 102
Pseudoprolactinoma, 171, 258
  therapy for, 277-278
Pterion, 7
Pterional craniotomy, 362-366
  to craniopharyngioma, 330
  positioning for, 356
Pterygoid canal, 3, 7
Pterygoid fossa, 7
Pterygoid plate
  lateral, 7
  medial, 3, 7
Pterygoid process, 7

Q

Quadrantanopsia
  bitemporal, from pituitary tumor, 126
  temporal, with craniopharyngioma, 325

R

Radiation
  directly ionizing, 404
  effects of
    on central nervous system, 410-412
    on normal pituitary, 409-410
    on tissues, 408-412
  electromagnetic, 402-403
    clinical use of, 408
  ionizing; see Ionizing radiation
  particulate, 403-404
  pathologic effects of, on pituitary adenomas, 410
  properties of, influencing biologic effects, 406-408
Radiation-induced brain injury, 426-427
Radiation therapy, 401-432
  for acromegaly, effects of, 416-419
  for craniopharyngiomas, effects of, 425-426
  for Cushing's disease, effects of, 420-421
  history of, 402
  for meningiomas, effects of, 424-425
  for Nelson's syndrome, effects of, 421-422
  for nonfunctional pituitary adenomas, effects of, 422-423
  for prolactinoma, effects of, 415-416
  results of, 414-426
  techniques and tumor dosages in, 412-414
Radioimmunoassay for peptide measurement, 51
Radioisotopes used for internal radiation, 414
Radiologic findings in pituitary adenomas, 163-174
Radiologic studies
  in acromegaly, 216-217
  of aneurysms, 192-193
  of arachnoid cysts, 191
  of chordomas, 188-189
  of craniopharyngiomas, 174-178, 327-329
  in Cushing's disease, 140, 238-239
  of "empty sella" syndrome, 198-199
  in histiocytosis X, 196-197
  of hypothalamic and optic gliomas, 184-187

Radiologic studies—cont'd
  of meningiomas, 179-183
  in nonfunctional pituitary adenomas, 283-287
  of non-neoplastic cysts, 190-191
  of pituitary abscesses, 194
  of prolactinomas, 259
  of Rathke's pouch cyst, 190
  in sarcoidosis, 195-196
Radionecrosis, cerebral, 426-427
Radiotherapy
  alpha particle, 413
  proton beam, 413
Rathke's pouch (cleft) cysts, 315-316
  pathology of, 109-110
  radiologic studies of, 190
Rathke's pouch, 9-10, 27-28
Recurrent acromegaly, 222
Recurrent hyperprolactinemia after treatment, 270-271
Recurrent prolactinoma after surgery, 271
Reflex(es)
  "milk let-down," 46
  neural, and vasopressin secretion, 45
  neuroendocrine, 36, 43
Regulatory peptides, 47-56
Releasing factors, 26
Retinopathy, diabetic, hypophysectomy for, 446
Rhinorrhea, cerebrospinal fluid, in "empty sella" syndrome, 199, 477
Rosenthal fibers, 102

S

Sampling
  petrosal sinus, 21, 160
Sarcoidosis, 112-113
  causing hypopituitarism, 456
  radiologic studies in, 195-196
Sarcoma(s), 94
  malignant, 306
Schwannomas, 108
Schwartz-Bartter syndrome, 468-470
Scotoma, junctional
  with craniopharyngioma, 325
  from pituitary tumor, 125, 127
Secondary portal system, 11
Secretin, 49
Secretion
  ACTH and cortisol, physiology of, 232
  of antidiuretic hormone (vasopressin)
    controls on, 46
    inppropriate, 468-470
    regulation of, 43-45
  glandular, neural control of, 24-26
  of growth hormone, regulation of, 204-205
  oxytocin, acetylcholine and, 46
Secretory cells, 24
Seizures, mass effect of, 124
Sella turcica, 1, 3
  anterior wall of, 5
  assessment of size and configuration of, in skull films, 148-150
  pituitary gland within, diagram of, 28
  skull film of, 147

Sellar area, gross abnormalities in, skull films to determine, 150-151
Sellar cysts, pathology of, 109-111
Sellar diaphragm, deficient; see "Empty sella" syndrome
Sellar polytomography, 154
Sellar region, pituitary gland and
  histology of, 65-66
  immunologic staining of, 67, 70
  microscopy of, 66-67
  pathology of, 64-114
Sellar type of sphenoid sinus, pneumatization of, 152, 153
Senile dementia, Alzheimer's-type, 52
Septae, sphenoid, 5
Septal cartilage, 9
Septum, nasal, 3, 7-9
  arterial supply to, 8
  nerve supply of, 9
  sagittal view of, 8
Serotonin
  and activity of neurosecretory cells, 46
  functions of, 40
  to innervate hypothalamus, 39-40
Serotonin antagonists for Cushing's disease, 243-244
"Set point" of neurohypophysial control, 44-45
Sex steroids, measurement of, 134
Sheehan's syndrome, 454, 463
Shunting, ventricular, in craniopharyngioma, 334
Shy-Drager syndrome, 56
SIADH: see Syndrome of inappropriate secretion of antidiuretic hormone
Sign, Marcus Gunn, 132, 311
"Silent" corticotroph cell adenomas, pathology of, 80, 81, 82
Sinus
  cavernous; see Cavernous sinus
  ethmoid, 4
  petrosal, sampling of, 160
  sphenoid; see Sphenoid sinus
Sinusitis from transsphenoidal surgery, 397
Skeletal origin, tumors of, in sellar and parasellar areas, 108
Skin changes in acromegaly, 212
Skull films, 146-153
  for acromegaly, 216
  of aneurysm, 192
  of chordomas, 188
  for craniopharyngiomas, 174, 175, 327, 332
  in Cushing's disease, 239
  in "empty sella" syndrome, 198, 478, 479
  in histiocytosis X, 196
  for hypothalamic and optic gliomas, 185
  of meningiomas, 179
  of pituitary adenomas, 163, 164-165
  in sarcoidosis, 195
Sleep peptide(s), 49
Soft tissue reactions to cranial radiation, 430
Somatocrinin and growth hormone, 204
Somatomedin-C levels in acromegaly, 136, 215
Somatomedins, 205

Somatostatin, 34, 35, 36, 49
  in Alzheimer's disease, 52, 53
  as brain-gut peptide, 48
  in cerebrospinal fluid, 56
  concentration of, in brain, 49
  evolutionary aspects of, 50
  and growth hormone, 204
  measurement of, 51
Somatostatin-like immunoreactivity in Alzheimer's disease, 52
Somatotropin release-inhibiting factor, 34
Sphenoid aperture, 3
Sphenoid bone, 1-7, 8
  anteroinferior aspect of, 3
  and associated bony structures, 1-7
  midline sagittal section through, 4
  superior aspect of, 2
  wings of, 2, 3, 6, 7
Sphenoid concha, 3
Sphenoid crest, 3, 4
Sphenoid ostia, 3
Sphenoid ridge, 7
Sphenoid rostrum, 6
Sphenoid septae, 5
Sphenoid sinus, 1, 3, 4, 5-6, 8, 13
  anatomic structures adjacent to, 6
  pneumatization of, skull films to determine, 151-153
Sphenopalatine foramen, 8
Spine
  ethmoid, of sphenoid bone, 1, 2
  nasal, posterior, 8
Spongioblastoma, 102, 103, 310
SRIF; see Somatotropin release–inhibiting factor
Staining, immunologic, of pituitary gland and sellar region, 67, 70
Stereotaxic cryohypophysectomy, 447
Stereotaxic radiofrequency lesioning, 447
Steroids, sex, measurement of, 134
Stress
  in neuroendocrine regulation, 43
  and vasopressin release, 45
Stress-induced diuresis, 46
Stria medullaris, 13
Subfrontal approach
  to craniopharyngioma, 330
  to surgery, 366-367
  positioning for, 357
Substance P, 47-48, 49, 50
  in Alzheimer's disease, 52
  in cerebrospinal fluid, 56
  in Huntington's disease, 53
  measurement of, 51
  in Parkinson's disease, 54-55
Substance P–like immunoreactivity in Parkinson's disease, 54-55
Subtemporal approach to surgery, 367
  positioning for, 357
Sulcus
  carotid, 2, 3
  chiasmatic, 2
  hypothalamic, 13

Superior hypophysial artery, 11, 12
Superior orbital fissure, 2, 6
Suprachiasmatic nucleus, 15, 40
Supraoptic-hypophysial nerve tract, 40
Supraoptic-hypophysial tract, 15-16
Supraoptic hypothalamic region, 15
Supraoptic neurons, excitatory and inhibitory cholinergic receptors in, 46
Supraoptic nucleus, 11, 15, 40
Suprapineal recess, 13
Suprasellar cysts, pathology of, 109-111
Surgery, 349-397
   for acromegaly, 218-220
   anesthesia considerations during, 354-358
   approaches to, 359
   assessment before, 354-355
   complications of, 385-397
   for craniopharyngioma, 330-335
      results of, 336-338
   for Cushing's disease, transsphenoidal, 240-241
   for "empty sella" syndrome, 480
   frontotemporal (pterional) approach, 362-366
   history of, 350-353
   monitoring during, 355
   for Nelson's syndrome, 246
   for nonfunctional pituitary adenomas, 287-293
   positioning for, 356-359
   for prolactinoma, 261-264, 271
      bromocriptine before, 274-276
   subfrontal approach, 366-367
   subtemporal approach, 367
   transcranial approaches, 360-367
   transsphenoidal; *see* Transsphenoidal surgery
Syncytial meningioma, pathology of, 101
Syndrome
   "cerebral salt wasting," 470
   Cushing's; *see* Cushing's disease
   "empty sella"; *see* "Empty sella" syndrome
   of inappropriate secretion of antidiuretic hormone, 468-470
   Nelson's; *see* Nelson's syndrome
   Schwartz-Bartter, 468-470
   Sheehan's, 454, 463
   Shy-Drager, 56
Syphilis causing hypopituitarism, 455

T

Tachykinins, 50
Tamoxifen for breast cancer, 448
Tanycytes, 14, 32, 33
Taveras and Wood method for measuring sella, 150
Teeth, damage to, from transsphenoidal surgery, 397
Temporal quadrantanopsia with craniopharyngioma, 325
Tentorium cerebelli, 3
Teratoid tumors, 312-313
   pathology of, 106-107
Terminal boutons of median eminence, 32
Test; *see also* Testing; specific disease; specific test
   of adrenal axis, 133
   of gonadal axis, 134
   of growth hormone, 134

Test—cont'd
   of prolactin, 134
   of thyroid axis, 133-134
Testing; *see also* Test
   endocrine; *see* Endocrine testing
   endrocrinologic, 132-142
   neuro-ophthalmologic, 131-132
   of vasopressin, 134
Testosterone, measurement of, 134
Third ventricle, 14, 16
Thyroid axis, endocrinologic testing of, 133-134
Thyroid replacement for hypopituitarism, 461
Thyroid-stimulating hormone–secreting adenoma, 130
Thyrotroph cell
   electron microscopy of, 68
   histology of, 65
Thyrotroph cell adenomas
   pathology of, 85-86
   of pituitary, 305
Thyrotropin, 35, 49
Thyrotropin-releasing hormone, 23, 34, 35, 49
   as brain-gut peptide, 48
   in Huntington's disease, 53
   measurement of, 51
Thyrotropin-releasing hormone stimulation test, 134
   for acromegaly, 136
   for prolactinomas, 141-142
Thyrotropin-secreting adenoma, 302-305
Thyroxine, serum, measurement of, 133-134
Tissues, effects of radiation on, 408-412
Tomography, computed; *see* Computed tomography
Toxins, adrenal, for Cushing's disease, 242-243
Transantral surgical approach, 385
Transcranial surgical approaches, 360-367
Transethmoidal surgical approach, 384-385
Transitional meningiomas, pathology of, 102
Transnasal alcohol injection for hypophysectomy, 447
Transnasal midline transsphenoidal approach to surgery, 384
Transsphenoidal surgery, 368-385
   for craniopharyngioma, 332-333
   for Cushing's disease, 240-241
   for "empty sella" syndrome, 480
   for hypophysectomy, 447
   for Nelson's syndrome, 246
   for nonfunctional pituitary adenomas, 287-293
   operative
      complications of, 389-397
      mortality from, 391, 397
   positioning for, 358
   for prolactinoma, 261-264
Transsphenoidal chiasmopexy, 480
Trauma causing hypopituitarism, 456
TRH; *see* Thyrotropin-releasing hormone
Trigeminal groove, 2
TSH; *see* Thyrotropin
Tuber cinereum, 13, 30
Tuberal hypothalamic region, 15
Tuberal nuclei, 14, 16
Tuberculosis causing hypopituitarism, 455

Tuberculum sella, 1, 2
  meningiomas of, 316
Tuberohypophysial tract, 16
Tuberoinfundibular dopamine system, 38
Tuberoinfundibular neurons, 33, 34
Tumor
  "collar button," 361
  granular cell, 95-96, 315
  causing hypopituitarism, 453-454
  hypothalamic, 310
  malignant, of pituitary, primary, 94
  "pearly," 104, 105, 315
  "physaliphorous," 104
  pituitary
    clinical and endocrinologic evaluation of patients with, 123-142
    clinical features of, 124-131
    uncommon, 301-309
    prolactin-secreting; see Prolactinomas
  of skeletal origin in sellar and parasellar areas, 108
  teratoid, 312-313
    pathology of, 106-107
  yolk sac, 312
Tumorigenesis, radiation-induced, 431-432
Tyrosine hydroxylase in Parkinson's disease, 54

U

Undifferentiated cell adenoma; see Null cell adenoma
Urinary free cortisol, measurement of, in Cushing's disease, 137

V

Vascular lesions and diabetes insipidus, 463-464
Vascular malformations, 111
Vasoactive intestinal polypeptide, 35, 49
  in Alzheimer's disease, 52
  in Huntington's disease, 54
  measurement of, 51
Vasopressin, 12, 25-26, 32, 40-43, 49
  arginine, in Alzheimer's disease, 52
  chemical structure of, 42
  drugs effecting release of, 462
  injectable, for diabetes insipidus, 466, 467
  lysine, 50

Vasopressin—cont'd
  measurement of, 134
  and morphine, 47
  neuropharmacology of, 46-47
  secretion of
    controls of, 46, 47
    inappropriate, 468-470
    regulation of, 43-45
Vasospasm, cerebral, from transsphenoidal surgery, 396
Vasotocin, 50
Vein, hypophysial, long, 11
Venography, cavernous sinus, 160, 161
Venous catheterization and sampling for ACTH in Cushing's disease, 239
Venous hemorrhage after transsphenoidal surgery, 394
Ventricle, third, 14, 16
Ventricular shunting in craniopharyngiomas, 334
Ventromedial hypothalmic nucleus, 15, 16
VIP; see Vasoactive intestinal peptide
Visual field defects, mass effects of, 124, 125
Volumetric increase in sella, skull films to measure, 149
Vomer, 4, 8, 9
von Willebrand's knee, 125

W

Water deprivation test, 134
  for diabetes insipidus, 464, 465
Water intoxication, 45, 47
Wings of sphenoid bone, 2, 3, 6, 7

X

X granule, 114
X-rays, 402-403

Y

Yolk sac tumors, 312
Yttrium-90 for internal radiation, 414
  for acromegaly, 419
  for Cushing's disease, 421

Z

Zones of median eminence, 32